Companion CD-ROM Contents

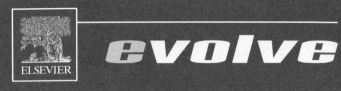

Health Assessment *for* Nursing Practice

4th Edition

Susan Fickertt Wilson, RN, PhD, FNP

Associate Professor
School of Nursing
College of Health and Social Welfare
University of Alaska
Anchorage, Alaska;
Emeritus Associate Professor
Harris College of Nursing and Health Sciences
Texas Christian University
Fort Worth, Texas

Jean Foret Giddens, RN, PhD, APRN, BC

Professor and Coordinator
MSN Nursing Education Concentration
College of Nursing
University of New Mexico
Albuquerque, New Mexico

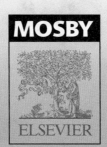

MOSBY

ELSEVIER

MOSBY
ELSEVIER

11830 Westline Industrial Drive
St. Louis, Missouri 63146

HEALTH ASSESSMENT FOR NURSING PRACTICE   ISBN: 978-0-323-05322-8
Copyright © 2009 by Mosby, Inc., an affiliate of Elsevier Inc.

Notice

Knowledge and best practice in this field are constantly changing. As new research and experience broaden our knowledge, changes in practice, treatment and drug therapy may become necessary or appropriate. Readers are advised to check the most current information provided (i) on procedures featured or (ii) by the manufacturer of each product to be administered, to verify the recommended dose or formula, the method and duration of administration, and contraindications. It is the responsibility of the practitioner, relying on their own experience and knowledge of the patient, to make diagnoses, to determine dosages and the best treatment for each individual patient, and to take all appropriate safety precautions. To the fullest extent of the law, neither the Publisher nor the Authors assumes any liability for any injury and/or damage to persons or property arising out of or related to any use of the material contained in this book.

The Publisher

Previous editions copyrighted 1996, 2001, 2005

Library of Congress Cataloging-in-Publication Data
Wilson, Susan Fickertt.
Health assessment for nursing practice / Susan Fickertt Wilson, Jean Foret Giddens. — 4th ed.
  p. ; cm.
Includes bibliographical references and index.
ISBN 978-0-323-05322-8 (hardcover : alk. paper) 1. Nursing assessment. I. Giddens, Jean. II. Title.
[DNLM: 1. Nursing Assessment—methods.   2. Medical History Taking.   3. Physical Examination. WY 100.4 W753h 2009]
RT48.W55 2008
616.07'5—dc22

                              2008025937

Executive Editor: Robin Carter
Developmental Editor: Deanna Davis
Publishing Services Manager: Deborah Vogel
Project Manager: Brandilyn Tidwell
Designer: Paula Catalano

Printed in Canada

Last digit is the print number: 9 8 7 6 5 4 3 2 1

To my daughter, Megan, for her continued love, patience,
and support; to June Thompson for giving me the opportunity to
publish; and to the faculty, colleagues, and students
who have challenged me through the years.
SFW

To my family, for their unconditional support of my
professional and personal goals; to my mentors and role models
for their guidance throughout my career; and to our nursing
students, the future of our profession.
JFG

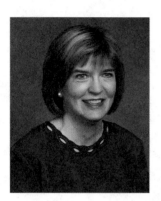

Susan Fickertt Wilson has 36 years of teaching experience, including 24 years teaching health assessment. She has cared for adult clients in critical care, general care, and rehabilitation units. Dr. Wilson has taught undergraduate and graduate students on the care of clients in a variety of settings. This text is a synthesis of all that she has learned about performing health assessment and teaching health assessment, as well as how to meet the challenges she knows students experience in learning health assessment.

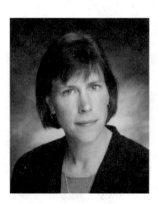

Jean Foret Giddens is a professor and coordinator for the MSN Nursing Education Concentration at the College of Nursing, University of New Mexico in Albuquerque. Dr. Giddens earned a Bachelor of Science in nursing from the University of Kansas, a Master of Science in nursing from the University of Texas at El Paso, and a doctorate in Education and Human Resource Studies from Colorado State University. Dr. Giddens has been involved with nursing education since 1984. Her teaching experience includes associate, baccalaureate, and master's degree programs in New Mexico, Texas, and Colorado. Her content areas in nursing education include adult health nursing, health assessment, nursing process, curriculum development, and innovative educational strategies.

Contributors and Consultants

Clinical Reasoning Special Consultant

Christine A. Tanner, PhD, RN
A.B. Youmans-Spaulding Distinguished Professor
Oregon Health & Science University
School of Nursing
Portland, Oregon

Chapter 20

Joanne Bartram, RN, MSN, FNP
Clinical Educator, Family Nurse Practitioner
University of New Mexico
Albuquerque, New Mexico

Carolyn Montoya, RN, MSN, PNP
Coordinator, Family Nurse Practitioner and Pediatric Nurse
Practitioner
Concentration College of Nursing
University of New Mexico
Albuquerque, New Mexico

Chapter 22

Mildred O. Hogstel, PhD, RN
Professor Emeritus of Nursing
Texas Christian University
Fort Worth, Texas

Reviewers

Jimmie Borum, RN, MS
Lecturer
Harris School of Nursing
Texas Christian University
Fort Worth, Texas

Ian Camera, RN, MSN, ND
Professor of Nursing
Holyoke Community College
Holyoke, Massachusetts

Connie Davis, RN, MSN
Geriatric Clinical Program Development Specialist
Fraser Health
Abbotsford, British Columbia
Canada

Catharine Muskus, MS, APRN, BC
Lecturer
Department of Nursing
University of Vermont
Burlington, Vermont

Janice Reilley, RN, MSN, EdD
Assistant Professor
Widener University
Chester, Pennsylvania

Patricia Rylander, RN, MSN
Department of Nursing
Central Texas College
Killeen, Texas

Mary B. Winton, MSN, RN, APRN, BC, ACNP
Instructor
School of Nursing
Tarleton State University
Stephenville, Texas

Student Focus Group Participants

Lauren Cardoni
University of New Hampshire
Durham, New Hampshire

Avani Contractor
University of New Hampshire
Durham, New Hampshire

Debby Fickling
Pensacola Junior College
Pensacola, Florida

Amy Fisher
Butler Community College
El Dorado, Kansas

Erica Gean
Butler Community College
El Dorado, Kansas

Nicole Kenyon
Pensacola Junior College
Pensacola, Florida

Amy Kliesner
Butler Community College
El Dorado, Kansas

Carole Ann Koger
University of Central Oklahoma
Edmond, Oklahoma

Jamie Manuele
University of Central Oklahoma
Edmond, Oklahoma

Kathleen O'Donnell
University of New Hampshire
Durham, New Hampshire

Amanda Patterson
University of Central Oklahoma
Edmond, Oklahoma

Beth Ramey
Butler Community College
El Dorado, Kansas

If a teacher is indeed wise, he does not bid you enter the house of his wisdom, but rather leads you to the threshold of your own mind.

Kahlil Gibran
The Prophet

Following this teaching we have revised this text *Health Assessment for Nursing Practice* to retain the strong features and add others. The underlying principles of the previous editions are steadfast. Like the previous editions, the fourth edition is based on the assumption that every client from neonate to older adult is an interactive, complex being who is more than a collection of his or her parts. Each client's health status depends on the interactions of physiological, psychological, sociocultural, and spiritual factors. These interactions occur within their physical environments (what they eat, drink, and breathe); what kind of activity and work they participate in and where they live; their social environments and health beliefs (friends, family, and support systems and when and how they seek healthcare); and their internal environments (what they eat and drink, how they sleep, and how often they exercise).

As faculty, we are challenged with several responsibilities toward our students:

1. Demonstrate caring and compassion when we interact with clients to act as role models for students.
2. Help students become knowledgeable and skilled in history-taking and physical assessment.
3. Model for students as well as teach them how to be objective and nonjudgmental.
4. Assist students to mobilize their resources to apply health assessment knowledge and skills to clients of all ages and from a multitude of cultures and ethnic groups.

We know that students will need this content for the remainder of their professional lives. This textbook is a toolbox of information and techniques. As a wise teacher, you lead students to the threshold.

ORGANIZATION

Health Assessment for Nursing Practice is organized into four units to assist students and faculty efficiently to find their areas of interest. Unit I, entitled **Foundations for Health Assessment**, includes Chapters 1 to 9, which provide a strong foundation for students, covering issues pertinent to nursing practice with all age groups such as *Why Health Assessment is Essential to Nursing Practice, Ethnic and Cultural Considerations, Interviewing to Obtain a Health History,* and *Equipment and Techniques for Physical Assessment.* Also included are chapters on *General Inspection and Vital Signs, Pain Assessment, Mental Health Assessment, Sleep Assessment,* and *Nutritional Assessment.*

Unit II, entitled **Health Assessment of the Adult**, contains Chapters 10 to 18, which are organized by body system. To facilitate learning and performance of a systematic assessment, the authors combined several chapters from the third edition into a chapter entitled *Head, Eyes, Ears, Nose and Throat.* Likewise, we combined chapters on female and male reproductive systems and perineum into one chapter called *Reproductive Systems and the Perineum.*

Each chapter in Unit II begins with a review of **Anatomy and Physiology**. This content begins the chapter because physical assessment techniques allow the student to answer the question, "How does this client's anatomy and physiology compare with that expected for his or her age and ethnic group?"

The **Health History** section that follows instructs the student on history data to collect by providing sample questions to ask the clients along with the reasons for asking those questions. The text below each question describes the variances that the student may find. Included in the Health History section are new headings for **Present Health Status**, **Past Medical History**, **Family History**, and **Problem-Based History**. Descriptions of how to assess clients with special needs and how to teach clients to improve their health and reduce their risks of illness or injury are retained from the third edition.

The **Examination** section begins with a table outlining procedures that are performed routinely, under special circumstances, or in advanced practice. Identified in this edition are **Core Examination Skills** based on data collected from nurses who use these skills daily in their professional nursing practice with clients. Performing these core skills provides an evidence-base for the practice of assessment. A list of the appropriate **Equipment** needed for these procedures is included in the table. This section sequentially guides the student in the techniques of performing a physical assessment of an adult, telling what to do, how to do it, and what to expect. Photographs are provided to enhance learning. The left column, **Procedures and Techniques with Normal Findings**, details the techniques of the assessment and the normal findings, and the right column describes **Abnormal Findings**. When applicable, a section on **Clients with Situational Variations** may include examinations of clients who are hearing-impaired or paralyzed.

Clinical Application and Clinical Reasoning, at the end of each chapter, contains Review Questions with answers in Appendix E. **Sample Documentation** of a client assessment for each body system is provided, first in raw data format as would be collected by a nurse, then with an example of how these data would appear in documentation form. **Case Studies** give subjective and objective data about a client and ask students to use clinical reasoning skills to answer questions about the client. Answers for these questions also are included in Appendix E to facilitate self-study.

Health Promotion content has been retained, and these special feature boxes follow the Health History section so that data are collected at the time of history-taking. From data collected, the student can identify teaching needed to help the client maintain health. Special **Risk Factors** boxes for disorders in each body system, along with the Health Promotion sections, remind students to discuss these behaviors with clients to help them maintain health and reduce risk of disease. The areas of risk factor identification and health promotion are unique to this text, indicating our commitment to not only teaching students how to gather data from the clients and examine clients' bodies to detect health and disease, but also to teach students how to attain and maintain a higher level of health. Also included throughout body system chapters are special **Ethnic and Cultural Variations** boxes that contain racial and cultural variations the nurse should consider when assessing clients. The **Common Problems and Conditions** section toward the end of each chapter has been updated, with new photographs added where appropriate

Unit III, entitled **Health Assessment Across the Life Span**, contains Chapters 19 to 22, which begins with an overview of growth and development and continues with chapters on *Assessment of the Infant and Child* (**new to the fourth edition**), *Assessment of the Pregnant Client*, and *Assessment of the Older Adult* (**new to the fourth edition**). These chapters describe how to individualize the examination for clients of different ages and in pregnancy. Each chapter includes a box that lists the differences in anatomy and physiology pertinent to those clients. Health history and examination follow along with procedures and techniques and normal and abnormal findings. The Common Problems and Conditions section toward the end of each chapter has been retained in these chapters as they pertain to the clients described.

Unit IV, entitled **Putting It All Together**, contains chapters 23 and 24, *How to Conduct a Head-to-Toe Assessment* and *Documenting the Health Assessment*. These chapters provide guidelines and photographs for putting all of the body system assessments together into one comprehensive examination and for communicating the findings for other health care professionals to use.

A **Glossary** at the end of the book provides definitions to enhance student comprehension of key concepts and terms.

Chapters were updated and revised based on the feedback from users, both faculty and students. Consider each chapter a different type of tool from the toolbox. Collectively they provide all that students need to perform a comprehensive health assessment.

SUMMARY OF SPECIAL FEATURES

- **Health Promotion** boxes provide *Healthy People 2010* objectives as well as data from national authorities that include recommendations for primary and secondary prevention to promote health and prevent disease.

- Special **Risk Factors** boxes are found at the beginning of each Health History section in the body system chapters and highlight information specific to various body systems and disorders.
- The **Examination** section in each body system chapter has a table outlining procedures that are performed routinely, under special circumstances, or in advanced practice.
- **Core Examination Skills** are identified in this edition based on data collected from nurses. Performing these core skills provides an evidence-based practice of assessment. Core skills are denoted with a symbol of a key to highlight this material.
- **Advanced Practice Skills** are distinguished from basic skills and identified with a special icon. This feature bridges the gap between undergraduate and advanced practice education. Advanced content is denoted with a symbol to highlight this material for advanced practice students without being obtrusive for undergraduate students.
- **Link to Concepts** boxes feature eight concepts in the context of health assessment and are found throughout the text. Featured concepts include: pain, sleep, oxygenation, perfusion, tissue integrity, motion, sensory, and intracranial regulation. The concept and interrelated concepts are shown along with an explanation of how these concepts are linked.
- **Clinical Reasoning Exemplars** are featured in select chapters throughout the text. This feature helps students gain the perspective of an expert nurse in the process of clinical judgment and decision making in the context of health assessment. Look for clinical reasoning boxes in Chapters 10-16.
- **Frequently Asked Questions** boxes answer common questions students have as they are learning health assessment. These "FAQs" appear throughout Unit II.
- Near the end of each chapter is a section on **Clinical Application and Clinical Reasoning**. Included are the Case Studies and Review Questions with answers to these exercises in Appendix E to help students evaluate their learning.
- At the beginning of each chapter is a description of the **Electronic Resources** found in corresponding chapters or the companion CD-ROM, packaged free with the fourth edition, and on the Evolve site.

TEACHING AND LEARNING AIDS

An **Interactive Companion CD-ROM**, packaged free with each text, offers a **variety of student activities** designed to provide a mechanism for application of concepts. Activities include multiple-choice questions, matching, crossword puzzles, risk factor exercises, anatomy activities, symptom analysis, and "A Day in the Clinic" activity. Also included are **Student Lab Guides**, thoroughly revised for the fourth edition, which can be printed by the student and brought to class as assigned for use in the laboratory setting. The

Student CD-ROM contains 27 **cardiac and respiratory sounds**, which can be used in conjunction with the heart and lung chapters. New to the fourth edition CD are the **Core Exam Skills Checklists**, which outline assessment procedures for the most frequently-used exam skills, and **Quick Challenge** activities, which are designed to test students' new assessment skills through case-study style questions and expert answer comparison. A special **CD icon** at the beginning of each textbook chapter indicates where related study questions or exercises can be found on the CD-ROM.

The **Evolve website** for this book contains extensive student and instructor resources and can be accessed at *http://evolve.elsevier.com/Wilson/assessment/*. This dynamic educational component allows students and faculty to access the most current information and resources for further study and research. The comprehensive **Evolve Instructor Resources** include an **Instructor's Manual** containing Chapter Focus, Key Terms, Learning Objectives, Chapter Outline and Teaching Strategies, and Learning Activities for use with classroom lectures. The ExamView **Test Bank** has been thoroughly revised and includes approximately 750 test questions. Also included is a comprehensive **Electronic Image Collection** to accompany the fourth edition of *Health Assessment for Nursing Practice*, which contains hundreds of full-color images that can be used to make transparencies or be imported into the **PowerPoint lecture slides** for use in classroom lectures. **Audience Response Questions** for i-clicker and other systems are also provided for each PowerPoint chapter presentation.

Evolve Student Resources include: Frequently Asked Questions, with expert answers; printable Student Lab Guides for easy evaluation of students' assessment skills; Core Exam Skills Checklists for more focused evaluation of essential skills; PDA-Downloadable Exam Checklists outlining both routine and special circumstance or advanced practice procedures; 27 heart and lung sounds; growth charts and health promotion links; and a Spanish assessment tool with key assessment terms and phrases. Look for the Evolve logo and web address at the beginning of each fourth edition chapter.

Contents

UNIT 3
HEALTH ASSESSMENT ACROSS THE LIFE SPAN

Why Learn Health Assessment?

Health assessment refers to a systematic method of collecting data. The nurse collects health data from the client and compares this to the ideal state of health, taking into account the client's age, gender, culture, ethnicity, and physical, psychologic, and socioeconomic status. Through the collection and analysis of data, the client's strengths, weaknesses, health problems, and deficits are identified. The nurse incorporates the client's knowledge, motivation, support systems, coping ability, and preferences to develop a plan of care that will help the client maximize his or her health potential.

The Standards of Practice identified by the American Nurses Association (ANA) (2004) are based on the nursing process. Components of the nursing process include assessment, diagnosis, outcomes identification, planning, implementation, and evaluation (Box 1-1). The first and foundational step is assessment. Assessment is the collection of "comprehensive data pertinent to the patient's health or the situation" (ANA, 2004, p. 21). The assessment and subsequent analysis of data are performed by nurses in all settings.

COMPONENTS OF HEALTH ASSESSMENT

The components of health assessment include conducting a health history (the collection of subjective data), performing a physical examination (the collection of objective data), and documenting the findings.

Health History

The health history consists of the subjective data nurses collect when interviewing clients. It includes information about clients' current state of health, the medications they take, their previous illnesses and surgeries, their family histories,

and a review of systems. A *symptom* is a report of what the client experiences associated with a problem, and is considered subjective data (Box 1-2). If the data are acquired from another individual (such as a family member), it is referred to as a secondary source of data. The amount of information collected by the nurse during a health history depends on the setting, context of care, client needs, and experience of the nurse. More information about conducting a health history is presented in Chapter 3.

Physical Examination

The physical examination involves the objective data collected by the nurse. Objective data are also referred to as *signs* (Box 1-2). During a physical examination, the nurse obtains objective data using the techniques of inspection, palpation, percussion, and auscultation. The nurse also measures the client's height, weight, blood pressure, temperature, and respiratory rate. The extent of the examination depends on the setting, context of care, client needs, and the nurse's experience. Specific physical examination skills and techniques are presented in chapters throughout this textbook.

Documentation of Data

Data collected from health assessment must be documented so that other health care providers can use the information. Complete, accurate, and descriptive documentation of health assessment data improves the effectiveness of the entire health care team. Documenting these data also prevents the client from having to provide the same information to another health care provider. The written record serves as a legal document and permanent record of the client's health status at the time of the nurse-client interaction. Thus, it

STANDARDS OF NURSING PRACTICE
The Nursing Process

Standard 1: Assessment
The registered nurse collects comprehensive data pertinent to the patient's health or the situation.

Standard 2: Diagnosis
The registered nurse analyzes the assessment data to determine the diagnoses or issues.

Standard 3: Outcome Identification
The registered nurse identifies expected outcomes for a plan individualized to the patient or the situation.

Standard 4: Planning
The registered nurse develops a plan that prescribes strategies and alternatives to attain expected outcomes.

Standard 5: Implementation
The registered nurse implements the identified plan.
- 5A: Coordination of Care—The registered nurse coordinates care delivery.
- 5B: Health Teaching and Health Promotion—The registered nurse employs strategies to promote health and a safe environment.
- 5C: Consultation—The APRN and the nursing role specialist provide consultation to influence the identified plan, enhance the ability of others, and effect change.
- 5D: Prescriptive Authority and Treatment—The APRN uses prescriptive authority, procedures, referrals, treatments, and therapies in accordance with state and federal laws and regulations.

Standard 6: Evaluation
The registered nurse evaluates progress toward attainment of outcomes.

From American Nurses Association: *Nursing: scope and standards of practice,* Washington, DC, 2004, American Nurses Association. Available at *nursesbooks.org.*
APRN, Advanced practice registered nurse

CLARIFICATION OF TERMS   *Signs & Symptoms and Clinical Manifestations*

Signs & Symptoms
Signs are objective data observed, felt, heard, or measured by the nurse. Examples of signs include rash, enlarged lymph nodes, and swelling of an extremity. **Symptoms** are subjective data the client or family tells the nurse. Examples of symptoms include pain, itching, and nausea. Occasionally data may fall into both categories. For example, a client may tell the nurse he "feels sweaty"—a symptom. At the same time the nurse may observe excessive sweating, or diaphoresis—a sign.

Clinical Manifestations
Clinical manifestations is a term often used to describe the presenting signs *and* symptoms experienced by a client.

Context of Care

The context of care refers to the circumstance or situation related to the health care delivery. This may be related to the setting or environment; it might relate to physical, psychological, or socioeconomic circumstances involving the client, or the expertise of the nurse. For this reason, different types of assessments are performed by nurses. Examples include a comprehensive health assessment, a problem-based or focused health assessment, an episodic assessment, and a screening assessment (Box 1-3). If you are initiating care for a new client in a well-client setting, you will collect comprehensive subjective and objective information. On the other hand, if you are working in an emergency department and the client has minor burns on her arm, a comprehensive history and examination are not indicated. It is important, however, to conduct a problem-based or focused assessment, ensuring that subjective and objective data are collected that may have direct or indirect impact on the management of the client's burn and potential risk for future injury. For example, it would be important to inquire about the client's last tetanus

serves as a baseline for evaluation or subsequent changes and decisions related to care. Using an outline and taking brief notes during the encounter facilitates documentation and increases accuracy (Fig. 1-1). A variety of forms are used in various health care settings to document assessment findings. Regardless of the format used, basic underlying principles of documentation are common to all. The nurse must record data accurately, concisely, legibly, and without bias or opinion. Health assessment documentation is discussed further in Chapter 24.

TYPES OF HEALTH ASSESSMENT

As mentioned previously, the amount of information gained during a health assessment depends on several factors including the context of care, the setting, patient needs, and the experience of the nurse.

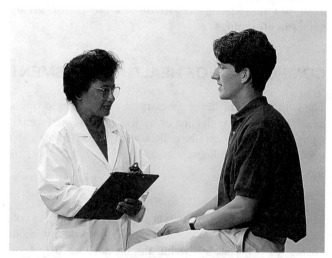

Fig. 1-1   The nurse may take notes while conducting a health assessment.

BOX 1-3 **TYPES OF HEALTH ASSESSMENT**

- **Comprehensive assessment:** This involves a detailed history and physical examination performed at the onset of care in a primary care setting or upon admission to a hospital or long-term care facility. The comprehensive assessment encompasses health problems experienced by the client, as well as health promotion, disease prevention, and assessment for problems associated with known risk factors, or assessment for age- and gender-specific health problems.
- **Problem-based/focused assessment:** The problem-based or problem-focused assessment involves a history and examination that is limited to a specific problem or complaint (e.g., a sprained ankle). This type of assessment is most commonly used in a walk-in clinic or emergency department, but it may also be applied in other outpatient settings. Although the focus of data collection is on a specific problem, the potential impact of the client's underlying health status also must be considered.
- **Episodic/follow-up assessment:** This type of assessment is usually done when a client is following up with a health care provider for a previously identified problem. For example, a patient treated by a health care provider for pneumonia might be asked to return for a follow-up visit after completion of antibiotics. An individual treated for an ongoing condition such as diabetes is asked to make regular visits to the clinic for episodic assessment. Another type of episodic assessment is the *shift assessment* performed by nurses in acute care facilities. The purpose of the shift assessment is to identify changes in condition from baseline; thus the focus of the assessment is largely based on the condition or problem the client is experiencing.
- **Screening assessment:** A screening assessment, or screening examination, is a short, usually inexpensive examination focused on disease detection. A screening examination might be performed in a health care provider's office (as part of a comprehensive examination) or at a health fair. Examples include blood pressure screening, glucose screening, cholesterol screening, and colorectal screening.

immunization, chronic medical conditions, and current medications. In addition, if you assess the client to be at risk or in need of further health evaluation, it is important that the client be referred to an appropriate site at a later date so that a comprehensive assessment may be completed.

Client Need

The type of health assessment performed by the nurse is also driven by client need. Because client needs can vary widely, the nurse must be prepared to conduct the appropriate level of assessment. The client's age, general level of health, presenting problems, knowledge level, and support systems are among many variables that impact client need. For example, a healthy 17-year-old male presenting for a sports physical to play on a high-school football team clearly has different needs than a 78-year-old, recently widowed, diabetic client presenting to a clinic with shortness of breath.

Expertise of the Nurse

The expertise of the nurse is another factor determining the type of assessment conducted. For example, a nurse working in an adult intensive care unit has expertise assessing a client with hemodynamic instability; a family nurse practitioner working in a women's clinic has expertise in performing routine pelvic examinations. Such expertise is gained with specialization within a given area of practice.

This textbook presents the process of health assessment from basic to advanced. It is not realistic for the beginning student to learn every assessment skill presented; in fact, few nurses apply all health assessment skills. Research involving the physical assessment skills utilized in clinical practice has shown that nurses incorporate some skills regularly and other skills less frequently. In a study representing a sample of 193 nurses across multiple areas of clinical practice, respondents reported only performing 30 of 124 examination skills on a routine basis; the remaining skills were reportedly performed occasionally or not performed at all (Giddens, 2007). Secrest, Norwood, and DuMont (2005) reported that 92.5% of physical assessment skills on a 120-item survey were taught and practiced in baccalaureate nursing programs, yet only 29% of nurses in clinical practice actually performed those skills on a regular basis. A major limitation in this study, however, was a small sample size (n=51). A survey of baccalaureate students in one nursing program found that fewer than half of the skills taught in the physical examination course were actually used in clinical practice (Barbarito, Carney, and Lynch, 1997). In all three studies, the large majority of the skills routinely performed by nurses represented inspection and auscultation involving cardiovascular and respiratory systems. These findings suggest the need to clearly differentiate skills that are more likely to be used in practice from those that are infrequently used. Box 1-4 presents *core* physical assessment skills identified through research. Throughout this textbook, techniques that are frequently performed by most nurses in most settings are differentiated from techniques that are less commonly performed by nurses or are indicated only in special situations. These core examination skills are indicated with the following symbol: ⚷. Furthermore, assessment techniques typically performed by an advanced practice nurse (such as a clinical nurse specialist, nurse practitioner, or certified nurse midwife) are indicated with the following "Advanced Practice" symbol: ★.

CLINICAL REASONING AND JUDGMENT

The outcome of a health assessment is a portrait of the client's physical status, strengths and weaknesses, abilities, support systems, health beliefs, and activities to maintain health, as well as his or her health problems and lack of resources for maintaining health. The nurse must analyze and interpret these data before initiating a plan of care.

BOX 1-4 CORE EXAMINATION SKILLS*

Skin
- Inspect skin
- Inspect skin lesions and wounds

Head, Eyes, Ears, Nose, Throat
- Inspect the face
- Inspect the oral cavity
- Assess hearing (based on conversation)
- Inspect external eyes
- Inspect pupils and response to light and accommodation

Chest & Lungs
- Inspect the chest
- Evaluate breathing effort
- Auscultate lung sounds

Cardiovascular
- Auscultate heart sounds and apical pulse
- Palpate distal pulses
- Palpate and inspect nails (capillary refill)
- Inspect and palpate extremities for edema
- Palpate extremities for temperature
- Inspect extremities for skin color and hair growth

Musculoskeletal
- Inspect upper and lower extremities for size and symmetry
- Palpate extremities for tenderness
- Observe range of motion
- Assess muscle strength
- Inspect the spine
- Assess gait

Abdomen
- Inspect abdomen
- Auscultate bowel sounds; aortic vascular sounds
- Palpate abdomen lightly (generalized tenderness and distension)

Neurologic
- Assess mental status and level of consciousness
- Evaluate speech

Genitalia
- Inspect male genitalia (penis/scrotum)
- Inspect female genitalia

Data from: Giddens, 2007; Secrest, et al, 2005.
*Find related Core Examination Skills Checklists for use in the lab or further study at *http://evolve.elsevier.com/Wilson/assessment/*.

Data Organization

After collecting data, nurses organize or cluster data so that the problems appear more clearly. Some assessment forms are organized under a body system format (e.g., cardiovascular, musculoskeletal, auditory, visual). Although organization of data in such a format is useful to nurses, it is incomplete because it does not include data from other important areas such as sleep, activity, or health promotion activities. Functional health patterns, developed by Gordon (1994), is a framework for organizing data by 11 areas of health status or function rather than body systems (Table 1-1). A similar format is the North American Nursing Diagnosis Association (NANDA) Taxonomy II (NANDA, 2007). The NANDA Taxonomy II (an adaptation

TABLE 1-1 Functional Health Pattern Organization

FUNCTIONAL HEALTH PATTERN	DESCRIPTION
• Health perception–health management	Client's perceived level of health, practices for maintaining health, and adherence to medical or nursing prescriptions
• Nutrition–metabolism	Pattern of foods and fluids consumed relative to the metabolic need, appetite and food preferences, weight loss/weight gain; also focuses on metabolic activity and tissue integrity
• Elimination	Patterns of bowel and urinary elimination, problems with control, and use of assistive devices; also explores skin excretion
• Activity–exercise	Client's level of activity, including leisure activities, exercise, level of energy with expenditure, ability to complete activities of daily living
• Sleep–rest	Client's routines and function related to sleep, resting, and relaxing
• Cognitive–perceptual	Client's comprehension and sensory abilities, such as vision, hearing and touch, pain, and decision-making abilities
• Self-perception–self-concept	Attitudes towards self, including body image, self-identity, and sense of self-worth and self-esteem
• Role–relationship	Patterns of relationships, satisfaction of relationships, and role responsibilities
• Sexuality–reproduction	Menstrual and reproductive history, sexual activity and function, and satisfaction with sexual activity
• Coping–stress tolerance	Client's perception of stress, response to stresses, and coping strategies
• Value–belief	Values and beliefs or goals held by the client and family and perceived conflicts with value system

From Gordon MJ: *Nursing diagnosis: process and application,* ed 3, St Louis, 1994, Mosby.

of Gordon's functional health patterns) is based on 13 domains (Table 1-2).

FREQUENTLY ASKED QUESTIONS

What do the Functional Health Patterns and the NANDA taxonomy have to do with health assessment?
Functional health patterns and NANDA Taxonomy II are classification systems for data and nursing diagnoses. These are used to organize data as well as other applications associated with health assessment such as documentation forms and care plans. These classification systems allow organization of data so that a portrait is revealed of how the client's deficits/problems affect his or her daily function or activities of daily living, rather than organizing data by body systems

Data Analysis, Interpretation, and Clinical Judgment

After collecting and organizing data, the nurse recognizes abnormal findings and identifies problems the client is experiencing through the process of analysis. The findings, however, must be correctly interpreted by the nurse to order to select appropriate nursing diagnoses and collaborative problems, and initiate an appropriate plan of care. A list of the current NANDA nursing diagnoses is presented in Appendix A of this text. The term *clinical judgment* is defined as "an interpretation or conclusion about a patient's needs, concerns, or health problems, and/or the decision to take action (or not), use or modify standard approaches, or improvise new ones as deemed appropriate by the patient's response" (Tanner, 2006, p. 204). Although clinical judgment requires accurate collection of assessment data, it is the interpretation

of data by the nurse that impacts the decisions made. According to Tanner, clinical judgment is influenced more by experiences, knowledge, attitudes, and perspectives of the nurse than the data alone. Consider the following situation:

A 50-year-old man arrives at a walk-in medical clinic with a gradual onset of cough and mild wheezing over the course of the day; he also states that he is nauseated. His vital signs and oxygen saturation are within normal limits. He states that his symptoms began while he was at work. He takes no medications and smokes one-half pack of cigarettes a day.

- An inexperienced nurse will collect and document these initial data, and inform the primary care provider that a client with a cough and wheezing is waiting to be seen.
- An experienced nurse has immediate grasp of the situation, recognizing possible problems based on his symptoms. This nurse intuitively collects additional information about each of the client's signs and symptoms, initiates appropriate interventions, determines the type of health care provider that may best assist the client, and ensures that the client receives appropriate immediate and follow-up care.

Both nurses in the preceding scenario had the same initial signs and symptoms: however, the analysis and interpretation of data differed, resulting in different nursing actions. These differences can partly be explained by clinical judgment. As described by Tanner (2006), the process of clinical judgment includes noticing (a perceptual grasp of the situation), interpreting (understanding the situation), responding (determining appropriate actions, if any), and reflecting (considering the appropriateness of patient outcomes) (Fig. 1-2). It is im-

TABLE 1-2 *NANDA Taxonomy II Domains*

DOMAIN	DESCRIPTION
• Health promotion	The awareness of well-being or normality of function and the strategies used to maintain control of and enhance that well-being or normality of function
• Nutrition	The activities of taking in, assimilating, and using nutrients for the purposes of tissue maintenance, tissue repair, and the production of energy
• Elimination/Exchange	Secretion and excretion of waste products from the body
• Activity/Rest	The production, conservation, expenditure, or balance of energy resources
• Perception/Cognition	The human information processing system, including attention, orientation, sensation, perception, cognition, and communication
• Self-Perception	Awareness about the self
• Role Relationship	The positive and negative connections or associations between persons or groups of persons and the means by which those connections are demonstrated
• Sexuality	Sexual identity, sexual function, and reproduction
• Coping/Stress Tolerance	Contending with life events/life processes
• Life Principles	Principles underlying conduct, thought, and behavior about acts, customs, or institutions viewed as being true or having intrinsic worth
• Safety/Protection	Freedom from danger, physical injury or immune system damage, preservation from loss, and protection of safety and security
• Comfort	Sense of mental, physical, or social well-being or ease
• Growth/Development	Age-appropriate increases in physical dimensions and organ systems; attainment of developmental milestones

From North American Nursing Diagnosis Association: *Nursing diagnoses: definitions and classification 2007-2008,* Philadelphia, 2007, North American Nursing Diagnosis Association.

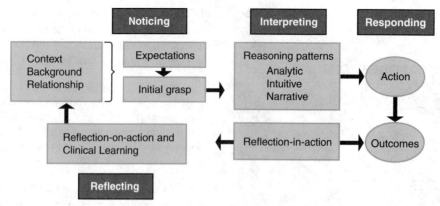

Fig. 1-2   Clinical Judgment Model. *Noticing* refers to the nurse's expectations and initial grasp of a situation. Noticing triggers reasoning patterns that allow the nurse to interpret the situation and respond with interventions. *Reflection-in-action* specifically relates to evaluating outcomes of interventions while *reflection-on-action* represents the contribution of an experience to a nurse's collective experiences. *(From Tanner C: Thinking like a nurse: A research-based model of clinical judgment in nursing,* J Nurs Educ *45:204-211, 2006.)*

portant to understand that although assessment is linked to noticing, the process of assessment in itself does not automatically lead to noticing. Noticing is based on expectations of the nurse associated with multiple variables, including clinical experience, knowledge, and the clinical context.

HEALTH PROMOTION AND HEALTH PROTECTION

A central component of nursing is the promotion of health. Health promotion begins with health assessment; thus health promotion and health protection are themes found throughout this textbook. Through the process of health assessment, the nurse assesses a client's current health status, health practices, and risk factors. Interpretation of such data allows the nurse to target appropriate health promotion needs for the client. *Health promotion* is behavior motivated by the desire to increase well-being and actualize human health potential. *Health protection* is behavior motivated by a desire to actively avoid illness, detect it early, or maintain functioning within the constraints of illness (Pender et al, 2006).

Three levels of health promotion—primary prevention, secondary prevention, and tertiary prevention—address the promotion of health regardless of a client's health status. Nurses are instrumental in providing education and care so that an individual's health promotion needs are met. The focus of *primary prevention* is to prevent a disease from developing through the promotion of a healthy lifestyle. *Secondary prevention* consists of screening efforts to promote early detection of disease. *Tertiary prevention* is directed toward minimizing the disability from acute or chronic disease or injury and helping the client to maximize his or her health. Table 1-3 clarifies these levels of health promotion further.

The framework for health promotion efforts in the United States is found in *Healthy People 2010: Understanding and Improving Health* (Department of Health and Human Services, 2000). This document contains the national health objectives that address the most significant preventable threats to health, and national goals to reduce such threats. The two overarching goals of *Healthy People 2010* are (1) increase the years of healthy life, and (2) eliminate health care disparities. The goals are supported by 467 detailed objectives in 28 focus areas. Ten leading health indicators are linked to the objectives and focus areas (Fig. 1-3). It is beyond the scope of this textbook to address all areas within this document; however, select areas are presented in health promotion boxes found throughout the text.

TABLE 1-3 *Levels of Health Promotion*		
LEVEL OF PREVENTION	**FOCUS**	**EXAMPLES**
Primary prevention	Protection to prevent occurrence of disease	Immunizations, pollution control, nutrition, exercise, etc.
Secondary prevention	Early identification of disease before it becomes symptomatic in order to halt the progression of the pathologic process	Screening examinations and self-examination practices (e.g., colorectal screening, mammography, blood pressure screening)
Tertiary prevention	Minimize severity and disability from disease through appropriate therapy for chronic disease	Diabetes mellitus management, cardiac rehabilitation, etc.

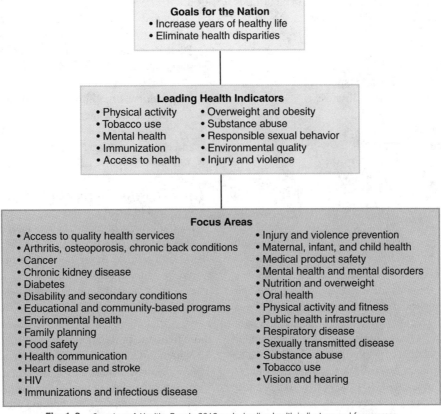

Fig. 1-3 Overview of *Healthy People 2010* goals, leading health indicators, and focus areas.

You are now challenged to diligently study this health assessment textbook. You need to be prepared to collect accurate health assessment data about the client, to make accurate clinical judgments about the client's situation, and to develop interventions that will improve the client's actual or potential health status. If you do this, the client's health has a higher probability of improving. Accurate health assessment is one of the cornerstones of the art and science of professional nursing.

CLINICAL APPLICATION & CLINICAL REASONING

See Appendix E for answers to exercises in this section.

REVIEW QUESTIONS

1 A 52-year-old client is admitted to the hospital with a new diagnosis of rectal cancer. The nurse will conduct which of the following on his admission?
    1 A comprehensive assessment.
    2 A problem-based health assessment.
    3 An episodic assessment.
    4 A screening assessment for colorectal cancer.
2 The formation of a plan of care for a client is initiated with:
    1 Data analysis.
    2 Data collection.
    3 Functional health patterns.
    4 Identification of nursing diagnoses.
3 During an interview, the nurse learns that a client has a 5-year history of hypertension. Health promotion interventions are geared toward:
    1 Teaching the client methods to prevent hypertension.
    2 Monitoring and minimizing the progression of disease.
    3 Establishing a screening schedule for disease detection.
    4 All of the above.

4 A client reports painful urination for 2 days. The urine is pink tinged and cloudy. These data represent:
   1 Subjective data.
   2 Objective data.
   3 Subjective and objective data, respectively.
   4 Objective and subjective data, respectively.
5 The process of clustering data facilitates:
   1 Data analysis.
   2 Collection of data.
   3 Implementing nursing care.
   4 Evaluating nursing care.

CASE STUDY 1

Sharon is a 42-year-old woman admitted to the hospital with a diagnosis of acute cholecystitis. Sharon tells the nurse the pain she is experiencing in her right upper abdomen feels like a knife and that it goes all the way to her shoulder. Sharon is also very nauseated. She tells the nurse that she is exhausted and has not slept for three nights because the pain keeps her awake. The nurse observes dark circles under Sharon's eyes. Her vital signs are as follows: blood pressure (BP), 132/90 mm Hg; heart rate, 104 beats/min; respiratory rate, 22 per minute; temperature, 101.8° F (38.8° C). A complete blood count laboratory test reveals that Sharon has an elevated white blood cell count. She lies in her bed in a fetal position and tells the nurse that it hurts too much to get up and move.
   1. List the subjective data described in Case Study 1.
   2. List the objective data described in Case Study 1.

CASE STUDY 2

Linda is a 41-year-old female on the orthopedic unit. Listed below are data collected by the nurse during an interview and assessment.

Interview Data

Linda states, "I fell off my horse while riding. The horse stepped on my leg and crushed the bone in my upper leg." She complains of pain in her right leg and states that the pain medication helps only a little. She wants to move but cannot because of the traction. Linda says, "My butt hurts because I can't move around." She tells the nurse, "I have not had a bowel movement for 3 days now; the last time I had a bowel movement the stool looked like hard, dry rabbit turds. Normally at home I go every day." Linda has not been hungry either. She says that "the food is horrible." Linda also complains that she is so bored she cannot stand it. "I am used to being active—being stuck in bed is driving me crazy. TV shows aren't worth watching."

Examination Data

- *Vital signs:* BP, 108/72 mm Hg; pulse, 88 beats/min; respiration, 16 per minute; temperature, 98.1° F (36.7° C); height, 5 ft 5 in (165 cm); weight, 135 lb (61 kg).
- *Medication:* Percocet 1 or 2 by mouth every 4 to 6 hours as needed for pain. She has taken 2 every 6 hours over the last several days.
- *Diet:* Regular diet. Has eaten, on average, 30% of meals. Fluid intake has averaged 1000 ml/day.
- *Activity:* Client is on complete bed rest.
- *Respiratory:* Breathing even/unlabored. Lungs are clear to auscultation bilaterally.
- *Cardiovascular:* All distal pulses palpable. Heart rate and rhythm regular. No peripheral edema.
- *Abdomen:* Slightly distended. Bowel sounds auscultated throughout abdomen.
- *Musculoskeletal:* Right leg in skeletal traction. Normal sensation to foot/toes, rapid capillary refill. Other extremities: full range of motion. No pain over joints and muscles.
- *Integument:* Skin warm and dry. Pin sites for traction without redness or drainage. Two-inch-diameter redness over sacrum. Skin intact.

The four nursing diagnoses listed below are applicable to Linda. List data presented in this case study that support each nursing diagnosis. Note: Some data may be placed under more than one problem.
1. Nursing diagnosis: *Acute pain* related to right leg injury
   a. Subjective data
   b. Objective data
2. Nursing diagnosis: *Constipation* related to inactivity and analgesics
   a. Subjective data
   b. Objective data
3. Nursing diagnosis: *Risk for impaired skin integrity* related to immobility
   a. Subjective data
   b. Objective data
4. Nursing diagnosis: *Deficient divisional activity* related to complete bed rest
   a. Subjective data
   b. Objective data

⊙ INTERACTIVE ACTIVITIES

Open the interactive student CD-ROM, click on Chapter 1, and choose from the following activities on the menu bar:

- **Multiple Choice Challenge.** Click on the best answer for each question. You will be given immediate feedback, rationale for incorrect answers, and a total score. Good luck!

- **Crossword Wizard.** Complete a crossword puzzle using the clues associated with health assessment concepts. It's a whiz!

- **Marvelous Matches.** Drag each word or phrase to the appropriate place on the screen. Test your ability to correctly match subjective and objective data.

- **Quick Challenge.** Use this critical thinking exercise to assess your skills through case study-style questions, then compare with expert answers!

CHAPTER 2

Ethnic and Cultural Considerations

ELECTRONIC RESOURCES

Additional information related to the content in Chapter 2 can be found

in the companion website at

evolve

http://evolve.elsevier.com/Wilson/assessment/

or on the interactive student CD-ROM.

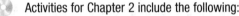 Activities for Chapter 2 include the following:
• Multiple Choice Challenge • Marvelous Matches
• Quick Challenge

We live in a country of many colors, many heritages, and many histories. Some refer to the United States as a "melting pot" because people from so many different cultures live here. At one end of the continuum are people who came to the United States from other countries and have not changed their behaviors or beliefs. They live in small communities with people who have a similar cultural heritage. At the other end of the continuum are people who came to the United States from other countries and changed from the "old country" beliefs and behaviors to those that better suit them. Between the two ends of this continuum are people with varying behaviors and beliefs that represent a blending of foreign and American influences. Culture is dynamic that results from human interactions among people of many beliefs. As individuals interact with people and their physical and social environments, they create ways of naming, understanding, and managing their worlds. As people interact with new individuals and new environments, their culture may change. People within a culture share values, beliefs, and expected behaviors that define what is right, normal, and appropriate as well as what is wrong, abnormal, and inappropriate (McNaughton, 2002). Belief systems act as lenses on the world through which we filter everything we view. When we gain new information that contradicts our beliefs, we may tend to disregard that information rather than change beliefs. Unfortunately, some our beliefs may be based on incorrect or incomplete information.

Diversity refers to differences in gender, age, culture, race, ethnicity, religion, sexual orientation, physical or mental disabilities, and social and economic status. As a health care professional, you are challenged with the responsibility to work with and care for diverse individuals who may not have the same skin color, language, health practices, beliefs,

and values as your own. When this occurs, the goal is not to force the client and his or her family to comply with your beliefs, values, and health practices but instead to meet the client where he or she is and to work with his or her belief and value system. The challenge occurs not when the client is of the same heritage and speaks the same language as the nurse, but when the cultures and languages are different. Consider the following scenario:

> You are caring for a 72-year-old Hispanic woman, Rosa Martinez, who speaks Spanish as her primary language. Conversing in broken English, she tells you that she has injured her lower back and now has continuing aches and stiffness. She does not want to be at the clinic but is here because her daughter forced her to come. She says that she hasn't seen a physician in years because Maria, her *curandera*, takes good care of her. When you inquire whether she has seen Maria for her back, she replies yes and then goes on to tell you that Maria had given her an herbal formula to take internally and had made herbal poultices to use at home. The client tells you that she believes that these remedies are working and she is not sure why her daughter made her come to the clinic.

The nurse caring for Mrs. Martinez is potentially challenged by three issues: (1) the language barrier; (2) an alternative health care provider, Maria, the *curandera,* in whom Mrs. Martinez has much confidence; and (3) the use of alternative folk remedies—the herbal formulas and poultices. How the nurse interacts with this client and her family will depend partly on the nurse's own heritage and culture and partly on her knowledge of and attitude toward other cultures and other cultural health beliefs and practices.

Nurses working together from diverse cultures may practice nursing in different ways. Some nurses who are Native American report that their nursing practice may be different from that of other nurses because they perceive life through a view that is different and that guides them in making their own sense of health care matters (Lowe and Struthers, 2001). As more nurses from other countries join the nursing profession in this country, the need for learning about how other cultures practice nursing gains new significance.

Because the diversity among us is so great, nurses are *not* responsible for knowing about the health beliefs, practices, and values of all of the cultural and racial groups other than our own, However, we are responsible for asking the client about his or her health beliefs, practices, and values because knowing this information is essential for individualizing care. A person may be from one of the major racial and cultural groups, such as Native American, African American, Asian, white American, or Hispanic, or one of the often unrecognized cultural groups, such as the homeless, migrant workers, gay men, or lesbians. To improve cultural awareness and sensitivity, you can ask questions to gather information about the unique beliefs and value systems of individuals of other cultures and backgrounds.

Culture, ethnicity, and *race* are terms that relate to cultural awareness. *Culture* is defined as all of the socially transmitted behavioral patterns, arts, beliefs, knowledge, values, morals, customs, life ways, and characteristics of a population that influence perception, behavior, and evaluation of the world. *Ethnicity* refers to a social group within a cultural and social system that shares a common social and cultural heritage, including language, history, lifestyle, and religion (Fig. 2-1). Cultural background is a fundamental component of one's ethnic background. Ethnicity is indicative of some of the following characteristics that a group may share in some combination: common geographic origin; race; language and dialect; religious beliefs; shared tradition, values, and symbols; literature, folklore, and music; food preferences; settlement and employment patterns; and an internal sense of distinctiveness (Spector, 2004). *Race* is genetic in origin and includes physical characteristics such as skin color, bone structure, eye color, and hair color. The Human Genome Project provides evidence that all human beings share a genetic code that is more than 99% identical. Although less

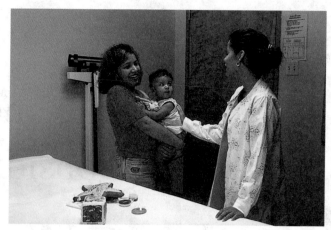

Fig. 2-2 Clients receive effective, understandable, and respectful care.

than 1% difference exists in genetic code, the differences are evident when performing health assessments. People from a given racial group do not necessarily share a common culture (Purnell & Paulanka, 2005).

To emphasize the importance of culturally and linguistically appropriate services in health care, the U.S. Department of Health and Human Services (USDHHS) Office of Minority Health (OMH) issued national standards to ensure that all people entering the health care system receive equitable and effective treatment (Fig. 2-2). These 14 standards provide for culturally and linguistically appropriate services (CLAS) to help eliminate racial and ethnic health disparities and to improve the health of all people who live in the United States of America. Although the CLAS standards are primarily directed at health care organizations, individuals in the health care systems are encouraged to use the standards to make their practices more culturally and linguistically accessible. The standards are organized around three themes: culturally competent care, language access services, and organizational supports for cultural competence. As a nurse, you are affected by Standard 1, which states that "healthcare organizations should ensure that clients/consumers receive from all staff members effective, understandable, and respectful care that is provided in a manner compatible with the cultural health beliefs and practices and preferred language" (USDHHS, OMH, 2001). Improving cultural awareness, as well as meeting Standard 1 of CLAS, requires that nurses take several steps: first, develop sensitivity to the differences between their own culture and the client's; second, avoid stereotyping; and third, develop a template that may be used for cultural assessment of the client and the family.

BECOME CULTURALLY COMPETENT

Cultural competence is the ability to communicate between and among cultures and to demonstrate skill in interacting with and understanding people from cultures other than your own. A culturally competent nurse communicates in a way that allows clients to explain what an illness means;

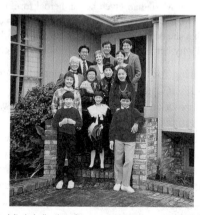

Fig. 2-1 Ethnicity is indicative of a common race, language, and dialect, as well as shared tradition.

BOX 2-1 WAYS TO ACHIEVE CULTURAL COMPETENCE

- Acknowledge that cultural diversity exists (Fig. 2-3).
- Recognize the uniqueness of and demonstrate respect for individuals and families of cultures other than your own (Fig. 2-4). Each person's cultural values are ingrained and are a part of who that person is.
- Demonstrate knowledge and understanding of the client's culture, health-related needs, and meanings of health and illness. When the client's culture is unfamiliar, ask the client about his or her culture using the template for assessment. Recognize that some cultural groups have definitions of health and illness that may differ from your own and thus use health and healing practices that may be different from your own.
- Respect the unfamiliar and learn more about it so that it is no longer unfamiliar. Be open to cultural encounters. Identify and explore your own cultural beliefs as you learn about those of others.
- Be willing to modify health care delivery to be more congruent with the client's cultural background.

Modified from Seidel et al, 2006; Purnell & Paulanka, 2003.

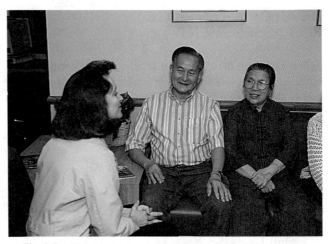

Fig. 2-3 When interviewing clients, recognize that cultural diversity exists.

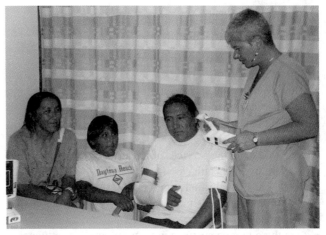

Fig. 2-4 It is important to develop sensitivity to the differences between your own culture and that of clients from another culture.

respects the concepts of time, space, and contact of the client; and respects physical and social activities of clients. This nurse respects systems of social organization and provides as much of a sense of environmental control as is possible (McNaughton, 2002). Box 2-1 describes ways to achieve cultural competence.

DON'T STEREOTYPE

Regardless of a person's skin color, physical features, cultural heritage, or social group, you must acknowledge that individual's uniqueness. Cultural heritage plays an important part in helping to identify the individual's "roots" and perhaps helps to explain attitudes, beliefs, and health practices. Each major cultural group, however, is made up of unique individuals and families who may have values and attitudes that differ from the cultural norm. Nurses must not assume that because individuals or families are Asian or Pacific Islander they all share culturally similar beliefs. For example, within the Asian or Pacific Islander people are Chinese, Filipino, Japanese, Asian Indian, Korean, Vietnamese, Cambodian, Thai, Bangladeshi, Burmese, Indonesian, Malayan, Laotian, Kampuchean, Pakistani, Sri Lankan, Hawaiian, Samoan, Tongon, Tahitian, Palauan, Fijian, and Northern Mariana Islanders, and each of these groups has a unique heritage and set of beliefs.

Personal beliefs and knowledge about other cultures in the United States have been influenced by stereotyped images and misinformation presented through the media, educational and political institutions, and family beliefs. Understanding how your beliefs were formed increases your receptiveness to different beliefs. Some common misbeliefs and stereotyped images include the following:

- All African Americans have large families.
- All welfare recipients are minorities.
- All Asians excel in math and science.
- All Native Americans live on reservations.
- All Hispanics speak Spanish.

If you learn nothing else from this text, learn that we are all unique individuals deserving of a unique and personalized assessment of our beliefs, our values, and our culture. Even people who share the same culture and background are not necessarily the same. Additionally, we may act one way in one role, but differently in another role.

To illustrate the fallacy of stereotyping, consider the analogy of assuming that all clients who have type 1 diabetes mellitus have renal failure, visual impairment, and an amputated extremity. You would assess those clients to determine their unique characteristics. Likewise, you do not assume that all people who are Catholics are opposed to divorce just because it is a belief of the religion (Dreher and MacNaughton, 2002). You would ask each client questions selected from a template for assessment that you thought were applicable.

DEVELOP A TEMPLATE FOR ASSESSMENT

When assessing the client and family, it is important to include a direct assessment of the health beliefs and practices that may reflect the client's cultural heritage. Knowing the risks of stereotyping, perform a focused interview that will provide information about the client's personal beliefs, values, and attitudes.

Introductory Questions

- Where were you born?
- With what particular cultural group (or groups) do you identify?
- What cultural practices are important to you?

What is the Client's Primary Language and Method of Communication?

- What is the language that is usually spoken in your home?
- How well do you speak, read, and write English?
- In what language do you think?
- Do you have to translate in your mind when communicating in English?
- Will you need the services of a translator during the time you are in this health care facility?
- Are there special rituals of communication in your family? (For example, is there someone special to whom questions should be directed?) Tell me about these.
- Are there unique customs in your culture that influence nonverbal or verbal communication? Tell me about them.
- What are some signs of indicating respect for others?
- What are appropriate ways to enter and leave situations?

What are the Client's Personal Beliefs about Health and Illness?

- How do you define health and illness?
- Do you believe that you have control over your health? If not, what or who do you believe controls your health?
- What are some of the practices or rituals that you believe will improve your health?
- Do you or have you used any of the alternative healing methods, such as acupuncture, acupressure, *ayurveda,* healing touch, or herbal products? If so, how effective was the treatment?
- Whom do you consult when you are ill?
- What are specific practices or rituals that you believe should be used to treat your health problem?
- What are your attitudes toward mental illness? Pain? Handicapping conditions? Chronic disease? Death? Dying?
- Who makes the health decisions in your family?
- What health topics do you feel uncomfortable talking about?
- What examination procedures do you feel modest about?

- What can the members of the health care team do to help you stay healthy (or become healthy again)?

What Religious or Spiritual Influences Affect the Client?

- Is there a particular religion that you practice?
- What are your spiritual needs?
- Whom do you look to for guidance and support?
- Are there any special religious practices or beliefs that are likely to feel supportive when you are ill?
- What events, rituals, and ceremonies are considered important within your life cycle, such as birth, baptism, puberty, marriage, and death?

What are the Roles of Individual People in the Family?

- Who makes the decisions in your family?
- What is the composition of your family? How many generations or family members live in your household?
- When the marriage custom is practiced, what is the attitude about separation and divorce?
- What is the role of and attitude toward children in the family?
- When the children are punished, how is it done, and who does it?
- What are the major important events in your family? How are they celebrated?
- Do you or the members of your family have special beliefs and practices surrounding conception, pregnancy, childbirth, lactation, and child rearing?

Does the Client have Special Dietary Practices?

- What is the main type of diet eaten in your home?
- Are there special types of foods that are forbidden by your culture or foods that are a cultural requirement in observance of a rite or ceremony? If so, what are they?
- Who in your family is responsible for food preparation?
- How is the food in your culture prepared?
- Are there specific beliefs or preferences concerning food, such as those believed to cause or cure illness?

REMEMBER . . .

The most important behaviors in cultural assessment are to be sensitive; to ask questions; to gather information specific to the individual client; to not stereotype; and to not assume that, just because you took care of a similar client last week, you know exactly how this client feels and what he or she believes.

Regardless of the client's race or cultural heritage, each individual is unique. Before you become involved in the detailed task of a physical assessment, first take the time to get to know the client and his or her family.

CLINICAL APPLICATION & CLINICAL REASONING

See Appendix E for answers to exercises in this section.

REVIEW QUESTIONS

1 A school nurse notices a boy with a bandage on his arm and black fluid under the edge of the bandage. She asks the teen what happened to his arm. He replies that his mother applied axle grease to a boil. The nurse responds by:
  1 Telling the teen to remove the bandage and wash his arm.
  2 Asking the teen what the boil looks like, what it feels like, and if the axle grease is helping it get better.
  3 Advising the teen to tell his mother to use antibiotic cream rather than axle grease.
  4 Suggesting that the teen see a health care provider because the axle grease will infect the boil.

2 The nurse is caring for a woman who has just been pronounced dead. Her adult children are in the room. To provide culturally competent care the nurse says:
  1 "Which funeral home would you like notified of your mother's death?"
  2 "We will be moving her to the morgue in about 30 minutes."
  3 "Would you like time alone with your mother for any specific ceremonies?"
  4 "Here are some of her personal belongings that were in the drawer."

3 A nurse is assessing a woman whose religious beliefs do not allow blood transfusions. She has severe anemia, is very weak, and has altered mental status. To provide effective care to this woman the nurse should:
  1 Examine his or her own feelings about the importance of religious beliefs in making decisions about life.
  2 Recognize that he or she cannot provide care to clients whose religious beliefs endanger their lives.
  3 Try to convince the client to have a blood transfusion to save her own life.

4 Determine whether the client is competent to make her own decisions about health care.

4 A nurse is teaching a family from Guatemala about the importance of exercise to reduce body weight. The husband asks, "What do we need to do now?" Considering the time orientation of this family, the nurse's most effective reply would be:
  1 "In the past, research has shown that walking 30 minutes most days of the week is best."
  2 "Is there an exercise you can do today for 30 minutes and make it part of your daily routine?"
  3 "If you will exercise 30 minutes most days of the week, you can lose weight by your next visit."
  4 "I have always found resistance weight training to be effective to do each day for 30 minutes."

INTERACTIVE ACTIVITIES

Open the interactive student CD-ROM, click on Chapter 2, and choose from the following activities on the menu bar:

- **Multiple Choice Challenge.** Click the best answer for each question. You will be given immediate feedback, rationale for incorrect answers, and a total score. Good luck!

- **Marvelous Matches.** Drag each word or phrase and drop it below the appropriate place on the screen. Test your ability to match the cultural description with its meaning.

- **Quick Challenge.** Use this critical thinking exercise to assess your skills through case study-like questions, then compare with expert answers!

CHAPTER 3

Interviewing to Obtain
a Health History

ELECTRONIC RESOURCES

Additional information related to the content in Chapter 3 can be found

in the companion website at

evolve

evolve: http://evolve.elsevier.com/Wilson/assessment/

or on the interactive student CD-ROM

Activities for Chapter 3 include the following:
- Multiple Choice Challenge • Quick Challenge
- Marvelous Matches • Printable Lab Guide

The two primary components of health assessment are the health history and the physical examination. Collection of assessment data is the first step in the nursing process and an expectation of nurses in clinical nursing practice (American Nurses Association, 2004). Together, the nurse and client use this database to create a plan to promote health, prevent disease, resolve acute health problems, and minimize limitations related to chronic health problems. Accomplishing this purpose involves meeting both the client's expectations for health and the nurse's expectations for the health of those clients.

The purpose of the health history is to obtain subjective data from clients. Information gathered includes how clients' define health and their beliefs about attaining and maintaining health, such as how they view their responsibility for their health, what health behaviors they currently practice, and which unhealthy behaviors they are willing to change. The clients' expectations for health are based on their life experiences, the experiences of their families and friends, and the culture in which they live. The nurse has a broader view of health and compares a client's current state of health to a standard needed to attain or maintain optimal health and then determines how far away the client is from the desired standard.

THE INTERVIEW

The health history is obtained through an interview process between the client and nurse. During the interview, the nurse's role is to facilitate discussion in order to collect and record data. The nurse may use an outline to prompt questions and take brief notes during the interview. Both practices are acceptable as long as they do not interfere with the communication process.

The nurse should learn about clients' health concerns and the social, economic, and cultural factors that influence their health and their responses to illness. Data generated from an interview provides the foundation for personalized and effective health care for each individual. In many settings, clients are asked to complete a health history questionnaire. This is a form that typically consists of a series of yes/no questions pertaining to specific problems or symptoms. Although a questionnaire is a useful tool for collecting a health history, it should only be considered adjunct data—it is never a substitute for an interview. Any past medical problems or symptoms identified by clients on a questionnaire should be further investigated by the nurse.

The interview typically consists of three phases: introduction, discussion, and summary (Box 3-1). To begin the introduction phase, introduce yourself to the clients and tell them your role in their care (Fig. 3-1). Address clients by their title (for example, Mr., Mrs., Miss, or Ms.) and surname. Avoid using the first name with clients unless they request it, except when clients are adolescents or children. Also avoid substituting the client's role for his or her name, such as referring to the client as "mom" or "grandpa." During the introduction phase you should also explain to clients what to expect during the interview and how long the process should take. Next, the interview moves into the discussion phase. During this phase you will collect the health history by facilitating a discussion regarding various aspects of clients' health. Although your role is to facilitate the direction of conversation, ideally the conversation is *client centered,* meaning that cli-

PHASES OF AN INTERVIEW

Introduction Phase
- Nurse introduces self to client
- Nurse describes the purpose of the interview
- Nurse describes the process of the interview so that client knows how long interview will take and what to expect

Discussion Phase
- Nurse facilitates discussion
- Discussion is client centered
- Nurse uses various communication techniques to collect data

Summary Phase
- Summarization of data
- Allows for clarification of data
- Provides validation to the client that nurse understands problems

ents are free to share their concerns, beliefs, and values in their own words (Smith, 2002). During the discussion phase, you will use a variety of communication skills and techniques to enhance the conversation and data collection. The summary phase is a time for closure. Summarize with clients the main points and emphasize data that have implications for health promotion, disease prevention, or resolving their health problems. The summary allows for clarification of data and provides validation to clients that you have an accurate understanding of their health issues, problems, and concerns.

Therapeutic Communication: The Foundation for Interviewing

Perhaps the single most important factor in the success of an interview is the communication skills of the nurse. Through the use of therapeutic communication skills, the nurse establishes client rapport. This rapport is necessary to gain clients' trust to share personal information. Numerous factors affect the interview and the therapeutic communication process,

including the physical setting, nurse behaviors, the type of questions asked, and how they are asked. Additionally, the personality and behavior of clients, how they are feeling at the time of the interview, and the nature of information being discussed or problem being confronted may affect the interview process.

The Physical Setting

Before conducting an interview, consider the physical setting, which can impact the exchange of information between the client and nurse. Ideally, an interview is conducted in a private, quiet, comfortable room free from environmental distractions.

The importance of privacy, especially when discussing issues that are highly personal, cannot be overemphasized. Clients may not be willing to share sensitive information openly and honestly if they are fearful of being overheard or in the presence of friends or family members. Consider, for example, the potentially compromising situation if you ask clients about drug use or sexual activity in the presence of family members. Privacy is best gained by conducting an interview in an unoccupied room, such as an examination room or a private hospital room. Unfortunately, the physical layout of many health care facilities makes it difficult to find a completely private place to conduct an interview; thus you must take measures to allow for as much privacy as possible. If the interview occurs in an environment with multiple treatment areas or in a semiprivate hospital room, drawing the curtains helps provide some degree of privacy and blocks out visual distractions.

Clients should be physically comfortable during an interview. When possible, allow clients to remain in street clothes and then have them change into a gown for the physical examination. The nurse and client should sit at a distance from each other that provides a comfortable flow of conversation. The client's comfort level is partly related to personal space, that is, the area that surrounds the person's body. How much space clients want will vary and is influenced by their culture and previous experiences in similar situations. Be attentive to how comfortable clients appear; if you are not sure, ask, "Is this a comfortable seating arrangement for you?" Also, if at all possible, be sure the room temperature is set at a comfortable level.

Finally, the interview should be conducted in a quiet setting without distractions. Interruptions by other individuals should be avoided. Ensure that unnecessary noise is eliminated and that unnecessary equipment is removed from the area or turned off if at all possible. Except for cases of an emergency, avoid answering cell phones or pagers while conducting an interview.

Professional Nursing Behavior

The first impression you make starts with the way you appear to the client. The way you are dressed and groomed is important in establishing a positive first impression. Modest dress, clean fingernails, and neat hair are imperative. Avoid ex-

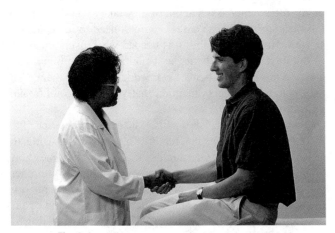

Fig. 3-1 Introduce yourself when you begin an interview.

tremes in dress and manner so that appearance does not become an obstacle or a distraction to the client's response.

The interpersonal skills of the nurse are instrumental to a successful interview. You must convey a professional yet warm demeanor. A stiff, formal attitude may inhibit communication, yet being too casual or displaying a "laid-back" attitude may fail to instill confidence. Actively listen to clients and project a genuine interest in them and in what they are saying. Clients have a need to feel understood; you should make every attempt to understand their point of view. Communicate acceptance and treat them with respect. Failure to do so jeopardizes the flow of information. The nurse must also avoid being careless with words. What may seem like an innocent comment to you may be interpreted differently by clients. Finally, nonverbal behavior is as important as your words. Avoid the extremes of reaction—startle, surprise, laughter, grimacing—as clients provide information.

Client-Related Variables

When conducting an interview, consider client variables such as age and physical, mental, and emotional status. Ideally, clients are mentally alert and in no physical or emotional discomfort. Conducting an interview with a client in physical or emotional distress is difficult. In such a case, limit the number and nature of the questions to what is absolutely necessary for the given situation, and save additional questions for a later time.

The Art of Asking Questions

The art of obtaining information from clients and listening carefully to their responses is an essential competency of nurses. Questions you ask must be clearly spoken and understood by clients. Define words clients may not understand, but do not use so many technical terms that the definitions become confusing. Use terms familiar to clients if possible. Slang words may be used if necessary to describe certain conditions. Adapt questions to a client's level of knowledge and understanding.

Encourage clients to be as specific as possible. For example, if you ask how many glasses of water the client drinks each day and he or she says, "Oh, a few," clarify what the client means by asking "How many is a few? Three? Four? Five?" This approach yields a more specific answer and provides the client's interpretation of "a few."

Ask one question at a time and wait for the reply before asking the next question. If you ask several questions at a time, the client may become confused about which question to answer, and you may be uncertain about which question the client is answering. For example, you ask, "Have you had immunizations for tetanus, hepatitis B, and influenza?" If the client answers yes, you are not sure if he or she means yes to all three or to one. If you become confused by something a client says, ask for clarification. The explanation may clear up the confusion, or it may indicate that the client has misinformation or some underlying emotional or thought processing difficulty that impairs understanding.

Be attentive to the feelings that accompany the client's responses to some questions. These responses may signify additional data you need to collect during this interview or a problem that needs to be addressed in the future. For example, if the client reports that her mother died of breast cancer and she begins to cry, this may indicate a future need to discuss coping or adjustment strategies with the client.

Some areas of questioning (such as sexuality, domestic violence, and use of alcohol or drugs) are more sensitive than others; furthermore, what is perceived as sensitive may vary from client to client. Asking questions about sensitive issues can be accomplished by explaining that you have personal or sensitive questions to ask, or using a technique referred to as *permission giving*. For example, you might say, "Many people have experimented with drugs; have you ever used street drugs?" or "Many young people your age have questions about sex. What questions or concerns do you have?" With the permission-giving technique, the nurse essentially communicates to the client that it is safe to discuss such topics.

Clients may ask you questions during the interview. Answer specific questions using terms that they understand. Avoid overburdening them with an in-depth answer that is more information than necessary to satisfy them. If clients ask broad questions, or questions you are not prepared to answer at the moment, you can get additional information regarding the situation by responding with, "Tell me more about what you are thinking." This will give you direction in answering the specific question. If you do not know the answer to the question, refer clients to the appropriate resources.

Types of Questions to Ask

Begin the interview with *open-ended questions,* such as "How have you been feeling?" This broadly stated question encourages a free-flowing, open response. The aim of an open-ended question is to elicit a response that is more than one or two words. Clients respond to this type of question by describing the onset of signs or symptoms in their own words and at their own pace. The open-ended question, however, should focus on the client's health. A question that is too broad, such as "Tell me a little about yourself," may be too general to get any useful information. The risk of asking open-ended questions is that clients may be unable to focus on the topic being asked about or may take excessive time to tell their story. In these cases, you will need to focus the interview. However, flexibility is needed when using this type of question because clients' associations may be important, and you must allow clients the freedom to pursue them. You may note topics clients mention that you want to follow up on later in the interview.

To gain more precise details, ask more direct, specific, *closed-ended questions* that require only one or two words to answer. For example, you might ask, "Do you become short of breath?" or "Do you frequently get bruises?" Another reason for using this type of question is to give clients options when answering questions, such as "Is the pain in your stomach sharp, dull, or aching?" This type of question is valuable in collecting data, but it must be used in combination with open-ended questions because failure to allow clients to describe their health in their own words may lead to inaccurate conclusions. *Directive questions* lead clients to focus on one set of thoughts. This type of question is most often used in reviewing systems or in evaluating functional status. An example would be "Describe the drainage you have had from your nose."

Techniques that Enhance Data Collection

The question-answer format is the essential tool used in obtaining a client history. Data collection can be facilitated by using the following techniques:

Active Listening

Active listening is performed by concentrating on what the client is saying and the subtleties of the message being conveyed. Active listening involves listening with a purpose to spoken words. It can also be described as concentrating on what someone is saying. Give your full attention to the client's response rather than formulating your next question. If you are concentrating on how you are going to word your next question, your attention is shifted away from the information that client is providing you. Also, avoid predicting how the client will respond to your question. When you make assumptions about how the client will respond to questions and plan your next question based on your assumptions, you may ask illogical questions based on incorrect assumptions.

Facilitation

Facilitation uses phrases to encourage clients to continue talking. These include verbal responses such as "Go on," "Uh-huh," and "Then?" and nonverbal responses such as head nodding and shifting forward in your seat with increased attention.

Clarification

Clarification is used to obtain more information about conflicting, vague, or ambiguous statements. Examples might be "What do you mean by 'you almost lost it'?" or "What do you think kept you from returning to work?"

Restatement

Restatement involves repeating what clients say using different words: it confirms your interpretation of what they said. For example, "Let me make sure I understand what you said. The pain in your stomach occurs before you eat and is relieved by eating. Is that correct?"

Reflection

Reflection is repeating a phrase or sentence the client just said. This encourages elaboration and indicates you are interested in more information.

> *Client:* "I got out of bed and I just didn't feel right."
> *Nurse:* "You didn't feel right?"
> *Client:* "Uh huh, I was dizzy and had to sit back on the bed before I fell over."

Confrontation

Confrontation is used when you notice inconsistencies between what the client reports and your observations or other data about the client. For example, "I'm confused here. You say you are staying on your diet and exercising three times a week, yet your weight has increased since your last visit. Can you help me to understand this?" Your tone of voice is important when using confrontation; use a tone that communicates confusion or misunderstanding, rather than one that is accusatory and angry.

Interpretation

Interpretation is used when you want to share with clients conclusions you have drawn from data they have given. After hearing your interpretation, clients can confirm, deny, or revise your interpretation. For example, "Let me share my thoughts about what you just told me. The week you were out of the office you exercised, felt no muscle tension, felt relaxed, and slept well. I wonder if your work environment is contributing to the anxiety you are experiencing."

Summary

A summary condenses and orders data obtained during the interview to help clarify a sequence of events. This is useful when interviewing a client who rambles or does not provide sequential data.

Techniques that Diminish Data Collection

The following communication techniques have been found to interrupt the flow of the interview, interfere with data collection, and possibly impair the client-nurse relationship. These techniques can be avoided by considering the interview from the client's perspective, such as how you would prefer the flow of the conversation to go and how you would want things explained to you.

Using Medical Terminology

You are using medical terminology when you use words or abbreviations not commonly known to clients. Some examples include saying "hypertension" instead of "high blood pressure," "dysphagia" rather than "difficulty in swallowing," "CVA" rather than "stroke," or "myocardial infarction" rather than "heart attack." Using these words may be confusing to the client. Clients may not understand the question and may feel too embarrassed to ask for clarification. Such a scenario can lead to inaccurate data collected by the nurse.

Expressing Value Judgments

Including value judgments in your questions is always a hindrance. For example, you should ask "What kind of protection do you use during intercourse, if any?" rather than saying "You do use protection during intercourse, don't you?" The latter question forces clients to respond in a way that is consistent with your values or causes them to feel guilty or defensive when they must answer to the contrary.

Interrupting the Client

Allow clients to finish sentences; do not become impatient and finish their sentences for them. The ending you add to a sentence may not be the ending that clients would have used. Associated with interrupting is changing the subject before clients have finished giving information about the last topic discussed. You may feel pressured for time and eager to move on to other topics, but allow clients an opportunity to complete their thoughts.

Being Authoritarian or Paternalistic

When you use the approach of "I know what is best for you, and you should do what I say," you risk alienating the client. Despite what you believe is best for clients, you must always remember that their health is their responsibility. They may choose to follow or ignore your advice and teaching.

Using "Why" Questions

Using "why" questions can be perceived as threatening and may put clients on the defensive (Riley, 2003). When clients are asked why they did something, the implication is that they must defend their choices. Instead of asking "Why didn't you take all the antibiotic?" you might say "I noticed you stopped taking the antibiotics before all the pills were gone" and then wait to see if the client offers an explanation. If no explanation is forthcoming, you can follow up with "I am curious about the reason for not taking all the antibiotic."

Managing Awkward Moments During an Interview

Answering Personal Questions

Clients may ask questions about you from time to time. They are curious about you and your life. Often a brief, direct answer satisfies the clients' curiosity. You may feel comfortable sharing certain experiences that may support clients, such as parenting issues or how you handle stress. Sharing these mutual experiences may enhance the relationship with clients and increase your credibility.

Silence

Silence can be awkward. You may have the urge to break the silence with a comment or question. Remember, however, that clients may need the silence as time to reflect or to gather courage. Some issues can be so painful to discuss that silence is necessary and should be accepted. Silence may indicate that they may not be ready to discuss this topic now or that your approach needs to be evaluated. Become comfortable with silence; it can be useful.

Displays of Emotion

Crying is a natural emotion and should be permitted. Saying "Don't cry" is not a therapeutic response. A more appropriate approach is to provide tissues and let clients know it is all right to cry by giving a response such as "Take all the time you need to express your feelings." Postpone further questioning until the client is ready. Crying may indicate a need that can be addressed at a later time. Compassionate response to a crying client demonstrates caring and may enhance the therapeutic relationship.

A client's anger may be uncomfortable. The most therapeutic approach is to deal with it directly by first identifying the source of the anger. You may say, "You seem angry; can you tell me the reason for your feelings?" If clients choose to discuss the anger, they may identify whether the anger is directed at someone else or at you. If clients are angry at someone else, you can discuss with them an approach for talking with that person about the reason for the angry feelings. When clients are angry with you, encourage them to discuss their feelings. Acknowledge their feelings and, if appropriate, apologize. You may be able to continue working with these clients after the angry feelings are discussed, but if clients would prefer to interact with another nurse, you should honor their request. Regardless of the outcome, you have modeled for the clients a healthy, appropriate approach to managing anger.

Challenges to the Interview

Managing the Overly Talkative Client

Occasionally, you encounter clients who are difficult to interview because they are overly talkative. Some clients feel a need to go into every detail of a problem or illness and get distracted as they tell their story. Some clients focus on remote past events with no apparent relevance to their present situation. Still others may want to discuss issues that do not relate directly to themselves, such as discussing other people or current world events. In such situations, it is sometimes very difficult to determine what is actually bothering them. Although each situation is unique, ideally you should tactfully redirect the conversation. The use of closed-ended questions may help to maintain direction and flow of the conversation.

Others in the Room

Clients are often accompanied by other individuals when seeking health care. Be careful not to assume relationships among the people present. It is best to ask, "What is your relationship?" The parent or guardian of a child usually answers interview questions on behalf of the child. When adults are unable to answer questions for themselves, it may be necessary to have other persons assist with the interview. However, all clients should be involved with the interview to the extent their mental or physical ability allows. When adult or adolescent clients are able to speak for themselves, it is best to interview them directly, and if at all possible in private. If other individuals are to remain present during the interview, be sure this is done with the client's permission.

At times, individuals who accompany clients are disruptive to an interview. For example, sometimes a parent, spouse, or friend answers questions for the client. Often these are individuals who are just trying to be helpful, but it may also suggest a dominant personality. Such situations can adversely affect the accuracy of your data, and you must validate with clients that the information is correct. If others persist in answering for a client, you may have to specifically request them to allow the client to answer, or ask them to leave until the end of the interview.

A disruptive interview also occurs when attempting to talk with mothers who have active children in the room causing constant distractions. If children are too young to wait in the waiting room, find developmentally appropriate activities for them to do while you complete the interview.

Language Barrier

When clients speak a different language than the nurse, a translator is needed for accurate communication. An objective observer who is the same gender as the client is a better translator than a family member who may alter the meaning of what is said and violates client confidentiality. Keep in mind that conducting an interview through a translator takes considerably more time than a typical interview because everything spoken must be repeated. For this reason, it is important to use your time well and focus on collecting the most important data.

Cultural Differences

Nurses work with clients from many cultural backgrounds. It is essential that the nurse develop cultural competence to identify cultural factors that may influence how a client behaves when ill. The health care system places accountability for cultural competence with the nurse and others who provide direct patient care (Dreher and MacNaughton, 2002). Furthermore, *Healthy People 2010* objectives include an emphasis on cultural competence as a component of health care delivery (U.S. Department of Health and Human Services, 2000). Cultural competence refers to "the ability to communicate between and among cultures and to demonstrate skill outside one's culture of origin" (Dunn, 2002, p. 106). To deliver culturally competent care, nurses must interact with each individual as a unique person who is a product of past experiences, beliefs, and values that have been learned and passed down from one generation to the next (Fig. 3-2). Remember, however, that all individuals within a specific cultural group do not think and behave in a similar manner. Avoid stereotyping clients because of their culture or ethnicity. There may be as much diversity within a cultural group as there is across cultural groups. Ask clients about experiences that illustrate what has been of value to them and that characterize their culture. This will increase your understanding and demonstrate to clients your interest in them as individuals (see Chapter 2).

THE HEALTH HISTORY

Types of Health Histories

The health history is the process of collecting and documenting subjective data about your client through an interview process. A history is typically taken with clients on every visit; the amount of data you collect for a history depends largely on the setting and the purpose of the visit. A history is a component of all assessments, including a comprehensive assessment, a problem-based or focused assessment, and an episodic or follow-up assessment.

The *comprehensive health history* includes biographic data, reason for seeking care, present health status, past medical history, family history, personal and psychosocial history, and a review of all body systems. This type of history may be done with a hospital admission, with an initial clinic or home visit, or when the client's reason for seeking care is for relief of generalized symptoms such as weight loss or fatigue. A comprehensive health history requires more time than other types of histories because a complete database is being established. The admission process for many hospitals includes obtaining a comprehensive database. The condition of the client, however, must be considered. A critically ill client, for example, is unable to participate in a comprehensive interview, and thus it is inappropriate to pursue. Family members may be of assistance in providing important information to the nurse while the client is seriously ill. Once the client is no longer critically ill, a comprehensive interview should be conducted. An example of a comprehensive health history for an adult is presented in Chapter 24.

The history for a problem-based or focused health assessment involves data that are limited in scope to a specific problem. However, the history must be detailed enough that the nurse is aware of other health-related data that might af-

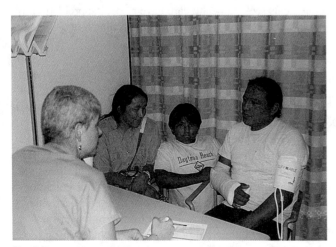

Fig. 3-2   Interact with the client as a unique person and be sensitive to cultural diversities.

FREQUENTLY ASKED QUESTIONS

It is confusing to see so much information for a health history. Do all those questions really need to be asked? What are the appropriate questions to ask?

The type of interview and amount of information you collect depend on the setting, the purpose of the visit, and individual client needs. Certain components of the history are included with all interviews, such as past medical history, current medical problems, medications the client is taking, allergies, and last menstrual period (for women of childbearing age). Some components of the history may be deferred. What is most important to remember is that the history must be individualized to the client so that unique aspects about his or her health care needs are understood by all.

fect the current problem. For example, the history for a client with a lacerated foot should include information about the incident and symptoms, but also medications the client is currently taking, medication allergies, other health problems that the client has, and immunization status. Imagine the disastrous result that could occur if this client had a history of diabetes mellitus and a severe allergy to penicillin, and this information was not discovered. A focused interview is also used when the client seeks help to address an urgent problem such as relief from asthma attacks or chest pain. Further data may be collected once the client is stabilized, particularly if the client will require ongoing care.

The history associated with an episodic or follow-up assessment generally focuses on the specific problem or problems that a client has already been receiving treatment for, or it could include well visits to an established health care provider. The nurse should assess for changes in the history since the last visit.

Regardless of the type of history taken, the nurse determines whether to ask or defer various questions on a health history because certain data are irrelevant in some situations. In addition, during an interview the nurse may uncover important data requiring further investigation. When this occurs, the nurse determines what additional questions will help clarify the data.

Components of the Health History

Because the scope of a health history varies with the type of health assessment to be conducted (comprehensive assessment, problem-based assessment, etc.), the nurse can expect variations in history format. However, many components are consistently found in all health histories. A comprehensive health history includes the following components:

- Biographic data
- Reason for seeking care
- History of present illness
- Present health status
- Past health history
- Family history
- Personal and psychosocial history
- Review of systems

Biographic Data

The biographic data are collected at the first visit and then updated as changes occur. These data begin to form a picture of the client as a unique individual. Box 3-2 lists the data to be obtained.

Reason for Seeking Health Care

The reason for seeking care (also called the *chief complaint* [CC] or *presenting problem*) is a brief statement of the client's purpose for requesting the services of a health care provider. The client's reason for seeking care is often recorded in direct quotes. Some clients will present for a routine examination or well visit and thus will not have a chief complaint or presenting problem. When clients have multiple complaints or problems, list them all and ask clients to indicate the priority of the

---

BOX 3-2   **BIOGRAPHIC DATA**
Name   Gender   Address and telephone number   Birth date   Birthplace (important when born in foreign country)   Race/ethnicity   Religion   Marital status   Occupation   Contact person   Source of data

---

problems. Some clients may initially be uncomfortable giving you the actual reason for seeking care. In this case, it is possible that they may not divulge the true reason they came until the end of the visit, after they begin to feel more comfortable. The client's condition dictates how the nurse proceeds. Urgency dictates expediency. Clients with severe pain, dyspnea, or injury should not be subjected to a prolonged history. Biographic data may be delayed to pursue the health concern. This approach enables the nurse to analyze the data quickly, identify the cause of the health concern, and plan how to alleviate the signs or symptoms. However, clients with depression may need to be given more time to freely divulge feelings and surrounding circumstances.

History of Present Illness

When clients seek health care for a specific problem, the nurse documents the present illness or problem as described previously but then should further investigate the history of the present problem. This is best accomplished by conducting a symptom analysis—a systematic way to collect data about the history and status of symptoms. There are several formats you can use to conduct a symptom analysis, but it should include all of the following variables: onset of symptoms, location and duration of symptoms, characteristics, severity of symptoms, related symptoms, alleviating factors, aggravating factors, and attempts at self-treatment (Box 3-3). Keep in mind that not all individuals seeking health care have a specific problem or illness, thus recording a history of present illness or a symptom analysis is not always indicated.

Present Health Status

An individual's present health status focuses on the client's conditions (acute and chronic), medications the client is currently taking, and allergies the client has experienced.

- *Health Conditions.* Examples include diabetes, hypertension, heart disease, sickle cell anemia, cancer, seizures, pulmonary disease, arthritis, mental illness. Ask the client how long they have had the condition, and the impact of the illness on their daily activities.
- *Medications.* Inquire about prescription, over-the-counter, and herbal preparations. Include reason for taking the medication, how long the client has been taking the medication, dose and frequency of medica-

BOX 3-3 MNEMONIC FOR SYMPTOM ANALYSIS *OLD CARTS*

Onset: When Did the Symptoms Begin?
- Did they develop suddenly or over a period of time? (Ask specific date, time, day of week if appropriate.)
- Where were you or what were you doing when the symptoms began?
- Does anyone else with whom you have been in contact have a similar symptom?

Location: Where Are the Symptoms?
- Is the location in a specific area?
- Vague and generalized?
- Does symptom radiate to another location?

Duration: How Long Do the Symptoms Last?
- Since they began, have the symptoms become worse? About the same?
- Are symptoms constant or intermittent (come and go)?
- If constant, does the severity of symptoms fluctuate?
- If intermittent, how many times a day, week, month do the symptoms occur? How do you feel in between episodes of the symptom?

Characteristics: Describe the Characteristics of the Symptom
- Describe what the symptoms feel like or look like.
- Describe the sensation: stabbing, dull, aching, throbbing, nagging, sharp, squeezing, itching.
- If applicable, describe the appearance: color, texture, composition, and odor.

Aggravating and Alleviating Factors: What Affects the Symptoms?
- What makes the symptoms worse? Is symptom aggravated by an activity (e.g., walking, climbing stairs, eating, a body position)? Are there psychologic or physical factors in the environment that may be causing the symptom (e.g., stress, smoke, chemicals)?
- What makes the symptoms better? Are there certain body positions that relieve the symptoms?

Related Symptoms: What Other Symptoms Are Present?
- Have you noticed other symptoms that have occurred at the same time (e.g., fever, nausea, pain)?

Treatment: Describe Self-Treatment Tried before Seeking Care
- What methods of self-treatment have you tried? Medications? (If so, ask the name of the medication, dosage, and time of last dose.) Heat applications? Cold applications?
- Have any of these methods been effective?

Severity: Describe the Severity of the Symptom
- Describe the size, extent, number, or amount.
- On a scale of 0 to 10, with 10 being most severe, how would you rate your symptom?
- Is the symptom so severe that it interrupts your activities (work, school, eating, sleeping, etc.)?

tion, any side effects, and the client's perception of the effectiveness of the medication.
- *Allergies.* Ask the client about allergies to foods, medications, environmental factors, and contact substances. Be sure to specifically ask about substances to which the client could be exposed in the health care setting, such as latex and iodine. When asking about allergies, be sure the client knows what is meant by the term *allergy.* Many people do not know the difference between a side effect (such as nausea) and a true allergic reaction. When the client indicates that he or she has an allergy to a medication or substance, ask the client to describe what happens with exposure to determine whether the client's reaction is a side effect or an allergic reaction.

Past Health History

The past health history is important, because past and present conditions may have some effect on the client's current health needs and problems. The following categories of data are included:
- *Childhood illnesses:* measles, mumps, rubella, chickenpox, pertussis, *Haemophilus influenzae* infection, streptococcal throat infection, otitis media. (Ask if there were complications in later years, such as rheumatic fever or glomerulonephritis that can occur after streptococcal throat infection.)
- *Surgeries:* type, date, outcome.

- *Hospitalizations:* illnesses, dates, outcome.
- *Accidents or injuries:* type (fractures, lacerations, loss of consciousness, burns, penetrating wounds), dates, outcome.
- *Immunizations:* tetanus, diphtheria, pertussis, mumps, rubella, poliomyelitis, hepatitis B, influenza, pneumococcal pneumonia, and varicella; for foreign-born clients: bacille Calmette-Guérin (BCG).
- *Last examinations:* type (physical, dental, vision, hearing, electrocardiogram [ECG], chest radiograph, skin test for tuberculosis; for women: Papanicolaou [Pap] smear, mammogram; for men: prostate examination), dates, and outcome.
- *Obstetric history:* number of pregnancies (gravidity), number of births (parity), and number of abortions/miscarriages if applicable. If working with a pregnant client or woman in child-bearing years, further information is recorded; see Chapter 21.

Family History

A family history of the client's blood relatives (biologic parents, aunts, uncles, and siblings), spouse, and children is obtained to identify illnesses of genetic, familial, or environmental nature that might affect the client's current or future health. Trace back at least two generations to parents and grandparents. Specifically ask about the presence of any of the following diseases among family members: Alzheimer's disease, cancer (all types), diabetes mellitus (specify type 1 or type 2), coronary artery disease (including myocardial infarction), hypertension, stroke, seizure disorders, mental illness (including depression, bipolar, schizophrenia), substance abuse, endocrine diseases (specify), and kidney disease. Documentation of the family history can be done in narrative form, or it can be illustrated. A genogram is a tool consisting of a family tree diagram depicting members within a family over several generations. This tool is useful in tracing diseases with genetic links. Symbols are used to indicate males and females, as well as those who are alive and deceased. Include the current ages of those who are alive and the cause of and age at death of those who are deceased (Fig. 3-3).

Personal and Psychosocial History

The personal and social history explores a variety of topics including information that affects and reflects the client's physical and mental health.

Personal Status. Ask the client for a general statement of feelings about self. Ask about cultural/religious affiliations and practices. Ask about education preparation; occupational history, satisfaction with work, and perception of adequate time for leisure and rest; and current hobbies and interests.

Family and Social Relationships. Ask about general satisfaction with interpersonal relationships, including significant others, persons with whom client lives, and the client's role within the family. Sometimes health information about significant others, sexual partners, and roommates is relevant to the client's health. Ask about the current state of health for these family members. Ask about social interactions with friends, participation in social organizations (community, school, work), and participation in spiritual or religious groups. If interactions are limited, find out what keeps the client from social interactions—perhaps this is by choice, or there could be an underlying problem. Be aware of issues

associated with domestic violence; make a point to screen all clients (Box 3-4).

Diet/Nutrition. Clients should describe their appetite and a typical daily dietary intake (or 24-hour dietary recall) for both food and fluids. Inquire about food preferences and dislikes, food intolerance, use of caffeine-containing beverages, and dietary restrictions, as well as use of dietary supplements such as vitamins or protein drinks. Ask about recent changes in appetite or weight, changes in the taste of food, or problems with nutritional intake (such as indigestion, pain or difficulty associated with eating, heartburn, bloating, difficulty chewing or swallowing). Also ask about overeating, sporadic eating, or intentional fasting.

Functional Ability. The functional ability (or functional assessment) focuses on a person's ability to perform self-care activities such as dressing, toileting, bathing, eating, and ambulating. Functional ability also includes a person's ability to perform skills needed for independent living such as shopping, cooking, housekeeping, and managing finances. Ask clients questions related to their perceived ability to complete these tasks. Assessment of functional ability is especially important for adults with physical or mental disabilities and for older adults.

Mental Health. Ask the client about personal stress and the source of stress. Common causes of stress include recent life changes such as divorce, moving, family illness, new baby, new job, and finances. Also ask the client about feelings of anxiety or nervousness, depression, irritability, or anger. Explore with the client about personal coping strategies for stressful situations and previous counseling or mental health care in the past.

Personal Habits. The habits most detrimental to health include tobacco use, excessive intake of alcohol, and use of illicit street drugs. Obtain specific information including the substance used, the amount of use, and the duration of the habit.

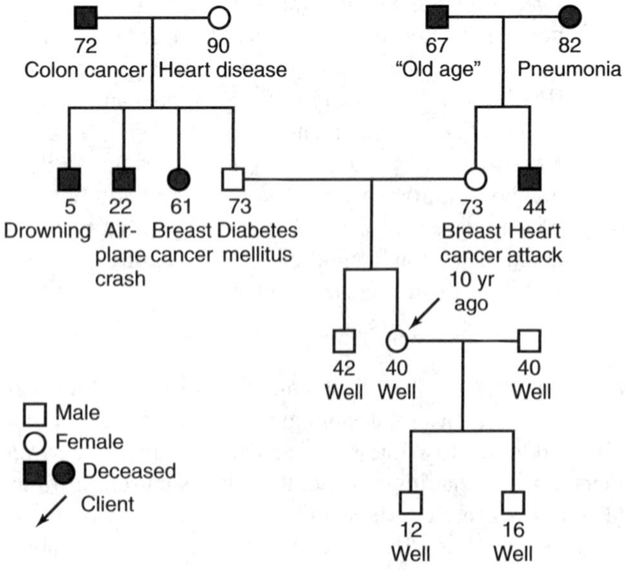

Fig. 3-3 Sample genogram identifying grandparents, parents, aunts and uncles, siblings, spouse, and children.

BOX 3-4 DOMESTIC VIOLENCE

Recognizing Domestic Violence
- *What:* Domestic violence can be either physical or emotional and occurs within the home.
- *Victims:* Usually women and children; men have been known to be victimized, although less frequently.
- *Perpetrators:* Most often an intimate partner or parent figure.
- *Contributing factors:* Domestic violence is often associated with drug or alcohol use (or both).

Screening Questions for Domestic Violence
Ask the client:
- Have you been physically injured (hit, kicked, punched) by someone in your home in the last year?
- Many women are victims of domestic violence. Do you feel safe in your current relationship with your husband or significant other?
- Are you fearful of an individual you have previously had a relationship with?

- *Tobacco:* identify type of tobacco used (cigarette, cigars, pipe, chewing tobacco) and frequency. For cigarette smokers, record the smoking history in *pack-years* (the number of packs per day times the number of years smoked). For example, a client who has smoked one-half pack a day for 20 years has a 10 pack-year smoking history.
- *Alcohol:* identify the type and amount of alcohol consumed. Ask how many alcoholic drinks are consumed in a day; if not daily use, then weekly or monthly. Ask about driving under the influence of alcohol. Screening questionnaires such as the Alcohol Use Disorders Identification Test (AUDIT) and the Cut down, Annoyed, Guilty, Eye opener (CAGE) screening test can be used to assess problem drinking and are discussed further in Chapter 7.
- *Illicit drug use:* for use of illicit drugs, specifically ask about use of marijuana, cocaine, crack cocaine, barbiturates, and amphetamines. Ask about high-risk behaviors such as sharing needles or driving under the influence of drugs.

Health Promotion Activities. Ask clients what activities they regularly perform to maintain health. Specifically ask about exercise, stress management, use of seat belts, routine examinations, and self-examinations (such as breast self-examinations or testicular self-examinations). Health promotion practices can be further assessed when reviewing specific body systems.

Environment. The history also includes data related to environmental health. Obtain a general statement of the client's assessment of environmental safety or concerns. Variables to consider include potential hazards within the home (concern about fire, smoke detector, stairs to climb, inadequate heat, open gas heaters, pest control, violent behaviors); hazards in the neighborhood or community (noise, water and air pollution, heavy traffic on surrounding streets, overcrowding, violence, firearms, sale/use of street drugs); and hazards associated with employment (inhalants, noise, heavy lifting, machinery, psychologic stress). Also ask clients about recent travel outside the United States (when and which countries visited, length of stay).

Review of Systems

Review of systems is conducted to inquire about the past and present health of each of the client's body systems. Conduct a symptom analysis when clients acknowledge the presence of symptoms. If the data collection from the present illness/present health status section has already provided sufficient data on a body system, you do not need to repeat those questions in this section. For example, if you completed a symptom analysis on "cough" when completing the present health status, you need not repeat questions about cough in the review of systems.

Symptoms are listed in this chapter using medical terms, but a brief definition is included as needed to facilitate your interpretation of the term to the client. For example, if you want to know if the client has dyspnea, you ask, "Do you become short of breath?" If the client says "No," you would

document "denies dyspnea" or "no dyspnea," but if the client says "Yes," you would use questions from the symptom analysis and document your findings. Therefore, you need to use medical terms for documentation and communication with other health care providers, but only use terms understood by the client during the interview. Although some health promotion data are included in the previous sections, additional information is collected during the review of systems.

Following is an outline, organized by body region or body system, of the symptoms you ask the client about. This list is not inclusive; rather it is an example of questions to ask. More detailed questions are presented in the chapters that follow. Remember, in a comprehensive health assessment, you ask most of the questions; in a focused health assessment, you ask about only those systems related to the reason for seeking care.

General Symptoms
- Pain; general fatigue, weakness; fever; problems with sleep; unexplained changes in weight

Integumentary System
- *Skin:* skin disease, problems, lesions (wounds, sores, growths); excessive dryness, diaphoresis (sweating), or odors; changes in temperature, texture, or pigmentation; discoloration; rashes, pruritus (itching); frequent bruising
- *Hair* (refers to all body hair, not just head and pubic area): changes in amount, texture, character, distribution; alopecia (loss of hair); scalp itching
- *Nails:* changes in texture, color, shape
- *Health Promotion:* measures taken to limit sun exposure; use of sunscreen; skin self-examination; type and frequency of nail care

Head and Neck
- *Head:* headaches; past significant trauma; vertigo (dizziness); syncope (brief lapse of consciousness)
- *Eyes:* discharge, redness, pruritus; excessive tearing; eye pain; changes in vision (generalized or vision field); difficulty reading; visual disturbances such as blurred vision, photophobia (sensitivity to light), blind spots, floaters, halos around lights, diplopia (double vision), or flashing lights; use of corrective or prosthetic devices; interference with activities of daily living
- *Ears:* pain; excessive cerumen (earwax); discharge; recurrent infections; changes in hearing (deceased hearing or increased sensitivity to environmental noises); tinnitus (ringing or crackling); use of prosthetic devices; change in balance; interference with activities of daily living
- *Nose, nasopharynx, and paranasal sinuses:* nasal discharge; frequent epistaxis (nosebleed); sneezing; obstruction; sinus pain; postnasal drip; change in ability to smell; snoring
- *Mouth and oropharynx:* sore throat; tongue or mouth lesion (abscess, sore, ulcer); bleeding gums; use of prosthetic devices (dentures, bridges); altered taste; dysphagia (difficulty swallowing); difficulty chewing; changes to voice or hoarseness
- *Neck:* lymph node enlargement; swelling, edema, or masses in neck; pain/tenderness; neck stiffness; limitation in movement

- *Health promotion:* use of protective headgear and protective eyewear; protection of ears from excessively loud noise; dental hygiene practices (brushing/flossing); dental care from dentist

Breasts

- *General:* Breast pain/tenderness; swelling or edema; breast lumps or masses, breast dimpling; nipple discharge; changes in nipples
- *Health promotion:* breast self-examination (frequency, method)

Respiratory System/Chest

- *General:* Cough (nonproductive or productive); hemoptysis (coughing up blood); frequent colds; dyspnea (shortness of breath); night sweats; wheezing; stridor (abnormal, high-pitched, musical sound); pain on inspiration or expiration; exposure to smoke or other respiratory irritants
- *Health promotion:* handwashing (reduction of respiratory infection); tuberculosis screening; wearing mask for occupational or environmental respiratory irritants or hazards, annual flu shots, smoking cessation, secondhand smoke

Cardiovascular System

- *Heart:* palpitations; chest pain; dyspnea (shortness of breath); orthopnea (person must sit to breathe); paroxysmal nocturnal dyspnea (periodic dyspnea during sleep)
- *Blood vessels:* coldness in extremities; numbness; edema; varicose veins; intermittent claudication (leg pain with exercise that ceases with rest); paresthesia (abnormal sensations); changes in color of extremities
- *Health promotion:* dietary practices to limit salt and fat intake; cholesterol screening; blood pressure screening; use of support hose if work involves standing; avoid crossing legs at the knees; exercise/activity

Gastrointestinal System

- *General abdominal symptoms:* abdominal pain; heartburn, nausea/vomiting; hematemesis (vomiting blood); jaundice (yellowish color to skin and sclera); ascites (abnormal intraperitoneal fluid accumulation)
- *Elimination:* bowel habits (frequency, appearance of stool); pain or difficulty with defecation; excessive flatus, change in stools (color, consistency); problems with diarrhea or constipation; presence of blood in stool; hemorrhoids; use of digestive or evacuation aids (stool softener, laxatives, enemas)
- *Health promotion:* dietary analysis (compare diet to food pyramid); use of dietary fiber supplements; colon cancer screening

Urinary System

- *General:* Characteristics of urine (color, contents, odor); hesitancy; frequency; urgency; change in urinary stream; nocturia (excessive urination at night); dysuria (painful urination); flank pain (posterior portion of body between ribs and iliac crest); hematuria (blood in the urine); dribbling or incontinence; polyuria (excessive excretion of urine); oliguria (decreased urination)
- *Health promotion:* measures to prevent urinary tract infections (females); Kegel exercises

Reproductive System

- *Male genitalia:* presence of lesions; penis or testicular pain or masses, penile discharge, hernia
- *Female genitalia:* presence of lesions, pain, discharge, odor; menstrual history (date of onset, last menstrual period [LMP], length of cycle); amenorrhea (absent menstruation); menorrhagia (excessive menstruation); dysmenorrhea (painful menstruation); metrorrhagia (irregular menstruation); pelvic pain
- *Sexual history:* ask about current and past involvement in sexual relationships; nature of sexual relationship(s) (heterosexual, homosexual, bisexual); type and frequency of sexual activity; number of sexual partners (past and present); satisfaction with sexual relationships; method of contraception used (if applicable); changes in sex drive; problems with infertility; exposure to sexually transmitted infections; females—dyspareunia (pain during intercourse); postcoital bleeding (bleeding after intercourse); males—impotence; premature ejaculation
- *Health promotion:* methods to prevent unwanted pregnancy; protection from sexually transmitted infections; testicular or vulvar self-examination; Papanicolaou (Pap) smear (females); prostate screening (males)

Musculoskeletal System

- *Muscles:* twitching; cramping; pain; weakness
- *Bones and joints:* joint swelling or edema; pain; redness; stiffness; deformity; crepitus (noise with joint movement); limitations in range of motion; arthritis; gout; interference with activities of daily living
- *Back:* back pain, pain down buttocks and into legs; limitations in range of motion; history of disk disease; interference with activities of daily living
- *Health promotion:* amount and kind of exercise per week; calcium intake; osteoporosis screening

Neurologic System

- *General:* syncope (fainting episodes); loss of consciousness; seizures (characteristics, how treated); cognitive changes; changes in memory (short-term, recent, long-term); disorientation (time, place, person)
- *Motor-gait:* loss of coordinated movements; ataxia (balance problems); paralysis (partial versus complete); paresis (weakness); tremor; spasm; interference with activities of daily living
- *Sensory:* paresthesia (abnormal sensations, e.g., "pins and needles," tingling, numbness); pain (describe)

Health History Based on Functional Health Patterns

Not all health histories are organized in a body systems format as previously described. Functional health patterns is a common interview format used by nurses in many areas. For example, it is the format used for the nursing admission history in many hospitals. Functional health patterns as a nursing database is briefly discussed in Chapter 1. In addition to biographic data and the reason for seeking care, a nursing history based on functional health patterns collects and organizes data in each of the following 11 areas (Gordon, 1994):

- Health perception–health management
- Nutrition-metabolism, nutrition-metabolic
- Elimination
- Activity-exercise
- Cognitive-perception
- Sleep-rest
- Self-perception–self-concept
- Role-relationship
- Sexuality-reproduction
- Coping–stress tolerance
- Values-belief

An example of a health history based on functional health patterns is presented in Appendix B.

AGE-RELATED VARIATIONS

This chapter discusses principles of interviewing and conducting a health history with adult clients. It is important to recognize that a health history may require a different approach and focus on different information depending on the age of the client.

Infants, Children, and Adolescents

The pediatric health history is similar to that of the adult, with the addition of questions regarding pregnancy, prenatal care, growth and development, and behavioral and school status, as applicable. Most data are obtained from the adult accompanying the child, but you should include the child as much as appropriate for his or her age. When obtaining a health history from an adolescent, the nurse determines if an adult or pediatric database and history format is more appropriate. Also a decision is made whether to interview the adolescent with the parent present or alone. Chapter 20 presents further information regarding conducting a health history from this age group.

Pregnancy

A comprehensive health history is obtained at the first prenatal visit to establish baseline data. It is similar to what has been presented in this chapter, but with a special emphasis on

data that could impact pregnancy outcomes. See Chapter 21 for further information.

Older Adults

The primary difference in conducting a health history with an older adult from that previously described is the incorporation of various age-related questions and questions involving functional status into the interview. Also, depending on the age of the older adult, it may not be necessary to collect data on childhood immunizations or develop a genogram. It is also important to remember that many older adults have multiple symptoms, conditions, medications, and a long past health history. For this reason, the amount of time needed to conduct the history may be significantly longer.

SUMMARY

Collecting a thorough history accomplishes several goals. It establishes a therapeutic relationship with the client. It also provides a picture of the client and identifies problems mentioned by the client that you can confirm or refute during the physical examination. Once data are collected they must be organized, synthesized, and documented. When you collect health history data in an organized manner, the documentation becomes easier.

CLINICAL APPLICATION & CLINICAL REASONING

See Appendix E for answers to exercises in this section.

REVIEW QUESTIONS

1 The nurse is interviewing an adult Navajo woman. Which of the following demonstrates cultural sensitivity and acceptance of the client?
   1 "How often do you visit the medicine man for your health care?"
   2 "Tell me about your health care beliefs and practices."
   3 "Many Navajo people are afraid of hospitals. Are you afraid?"
   4 "Have you ever had a physical exam with a physician or a nurse practitioner?"

2 The nurse is conducting an interview with Jeremy, a 17-year-old accompanied by his mother. Which statement by the nurse is an age-appropriate adjustment when conducting a health history on an adolescent?

1 "Are you sexually active yet?"

2 "Mrs. Williams, is your son sexually active yet?"

3 "Jeremy, you are not sexually active, are you?"

4 "Mrs. Williams, would you mind waiting outside for a few minutes while I discuss a few things with Jeremy?"

3 During an interview, an elderly client tells the nurse that she has periodic problems keeping her balance. The nurse asks her what she is doing when the episodes occur. In this situation, the nurse is pursuing a symptom analysis in the area of:

1 Severity.

2 Frequency.

3 Aggravating factors.

4 Location.

4 Which of the following communication techniques conveys genuine interest in what the client has to say?

1 Active listening.

2 Sitting close to the client.

3 Maintaining professional dress and conduct.

4 Holding the client's hand during the interview.

5 A 62-year-old client tells the nurse that he is in excellent health and does not take any medications. The best follow-up question or statement is:

1 "Do you have an aversion to taking drugs?"

2 "What medications have you taken in the past?"

3 "That is hard to believe. Most men your age take medications."

4 "Do you use over-the-counter medications or herbal preparations?"

CASE STUDY

During an interview, Jean provides the following family history. She is 37 years old, married, and in good health. Her husband is 43, also in good health. The couple have a 12-year-old son, an 11-year-old daughter, and a 10-year-old son, all in good health. Jean has a 42-year-old brother and three sisters who are 32, 36, and 40 years old. All of her siblings are in good health. Both of Jean's parents are alive. Her 70-year-old father has mild emphysema and is an only child. Her mother is 66 and has hypertension. Jean's mother has three siblings. The oldest brother (Jean's uncle) is 74 and suffers from glaucoma. Another brother is 72 and is in good health. A sister is 69 and has osteoarthritis. All of Jean's grandparents are deceased. Her paternal grandfather died at age 89 of prostate cancer. Her paternal grandmother died of heart failure at age 91. Jean's maternal grandfather died at age 86 of prostate cancer; her maternal grandmother died of "old age" at age 96.

Questions

Draw a genogram for Jean's family history with the information provided.

🔘 INTERACTIVE ACTIVITIES

Open the interactive student CD-ROM, click on Chapter 3, and choose from the following activities on the menu bar:

- **Multiple Choice Challenge.** Click on the best answer for each question. You will be given immediate feedback, rationale for incorrect answers, and a total score. Good luck!

- **Quick Challenge.** Use this critical thinking exercise to assess your skills through case study-like questions, then compare with expert answers!

- **Marvelous Matches.** Drag each word or phrase to the appropriate place on the screen. Test your ability to match an interview technique to the clue provided.

- **Printable Lab Guide.** Locate the Lab Guide for Chapter 3, and print and use it (as many times as needed) to help you apply your assessment skills. These guides may also be filled in electronically and then saved and e-mailed to your instructor!

CHAPTER 4

Techniques and Equipment
for Physical Assessment

ELECTRONIC RESOURCES

Additional information related to the content in Chapter 4 can be found

in the companion website at

evolve

evolve: http://evolve.elsevier.com/Wilson/assessment/

or on the interactive student CD-ROM

Activities for Chapter 4 include the following:
- Multiple Choice Challenge • Marvelous Matches
- Printable Lab Guide • Quick Challenge

Before conducting an examination, you must become familiar with assessment techniques, optimal client positions for examination, equipment used to perform the examination, and infection control measures. Correct technique and proper use of equipment are essential to accurate data collection.

TECHNIQUES OF PHYSICAL ASSESSMENT

Data for physical assessment are collected using four basic assessment techniques: inspection, palpation, percussion, and auscultation.

Inspection

Physical examinations begin with inspection. The term *inspection* refers to a visual examination of the body, including body movement and posture. Data obtained by smell are also a part of inspection. Examination of every body system includes the technique of inspection. For example, when examining the lungs and respiratory system, inspection includes observing the shape of the chest; observing breathing (noting the rate, depth, and effort of respirations); and observing the overall color of the skin, lips, and nail beds. During inspection, the client is draped appropriately to maintain modesty while allowing sufficient exposure for examination; adequate lighting is essential.

Inspection can be hindered by preconceived assumptions nurses have about clients; thus it is important that the client is thoroughly observed with a critical eye. By concentrating on the client without being distracted, the nurse will not overlook potentially important data. Although inspection at first may seem like an easy assessment technique to master, practice is necessary to develop this skill.

Sometimes the use of equipment facilitates inspection of certain body systems. A penlight, for example, may be used to increase the light on a specific location (looking in a mouth, looking at a skin lesion) or may be used to create shadows by directing light at right angles to the area being inspected-a technique referred to as *tangential lighting* (Fig. 4-1). Other instruments, such as an otoscope, an ophthalmoscope, or a vaginal speculum, are used to enhance inspection for specific body systems. Equipment used to facilitate inspection is presented later in this chapter.

Palpation

Palpation involves using the hands to feel texture, size, shape, consistency, pulsations, and location of certain parts of the client's body and also to identify areas the client reports as being tender or painful. This technique requires the nurse to move into the client's personal space. It is important that the touch is gentle, hands are warm, and nails are short to prevent discomfort or injury to the client. Touch has cultural significance and symbolism. Each culture has its own understanding about the uses and meanings of touch. As a result, it is of utmost importance that nurses tell clients the purpose of their touch (e.g., "I'm feeling for lymph nodes now") and manner and location of touch (e.g., "I'm going to press deeply on your abdomen to feel the organs"). Gloves are worn when palpating mucous membranes or any other area where contact with body fluids is possible.

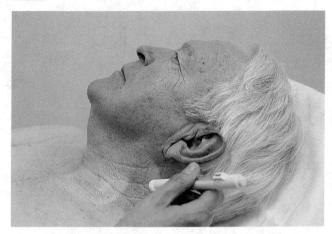

Fig. 4-1 Tangential light used to inspect jugular vein pulsation.

The palmar surfaces of fingers and finger pads are more sensitive than the fingertips; thus they are better for determining position, texture, size, consistency, masses, fluid, and crepitus. The ulnar surface of the hand extending to the fifth finger is the most sensitive to vibration, whereas the dorsal surface of the hand is better for assessing temperature.

Palpation using the palmar surfaces of the fingers may be light or deep and is controlled by the amount of pressure applied. Light palpation is accomplished by pressing up to a depth of approximately 1 cm and is used to assess skin, pulsations, and tenderness (Fig. 4-2, A). Deep palpation is accomplished by pressing up to a depth of 4 cm with one or two hands and is used to determine organ size and contour (Fig. 4-2, B). A bimanual technique of palpation uses both hands, one anterior and one posterior, to entrap an organ (such as the uterus, or large breasts) or mass between the fingertips to assess size and shape. Light palpation should always precede deep palpation because palpation may cause tenderness or disrupt fluid, which could interfere with collecting data by light palpation.

Percussion

Percussion is performed to evaluate the size, borders, and consistency of internal organs, to detect tenderness, and to determine the extent of fluid in a body cavity. There are two percussion techniques: direct and indirect.

Direct Percussion

Direct percussion involves striking a finger or hand directly against the client's body. The nurse may use direct percussion technique to evaluate the sinus of an adult by tapping a finger over the sinus, or to elicit tenderness over the kidney by striking the costovertebral angle (CVA) directly with a fist (Fig. 4-3). This technique is discussed in Chapter 14.

Indirect Percussion

Indirect percussion requires both hands and is done by different methods depending on which body system is being assessed. It is an awkward technique at first but can be mastered with practice. Indirect fist percussion of the kidney, for example, involves placing the nondominant hand palm down (with fingers together) over the CVA and gently striking the fingers with the lateral aspect of the fist of the dominant hand.

Indirect percussion of the thorax or abdomen is performed by placing the distal aspect of the middle finger of the nondominant hand against the skin over the organ being percussed, or between the ribs when percussing the thorax. This finger is sometimes referred to as the *pleximeter*. The other fingers of that hand are spread apart and slightly elevated off the client's skin so that they do not dampen the vibration. With the tip of the middle finger of the dominant hand (the *plexor*), the nurse strikes the distal interphalangeal joint, or just distal to the joint, that lies against the client's skin (Fig. 4-4). The tip of the striking finger hits the middle finger, which is against the skin, between the cuticle and first joint. Some nurses use both the index and the middle fingers as plexors. The force of the downward snap of the striking finger(s) comes from rapid flexion of the wrist. The wrist must be relaxed and loose while the forearm remains stationary. Rebound the plexor finger as soon as it strikes the pleximeter so that the vibration is not muffled. Listen for the vibrations created by one finger striking another.

The tapping produces a vibration 1.5 to 2 inches (4 to 5 cm) deep in body tissue and subsequent sound waves. Percuss two

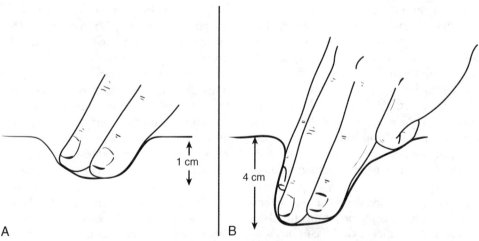

Fig. 4-2 **Palpation.** **A,** Superficial palpation. **B,** Deep palpation.

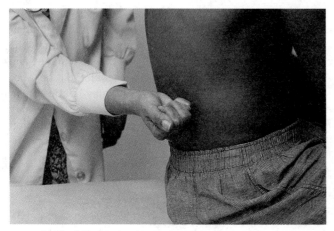

Fig. 4-3 Hand position for direct fist percussion of kidney.

or three times in one location before moving to another. Stronger percussion is needed for obese or very muscular clients, because thickness of tissue can impair the vibrations; the denser the tissue, the quieter the percussion tones. Five percussion tones are described in Table 4-1. *Tympany* is a loud, high-pitched sound heard over the abdomen. *Resonance* is heard over normal lung tissue, whereas *hyperresonance* is heard in overinflated lungs (as in emphysema). *Dullness* is heard over the liver, and *flatness* is heard over bones and muscle. Detecting sound changes is easier when moving from resonance to dullness (e.g., from the lung to the liver).

FREQUENTLY ASKED QUESTIONS

I am having difficulty hearing percussion tones. How can I improve my technique?

With beginning learners the two technique errors seen most often during indirect percussion are contact of the nondominant hand and the delivery of the plexor finger.

- Only the middle finger of the nondominant hand should be in contact with the percussion surface. Students tend to allow all the fingers to be in contact. Get those fingers off!
- The plexor (striking finger) must get wrist action for a quick, snappy, forceful strike. The strike should occur with the fingertip, not the finger pad.

Auscultation

Auscultation is the act of listening to sounds within the body. Although some sounds are audible to the ear without the use

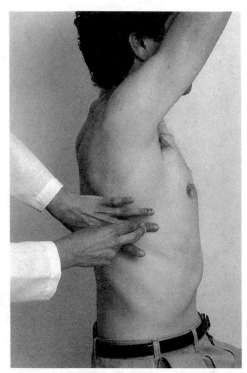

Fig. 4-4 Indirect percussion of lateral chest wall.

of special equipment (e.g., respiratory stridor, severe wheezing, and abdominal gurgling), the nurse most commonly uses a stethoscope to facilitate auscultation.

A stethoscope is used for auscultation to block out extraneous sounds when evaluating the condition of the heart, blood vessels, lungs, and intestines (Fig. 4-5). Listen for the sound and also its characteristics: intensity, pitch, duration, and quality (Box 4-1). Nurses concentrate as they listen because sounds may be transitory or subtle. Closing the eyes may improve listening because it reduces distracting visual stimuli. The isolation of specific sounds, such as sounds of air during inspiration or a single heart sound, is referred to as selective listening.

The nurse should take measures to optimize the quality of auscultation findings. It is best to perform auscultation in a quiet room because environmental noise can interfere with auscultation. The stethoscope must be placed directly on the skin because clothes obscure or alter sounds. Be sure to warm the head of the stethoscope before placing it on the client. If the client becomes cold and shivers, involuntary muscle contractions could interfere with normal sounds. The

TABLE 4-1 *Percussion Tones*

AREA PERCUSSED	TONE	INTENSITY	PITCH	DURATION	QUALITY
Lungs	Resonant	Loud	Low	Long	Hollow
Bone and muscle	Flat	Soft	High	Short	Extremely dull
Viscera and liver borders	Dull	Medium	Medium high	Medium	Thudlike
Stomach and gas bubbles in intestines	Tympanic	Loud	High	Medium	Drumlike
Air trapped in lung (emphysema)	Hyperresonant	Very loud	Very low	Longer	Booming

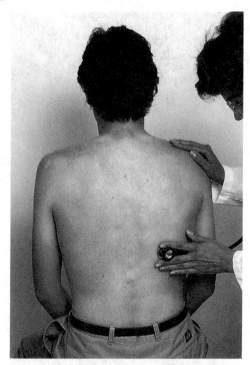

Fig. 4-5 The diaphragm of the stethoscope is stabilized between the index and middle fingers.

BOX 4-1	CHARACTERISTICS OF SOUNDS HEARD BY AUSCULTATION

- *Intensity* is the loudness of the sound, described as soft, medium, or loud.
- *Pitch* is the frequency or number of sound waves generated per second. High-pitched sounds have high frequencies. Expected high-pitched sounds are breath sounds, whereas cardiac sounds are low pitched.
- *Duration of sound vibrations* is short, medium, or long. Layers of soft tissue dampen the duration of sound from deep organs.
- *Quality* refers to the description of the sounds (e.g., hollow, dull, crackle).

---

friction of body hair rubbing against the diaphragm of the stethoscope could be mistaken for abnormal lung sounds (crackles). If the stethoscope tubing is bumped while auscultating, the nurse will hear a loud tapping sound that will obscure underlying auscultation findings.

POSITIONING

The client may assume a number of positions during the process of examination; the positions depend on the type of examination to be done and the condition of the patient. The sitting and supine positions are the most common during the examination. Various positions for examination are presented in Table 4-2. It is also important to note the need

to drape the client appropriately. The goal is to provide for modesty, while allowing exposure needed for the examination. The inability of a client to assume a position may be a significant finding about the client's physical status, and requires the nurse making necessary accommodations. For example, a client who is short of breath may not be able to tolerate a supine position. In this situation, the nurse may be required to elevate the head of the bed or examination table for certain aspects of the examination (e.g., abdominal assessment).

EQUIPMENT USED DURING THE EXAMINATION PROCESS

Examination equipment is used to facilitate the collection of data. Keep in mind that not all equipment presented in this chapter is used for all examinations. The type of equipment used varies depending on the type of examination and the problem being assessed. Like a carpenter who chooses tools from a toolbox based on the job to be performed, the nurse chooses equipment based on the examination performed. Most equipment used in a physical examination either provides a measurement (e.g., body temperature, body weight, visual acuity) or facilitates an examination technique (e.g., inspection, auscultation, percussion, or palpation).

Thermometers (Temperature Measurement)

Purpose: To measure body temperature.

The two most common thermometers used in health care settings are the electronic and tympanic thermometers.

The electronic thermometer (Fig. 4-6, *A*) consists of a battery-powered display unit, a thin wire cord, and a temperature-sensitive probe. The probe must be covered with a disposable sheath before use and placed under the tongue; the probe measures the temperature of the blood flowing under the tongue. The electronic thermometer calculates and displays the temperature on a digital screen within 15 to 30 seconds. Many electronic thermometers have a switch on the unit to permit the measurement of temperature in either Fahrenheit or Celsius.

The tympanic thermometer (Fig. 4-6, *B*) has become increasingly popular in all clinical settings because it provides a reading very quickly; taking the client's temperature with this device requires less than 5 seconds. The device works when the temperature-sensitive probe, covered with a disposable sheath, is inserted into the client's ear; the probe measures the temperature of the blood flowing near the tympanic membrane. This provides an accurate measurement of core body temperature. Like the electronic thermometer, tympanic thermometers may be programmed to measure temperature in either Fahrenheit or Celsius. Multiple studies have been conducted evaluating the accuracy of tympanic thermometers with widely varied results (El-Rahdi, 2006; Farnell, 2005; Leon, 2005), thus the evidence for accuracy remains in question.

TABLE 4-2 *Positions for Examination*

POSITION		AREAS ASSESSED	RATIONALE	LIMITATIONS
Sitting		Head and neck, back, posterior thorax and lungs, anterior thorax and lungs, breasts, axilla, heart, vital signs, and upper extremities	Sitting upright provides full expansion of lungs and provides better visualization of symmetry of upper body parts.	Physically weakened client may be unable to sit. Examiner should use supine position with head of bed elevated instead.
Supine		Head and neck, anterior thorax and lungs, breasts, axilla, heart, abdomen, extremities, pulses	This is the most normally relaxed position. It provides easy access to pulse sites.	If client becomes short of breath easily, examiner may need to raise head of bed.
Dorsal recumbent		Head and neck, anterior thorax and lungs, breasts, axilla, heart, abdomen	This position is used for abdominal assessment because it promotes relaxation of abdominal muscles.	Clients with painful disorders are more comfortable with knees flexed.
Lithotomy*		Female genitalia and genital tract	This position provides maximal exposure of genitalia and facilitates insertion of vaginal speculum.	Lithotomy position is embarrassing and uncomfortable, so examiner minimizes time that client spends in it. Client is kept well draped.
Sims		Rectum and vagina	Flexion of hip and knee improves exposure of rectal area.	Joint deformities may hinder client's ability to bend hip and knee.
Prone		Musculoskeletal system	This position is used only to assess extension of hip joint.	This position is poorly tolerated in clients with respiratory difficulties.
Lateral recumbent		Heart	This position aids in detecting murmurs.	This position is poorly tolerated in clients with respiratory difficulties.
Knee-chest*		Rectum	This position provides maximal exposure of rectal area.	This position is embarrassing and uncomfortable.

From Potter PA, Perry AG: *Basic nursing: essentials for practice,* ed 6, St Louis, 2006, Mosby.

*Clients with arthritis or other joint deformities may be unable to assume this position.

Two common devices to measure temperatures in children include pacifier thermometers and chemical dot thermometers. Pacifier thermometers have gained in popularity in recent years because they are less invasive, are well tolerated by children, and have been shown to be comparable in accuracy to adjusted core temperature gained by rectal measurement (Braun, 2006). Chemical dot thermometers have been shown to under measure body temperature compared to electronic thermometers and are not considered accurate (Fallis, et al., 2006).

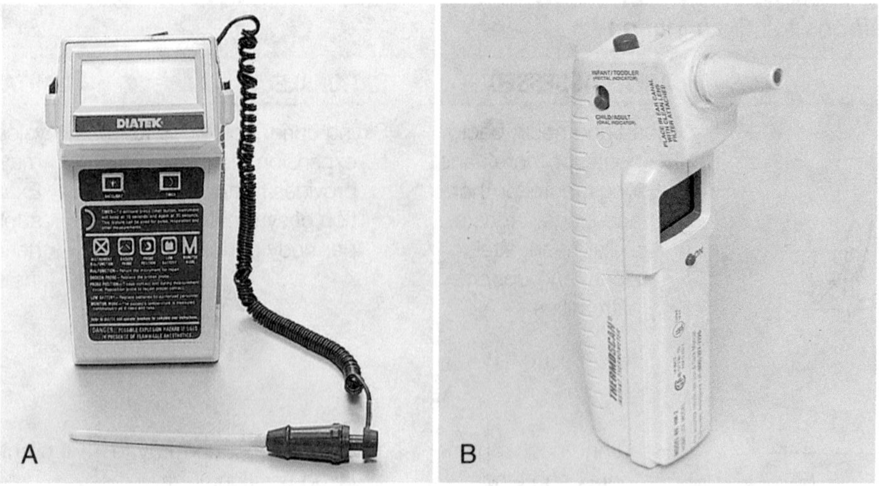

![Electronic thermometer and tympanic thermometer]

Fig. 4-6   **A,** Electronic thermometer. **B,** Tympanic thermometer. *(B, From Seidel et al, 2006.)*

Stethoscope

Purpose: To auscultate sounds within the body that are not audible with the naked ear.

As discussed previously, auscultation is usually performed with a stethoscope. Although there are several types of stethoscopes (acoustic, magnetic, electronic, and stereophonic), the acoustic stethoscope is routinely used for health assessment (Fig. 4-7, *A*).

The acoustic stethoscope is a closed cylinder that transmits sound waves from the source through the tube to the ears. It does not magnify sounds, but by blocking out extraneous room noise, it permits difficult-to-hear sounds to be more easily heard. The stethoscope consists of four components: the earpieces, the binaurals, the tubing, and the head.

The earpieces, which may be hard or soft, should fit snugly and completely fill the ear canal. The binaurals are tubes of metal that connect the stethoscope tubing to the ear pieces. They allow the ear pieces to be angled toward the nose so that sound is projected toward the tympanic membrane. The tubing of the stethoscope is usually a firm polyvinyl material that is no longer than 12 to 18 inches (30 to 46 cm). If the tubing is longer than 18 inches, the sounds may become distorted. Some health care workers place a soft and decorative fabric cover over the tubing (usually extending from just above the head to near the earpieces) to reduce irritation caused by the tubing when worn across the back of the neck, and also to personalize their stethoscope. These fabric covers, however, have been found to be a potential source of

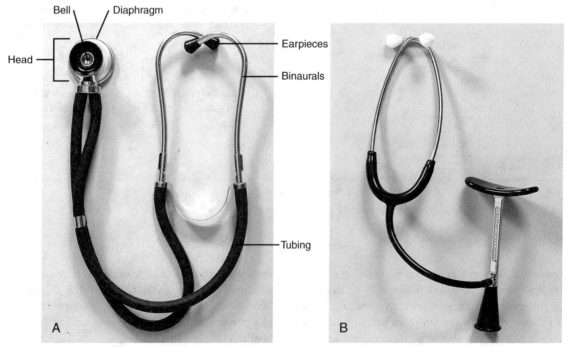

Fig. 4-7   **A,** Acoustic stethoscope. **B,** Fetoscope. *(From Seidel et al, 2006.)*

infection, and thus they are not appropriate for use in health care settings (Milam et al, 2001).

The head of the stethoscope consists of two components: the diaphragm and the bell. The head of the stethoscope should be heavy enough to lie firmly on the body surface without being held. This piece is configured by a closure valve so that only the diaphragm or the bell may be activated at any one time. The diaphragm consists of a flat surface with a rubber or plastic ring edge. It is used to hear *high-pitched* sounds such as breath sounds, bowel sounds, and normal heart sounds. Its structure screens out low-pitched sounds. The diaphragm is held firmly against the client's skin, stabilizing it between the index and middle fingers (See Fig. 4-5). The bell of the stethoscope is constructed in a concave shape. It should be used to hear soft, *low-pitched* sounds such as extra heart sounds or vascular sounds (bruit). When the bell is used, it should be pressed lightly on the skin with just enough pressure to ensure that a complete seal exists around the bell. If the bell is pressed too firmly on the skin, the concave surface is filled with skin, and the bell will function as a diaphragm and inhibits vibrations. Some stethoscopes have varying sizes of heads that are interchangeable. When examining an infant or young child, use a pediatric stethoscope which has a small head. The diaphragm and bell should span one intercostal space.

A special type of acoustic stethoscope known as a fetoscope (Fig. 4-7, *B*) is used to auscultate the fetal heart. The fetoscope has a metal attachment that rests against the head of the nurse. This metal piece aids in the conduction of sound so that heart tones are heard more easily.

Equipment to Measure Blood Pressure

Purpose: To measure the arterial blood pressure.

Blood pressure is most commonly measured indirectly (noninvasively) using a manual sphygmomanometer or an electronic noninvasive blood pressure (NIBP) monitor.

The sphygmomanometer consists of the gauge to measure the pressure (manometer), a blood pressure cuff that encloses an inflatable bladder, and a pressure bulb with valve used to manually inflate and deflate the bladder within the cuff (Fig. 4-8, *A*). A stethoscope is used in conjunction with the sphygmomanometer to auscultate the blood pressure.

The NIBP monitor is an electronic device attached to a blood pressure cuff (Fig. 4-8, *B*). It operates by sensing circulating blood flow vibrations through a blood pressure cuff sensor and converting these vibrations into electric impulses. These impulses are translated to a digital readout. The readout generally consists of blood pressure, mean arterial pressure, and pulse rate. The device is not capable of determining quality of the pulse, such as rhythm or intensity. The device may be programmed to repeat the measurements on a scheduled periodic basis and to alarm if the measurements are outside of the desired limits. This feature is especially useful for clients requiring frequent blood pressure monitoring. A stethoscope is not required when the electronic device is used.

Blood pressure cuffs come in a variety of sizes and are either reusable (occlusive cloth shell) or disposable (an inexpensive vinyl material) (Fig. 4-9). Both have a Velcro-type material on one end used to secure the cuff when wrapped on the arm. It is important to select a blood pressure cuff that is the correct size for the client. Only 43% of nurses participating in a recent study correctly answered questions regarding assessment of cuff size (Armstrong, 2002). If the cuff is too wide, it will underestimate the blood pressure; if it is too narrow, it will overestimate the blood pressure. Ideally the cuff width should be 40% of the circumference of the limb to be used. The bladder within the cuff should encircle at least 80% of the upper arm (National Institutes of Health, 2003). The American Heart Association recommends cuff sizes based on arm circumference (Table 4-3). On most cuffs, range lines are indicated to assess proper size. When a correctly sized cuff is applied, the cuff edge should lie between the range lines (see Fig. 4-9). Adult cuffs come in two

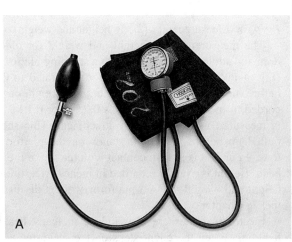
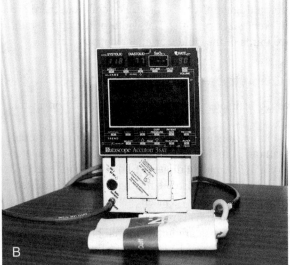

Fig. 4-8 **A,** Aneroid sphygmomanometer. **B,** Noninvasive blood pressure (NIBP) monitor with disposable blood pressure cuff.

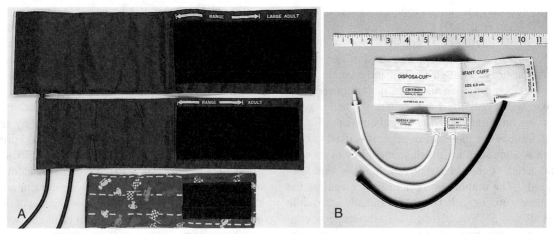

Fig. 4-9 **Blood pressure cuffs in various sizes.** **A,** Reusable cuffs in large adult *(top)*, adult *(middle)*, and child *(bottom)* sizes. Note the range lines above the Velcro material on the right side of each cuff. **B,** Disposable infant *(top)* and neonatal *(bottom)* cuffs. *(B, From Seidel et al, 2006.)*

TABLE 4-3 *Sizes for Blood Pressure Cuffs Based on Arm Circumference**

CIRCUMFERENCE OF EXTREMITY (MEASURED AT MIDDLE OF ARM OR THIGH)	SIZE OF CUFF (BY NAME)
5-7.5 cm	Newborn
7.5-13 cm	Infant
13-20 cm	Child
17-25 cm	Small adult
24-32 cm	Adult
32-42 cm	Wide/large adult
42-50 cm	Thigh

*Based on American Heart Association Recommendations (Frohlich, Grim, Labarthe et al, 1988).

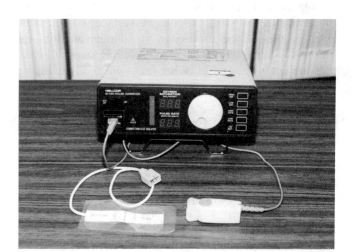

Fig. 4-10 Pulse oximeter shown with a clip and tape sensor probe.

widths. The standard cuff (4⅔ to 5⅙ inches) is adequate for most adults. If the adult is large or obese, an oversized cuff (6 to 6⅓ inches) may be used. If the adult has an extremely obese arm, a thigh cuff can be used. For children, there are many different sizes of cuffs. The width of the cuff should cover two thirds of the child's or infant's upper arm.

Pulse Oximetry

Purpose: To estimate the arterial oxygen saturation in the blood.

Pulse oximetry is a noninvasive measurement of arterial oxygen saturation in the blood (Fig. 4-10). A pulse oximeter consists of a light-emitting diode (LED) probe connected by a cable to a monitor. The LED emits light waves that reflect off oxygenated and deoxygenated hemoglobin molecules circulating in the blood. This reflection is used to estimate the percentage of oxygen saturation in arterial blood, as well as a pulse rate. The sensor probe is taped or clipped to a highly vascular area—typically a digit (finger or toe), an earlobe, or the bridge of the nose. Pulse oximetry is considered highly

accurate in the measurement of oxygen saturation over the range of 70% to 100%. In many settings, it is sometimes referred to as the "fifth vital sign."

Scales

Purpose: Measurement of body height and weight.

The measurement of height and weight for older children and adults is performed with a standing platform scale (Fig. 4-11, *A*). The scale should be calibrated to 0 (zero) before measuring a client's weight. The weight can be recorded in increments as small as 0.25 lb or 0.1 kg. Height is measured using the height attachment. This should be pulled up before the client stands on the platform, then lowered until it is in firm contact with the top of the client's head. Height is usually recorded in inches. Measurement of height and weight using a platform scale is discussed further in Chapter 5.

Electronic scales are also in use in many health care facilities. When the client steps on the scale, the weight is calculated and a digital readout of the client's weight (in either pounds or kilograms) is provided. Calibration of these scales occurs automatically with each use.

Infants are measured using an infant platform scale (Fig. 4-11, *B*). These work similarly to the adult platform scale, but can measure weight in ounces or grams. The child may sit or lie on the platform while the weight is measured. Because the infant platform scale does not have a height attachment, height (length) is measured using a mat or board. This is discussed further in Chapter 5.

Visual Acuity and Screening

Purpose: Used as a screening examination for visual acuity, color perception, and field perception. Several types of charts may be used for visual assessment.

Snellen's Chart

Snellen's chart is a large wall chart hung at a distance of 20 feet from the client (Fig. 4-12, *A*). The chart consists of

11 lines of letters of decreasing size. The letter size indicates the degree of visual acuity when read from a distance of 20 feet. The client should be tested one eye at a time. Beside each line of letters is the corresponding acuity rating that should be recorded (e.g., 20/40, 20/100). The top number of the recording indicates the distance between the client and the chart, and the bottom number indicates the distance at which a person with normal vision should be able to read that line of the chart. Ask the client to name the colors of the horizontal lines as a screening for color perception. The top line is green, and the bottom line is red. Also ask the client which line is longer as a screening for field perception measurement. The green line is longer.

For young children or non–English-speaking individuals, the "E" chart may be used (Fig. 4-12, *B*). The nurse describes the "E" as a table with legs and asks the client to point in the direction that the legs of the table point. The scoring of the "E" chart is the same as that of Snellen's chart. See Chapter 11 for further information regarding assessment of visual acuity.

Jaeger and Rosenbaum Charts

Two charts, the Jaeger and the Rosenbaum, are commonly used to evaluate near vision. The Rosenbaum chart consists of a series of numbers, *E*'s, *X*'s, and *O*'s in graduated sizes (Fig. 4-13). The client should hold the chart 14 inches from the face. Each eye should be individually evaluated for visual acuity. Visual acuity is measured in the same distance equivalents as the far-vision acuity charts, such as 20/20. The Jaeger equivalent is also shown on the Rosenbaum card.

Ophthalmoscope

Purpose: To inspect the internal structures of the eye.

The ophthalmoscope is an instrument that consists of a series of lenses, mirrors, and light apertures permitting inspection of the internal structures of the eye (Fig. 4-14). The ophthalmoscope consists of a head and a handle; the handle

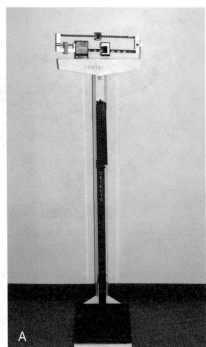

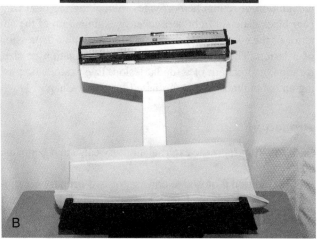

Fig. 4-11 **A,** Adult platform scale. **B,** Infant platform scale.

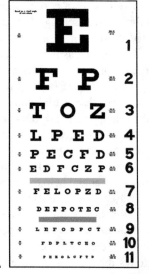

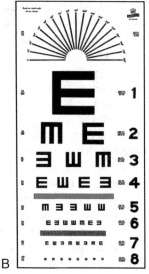

Fig. 4-12 **A,** Snellen's visual acuity chart. **B,** "E" chart. *(From Seidel et al, 2006.)*

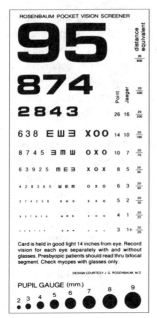

Fig. 4-13   Rosenbaum near-vision chart. *(From Seidel et al., 2006.)*

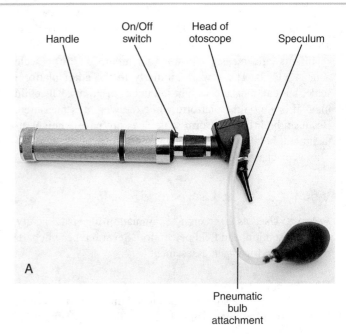

Fig. 4-15   **A,** Traditional otoscope with pneumatic bulb. **B,** MacroView ototscope.

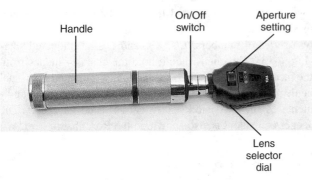

Fig. 4-14   Ophthalmoscope.

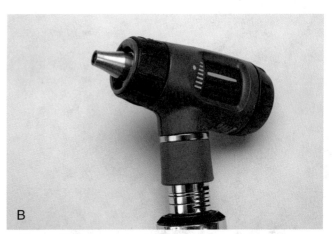

is a power source that contains batteries or connects to a wall-mounted electrical source. The head and handle fit together by a turn-and-lock system.

The head of the ophthalmoscope consists of two movable parts: the lens selector dial and the aperture setting. The lens selector dial allows the nurse to adjust a set of lenses that control focus. The unit of strength for each lens is referred to as a *diopter.* When the lens selector dial is turned clockwise, the positive, or black-number-sphere, lenses are brought into place. The black numbers on the lens selector dial indicate increasingly positive diopter; these help the nurse focus on near objects within the client's eye. Likewise, when the lens selector disk is turned counterclockwise, the negative, or red-number-sphere, lenses are brought into place. The red numbers indicate increasingly negative diopter and help the nurse focus on objects that are further away within the client's eye. The positive and negative lenses compensate for myopia or hyperopia in both the nurse's and client's eyes and also permit focusing at different places within the client's eye.

The aperture has several settings that permit light variations during the examination. If the client's pupils have been dilated, the large light may be used for the internal eye examination. The small light may be used if the client's pupils are very small or if the pupils have not been dilated. The red-free filter actually shines a green beam of light. The filter facilitates the identification of pallor of the disc and permits the recognition of retinal hemorrhages by making the blood appear black. The slit light permits easy examination of the anterior of the eye and determination of elevation or depression of a lesion. The grid light facilitates an estimation of size, location, and pattern of a fundal lesion. Eye examination using an ophthalmoscope is discussed further in Chapter 11.

Otoscope

Purpose: To inspect the external auditory canal and tympanic membrane.

The traditional otoscope consists of two primary components: the head and the handle. Some otoscopes also have a pneumatic attachment (Fig. 4-15, *A*). The head of the otoscope consists of a magnification lens, a light source, and a speculum that is inserted into the auditory canal. On newer models of otoscopes, such as the MacroView otoscope, an adjustable focus allows greater magnification and field of view compared to traditional otoscopes (Fig. 4-15, *B*). Specula come in various sizes. Choose the largest size speculum that fits into the client's ear canal. The handle of the otoscope is the power source; it either contains batteries or connects to a wall-mounted electrical source. The pneumatic attachment, used to evaluate the fluctuation of the tympanic membrane in children, consists of a small rubber tube with a bulb attached to the head of the otoscope. When the bulb is squeezed, it produces small puffs of air against the tympanic membrane, causing the membrane to move. No fluctuation of the membrane may indicate pressure from behind the membrane. See Chapter 11 for further discussion regarding use of the otoscope.

Penlight

Purpose: To provide a focused light source to facilitate inspection.

The penlight has many uses during a physical assessment (Fig. 4-16). It may be used to illuminate the inside of the mouth or nose, highlight a lesion, or evaluate pupillary constriction. It is most important that the penlight have a bright light source. If the nurse does not have a penlight, the light transmitted from the otoscope may be substituted as a focused light source.

Ruler and Tape Measure

Purpose: To provide accurate measurement of various findings.

A small metric ruler that has both millimeter and centimeter markings is useful for measuring lesions or other marks on the skin (Fig. 4-17). Ideally, use a ruler that is transparent. A disposable paper tape measure is useful in various situations such as measuring the length of an infant or the circumference of an extremity. A tape measure that has inches on one side and centimeters on the reverse side is ideal.

Nasal Speculum

Purpose: To spread the opening of the nares so the internal surfaces of the nose may be inspected.

Two instruments may be used as a nasal speculum. The simple nasal speculum is used in conjunction with a penlight to visualize the lower and middle turbinates of the nose (Fig. 4-18). The instrument is used by gently squeezing the handle of the speculum, causing the blades of the speculum to open and spread the nares, which permits inspection of the internal nose. The second type of nasal speculum is a broad-tipped, cone-shaped device that is placed on the end of an otoscope. The nasal cavity may be inspected by using the light source and viewing lens of the otoscope.

Tuning Fork

Purpose: The tuning fork has two purposes in physical assessment: auditory screening and assessment of vibratory sensation.

For auditory evaluation, a high-pitched tuning fork with a frequency of 500 to 1000 Hz should be used (Fig. 4-19). A fork that vibrates in this frequency range can estimate hearing loss in the range of normal speech (300 to 3000 Hz). If a lower-frequency fork were used, overestimation of hearing ability could result. For neurologic vibratory evaluation, a tuning fork with a pitch between 100 and 400 Hz should be used. To engage, sharply strike the tuning fork on the heel of the hand. See Chapters 11 and 16 for further information on this assessment technique.

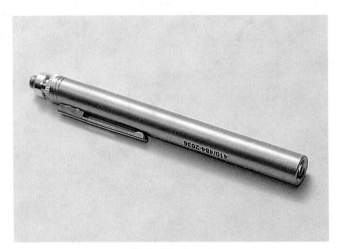

Fig. 4-16   Penlight.

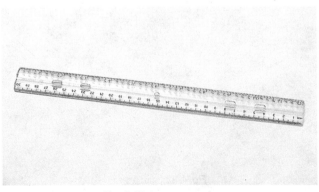

Fig. 4-17   Centimeter ruler.

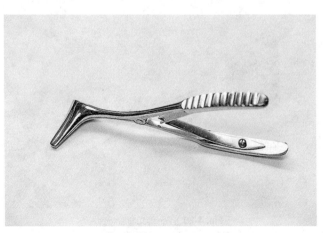

Fig. 4-18   Nasal speculum.

Percussion, or Reflex, Hammer

Purpose: To test deep tendon reflexes.

The percussion (reflex) hammer consists of a triangular rubber component on the end of a metal handle (Fig. 4-20). The hammer is configured so that either flat or pointed surfaces may be used to elicit the reflex response. The flat surface is more commonly used when striking the tendon directly. The pointed surface may be used either to strike the tendon directly or to strike the nurse's finger, which is placed on a small tendon such as the client's biceps tendon. A neurologic hammer can also be used to test deep tendon reflexes. It is similar to a percussion hammer, but the rubber striking end is rounded on both sides. The technique to assess deep tendon reflexes is found in Chapter 16.

Doppler

Purpose: To amplify sounds that are difficult to hear with an acoustic stethoscope.

The Doppler uses ultrasonic waves to detect difficult-to-hear vascular sounds, such as fetal heart tones or peripheral pulses (Fig. 4-21). To use the device, coupling gel is applied to the client's skin; then the transducer is slid over the skin surface until the blood flow source is heard in the nurses's earpieces. As blood in the vessels ebbs and flows, the probe on the distal end of the Doppler picks up and amplifies the subtle changes in pitch. The resulting sound that the nurse hears is a swishing, pulsating sound. A volume control helps amplify the sound further.

Goniometer

Purpose: To determine the degree of flexion or extension of a joint.

The goniometer is a two-piece ruler that is jointed in the middle with a protractor-type measuring device (Fig. 4-22). The goniometer is placed over a joint; as the individual extends or flexes the joint, the degrees of flexion and extension are measured on the protractor. This is discussed further in Chapter 15.

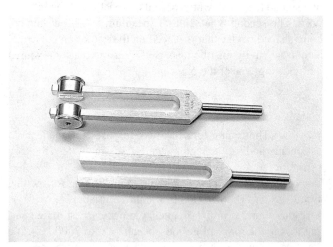

Fig. 4-19   Tuning forks for vibratory sensation *(top)* and auditory screening *(bottom).*

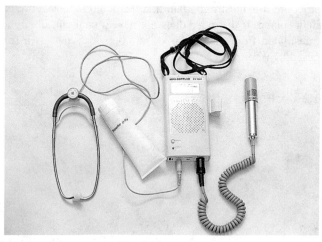

Fig. 4-21   Doppler.

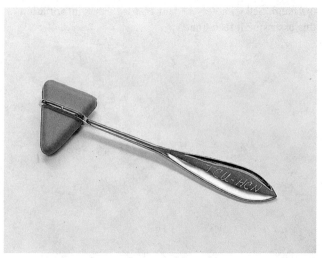

Fig. 4-20   Percussion hammer.

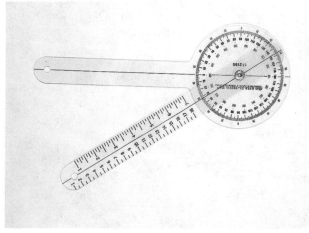

Fig. 4-22   Goniometer.

Calipers for Skinfold Thickness

Purpose: To measure the thickness of subcutaneous tissue to estimate the amount of body fat.

Different models of calipers (e.g., Lang or Herpendem) may be used to measure the thickness of subcutaneous tissue at different points on the body (Fig. 4-23). The most frequent location for thickness evaluation is the posterior aspect of the triceps. Use of calipers to measure skinfold thickness is discussed further in Chapter 9.

Vaginal Speculum

Purpose: To spread the walls of the vaginal canal so that the vaginal walls and cervix can be inspected.

There are three types of vaginal specula: the Graves' speculum, the Pederson speculum, and the pediatric or virginal speculum. All of the specula are composed of two blades and a handle and are available as either reusable metal or disposable plastic models (Fig. 4-24). The Graves' speculum is available in a variety of sizes, with blades ranging from 3.5 to 5.0 inches in length and 0.75 to 1.25 inch in width. The bottom blade is slightly longer than the top blade.

This conforms to the longer posterior vaginal wall and aids with visualization. The Pederson speculum has blades that are as long as the Graves' speculum but are much narrower and flatter. The pediatric or virginal speculum is smaller in all dimensions of width and length.

Plastic and metal specula differ slightly in ease of use and positioning. The metal speculum has two positioning devices. The top blade is hinged and has a thumb lever attached. When the thumb lever is pressed down, the distal end of the top blade rises, thus opening the speculum. The blade may be locked open at that point by tightening the screw on the thumb lever. The proximal end of the speculum may also be opened wider if necessary by loosening and then tightening another thumbscrew on the handle.

The bottom blade of the disposable plastic speculum is fixed to a posterior handle and the upper blade is fixed to the anterior lever handle. When the lever is pressed, the distal end of the top blade opens and, at the same time, the base of the speculum widens. As the speculum opens, it goes through a series of clicking sounds until it snaps into the desired position. The client should be forewarned about the clicking and snapping sounds. In addition, some of the plastic models have a port where a light source may be inserted directly into the speculum. See Chapter 18 for further discussion on use of the speculum.

Audioscope

Purpose: To perform basic screening for hearing acuity.

The handheld, battery-operated audioscope (Fig. 4-25) provides a fast, simple test to detect hearing problems. The audioscope systematically and automatically creates tones at the different frequencies: 1000, 2000, 4000, and 5000 Hz. A

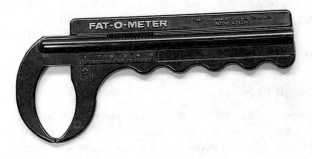

Fig. 4-23 Skinfold calipers.

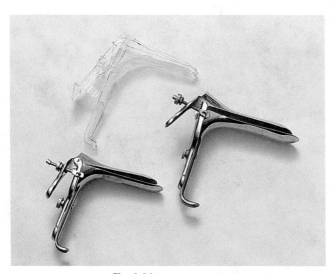

Fig. 4-24 Vaginal specula.

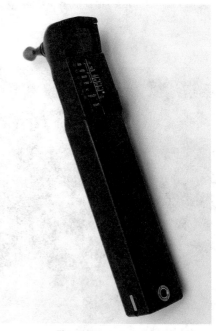

Fig. 4-25 Audioscope.

light appears on the audioscope when the specific tone at a given frequency is sounded. The client's raised index finger, indicating perception of a tone, should correspond to the light seen by the nurse on the audiometer. Hearing assessment is discussed further in Chapter 11.

Monofilament

Purpose: Test for sensation on lower extremities.

The monofilament is a small, flexible wire–like device attached to a handle (Fig. 4-26). The wire is placed on the skin surface and then bent (the wire bends at 10 grams of liner pressure). The client should indicate when and where the monofilament is felt. Clients who are unable to feel the monofilament when it is bent have reduced peripheral sensation. Typically the monofilament is used to assess sensation to the foot in several locations, including the plantar

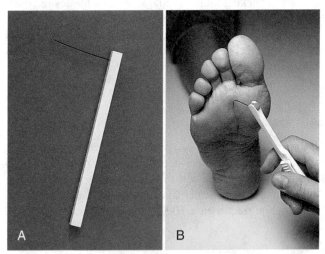

Fig. 4-26   A, Monofilament. **B,** Assessing peripheral sensation. *(From Seidel et al, 2006.)*

aspect of the foot, great toe, heel, and the ball of the foot. It is used only over areas with intact skin. Examination of peripheral sensation with a monofilament is discussed further in Chapter 16.

Transilluminator

Purpose: To differentiate the characteristics of tissue, fluid, and air within a specific body cavity.

A transilluminator consists of a strong light source with a narrow beam at the distal section of the light (Fig. 4-27). When the examination room is darkened and the light is placed directly against the skin over a body cavity such as a sinus area, the transilluminator disseminates its light source under the surface of the skin. Based on the character of the glowing light tones, the nurse can determine if the area under the surface is filled with air, fluid, or tissue.

Wood's Lamp

Purpose: To detect fungal infections of the skin or to detect corneal abrasions.

The Wood's lamp produces a black-light effect. The examination room should be darkened to enhance the clinical interpretation of the lesion color. Skin lesions caused by a fungal infection exhibit a fluorescent yellow-green or blue-green color when examined with a Wood's lamp (Fig. 4-28). When fluorescein dye is placed in the eye, the Wood's lamp can also detect scratches or abrasions to the surface of the eye.

Magnification Device

Purpose: To assist with the identification of skin lesions.

Many health care providers use a small handheld magnification device to assist with inspection. Some of these devices come with a battery-powered light source. Magnification and lighting facilitate the inspection of wounds, skin lesions, and parasites.

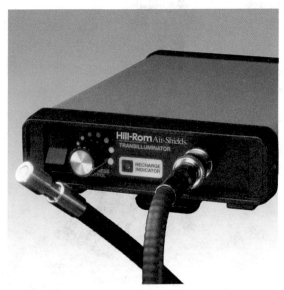

Fig. 4-27   Transilluminator. *(Courtesy, Draeger Medical, Inc., Telford, PA.)*

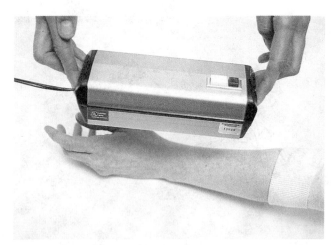

Fig. 4-28   Wood's lamp. The purple color on the skin indicates that no fungal infection is present.

APPLICATION OF INFECTION CONTROL PRINCIPLES

As a health care provider, you are expected to incorporate infection control principles in your practice. Infection control measures are referred to as *Standard Precautions*. Standard Precaution guidelines are published by the Centers for Disease Control and Prevention (CDC). These guidelines set the standard of care for infection control practice and are periodically updated. Standard Precautions reduce the risk of transmission from both recognized and unrecognized sources of infection. Guidelines that are specifically related to health examination includes hand hygiene, use of personal protective equipment, and management of equipment used on clients. CDC guidelines for hand hygiene are presented in Box 4-2. Personal protective equipment and management of patient care equipment are discussed in Box 4-3.

Standard precautions apply to all clients in all health care settings. Although health assessment is a relatively safe activity, the potential for infection transmission exists. Infection transmission can occur from the client to the health care worker, from the health care worker to the client, or from client to client via the hands of the health care provider or by equipment used by the health care provider.

Latex Allergy

It is important to note that the incidence of latex allergy has increased significantly in recent years. A latex allergy is a reaction to proteins in latex rubber. The amount of exposure needed to produce a latex allergy reaction is unknown, but it is known that frequent exposure increases the risk of developing allergic symptoms (National Institute for Occupational Safety and Health [NIOSH], 1998). Latex is found in gloves and many types of equipment and supplies. Health care professionals are at risk for developing latex allergy because of their frequent exposure to latex. NIOSH recommendations to prevent latex allergy for health care workers are summarized in Box 4-4. A variety of nonlatex gloves have been intro-

---

BOX 4-2 **STANDARD PRECAUTION GUIDELINES** *Hand Hygiene*

Hand hygiene is considered to be the single most important measure to reduce transmission of infection and is considered an essential element of Standard Precautions. Hand hygiene includes hand washing with soap and water and the use of alcohol-based products that do not require the use of water. Specific recommendations for hand hygiene issued by the Centers for Disease Control and Prevention that apply to physical examination include the following:

1. Hand hygiene technique:
   a. When decontaminating hands by washing with soap and water: wet hands, then apply soap to hands and rub vigorously for at least 15 seconds, covering all surfaces of the hands and fingers. Rinse hands with water and dry thoroughly with a disposable towel. Turn faucet off using towel.
   b. When decontaminating hands using alcohol-based hand rub: apply the product to the palm of one hand and rub hands together, covering all surfaces of the hands and fingers until hands are dry.
2. Indications for hand hygiene:
   a. Decontaminate hands when visibly dirty or contaminated with proteinaceous material or soiled with blood or other body fluids by washing hands with either a non-antimicrobial soap and water or an antimicrobial soap and water.
   b. If hands are not visibly soiled, decontaminate hands with an alcohol-based hand rub or, alternatively, wash hands with soap (either a non-antimicrobial or an antimicrobial soap) and water.
   c. Wash hands with soap (either non-antimicrobial or antimicrobial) and water before eating and after using a restroom.

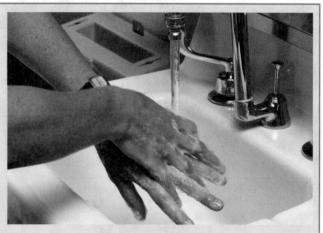

   d. Decontaminate hands in the following situations:
      • Before having direct contact with patients.
      • After having direct contact with a patient's intact skin.
      • After contact with body fluids, excretions, mucous membranes, nonintact skin, and wound dressings.
      • If moving from a contaminated body site (such as perineal area, mouth, etc.) to a clean body site.
      • After contact with objects (such as medical equipment, table tops, linens) in the immediate vicinity of the patient.
      • After removing gloves.

From Centers for Disease Control and Prevention: Guideline for hand hygiene in health-care settings: recommendations of the Healthcare Infection Control Practices Advisory Committee and the HICPAC/SHEA/APIC/IDSA Hand Hygiene Task Force, *MMWR* 51(RR016):1-45, 2002; and Siegel JD, Rhinehart E, Jackson M, Chiarello L, and the Healthcare Infection Control Practices Advisory Committee: *2007 Guideline for Isolation Precautions: Preventing Transmission of Infectious Agents in Healthcare Settings,* June 2007. Available at *www.cdc.gov/ncidod/dhqp/pdf/isolation2007.pdf.*

BOX 4-3 **STANDARD PRECAUTION GUIDELINES** *Personal Protective Equipment*

Gloves

Gloves should be worn when contact with a client's blood or other body fluid is possible. Specifically, this applies to contact with blood, body fluids (urine, feces, sputum, wound drainage, etc.), nonintact skin, and mucous membranes. Gloves should also be worn if handling equipment contaminated with blood or other body fluids. Gloves are worn for three primary reasons:

- To protect the health care worker from exposure to blood-borne pathogens carried by the client
- To protect the client from microorganisms on the hands of the health care worker
- To reduce the potential of infection transmission from one client to another client via the hands of the health care worker

The use of gloves does not reduce the frequency or importance of hand hygiene. Hands must be washed before performing a procedure even when gloves are worn, and then again immediately after removal of gloves. Gloves should be changed between procedures on the same client if the gloves have become contaminated to prevent cross contamination. If a glove breaks during a procedure, it should be removed promptly and replaced with a new glove. Gloves should be discarded after all procedures; they should never be washed and reused.

If gloves are used in combination with other personal protective equipment, they are put on last. Ideally the cuff of the glove fits snugly over the gown on the wrists to provide a more reliable, continuous barrier for the hands, wrists, and arms.

Masks, Eye Protection, Face Shields

The nurse should wear a mask with eye protection or a face shield during procedures that may result in splashes or sprays of the client's blood, body fluids, secretions, or excretions. Such equipment protects the mucous membranes of the eyes, nose, and mouth from contact, thus reducing the likelihood of pathogen transmission. Although not routinely needed for health assessment, situations may occur in which this equipment becomes necessary.

Gown

A gown should be worn to protect the health care worker's arms and other exposed skin surfaces, and to prevent contamination of clothing during procedures with the client's blood or other body fluids, or contact with other potentially infectious material. When applying Standard Precautions, a gown is only needed when contamination described above is anticipated. However, when Contact Precautions are used, use of an isolation gown and gloves is indicated. When a gown is to be worn, it should be donned first. Removal of a gown after patient contact is done in a manner to prevent contamination of clothing or skin surfaces.

Patient Care Equipment

The nurse should avoid touching equipment contaminated with blood or other body fluids unless gloves are worn. Multiple-use patient equipment that has been soiled with blood or other body fluids (e.g., a vaginal speculum) should not be reused until it has been adequately cleaned and reprocessed. Single-use items must be properly disposed of after client use. The nurse must take caution when handling contaminated sharp equipment. (Gloves will not provide protection from a sharp injury such as a needle stick.) Appropriate handling of sharps involves the following principles:

- Never recap a needle after client use.
- Never attempt to remove a needle from a disposable syringe by hand.
- After client use, place disposable syringes and needles directly into a "sharps container"—a puncture-resistant container designated for contaminated sharp items.

From Siegel JD, Rhinehart E, Jackson M, Chiarello L, and the Healthcare Infection Control Practices Advisory Committee, *2007 Guideline for Isolation Precautions: Preventing Transmission of Infectious Agents in Healthcare Settings,* June 2007. Available at *www.cdc.gov/ncidod/dhqp/pdf/isolation2007.pdf.*

BOX 4-4 **PREVENTING LATEX ALLERGY**

- Use nonlatex gloves for activities that are not likely to involve contact with infectious materials.
- If latex gloves are to be used, use a powder-free, low-allergen glove, if possible.
- Do not use oil-based hand lotions when wearing latex gloves.
- Immediately after removing latex gloves, wash hands with mild soap and dry thoroughly.

- If you develop latex allergy symptoms, avoid direct contact with latex products and see a health care provider knowledgeable about latex allergy. Early symptoms of latex allergy are similar to contact dermatitis (dry, itching, irritated areas on the hands or skin in contact with latex). A more severe symptom is a delayed hypersensitivity dermatitis. Lesions resembling poison ivy may appear 1 to 2 days after contact. The lesions can progress to oozing blisters.

From National Institute for Occupational Safety and Health: *NIOSH alert preventing allergic reactions to natural rubber latex in the workplace,* NIOSH pub no 97-135, Cincinnati, 1997; National Institute for Occupational Safety and Health: *Latex allergy: a prevention guide,* NIOSH pub no 98-113, Cincinnati, 1998.

duced into the health care environment over the last several years. It has been reported that nitrile examination gloves provide comparable barrier protection to latex and thus are a suitable alternative to latex gloves. Vinyl and copolymer examination gloves were found to be less effective barriers compared with latex (Korniewicz et al, 2002; Rego and Roley, 1999).

Clients may also have a latex allergy; particularly at risk are children with spina bifida and people who have had multiple medical procedures and surgeries, especially genitourinary surgery. For this reason nurses should routinely ask clients about latex allergy, and if it exists protect the client from coming in contact with latex gloves and other medical equipment made of latex, such as urinary catheters and feeding devices.

CLINICAL APPLICATION & CLINICAL REASONING

See Appendix E for answers to exercises in this section.

REVIEW QUESTIONS

1 The nurse is caring for a client with a femur fracture. The leg was placed in a cast a few hours ago. The nurse will palpate the foot distal to the cast in order to make which of the following determinations?
 1 Amount of drainage from the wound.
 2 Adequacy of blood perfusion to the foot.
 3 Presence of air in the underlying tissue.
 4 Range of motion to the foot.
2 Auscultation is a component of which of the following examination techniques?
 1 Blood pressure measurement.
 2 Visual acuity.
 3 Examination of the ears.
 4 Measurement of oxygen saturation.
3 According to CDC guidelines, the infection control intervention that should be used most frequently is:
 1 Wearing gloves.
 2 Using masks and face shields.
 3 Asking clients to change hospital gowns daily.
 4 Hand hygiene.
4 Which of the following is the correct application of a goniometer?
 1 Auscultation of fetal heart tones.
 2 Inspection of the cervix.
 3 Measurement of joint flexion.
 4 Assessment of hearing.
5 While examining a client with an infected abdominal incision, the nurse notices that it is very malodorous. Which technique does this represent?
 1 Inspection.
 2 Palpation.
 3 Auscultation.
 4 Percussion.

INTERACTIVE ACTIVITIES

Open the interactive student CD-ROM, click on Chapter 4, and choose from the following activities on the menu bar:

* **Multiple Choice Challenge.** Click on the best answer for each question. You will be given immediate feedback, rationale for incorrect answers, and a total score. Good luck!

* **Marvelous Matches.** Drag each word or phrase to the appropriate place on the screen. Test your ability to match techniques and equipment to the clue provided.

* **Printable Lab Guide.** Locate the Lab Guide for Chapter 4, and print and use it (as many times as needed) to help you apply your assessment skills. These guides may also be filled in electronically and then saved and e-mailed to your instructor!

* **Quick Challenge.** Use this critical thinking exercise to assess your skills through case study-style questions, then compare with expert answers!

CHAPTER 5

General Inspection and Measurement of Vital Signs

Initial data are collected before examining specific body systems. These initial data are often referred to as *general inspection* and typically include initial observations made by the nurse. Other terms include *general survey, general observations,* and *initial observations.* In addition to a general inspection, other baseline data typically collected by the nurse include vital signs, height, and weight.

GENERAL INSPECTION

Begin the general inspection the moment you meet the client. This involves observation of the client's physical appearance and hygiene, body structure, body movement, emotional and mental status, and behavior (Fig. 5-1). It requires attention to detail and provides clues regarding possible problems the client may be experiencing. Initial impressions gained from these preliminary observations direct the nurse for further examination in areas that do not initially appear normal.

Physical Appearance and Hygiene

The physical appearance includes a variety of general observations about the client, including general appearance, age, skin, and hygiene. Consider the client's general appearance. Does the client appear healthy? Are there any obvious findings you notice immediately (such as tremors or facial drooping)? Does the client appear close to his or her stated age? Some clients appear older or younger than their stated age as a result of a number of factors, such as drug and alcohol use, excessive sun exposure, chronic disease, and endocrine disorders (altered growth pat-

terns or altered sexual development). Notice the color and condition of the client's skin. Are there any variations in color or obvious presence of lesions? What is the general hygiene of the client? Is the client clean and well groomed? Does the client have a disheveled appearance? Are any odors detected? When unpleasant odors are detected, you must try to suppress reactions that may be communicated through facial expressions.

Body Structure and Position

Observations involving body structure include inspecting stature, general impression of nutritional status (well nourished, cachectic, or obese), and body symmetry (right and left sides of the body appear similar in size). Also note the client's position or posture. Does the client sit up and stand up straight? A client with spinal deformities or back pain, for example, may have a slumped posture when standing or sitting. A client who is having difficulty breathing may sit slightly forward bracing the arms on his or her knees in what is referred to as a *tripod position.* A client who is in pain may exhibit guarding or may assume a *fetal position* while lying down.

Body Movement

Note how the client moves. Does the client walk with ease? Is the gait balanced and smooth with symmetric movement of all extremities? Note the use of assistive devices for ambulation such as a cane or walker. Note the ease of movement from standing to sitting and from sitting to lying. Does the client move all extremities? Are there any limitations in range of motion of any of the extremities? Does the client

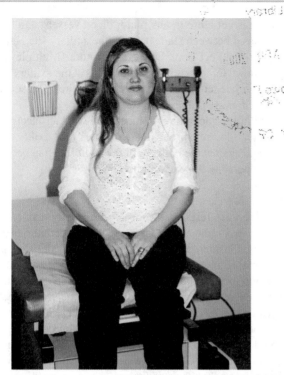

Fig. 5-1 General inspection begins immediately on meeting the client. Note physical appearance, hygiene, body structure, movement, posture, emotional status, and behavior.

seem to guard extremities or show evidence of pain with movement? Also observe for the presence of involuntary movements such as a tremor or tic.

Emotional and Mental Status and Behavior

Emotional and mental status are evaluated by noting alertness, facial expressions, tone of voice, and affect. Does the client maintain eye contact? Does the client converse appropriately? Are the facial expressions and body language appropriate for the conversation? Is the clothing appropriate for the weather? Is the behavior appropriate?

MEASUREMENT OF VITAL SIGNS, HEIGHT, AND WEIGHT

Baseline indicators of a client's health status include the measurement of vital signs (temperature, heart rate, respiratory rate, blood pressure, and oxygen saturation), height, and weight. Assessing the presence of pain is also considered standard baseline data to be collected on all clients and is often included with assessment of vital signs. Vital signs, pain assessment, height, and weight are usually assessed at the onset of the physical examination; however, they may also be integrated into the examination.

Temperature

Body temperature is regulated by the hypothalamus. Heat is gained through the processes of metabolism and exercise and lost through radiation, convection, conduction, and evapora-

tion. The expected temperature ranges from 96.4° to 99.1° F (35.8° to 37.3° C) with an average of 98.6° F (37° C). This is the stable core temperature at which cellular metabolism is most efficient.

FREQUENTLY ASKED QUESTIONS

The measurement of body temperature is a little confusing because there are so many routes and devices to choose from. Which device and route are the best to use?
Within the nursing literature there are many opinions regarding measurement of body temperature. The most accurate measurement of body temperature is gained from an internal (core) temperature reading. That being said, the most accurate measurement of core body temperature comes from the measurements gained from a hemodynamic monitoring line (such as a pulmonary artery catheter). Because these devices are found only in critical care settings, it is unlikely you would be using such a device for routine temperature measurement. Unfortunately, there is a fair amount of variability in all other temperature measurement devices. Generally speaking, internal measurements gained from the rectal and tympanic routes are considered to be more accurate than measurements taken by the oral and axillary routes, regardless of the type of device used.

Temperature changes occur as a result of normal variations and activities. Diurnal variations of 1° to 1.5° F (0.6° to 0.9° C) occur, with the lowest temperature early in the morning and the highest in the late afternoon and early evening. During the menstrual cycle, a woman's temperature increases 0.5° to 1.0° F (0.3° to 0.6° C) at ovulation and remains elevated until menses ceases. This elevation is due to progesterone secretion. Moderate to vigorous exercise increases temperature.

Temperature is measured by several routes: oral, tympanic, axillary, and rectal. Thermometers measure body temperature in Fahrenheit or Celsius; some devices measure in both. Conversion between the two measurements is easily done using a simple formula (Box 5-1).

Oral Temperature
Temperature measurement by the oral route is safe and relatively accurate. Oral measurement is usually taken with an electronic thermometer. Smoking or the ingestion of hot or

---

BOX 5-1 **CONVERSIONS BETWEEN FAHRENHEIT AND CELSIUS**

To convert Fahrenheit to Celsius:
(Fahrenheit temperature − 32) × 5/9
Example: (100.4° F − 32) × 5/9
   = 68.4 × 0.555
   = 37.96° C

To convert Celsius to Fahrenheit:
(Celsius temperature × 9/5) + 32
Example: (38.5° C × 9/5) + 32
   = 69.3 + 32
   = 101.3° F

cold liquids or food impacts the accuracy of measurement (Lockwood, Conroy-Hiller, & Paige, 2004); thus delay taking oral temperature readings for at least 10 minutes in such situations.

When using an electronic thermometer, cover the probe with a disposable sheath. Place the probe under the client's tongue in the right or left posterior sublingual pocket. This location receives its blood supply from the carotid artery; thus it indirectly reflects inner core temperature. Ask the client to keep the mouth closed while temperature is being measured. An electronic oral thermometer remains in place for 15 to 30 seconds until the audible signal occurs and the temperature registers on the display screen. Because the plastic sheath does not break, assessment of oral temperature with an electronic thermometer is safe for use with children or confused adults.

Tympanic Membrane Temperature

Tympanic thermometers measure temperature from the tympanic membrane within the ear. The probe is covered with a protective sheath and placed inside the external ear canal with firm but gentle pressure (Fig. 5-2). The probe must come in contact with all sides of the ear canal. (*Note:* The probe does not extend all the way to the tympanic membrane.) An ear tug in an upward direction for adults (downward direction in infants and children) should be used to help straighten the external auditory canal to ensure measurement accuracy; the presence of impacted cerumen will result in an inaccurate temperature measurement (Lockwood, Conroy-Hiller, & Paige, 2004). The thermometer is removed after the audible signal occurs (about 2 to 3 seconds) and the temperature reading is displayed.

Axillary Temperature

The axilla is a common site for temperature measurement on infants and children; however, it is an infrequently used site for adult temperature measurement. Results from research raise questions regarding the accuracy in measurement. Because it is not close to any major blood vessels, and because it is placed between skin surfaces, the axillary site is thought to poorly reflect core body temperature. Multiple studies have shown temperature measurements at the axillary site are less accurate compared to alternative sites (Jensen et al, 2002; Thomas et al, 2004).

Axillary temperature is measured with an electric thermometer. Place the probe in the middle of the axilla, with the arm held against the body, until the audible signal occurs and the temperature appears on the screen.

Rectal Temperature

Rectal temperatures are taken less frequently than tympanic or oral measurements. Although rectal temperature measurement is considered safe and accurate for adults, it is less comfortable, requires more time, and has an increased risk of infection transmission compared to other routes. Rectal temperature can be measured with an electronic thermometer.

To take a rectal temperature, place the client in a Sims' position with the upper leg flexed. Appropriate privacy should be provided. Insert a disposable sheath over the thermometer probe and apply a water-soluble lubricant. Wearing gloves, insert the lubricated thermometer probe in the rectum 1 to 1.5 inches (2.5 to 3.8 cm), and hold in place until the audible signal occurs and the temperature is displayed on the screen.

Heart Rate

Palpation of arterial pulses provides valuable information about the cardiovascular system. When assessing vital signs, the pulse is taken to determine heart rate and rhythm. The heart rate is most commonly assessed by palpating a pulse. Contraction of the heart results in ejection of blood into the peripheral vascular system; thus when a pulsation is felt, it is an indirect reflection of the heart contraction. The pulse rate is the number of times in a minute the pulsation is felt. The rhythm refers to the regularity of the pulsations, that is, the time between each beat. The palpation of pulses also provides important information regarding the strength of the pulse and perfusion of blood to various parts of the body. This is discussed further in Chapter 13.

To take a pulse, place your fingers over the artery and feel for the pulsations and the rhythm. Pulses are palpated using the finger pads of the index and middle fingers. Firm pressure is applied over the pulse, but not so hard that the pulsation is occluded. If the pulse is difficult to locate, vary the amount of pressure and palpate the location where you expect to find the pulse. If the rhythm is regular (time between each beat is consistent), count the number of pulsations palpated for 30 seconds and multiply by 2 or count for 15 seconds and multiply by 4. If the pulse rhythm feels irregular (time between each beat varies), note whether there is a regularity to the rhythm (e.g., a skip every fourth pulsation) or if the rhythm lacks regularity. Count the number of pulsations for a full minute. Document an irregular pulse when recording vital signs. Expected heart rates for various age groups are listed in Table 5-1.

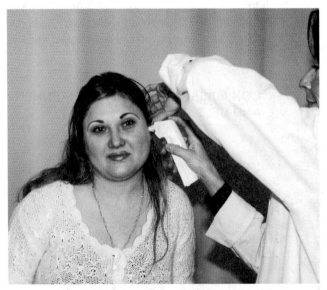

Fig. 5-2   Taking a tympanic membrane temperature.

TABLE 5-1 *Average Vital Signs Throughout the Life Span*

Vital Sign	Newborn	Toddler	School-Age Child	Adolescent	Adult
Heart rate (beats/min)					
• Range	120-160	90-140	75-100	60-90	60-100
• Average	140	110	85	70	70
Respiratory rate (breaths/min)	30-60	24-40	18-30	12-16	12-20
Blood pressure (mm Hg)					
• Systolic range	60-90	80-112	84-120	94-140	110-140
• Diastolic range	20-60	50-80	54-80	62-88	60-90

Although a pulse can be taken in many areas, the radial artery is most frequently used to measure heart rate because it is accessible and easily palpated. The radial pulse is found at the radial side of the forearm at the wrist (Fig. 5-3). The brachial and carotid arteries are common alternative sites to assess pulse rate. The brachial pulse is located in the groove between the biceps and triceps muscle just medial to the biceps tendon at the antecubital fossa (in the bend of the elbow) (Fig. 5-4). The carotid pulse is found by palpating along the medial edge of the sternocleidomastoid muscle in the lower third of the neck (Fig. 5-5). The heart rate can also be assessed by auscultating the heart (known as the apical pulse) and counting the heart sounds for 1 minute. Auscultation of the heart is discussed further in Chapter 13.

Respiratory Rate

Assessment of the respiratory rate involves counting the number of times the client completes a ventilatory cycle (inhalation and exhalation) each minute. Men usually breathe diaphragmatically, which increases the movement of the abdomen, whereas women tend to be thoracic breathers, which is noted with movement of the chest. It is best to count the respiratory rate when the client is unaware you are doing so; this will prevent the client from becoming self-conscious of the assessment and perhaps changing the breathing rate or pattern. Many nurses count respirations immediately after obtaining the pulse, but while maintaining their finger position on the pulse site. Respiratory rates vary with age (see Table 5-1). Other factors that increase respiratory rate are fever, anxiety, exercise, and increased altitude.

In addition to assessing the rate, note the rhythm, depth, and effort of breathing. Rhythm is the pattern or regularity of breathing and is described as regular or irregular. Depth is assessed by observing the excursion or movement of the chest wall. Depth is described as deep (full lung expansion with full exhalation), normal, or shallow. Shallow breathing (small volume of air movement in and out of lungs) may be difficult to observe. The effort that goes into breathing is also

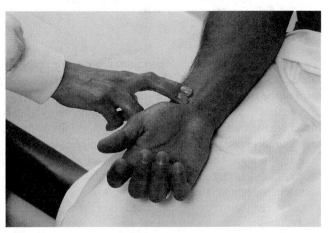

Fig. 5-3 Radial pulse.

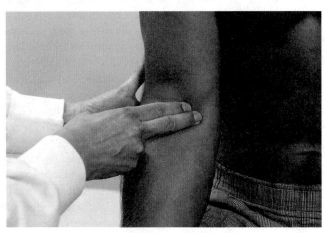

Fig. 5-4 Brachial pulse.

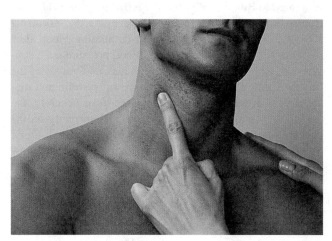

Fig. 5-5 Carotid pulse.

observed. Normally, breathing should be even, quiet, and effortless when the client is sitting or lying down.

Blood Pressure

Blood pressure is the force of blood against the arterial walls. It reflects the relationship between cardiac output and peripheral resistance. The cardiac output is the volume of blood ejected from the heart each minute. Peripheral resistance is the force that opposes the flow of blood through vessels. For example, when the arteries are narrow, the peripheral resistance to blood flow is high, which is reflected in an elevated blood pressure. Blood pressure depends on the velocity of the blood, intravascular blood volume, and elasticity of the vessel walls.

Blood pressure is measured in millimeters of mercury (mm Hg). *Systolic blood pressure* is the maximum pressure exerted on arteries when the ventricles eject blood from the heart. By contrast, *diastolic blood pressure* represents the minimum amount of pressure exerted on the vessels; this occurs when the ventricles of the heart relax. Blood pressure is recorded with the systolic pressure written on top of the diastolic pressure (e.g., 130/76), but it is not a fraction. The difference between the systolic and diastolic pressure is called the *pulse pressure,* which normally ranges from 30 to 40 mm Hg. Expected blood pressure ranges are shown in Table 5-1.

Measurement of Blood Pressure

Blood pressure can be measured directly or indirectly. Direct measurement is accomplished by inserting a small catheter into an artery that provides continuous blood pressure measurements and arterial waveforms. This direct measurement is done in the critical care setting when continuous monitoring is required. In all other settings, blood pressure is indirectly measured either by auscultation using a sphygmomanometer and a stethoscope (Fig. 5-6) or using a noninvasive blood pressure monitor (see Chapter 4).

The procedure for measuring blood pressure by auscultation is described in detail in Box 5-2. The procedure for measuring blood pressure with a noninvasive blood pressure (NIBP) monitor differs somewhat from the procedure presented in Box 5-2. Because the NIBP monitor is an electronic device, the nurse does not auscultate the Korotkoff sounds. The NIBP monitor senses circulating blood flow vibrations through a sensor in the blood pressure cuff, converts the vibrations into electric impulses, and translates the impulses into a digital readout indicating systolic and diastolic pressures. For the NIBP monitor to be accurate, the cuff must fit properly and must be placed correctly on the arm so that the sensor is directly over the brachial artery. The nurse must be familiar with the equipment and follow manufacturer guidelines before use. If there is any doubt about the blood pressure measurement obtained with an NIBP monitor, the blood pressure is rechecked by auscultation as described in Box 5-2.

Although the upper arm is the most common site to measure blood pressure, an acceptable alternative site is

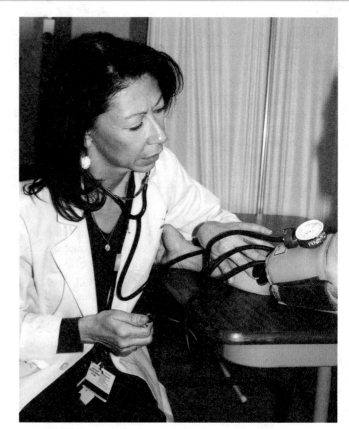

Fig. 5-6 Auscultating Korotkoff sounds to measure blood pressure.

the thigh. To take a thigh blood pressure reading, wrap a large cuff 7 to 7.9 inches (18 to 20 cm) around the lower third of the thigh, centering the bladder of the cuff over the popliteal artery. Follow the same procedure for taking a blood pressure measurement in the arm. Normally the systolic blood pressure is 10 to 40 mm Hg higher in the leg than in the arm. The diastolic pressures of arms and legs are similar. Another alternative site for blood pressure assessment using an NIBP monitor is the wrist, although this site has been shown to overestimate blood pressure (Angeli et al, 2006).

Mechanism of Blood Pressure Measurement

Blood flows freely through the artery until the inflated cuff occludes the artery enough to interrupt blood flow. As the cuff pressure is slowly released, the nurse listens for the sounds of the blood pulsating through the artery again. The initial sound is called the first *Korotkoff* sound (named for the Russian physician who first described it) and is characterized by a clear, rhythmic thumping corresponding to the pulse rate that gradually increases in intensity (Fig. 5-7). The pressure reading at which this sound is first heard indicates the systolic pressure. A swishing sound heard as the cuff continues to deflate is the second Korotkoff sound. The third Korotkoff sound is a softer thump than the first; the fourth Korotkoff sound is muffled and low pitched as the cuff is further deflated. The fifth Korotkoff sound actually marks the cessation of sound and indicates that the artery is completely open. The manometer pressure noted at the fifth Korotkoff sound is

BOX 5-2 **PROCEDURE FOR MEASURING BLOOD PRESSURE (AUSCULTATION METHOD)**

- With the client sitting or lying down, position the client's upper arm slightly flexed at heart level with the palm turned up. The arm should be free of clothing.
- Palpate the brachial pulse in the antecubital space. Apply an appropriately sized blood pressure cuff (see Chapter 4) 1 inch (2.5 cm) above the site of brachial pulsation. The bladder of the cuff should be centered over the artery. The cuff should fit evenly and snugly around the arm.
- Position the sphygmomanometer at eye level no more than 3 feet (1 meter) away. Close the valve on the pressure bulb clockwise until it is tight but easily releasable with one hand.
- Palpate the brachial or radial pulse with the fingertips of one hand while inflating the cuff rapidly; note the point at which you no longer feel the pulse, and continue to inflate 20 to 30 mm Hg above this point. Slowly release the valve to deflate the cuff and note the point at which the pulse reappears; this is the palpated systolic pressure. Immediately deflate the cuff completely.
- After waiting for 30 seconds, place the stethoscope over the brachial pulse, and inflate the cuff to 30 mm Hg above the palpated systolic pressure. Release the valve and allow the cuff to deflate slowly at a rate of 2 to 3 mm Hg per second.
- Note the pressure reading on the sphygmomanometer when the first Korotkoff sound is heard: this is the systolic pressure. Continue to deflate the cuff slowly and note the point at which the sounds disappear: this is the diastolic pressure.
- Deflate the cuff completely and remove it from the client's arm. Record the measurement.
- This procedure may be repeated on the other arm for comparison purposes. A series of blood pressure measurements may also be taken when the client is in a lying, sitting, and standing position to assess for *orthostatic hypotension.* (A 20- to 30-mm Hg drop in blood pressure when the client goes from a lying or sitting position to standing is indicative of orthostatic hypotension.)

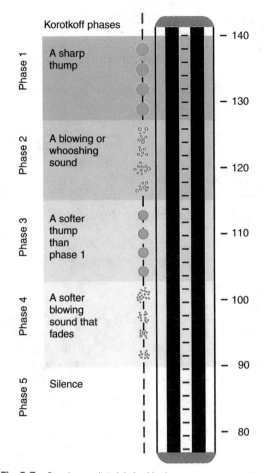

Fig. 5-7 Sounds auscultated during blood pressure measurement can be differentiated into five Korotkoff phases. In this example the blood pressure is 140/90. *(From Perry and Potter, 2006.)*

- *Race:* The incidence of hypertension is twice as high in African Americans as in whites.
- *Diurnal variations:* Blood pressure is lower in the early morning and peaks in later afternoon or early evening.
- *Emotions:* Feeling anxious, angry, or stressed may increase the blood pressure.
- *Pain:* Experiencing acute pain can increase blood pressure.
- *Personal habits:* Ingesting caffeine or smoking a cigarette within 30 minutes before measurement may increase blood pressure.
- *Weight:* Obese clients tend to have higher blood pressures than nonobese clients.

the diastolic pressure. It takes a great deal of practice to differentiate all five sounds. However, differentiation of the five sounds is ordinarily not necessary—in most cases only the first (systolic) and fifth (diastolic) Korotkoff sounds are recorded.

Physiologic Factors that Affect Blood Pressure Measurements

A number of client-related factors affect blood pressure and should be kept in mind when interpreting blood pressure measurements.

- *Age:* From childhood to adulthood there is a gradual rise.
- *Gender:* After puberty, females usually have a lower blood pressure than males; however, after menopause, women's blood pressure may be higher than men's.

Common Errors Associated with Blood Pressure Measurement

The accuracy of blood pressure measurement is significantly affected by the nurse's technique. Research has found that many health care providers demonstrate incorrect technique or lack of knowledge associated with blood pressure measurement (Armstrong, 2002; Carney, 1999). Incorrect technique can result in false-low or false-high measurements. Box 5-3 presents common errors in blood pressure measurement. Many of the errors are associated

BOX 5-3 ERRORS IN BLOOD PRESSURE MEASUREMENT

Errors Resulting in False-High Blood Pressure Measurement
- Positioning client's arm above the level of the heart
- Using a cuff that is too narrow for the extremity
- Wrapping the cuff too loosely or unevenly
- Deflating the cuff too slowly (slower than 2 to 3 mm Hg per second)
- Reinflating the cuff without completely deflating the cuff
- Failure to wait 1 to 2 minutes before obtaining a repeat measurement

Errors Resulting in False-Low Blood Pressure Measurement
- Positioning client's arm below the level of the heart
- Positioning the manometer higher than the client's heart
- Using a cuff that is too wide
- Not inflating the cuff enough
- Deflating the cuff too rapidly (faster than 2 to 3 mm Hg per second)
- Pressing the diaphragm too firmly on the brachial artery

with improper cuff size. Determination of proper cuff size is discussed in Chapter 4.

Oxygen Saturation

In many settings, measurement of the oxygen saturation is routinely included with vital signs. As discussed in Chapter 4, oxygen saturation is measured by a pulse oximeter—a device that estimates the oxygen saturation of hemoglobin in the blood. The probe is usually either clipped or taped to the client's fingertip; the toe, earlobe, and nose are alternative sites. The oxygen saturation appears as a digital readout within 10 to 15 seconds after the oximeter is placed. Oxygen saturation levels lower than 90% are considered abnormal and require further evaluation. Although this is considered an easy procedure, deficiencies in health care provider knowledge of pulse oximetry measurement and interpretation of results have been reported (Howell, 2002).

Pain

Routine assessment of a client's pain or comfort level is standard practice in all health care settings and is often assessed with vital sign measurement. An in-depth discussion of pain assessment is presented in Chapter 6.

Weight

Body weight or mass is influenced by a number of factors, including genetics, dietary intake, exercise, and fluid volume. Genetics influence height and body size, including bone structure, muscle mass, and gender. Body weight is important for nutritional assessment, to determine changes in weight over time (if previous body weight measurements are available), and in some situations to calculate medication dosage. An unintentional change in weight can be a significant finding. For example, an increase in weight may be the first sign of fluid retention. For every liter of fluid retained (1000 ml, or about 1 quart), weight increases 2.2 lb (1 kg). Also, unexplained weight loss may be one indication of suspected malignancy or disease process. Nutritional assessment is discussed further in Chapter 9.

Measure weight using a balance scale by asking the client to stand in the middle of the scale platform while the large and small weights are balanced. The scale uses a counterbalance system of adding or subtracting weights in increments as small as 0.25 lb (0.1 kg) to achieve a level horizontal balance beam on the scale. Move the larger weight to the 50 lb (22.7 kg) increment less than the client's weight. Adjust the smaller weight to balance the scale. Read the weight to the nearest 0.25 lb (0.1 kg).

Height

Height is also influenced by genetics and dietary intake. Height is measured on a platform scale with a height attachment. The height attachment is pulled up and the horizontal headpiece extended before the client steps on the scale to avoid poking the client as the headpiece is extended. Ask the client to stand on the scale (without shoes); then lower the attachment until the horizontal headpiece touches the top of the client's head (Fig. 5-8). The vertical measuring scale can measure in inches or centimeters. Adult height is attained between ages 18 and 20.

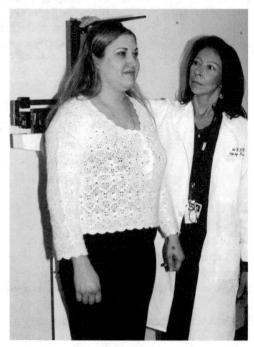

Fig. 5-8 Assessment of height using a platform scale.

AGE-RELATED VARIATONS

This chapter discusses conducting a general inspection and measurement of vital signs with adult clients. These data are important to assess for individuals of all ages, but the approach and techniques used to collect the information may vary depending on the client's age.

Infants and Children

The measurement of height (recumbent length), weight, head and chest circumference are important indicators of growth. These data are plotted on growth charts to assess growth patterns of the infant and child, and to compare growth to infants and children of the same age and gender. Although the same general process for general inspection and vital signs measurement among infants and children is followed as previously described, specific differences in the approach and techniques are presented in Chapter 20.

Older Adults

The measurement of height, weight, and vital signs in the older adult is the same as previously described.

CLINICAL APPLICATION & CLINICAL REASONING

See Appendix E for answers to exercises in this section.

REVIEW QUESTIONS

1 The nurse obtains vital signs on a 42-year-old man having his annual physical examination. He has no medical conditions and states that his health is excellent. The blood pressure recorded by the NIBP monitor is 62/40. Which of the following actions by the nurse is most reasonable?
   1 Obtain a different cuff.
   2 Reposition the cuff, ensuring that the sensor is over the brachial artery.
   3 Place the patient in a prone position and take the pressure on the leg.
   4 Record the blood pressure, and continue with the examination.
2 Which of the following sets of vital signs should the nurse recognize as out of the expected range?
   1 42-year-old male: BP 114/82; HR 74; RR 16; Temp 36.8° C.
   2 11-year-old girl: HR 88; RR 22; Temp 36.7° C.
   3 3-year-old boy: HR 130; RR 40; Temp 36.7° C.
   4 1-month-old girl: HR 120; RR 42; Temp 36.7° C.
3 The nurse records the following general inspection findings on a patient: "41-year-old Hispanic male in no distress; very thin, skin tone slightly jaundice, disheveled appearance, appears older than stated age. Client with flat affect and makes minimal eye contact." Additional information that should be added to this general inspection includes:
   1 Body movement.
   2 Family history.
   3 Estimated size of his liver.
   4 Palpation of pulses.

4 A patient is brought to the emergency department with severe respiratory distress. Which of the following methods of temperature measurement would be most appropriate?
   1 Oral temperature measurement with an electric thermometer.
   2 Axillary measurement with an electronic thermometer.
   3 Tympanic membrane measurement.
   4 Rectal temperature measurement.
5 A 62-year-old client tells the nurse he has recently had frequent fainting spells. After palpating the radial pulse, 13 pulsations are counted in 15 seconds. The nurse determines that he has a pulse rate of 52, with an irregular rhythm. In this situation the nurse will:
   1 Reassess the pulse rate after he walks around the room for several minutes.
   2 Reassess the pulse rate for 15 seconds using the carotid artery.
   3 Take an apical pulse for 5 full minutes, counting the number of skipped beats.
   4 Palpate the pulse for a full minute, and note whether there is a pattern to the irregularity.

INTERACTIVE ACTIVITIES

Open the interactive student CD-ROM, click on Chapter 5, and choose from the following activities on the menu bar:

- **Multiple Choice Challenge.** Click on the best answer for each question. You will be given immediate feedback, rationale for incorrect answers, and a total score. Good luck!

- **Crossword Wizard.** Complete a crossword puzzle using clues associated with health assessment concepts. It's a whiz!

- **Marvelous Matches.** Show your mastery of concepts. Match terms to clues provided.

- **Printable Lab Guide.** Locate the Lab Guide for Chapter 5, and print and use it (as many times as needed) to help you apply your assessment skills. These guides may also be filled in electronically and then saved and e-mailed to your instructor!

- **Quick Challenge.** Use this critical thinking exercise to assess your skills through case study-style questions, then compare with expert answers!

CHAPTER 6

Pain Assessment

ELECTRONIC RESOURCES

Additional information related to the content in Chapter 6 can be found

in the companion website at

evolve

evolve: http://evolve.elsevier.com/Wilson/assessment/

or on the interactive student CD-ROM

 Activities for Chapter 6 include the following:
- Multiple Choice Challenge • Marvelous Matches
- Printable Lab Guide • Quick Challenge

Working with clients to relieve pain is a primary responsibility of all nurses. Thus assessing the client's pain is the first step in achieving the goal of pain relief. Because of the importance of pain assessment and management, many refer to pain as the fifth vital sign after temperature, blood pressure, pulse, and respiration.

The most widely accepted definition of pain is the one adopted by the American Pain Society (APS), which states that pain is an unpleasant sensory and emotional experience associated with actual or potential tissue damage (APS, 1992). A practical definition of pain is that of Margo McCaffery, who believes that pain is whatever and wherever the person says it is (McCaffery and Pasero, 1999). This definition represents the belief that one person cannot judge the perception or meaning of pain of another person.

Although pain occurs when tissues are damaged, there is no correlation between the amount of tissue damage and the degree or intensity of pain experienced. For example, a client with extensive traumatic injuries may not report the intensity of pain expected, whereas a client with chronic cancer pain may experience intense pain for which no tissue damage can be found. The client's previous experiences with pain, as well as the client's current physical and mental status, affect pain perception and response.

Culture also influences people's response to pain. In some cultures people may express their pain loudly and overtly, whereas those in other cultures may be stoic about pain and remain silent about their pain or they may even smile. Another example is the differences in the expectations of pain. In some cultures people grow up not expecting a great deal of pain relief, because they believe that having pain is a part of the healing process. When caring for clients who have a low expectation for pain relief, the nurse asks about the clients' beliefs about pain and satisfaction with current pain level. The nurse teaches these clients that pain relief is available if desired and that it is the nurse's goal for the client to be comfortable. The nurse does not assume that the client has the same expectation of pain relief as the nurse would have in a similar situation. The client's satisfaction with pain relief is assessed, and both nonpharmacologic and pharmacologic interventions are offered to achieve the desired pain rating.

In 2000, The Joint Commission (TJC) issued pain standards as a criterion for accreditation of hospitals. In 2001, TJC began scoring this standard as a part of its on-site surveys for accreditation. One of the standards is that clients have the right to appropriate assessment and management of pain. This standard includes the following: (1) initial assessment and regular reassessment of pain, taking into account personal, cultural, spiritual, and ethnic beliefs; (2) education of all relevant providers in pain assessment and management; and (3) education of clients and families regarding their roles in managing pain, as well as the potential limitations and side effects of pain treatments. Another TJC standard is that pain is assessed in all clients. Examples of implementing this standard are assessing pain intensity, location, quality, onset, duration, and alleviating and aggravating factors and determining the effects of pain on the client's life (e.g., daily function) and the client's pain goal (*www.jointcommission.org*, 2000).

Pain is categorized in several ways, but a clear distinction among types of pain may not always be possible (McCaffery and Pasero, 1999). One categorization distinguishes acute from chronic pain. Acute pain has a recent onset (less than 6 months) and results from tissue damage, is usually self-limiting, and ends when the tissue heals. Acute pain is a stressor that initiates a generalized stress response, causing physiologic signs associated with pain. The sympathetic nervous system responds to acute pain of low to moderate intensity and superficial pain by increasing heart rate, increasing blood pressure, causing

53

diaphoresis, increasing respiratory rate, increasing muscle tension, dilating pupils, and decreasing gastrointestinal motility. The parasympathetic nervous system responds to severe or deep pain by causing pallor, muscle tension, and decreased heart rate; rapid, irregular breathing; nausea and vomiting; and weakness or exhaustion.

By contrast, chronic pain may be intermittent or continuous pain lasting more than 6 months. Clinical manifestations of chronic pain are not those of physiologic stress because the client adapts to the pain. The client reports symptoms of irritability, depression, withdrawal, and insomnia.

Another way to categorize pain is in terms of the inferred pathology, that is, nociceptive and neuropathic pain. Nociceptive pain arises from stimulation of somatic or visceral structures, whereas neuropathic pain occurs due to abnormal processing of sensory input by the central or peripheral nervous systems. Nociceptive pain and neuropathic pain are explained in Fig. 6-1.

Referred pain is pain felt at a site different from that of an injured or diseased organ. It commonly occurs during visceral pain because many organs have no pain receptors; thus when afferent nerves enter the spinal cord, they stimulate sensory nerves from unaffected organs in the same spinal cord segment as those neurons in areas where injury or disease is located. For example, gallbladder disease may cause referred pain to the right shoulder, and myocardial infarction may cause referred pain to the left shoulder, arm, or jaw.

Phantom pain is pain that a person feels in an amputated extremity after the residual limb has healed. It commonly occurs in a person who experienced pain in that limb before amputation. If the nerve pathway from the amputated extremity is stimulated anywhere along the pathway, nerve impulses ascend to the cerebral cortex so that the person perceives pain even though the limb is no longer there. Phantom pain also is influenced by emotions and sympathetic stimulation (Huether and McCance, 2004).

The concepts of pain threshold and pain tolerance affect the client's pain experience. *Pain threshold* is the point at which a stimulus is perceived as pain. This threshold does not vary significantly among people or in the same person over time. In contrast, *pain tolerance* is the duration or intensity of pain a person will endure before outwardly responding. A person's culture, pain experience, expectations, role behaviors, and physical and emotional health influence pain tolerance. Pain tolerance decreases with repeated exposure to pain, fatigue, anger, boredom, apprehension, and sleep deprivation. Tolerance increases after alcohol consumption, medications, hypnosis, warmth, distracting activities, and strong faith beliefs (Huether and McCance, 2004).

CLASSIFICATION OF PAIN BY INFERRED PATHOPHYSIOLOGY

Two Major Types of Pain

I. Nociceptive Pain	**II. Neuropathic Pain**
A. Somatic Pain B. Visceral Pain	A. Centrally Generated Pain B. Peripherally Generated Pain

I. Nociceptive Pain: Normal processing of stimuli that damages normal tissues or has the potential to do so if prolonged; usually responsive to nonopioids and/or opioids.
A. Somatic Pain: Arises from bone, joint, muscle, skin, or connective tissue. It is usually aching or throbbing in quality and is well localized.
B. Visceral Pain: Arises from visceral organs, such as the GI tract and pancreas. This may be subdivided:
1. Tumor involvement of the organ capsule that causes aching and fairly well-localized pain.
2. Obstruction of hollow viscus, which causes intermittent cramping and poorly localized pain.

II. Neuropathic Pain: Abnormal processing of sensory input by the peripheral or central nervous system; treatment usually includes adjuvant analgesics.
A. Centrally Generated Pain
1. Deafferentation pain. Injury to either the peripheral or central nervous system. Examples: Phantom pain may reflect injury to the peripheral nervous system; burning pain below the level of a spinal cord lesion reflects injury to the central nervous system.
2. Sympathetically maintained pain. Associated with dysregulation of the autonomic nervous system. Examples: May include some of the pain associated with reflex sympathetic dystrophy/causalgia (complex regional pain syndrome, type I, type II).
B. Peripherally Generated Pain
1. Painful polyneuropathies. Pain is felt along the distribution of many peripheral nerves. Examples: diabetic neuropathy, alcohol-nutritional neuropathy, and those associated with Guillain-Barré syndrome.
2. Painful mononeuropathies. Usually associated with a known peripheral nerve injury, and pain is felt at least partly along the distribution of the damaged nerve. Examples: nerve root compression, nerve entrapment, trigeminal neuralgia.

Fig. 6-1 A method of classifying pain is by the pathophysiology involved. *I,* Nociceptive pain (stimuli from somatic and visceral structures). *II,* Neuropathic pain (stimuli abnormally processed by nervous system). *(From McCaffery and Pasero, 1999.)*

ANATOMY & PHYSIOLOGY

The physiology of pain involves a journey from the site of stimulation of peripheral receptors to the spinal cord (transduction), up the spinal cord (transmission) to the cerebral cortex (perception), and back down the spinal cord (modulation).

The first step in the pain process is transduction. It is conversion of mechanical, thermal, chemical, or electrical stimuli that damage tissues. Table 6-1 lists examples of these stimuli and the pathophysiologic processes by which they produce pain. Numerous chemical substances found in an area of tissue damage stimulate nociceptors. These chemicals include prostaglandins (PGs), bradykinin (BK), serotonin (5HT), substance P (SP), and histamine (H). These nociceptors are located at the ends of small, thinly myelinated or unmyelinated fibers and are found in tendon bundles, muscle spindles, subcutaneous tissue (called Pacini's corpuscles), epidermis (called Meissner's corpuscles), dermis, and skeletal muscles. The activation of nociceptors by these chemicals generates an action potential (Fig. 6-2) (McCaffery and Pasero, 1999).

The next step in the journey is transmission, beginning with stimulation of afferent nerves by the nociceptors (Fig. 6-3). There are four different afferent nerve fibers: small myelinated A-delta fibers, small unmyelinated C fibers, large myelinated A-alpha fibers, and large myelinated A-beta fibers. The A-delta fibers and C fibers are stimulated by nociceptors that initiate an action potential that travels along these nerves

LINK TO CONCEPTS *Pain*

The feature concept for this chapter is *Pain.* This concept represents an unpleasant sensory and emotional experience associated with actual or potential tissue damage, or pain processing.

Two types of pain described in this chapter are nociceptive pain (pain related to damaged tissues) and neuropathic pain (pain associated with abnormal pain processing). Many concepts in this book potentially cause nociceptive-related pain. Pain (regardless of the cause) links to several other concepts presented in this book; this relationship is presented in the Pain Cause and Effect Model.

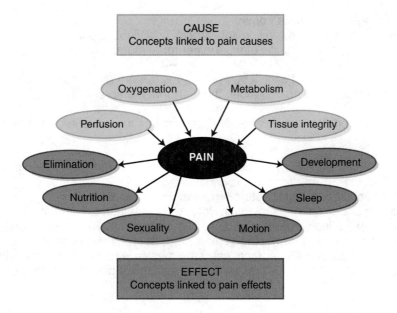

This model shows the potentially sweeping effects of pain on an individual. As an example, an individual with poor peripheral perfusion experiences pain because of inadequate oxygenation to the affected tissues (typically in the extremities). The effect of this pain can include reduced mobility, impaired sleep, and a loss of appetite. An individual taking narcotic pain medications may experience a change in elimination patterns (constipation). Having an understanding of the interrelationship of these concepts helps the nurse recognize risk factors and thus increases awareness when conducting a health assessment.

TABLE 6-1 *Examples of How Various Stimuli Produce Pain*

TYPE OF STIMULUS	EXAMPLE	PATHOPHYSIOLOGIC PROCESS
Mechanical	Alteration in body fluids	Edema distending body tissues
	Duct distention	Overstretching of duct's narrow lumen (e.g., passage of kidney stone through ureter)
	Space-occupying lesion (tumor)	Irritation of peripheral nerves by growth of lesion within confined space
Chemical	Perforated visceral organ	Chemical irritation by secretions on sensitive nerve endings (e.g., ruptured appendix, duodenal ulcer)
Thermal	Burn (heat or extreme cold)	Inflammation or loss of superficial layers of epidermis, causing increased sensitivity of nerve endings
Electrical	Burn	Skin layers burned with muscle and subcutaneous tissue injury, causing injury to nerve endings

From Potter PA, Perry AG: *Basic nursing: a critical thinking approach,* ed 4, St Louis, 1999, Mosby.

NOCICEPTION: BASIC PROCESS OF NORMAL PAIN TRANSMISSION

1 **Transduction:** Conversion of one energy from another. This process occurs in the periphery when a noxious stimulus causes tissue damage. The damaged cells release substances that activate or sensitize nociceptors. This activation leads to the generation of an action potential.

A. **Sensitizing substances** released by damaged cells:
- Prostaglandins (PG)
- Bradykinin (BK)
- Serotonin (5HT)
- Substance P (SP)
- Histamine (H)

B. An **action potential** results from:
- Release of the above sensitizing substances (nociceptive pain)
  + a change in the charge along the neuronal membrane
  or
- Abnormal processing of stimuli by the nervous system (neuropathic pain)
  + a change in the charge along the neuronal membrane

The change in charge occurs when Na^+ moves into the cell and other ion transfers occur.

2 **Transmission:** The action potential continues from the site of damage to the spinal cord and ascends to higher centers. Transmission may be considered in three phases:
- Injury site to spinal cord. Nociceptors terminate in the spinal cord.
- Spinal cord to brainstem and thalamus. Release of substance P and other neurotransmitters continues the impulse across the synaptic cleft between the nociceptors and the dorsal horn neurons. From the dorsal horn of the spinal cord, neurons such as the spinothalamic tract ascend to the thalamus. Other tracts carry the message to different centers in the brain.
- Thalamus to cortex. Thalamus acts as a relay station sending the impulse to central structures for processing.

3 **Perception of pain:** Conscious experience of pain.

4 **Modulation:** Inhibition of nociceptive impulses. Neurons originating in the brain stem descend to the spinal cord and release substances such as endogenous opioids, serotonin (5HT), and norepinephrine (NE) that inhibit the transmission of nociceptive impulses.

Fig. 6-2 Outlines the four basic processes involved in nociception: *1,* transduction; *2,* transmission; *3,* perception; and *4,* modulation. *(From McCaffery and Pasero, 1999.)*

to the dorsal horn of the spinal cord. Located in the dorsal horn is the substantia gelatinosa, called the "gate," which controls the stimulation of sensory tracts within the spinal cord. According to the gate theory of pain, when the "gate" is opened, pain impulses enter the spinal cord and ascend in the spinothalamic tract to the thalamus, which is a relay station for most sensory serves. The "gate" is opened by stimulation from A-delta fibers and C fibers. The A-delta fibers are associated with sharp, pricking, acute, well-localized pain of short duration. The C fibers are associated with a dull, aching, throbbing, or burning sensation that has a diffuse nature, slow onset, and relatively long duration. The "gate" can be closed by impulses from A-alpha and A-beta fibers. Massage and vibration are mechanical stimuli that close the gate by stimulating these A-alpha and A-beta myelinated nerves. A pharmacologic intervention to close the gate is the administration of opioid analgesics that block opioid receptors and the release of neurotransmitters; especially substance P. Diffuse

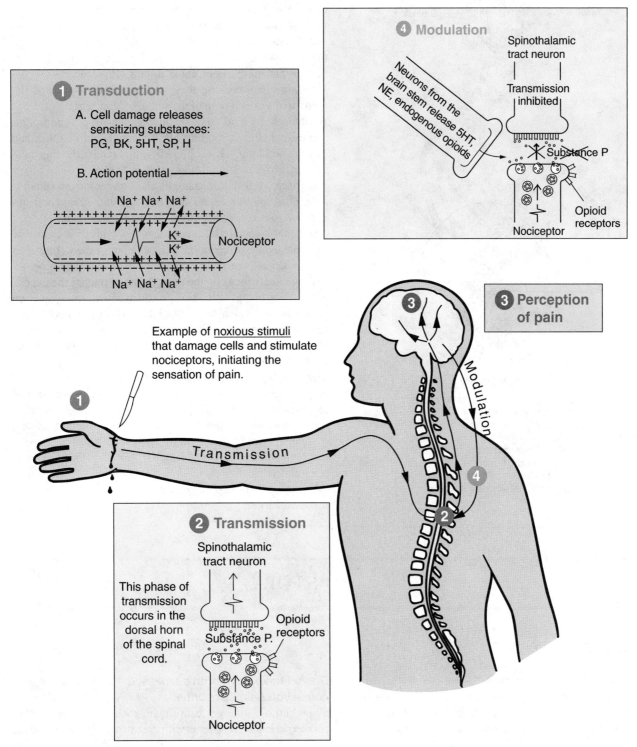

Fig. 6-2, cont'd

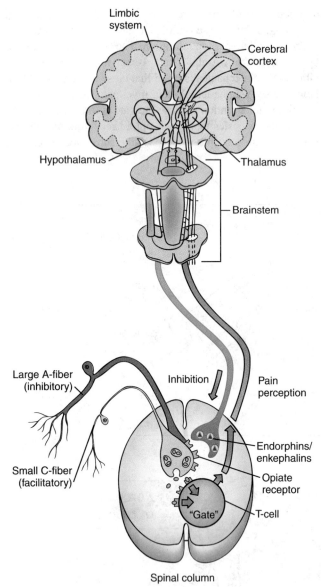

Limbic system

Cerebral cortex

Hypothalamus

Thalamus

Brainstem

Large A-fiber (inhibitory)

Inhibition

Pain perception

Small C-fiber (facilitatory)

Endorphins/ enkephalins

Opiate receptor

"Gate"

T-cell

Spinal column

Fig. 6-3 Illustrates the four steps involved in the pain process: transduction, when nociceptors stimulate the free nerve endings; transmission, when nociceptor stimulation initiates action potentials along A-delta or C fibers to open the gate in the substantia gelatinosa and ascend to the brain in the spinothalamic tract through the thalamus (or stimulate A-alpha or A-beta fibers that close the gate); perception, when impulses move from the thalamus to the parietal lobe, where pain is felt, and to the limbic system, which derives the emotional response to pain; and modulation, when the body produces endorphins and enkephalins to occupy the opiate receptor sites to close the gate.

pain that is transmitted by C fibers is highly sensitive to opioids (McCaffery and Pasero, 1999).

The third step in the journey is perception. The thalamus receives impulses from the spinothalamic tract and then sends these impulses to the parietal lobe of the cerebral cortex and to the limbic system. When impulses reach the parietal lobe, the client feels the pain. Although the journey of the pain stimulus takes a fraction of a second to reach the brain, people do not know they hurt until the parietal lobe is stimulated. Stimulation of the limbic system generates the emotional response to the pain, such as crying or anger.

The pain journey ends with *modulation,* defined as an alteration in the magnitude of electrical current; that is, the body produces substances to reduce pain perception. On the way to the thalamus, afferent nerve fibers travel through the brainstem, where they stimulate efferent (descending) nerves that inhibit nociceptor stimuli. These nerves are descending fibers because they start in the brainstem and descend to the dorsal horn of the spinal cord, where they release substances such as endogenous opioids (e.g., endorphins and enkephalin), serotonin (5HT), norepinephrine (NE), and gamma-aminobutyric acid (GABA) that inhibit the transmission of noxious stimuli and produce analgesia (McCaffery and Pasero, 1999). For example, endorphins and enkephalins act on the opioid receptor sites throughout the brain and spinal cord to decrease the afferent stimulation of pain.

Clients associate different meanings with their pain. For example, some perceive the pain as a punishment, threat, or loss, whereas others view pain as a challenge. The more attention clients focus on the pain, the more intense the experience. Thus using distraction to divert attention away from pain may be a valuable pain-relief intervention. Anxiety and fatigue are known to increase the pain perception. When clients are anxious about their disease process, they may report more intense pain than they report after they know the diagnosis and treatment plan. Previous experience with pain may influence the response. If clients have had a similar type of pain experience in the past, they are more likely to know how to relieve the pain, they are less anxious, and they feel more in control of their pain. In contrast, clients may experience more intense pain if they have not previously experienced intense pain and have no past coping skills to use or if they have a pain experience that is different from the ones they had earlier.

HEALTH HISTORY

HEALTH HISTORY

Because pain is a complex, multidimensional, subjective experience, the history contains questions about the clients' descriptions of the pain in a symptom analysis, but also about how they react emotionally to the pain and how it affects their lives.

Present Health Status

Do you have any chronic illnesses? If so, do they cause you pain? Describe.

Some chronic illnesses cause pain, such as the neuropathic pain experienced by clients with diabetes mellitus. The client may have chronic pain, as well as acute pain from a current disorder.

Do you take any medications? If so, what do you take and how often? How well do they relieve your pain? Are you allergic to any medications? If yes, what kind of allergic reaction do you have from these medications?

Both prescription and over-the-counter medications should be noted. Ineffective medications should be reevaluated by the health care provider. Allergies are always noted so that the client will not be given a medication that would cause an allergic reaction. Clients are asked to describe the reaction because sometimes what the client reports as allergic is actually a side effect.

DESCRIPTION OF PAIN

Location

Where is your pain? Can you point to the location(s)?

Location may provide information about the cause of pain and its type (e.g., somatic versus visceral) (see Fig. 6-1). Referred pain, however, may cause the client to describe pain location away for the site of pathology.

Quality

Can you describe what the pain feels like?

Fig. 6-4 is the McGill Pain Questionnaire, which helps clients describe their pain. Somatic pain is usually aching or throbbing in quality. Visceral pain is aching and well localized if from tumor or the pain may be described as intermittent, cramping, and poorly localized if from obstruction.

Quantity

How would you describe the intensity, strength, or severity of the pain on a scale of 0 to 10, with 0 being no pain and 10 being the most intense pain possible?

Figs. 6-5 *A*, *B*, and *C* and 6-6 provide scales and instruments to measure perception of pain intensity and quality.

This provides further description of how "bad" the pain feels to the client. The client's rating is subjective because pain is a personal experience, but scales allow the client to communicate how severe the pain feels (pain quantity) and can be used as a subjective measure of pain relief after interventions are implemented.

At what point on this scale of 0 to 10 do you usually take medication for your pain?

This question seeks knowledge about the client's pain tolerance, which is influenced by one's culture, pain experience, expectations of pain, and its ability to be relieved.

Chronology

When does the pain occur? During activity? Before or after eating?

The answer helps determine the source of the pain. Physical activity may aggravate pain. Eating may increase peptic ulcer pain.

Does the pain occur suddenly or gradually?

Acute pain has a sudden onset. Ischemic pain gradually increases in intensity.

Setting

Where are you when the pain occurs? Does the pain change if you change locations? Are there any factors in the environment that contribute to the pain?

These questions are trying to determine if environment contributes to pain, such as chemicals or gases in the air or a hot, dry environment versus a cold and damp one.

Associated Manifestations

What other symptoms do you have during the pain, such as nausea, vomiting, palpitations, shortness of breath, or sweating?

Acute pain stimulates the sympathetic nervous system, which can cause physiologic symptoms that may accompany the pain.

Alleviating Factors

How have you tried to relieve the pain (e.g., medication, certain position, distraction, rest, restricted activity, deep breathing)? How effective have these measures been at relieving your pain?

The answer may help determine the cause and the treatment.

Aggravating Factors

What makes the pain worse?

The answer may help determine the cause of the pain or help understand the impact pain may have on the client.

RESPONSE TO PAIN

How do you react to your pain? How do you express your pain (e.g., anger, frustration, crying, or no expression at all)?

Pain can affect people physically, psychologically, socially, and spiritually. Clients' responses to pain may be influenced by culture and previous experience with pain. Clients may feel anger, fear, depression, or anxiety. The nurse acknowledges these feelings as the client's personal response to pain without trying to change the client's feelings about the pain experienced.

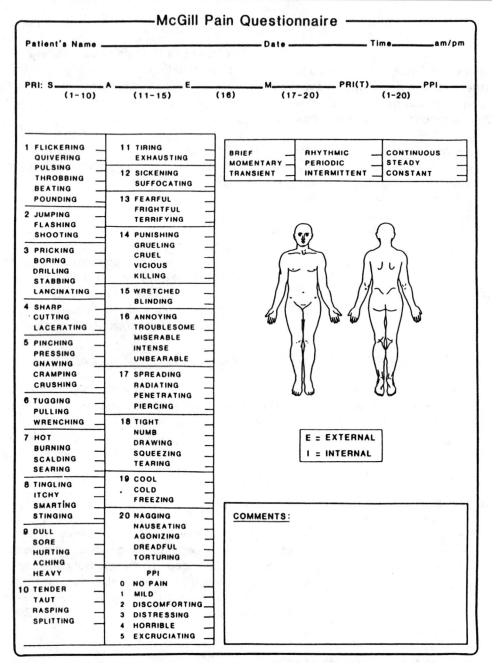

McGill Pain Questionnaire

Patient's Name _____ Date _____ Time_____am/pm

PRI: S_____ A_____ E_____ M_____ PRI(T)_____ PPI_____
      (1–10)   (11–15)   (16)   (17–20)   (1–20)

1 FLICKERING QUIVERING PULSING THROBBING BEATING POUNDING	11 TIRING EXHAUSTING
2 JUMPING FLASHING SHOOTING	12 SICKENING SUFFOCATING
3 PRICKING BORING DRILLING STABBING LANCINATING	13 FEARFUL FRIGHTFUL TERRIFYING
4 SHARP CUTTING LACERATING	14 PUNISHING GRUELING CRUEL VICIOUS KILLING
5 PINCHING PRESSING GNAWING CRAMPING CRUSHING	15 WRETCHED BLINDING
6 TUGGING PULLING WRENCHING	16 ANNOYING TROUBLESOME MISERABLE INTENSE UNBEARABLE
7 HOT BURNING SCALDING SEARING	17 SPREADING RADIATING PENETRATING PIERCING
8 TINGLING ITCHY SMARTING STINGING	18 TIGHT NUMB DRAWING SQUEEZING TEARING
9 DULL SORE HURTING ACHING HEAVY	19 COOL COLD FREEZING
10 TENDER TAUT RASPING SPLITTING	20 NAGGING NAUSEATING AGONIZING DREADFUL TORTURING

BRIEF MOMENTARY TRANSIENT — RHYTHMIC PERIODIC INTERMITTENT — CONTINUOUS STEADY CONSTANT

E = EXTERNAL
I = INTERNAL

PPI
0 NO PAIN
1 MILD
2 DISCOMFORTING
3 DISTRESSING
4 HORRIBLE
5 EXCRUCIATING

COMMENTS:

Fig. 6-4   McGill Pain Questionnaire. The descriptors fall into four major groups: sensory, 1 to 10; affective, 11 to 15; evaluative, 16; and miscellaneous, 17 to 20. The rank value of each descriptor is based on its position in the word set. The sum of the rank values is the pain rating index (PRI). The present pain intensity (PPI) is based on a scale of 0 to 5. *(From Melzack and Katz, 1994.)*

Does this pain have any particular meaning for you? If so, what is it?

The meaning of pain is unique for each person. For some people the meaning is that they should not have behaved in the way that hurt them (e.g., "I should not have tried to steal home base"). To others the meaning of pain is spiritual or psychologic. For example they may believe that they are being punished or that they have had impure thoughts. Know-

ing the meaning of the pain helps the nurse understand the client's subjective experience of pain.

What has been your past experience with pain and pain relief? What are your expectations for pain relief?

These questions address the cognitive response to pain. Clients use their past experiences to respond to pain. When

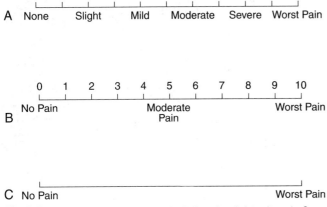

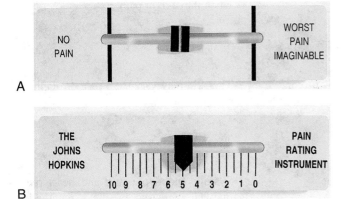

Fig. 6-5 **A,** Descriptive pain intensity scale; **B,** Numeric pain intensity scale; **C,** Visual analog scale. *(From Seidel et al, 2006.)*

Fig. 6-6 Self-contained, portable, pain-rating instrument that can provide immediate assessment of pain. It is a 5 × 20 cm plastic visual analog scale with a sliding marker that moves within a 10 cm groove. The side facing the client **(A)** resembles a traditional analog scale, whereas the opposite side **(B)** is marked in centimeters to quantify pain intensity. The tool has been shown to be valid to measure pain intensity. *(From Grossman SA et al: A comparison of the Hopkins pain rating scales in patients with standard visual analogue and verbal descriptor scales in patients with cancer pain, J Pain Symptom Manage 7:196-203, 1992. Copyright 1992 Elsevier Science. Reprinted from Journal of Pain and Symptom Management with permission from Elsevier Science.)*

nurses know what those past experiences are, they can be more therapeutic in assisting clients relieve their pain.

Do you have any concerns about taking medications for pain relief?
Some clients will not ask for pain relief medication because they fear it will cause an addiction. This misconception can be remedied by appropriate client education.

For clients with chronic pain: How has the pain affected your quality of life? How has your life been altered by the pain?
Those with chronic pain who have compensated for or adjusted to its persistence may perceive a higher quality of life than those who have not adjusted to the pain. However, chronic pain is often associated with a sense of hopelessness and helplessness. Clients with chronic pain may report depression, difficulty sleeping and eating, and preoccupation with the pain (Huether & McCance, 2004).

FREQUENTLY ASKED QUESTIONS

Today the nurse cared for a client who had her gallbladder out yesterday. She has a history of drug abuse. The nurse said the client was drug seeking and just wanted narcotic analgesics to "feed her habit." How can the nurse tell if the client is really in pain or abusing drugs?

Any client who had abdominal surgery yesterday will probably need narcotic analgesic pain relief. Remember that one of the definitions of pain is that pain is anything the client says it is. If the client says she is in pain and has a PRN order for narcotic analgesics that can be given now, the narcotic analgesic should be given now. Nurses cannot judge the presence, location, or intensity of pain of clients. For clients with a history of drug abuse, the postoperative period is not the time to be concerned with drug rehabilitation.

EXAMINATION

PROCEDURE AND TECHNIQUES WITH NORMAL FINDINGS

OBSERVE client for posture and behavior to relieve pain.

Posture should be erect, and no movement to relieve pain should be evident.

ABNORMAL FINDINGS

Guarding of a painful body part, rubbing or pressing the painful area, distorted posture, or fixed or continuous movement may indicate acute pain. Clients may lie very still to avoid movement or may be restless. Head rocking, pacing, or inability to keep hands still may be other signs of acute pain.

PROCEDURE AND TECHNIQUES WITH NORMAL FINDINGS	ABNORMAL FINDINGS

OBSERVE facial expressions.

The face should be relaxed with a neutral or pleasant expression.

Acute pain may be manifested by wrinkled forehead, tightly closed eyes, lackluster eyes, grimace, clenched teeth, or lip biting.

LISTEN for sounds the client makes.

Sounds other than those of conversation are not expected.

Moaning, grunting, screaming, crying, or gasping may indicate acute pain, but some clients make no verbal sounds when they are in pain.

☞ INSPECT AND PALPATE skin for color, temperature, and moisture.

Skin should be expected color for race, warm, and dry with elastic turgor.

The skin may vary from pale or diaphoretic to warm and dry.

☞ MEASURE blood pressure and pulse.

Blood pressure and pulse should be within expected limits for age.

Systolic blood pressure and heart rate may be increased by the sympathetic stimulation during acute pain.

☞ ASSESS respiratory rate and pattern.

Respirations should be within expected limits for age.

Respiratory rate and pattern may vary from slow and deep to rapid and shallow depending on which provides more comfort to the client. Some clients may use slow, deep breathing to relax as a pain-relieving strategy.

☞ OBSERVE pupillary size.

Pupils should be 3 to 5 mm in diameter and equal.

Pupils may be dilated or constricted from the effects of the autonomic nervous system or analgesia given to relieve pain.

☞ = core examination skill

AGE-RELATED VARIATIONS

Infants & Children

Nurses find different responses to pain depending on the age of the client. Neonates respond to pain in a global response as evidenced by increased heart rate, hypertension, decreased oxygenation saturation, pallor and sweating (Hockenberry et al, 2003). Young children have difficulty understanding pain and the procedures that cause pain; however, they have developed a basic ability to describe pain and its location. School-age children are better able to understand pain and to describe pain location. Chapter 20 presents further information regarding the pain assessment for this age group.

Older Adults

Although transmission and perception of pain may be slowed in the older person, the pain felt is no different from that of any other adult. Many older adults have a lifetime of experience in coping with pain, but pain is not an expected part of aging. Chapter 22 presents further information regarding the pain assessment from this age group.

CLINICAL APPLICATION & CLINICAL REASONING

See Appendix E for answers to exercises in this section.

REVIEW QUESTIONS

1 Before any medication, the body attempts to relieve pain by inhibiting the transmission of nociceptor stimuli by releasing:
   1 Endorphins to occupy the opiate receptor sites.
   2 Prostaglandins to open the gate in the spinal cord.
   3 Bradykinin to close the gate in the spinal cord.
   4 Histamine to stimulate C fibers at peripheral sites.
2 A client who has had a knee replaced because of arthritis reports that he has not slept well in several nights. He states that he cannot get comfortable. Today he is asking for pain medication more often. The nurse understands that a possible reason for this increase in pain is that:
   1 Arthritis pain is variable; it can be mild one day and severe the next.
   2 Pain tolerance decreases with sleep deprivation.
   3 The anesthesia from surgery is wearing off.
   4 The client is using the pain medication to help him sleep during the day.
3 When a client complains of chest pain, what question is pertinent to ask to gain additional information?
   1 "What were you doing when the pain first occurred?"
   2 "What does the pain feel like?"
   3 "Do you have shortness of breath with the chest pain?"
   4 "Has anyone in your family ever had similar pain?"
4 When a client complains of leg pain, what question is pertinent to ask to gain additional information?
   1 "What were you doing when the pain first occurred?"
   2 "How do you feel about having this pain?"
   3 "Do you think the pain is caused by a cramp?"
   4 "Has anyone in your family ever had similar pain?"
5 When caring for a client with pain that has lasted 7 days, what would the nurse expect to find during pain assessment?
   1 Signs of irritability, depression, or insomnia.
   2 Signs of decreased blood pressure, nausea, and vomiting.
   3 Signs of increased heart rate and respiratory rate with diaphoresis.
   4 Signs of fever, muscle weakness, and fatigue.

SAMPLE DOCUMENTATION

Review the data obtained during an interview and examination by the nurse below.

Ms. L. C. is a 50-year-old black woman who has breast cancer with metastasis to the bone and lung. She had a mastectomy 7 months ago and has had radiation therapy. Her vital signs are as follows: temperature 98.0° F (36.7° C), blood pressure 120/80, heart rate 80 beats per minute, and respirations 20 breaths per minute. She rates her pain as 8 on a scale of 0 to 10 before taking pain medication and 3 out of 10 after taking pain medication. She weighs 100 lb (45.5 kg) and says she is 5 feet 6 inches tall (102 cm). She says that she has been having difficulty sleeping and has felt sad because of all that has happened to her. She has stopped playing bridge with her friends twice a week and has stopped going to church because she "just does not feel like going anywhere." She has a well-healed incision on her left breast, where the mastectomy was performed. On auscultation, rhonchi were heard on both of her lungs. Both S_1 and S_2 heart sounds are heard without murmur. She quit smoking last year. She drinks a glass of red wine each evening before dinner. She has full range of motion in each of her shoulders. She has hypertension. She has had tonsillectomy, cholecystectomy, and appendectomy. She is allergic to lisinopril. Currently she is taking aspirin, sertraline (Zoloft), hydrochlorothiazine (Diuril), atenolol (Tenormin), and oxycontin.

Below, note how the nurse recorded these same data in a documentation format and identified appropriate nursing diagnoses from the data.

50-yr-old BF. CC: having difficulty sleeping and has felt sad by all that has happened to her. Medical Hx: breast CA c̄ metastasis to lungs and bone; HTN Surg; Hx. Mastectomy 7 mo ago followed by radiation therapy; tonsillectomy, cholecystectomy, appendectomy. Allergy: lisinopril. Meds: ASA, sertraline (Zoloft), hydrochlorothiazine (Diuril), atenolol (Tenormin), and oxycontin.

SUBJECTIVE DATA

She rates her pain as 8/10 p̄ taking pain med and 3/10 taking pain med. Stopped playing bridge and going to church—"just does not feel like going anywhere." She does enjoy visiting with her grandchildren each week. Quit smoking last year, drinks a glass of wine daily.

OBJECTIVE DATA

General survey: VS: T 98.0° F (36.7° C), BP 120/80, HR 80 bpm, RR 20 per min. Measured wt 100 lb (45.5 kg), stated ht. 5 ft. 6 in. (102 cm).
Skin: Well-healed incision Ⓛ breast.
Lungs: Rhonchi bil.
Heart: S_1 and S_2 present murmur
Musculoskeletal: Full ROM Ⓛ and Ⓡ shoulder.

CASE STUDY

Mr. M. is a 46-year-old man who comes to the emergency department with a chief complaint of severe right abdominal and flank pain.

Interview Data

Mr. M. tells the nurse, "The pain came on rather suddenly about an hour ago; I was doing some work at my desk, and it suddenly started." He points to the right flank areas as the location of the pain, but it extends into the right lower abdominal area as well. Mr. M. describes the pain as "severe," sharp pain. On a scale of 0 to 10, Mr. M. states, "This is off your pain scale—at least a 12." The pain is described as constant, with intensity being intermittent as it may lighten slightly and intensify again. The other symptom Mr. M. describes is nausea.

Examination Data

- *General survey:* Temperature, 101.8° F (38.8° C); pulse rate, 108 beats/min; blood pressure, 128/96 mm Hg; respirations, 24 breaths per minute. Client is curled up on a stretcher in the fetal position; appears uncomfortable, groaning.
- *Skin:* Skin is pale, diaphoretic, and warm to touch.
- *Abdomen:* Flat, no scars observed; bowel sounds are active in all four quadrants; soft, nontender to palpation.

Clinical Reasoning

1. What data deviate from normal findings, suggesting a need for further investigation?
2. What additional information should the nurse ask or assess for?
3. Based on these data, what recommendations for health promotion would you make for this client?
4. What nursing diagnoses and collaborative problems should be considered for this situation?

🔵 INTERACTIVE ACTIVITIES

Open the interactive student CD-ROM, click on Chapter 6, and choose from the following activities on the menu bar:

- **Multiple Choice Challenge.** Click on the best answer for each question. You will be given immediate feedback, rationale for incorrect answers, and a total score. Good luck!

- **Marvelous Matches.** First, drag each phrase and place it under the appropriate age-group on the screen. Test your ability to match the perception of pain with each age-group. Second, drag each phrase and place it below the appropriate item on the screen. Test your ability to match the process of pain journey with the description of what occurs during that part of the process.

- **Printable Lab Guide.** Locate the Lab Guide for Chapter 6, and print and use it (as many times as needed) to help you apply your assessment skills. These guides may also be filled in electronically and then saved and e-mailed to your instructor!

- **Quick Challenge.** Use this critical thinking exercise to assess your skills through case study-style questions, then compare with expert answers!

CHAPTER 7

Mental Health and Mental Status Assessment

A comprehensive assessment of an individual includes mental and emotional health as well as physical health. *Mental health* is defined as a relative state of mind in which a person who is healthy is able to cope with and adjust to daily stresses in an acceptable way. It is an elusive concept because data are based on a description of an individual's behavior by the health professional performing the assessment. Furthermore, the issue of persistence of behavior must be considered. How long must a person engage in a particular behavior or mood before health professionals determine that the person has a mental illness? These issues make quantifying mental health assessment a challenge. Changes in clients' lives may affect their mental health, requiring periodic mental health and mental status assessment. *Mental status* is defined as the degree of competence that a person shows in intellectual, emotional, psychologic, and personality functioning. The purpose of this chapter is to describe procedures and techniques to assess for mental health and identify the abnormal findings

that may indicate the need for a referral to a mental health professional. Factors influencing mental health and mental illness include self-concept, interpersonal relationships, stress management abilities, spiritual and belief systems, genetic factors, and physiologic functioning of the limbic system and neurotransmitters.

Researchers have found that it is the *perception* of a recent life event that determines a person's emotional or psychologic reaction to it. Each culture influences how a stressful event is perceived and the acceptable ways that people of that culture are expected to respond. Some cultures allow a verbal or physical response, whereas others refrain from any outward reaction at all. The Western European and North American cultures believe that stress from an emotional state can lead to somatic illness. Because some cultures do not believe that stress contributes to disease, their members would not understand the need for stress management (Varcarolis, 2002).

ANATOMY & PHYSIOLOGY

The limbic system is called the *emotional brain* because it regulates memory and basic emotions such as fear, anger, and sex drive. The structures of the limbic system surround the corpus callosum and include the limbic lobe, cingulate gyrus, hippocampus, amygdala, thalamus, and portions of the hypothalamus (Fig. 7-1). The structures of the limbic system are

linked to the lobes of the cerebral cortex. These links provide communication between the limbic system and cerebral cortex. For example, when a person sees something that jogs the memory about a happy event, there is communication among the occipital lobe for vision, prefrontal lobe for memory, and limbic system for the happy emotion and the memory.

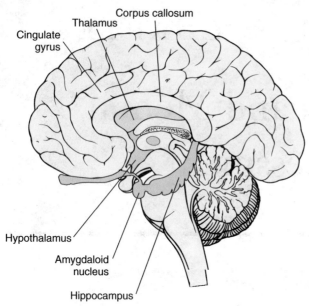

Fig. 7-1 The limbic system. *(From McKenry and Salerno, 2003)*

Several neurotransmitters are associated with mental health. Neurotransmitters are substances that carry messages from neuron to neuron or from neuron to muscle cell. They are synthesized in neurons, released in the synaptic cleft, and bind to receptor sites on other neurons or effector cells. Three neurotransmitters facilitate or initiate activity: norepinephrine, serotonin, and dopamine. Norepinephrine is thought to help regulate mood and maintain arousal. Cocaine and amphetamines increase release and block the reuptake of norepinephrine, causing overstimulation of the postsynaptic neurons. Serotonin pathways are similar to norepinephrine and have similar effects. Levels of serotonin are elevated in schizophrenia, contributing to delusions, hallucinations, and withdrawal. Dopamine acts in the midbrain on emotions and memory and in the hypothalamus and pituitary gland, affecting emotional responses and stress reactions. Gamma-aminobutyric acid (GABA) is an inhibitory neurotransmitter that suppresses activity; insufficient GABA may contribute to anxiety.

ETHNIC & CULTURAL VARIATIONS

Culturally Relevant Phenomena in Mental Health Nursing

Mental health is the degree to which a person is able to fulfill the cultural expectations of his or her society. Thus mental health and deviance from mental health are derived from cultural expectations (Arnault, 2002).

Phenomena include the following:

- *Perception of reality*—may be culturally prescribed, spiritually induced in a traditional healing system, or otherwise sanctioned by the cultural group. For example, a Native American client may appear to a white American to have lost touch with reality, but the Native American is practicing his or her spiritual healing ritual, which is important to attain or maintain health.

- *Needs, feelings, thoughts of others and self*—clients need to attend to their needs, feelings, and thoughts of self and others, whether they are internal or external. Events considered as stressors vary from one culture to another. For example, Kenyans are taught not to discuss or show their feelings of sadness or pain. If a Kenyan was seen by an American health care provider for a suspected mental health disorder, he or she would not willingly share feelings, which is a large part of the health history for mental health nursing. This client may be seen as uncooperative, when in fact he or she is complying with the Kenyan culture.

- *Decision making*—the ability to make decisions may be culturally prescribed so that families and cultures designate decision makers, which may include health care decisions. Inability to make decisions is a clinical manifestation of depression and anxiety. For example, in traditional Vietnamese families, the oldest male makes decisions about health care. As a result, a female client may delay seeking health care until she consults with the oldest male in the family.

Data from Arnault DS: Framework for culturally relevant psychiatric nursing. In Varcarolis EM: *Foundations of psychiatric mental health nursing,* ed 4, Philadelphia, 2002, WB Saunders.

HEALTH HISTORY

RISK FACTORS   *Depression and Anxiety*

As you conduct a health history related to mental health, it is important to consider common risk factors associated with depression and anxiety and follow up with additional questions should these risks exist.

Risk Factors for Depression
- *Gender:* Women are at risk for depression 2:1 over men.
- *Age:* Adolescents are at risk for depression and anxiety because of peer pressure and desire to fit in and to be independent of parents. In adults the onset is typically between 24 and 44 years of age.
- *Genetics:* Children of parents who have depression are likely to develop the disorder. A person has a 27% chance of inheriting a mood disorder from one parent, and this doubles if both parents are affected.
- *Psychosocial environment:* People who have a history of trauma, sexual abuse, physical abuse, physical disability, alcoholism, or loss of a spouse are at increased risk of developing depression.
- *Personal characteristics:* Low self-esteem, distorted perception of others' views, inability to acknowledge personal accomplishment, pessimistic outlook. (M)

Risk Factors for Anxiety
- *Genetics:* There is a 20% risk for general anxiety disorder in blood relatives of people with the disorder and a 10% risk among relatives with depression.
- *Physical health:* Sleep deprivation. (M)
- *Psychosocial environment:* Financial concerns, health, relationships, school or work problems. (M)

Data from *www.mentalhealthchannel.net,* 2002, 2003.
M = modifiable risk factor.

GENERAL HEALTH HISTORY

Because most of the data needed for a mental health assessment are collected by talking with the client, the nurse collects data about mental status during the history. This is a deviation from assessments of specific body systems, when data collection for the history is performed prior to the examination. During a mental health history, the nurse determines how the client's appearance, behavior, and cognitive function compare with the characteristics of a healthy personality. Data collection begins when the nurse first sees the client. Is the client dressed appropriately for the weather? Does his or her mood seem appropriate? Is the affect (emotional state) appropriate? What is the client's body posture? Is the client slumped over and looking at the ground with a sad facial expression, or walking tall with a brisk step and a smiling face? What is the client's tone of voice? Does he or she talk in a monotone or a happy, expressive tone? Does the client's conversation flow in a logical sequence? Table 7-1 lists conversational styles consistent with alterations in thought processes.

Present Health Status

How have you been feeling about yourself? Do you consider your present feelings to be a problem in your daily life? If so, do you feel the problem is temporary or curable?

This invites the client to discuss feelings and may help to begin to identify problems (e.g., depression, stress, anger).

Are you having any medical problems?

Some medical problems may cause changes in mood or behavior (e.g., endocrine disorders such as hypothyroidism or adrenal insufficiency).

What medications are you taking?

Side effects of some medications may cause changes in mood and behavior. Also the nurse needs to know if the client is taking medications for mental health disorders.

Self-Concept

How would you describe yourself to others? What are your best characteristics? What do you like about yourself?

This determines how clients perceive themselves. Those with positive self-esteem regard themselves favorably and can name their positive attributes. Those with negative self-esteem tend to list primarily negative attributes and may be at risk for depression.

TABLE 7-1 *Problems of Word Usage Associated with Alterations in Thought Processes*

DEFINITION	EXAMPLE
Blocking occurs with thought disorganization when clients have difficulty articulating a response or stop in midsentence as if they were stuck.	"I work as a computer programmer for . . . I can't think of my company's name."
Confabulation is a fabrication of experiences or situations, explained in detailed and plausible ways to cover up gaps in memory. Often used as a defense mechanism by persons with head injuries, dementia, lead poisoning, or alcoholism.	The nurse asks, "What brought you to the clinic today?" The client responds, "I turned my ankle. I was running a new pass pattern with John. He was right on target, a 30-yard pass, but another player got in my way, and I fell."
Neologism is a word or term used with a new meaning known only to the client, who is often delusional, psychotic, or delirious.	"I turned the corner and there was a huge *combaster* headed right for me. Well, you can imagine how I felt."
Circumstantiality is a speech pattern in which a client has difficulty separating relevant from irrelevant information. While describing an event, the client uses so much detail that the original thought becomes lost. Circumstantiality may be a sign of chronic brain syndrome.	The nurse says, "How did you feel when you won the award?" The client responds, "Well, I jumped out of my chair, I wore the black backless gown, but I seriously considered wearing the red sequin gown, with diamond stud earrings and necklace, but the shoes were uncomfortable, you know, with 3-inch heels, I would just fall over getting up to get my award, but then I could have borrowed shoes from Lisa, her apartment is so well decorated with the country look . . . ."
Loosening (loose association) is a disturbance in thinking in which the association of ideas and thought patterns becomes so vague, diffuse, and unfocused as to lack any logical sequence or relationship to any preceding topics of conversation.	"I have three sisters . . . living in the north is so cold . . . but typing is what I do best . . . so when I started the car I heard a funny noise . . . you know."
Flight of ideas is a continuous talking in which the client switches rapidly from one topic to another with each topic being incoherent or unrelated to the previous one or stimulated by some environmental stimuli. Flight of ideas is a frequent symptom of manic states and schizophrenia.	"Hi, I came in today . . . that coffee smells great, but the caffeine . . . chocolate has caffeine, but so much fat . . . need to walk 3 miles every day to keep the weight off . . . I bought a new swim suit, it's a two-piece."
Word salad is a jumble of words and phrases that lacks logical coherence and meaning. Word salad occurs when clients are disoriented or have schizophrenia.	"Dog bark . . . sunshine today . . . fill . . . form . . . reclining chair . . . grass . . . hamburger . . . flowers . . . vacation . . . steamship."
Perseveration is the involuntary and pathologic persistent repetition of words, ideas, and phrases regardless of the stimulus or its duration. This is consistent with clients who have brain damage or organic mental disorders, although it may appear in schizophrenia.	Nurse: "Ready to see your family?" *Client:* "Ready set go." *Nurse:* "They are in the snack bar." *Client:* "Ready set go."
Echolalia is the automatic and meaningless repetition of another's words or phrases, seen in clients with schizophrenia.	Nurse: "Ready to see your family?" *Client:* "See your family, see your family, see your family."
Clanging (clang association) is the mental connection between dissociated ideas made because of similarity in the sounds of the words used to describe ideas. This occurs frequently in the manic phases of bipolar disorder.	"I went to bed . . . head on straight . . . wait . . . full . . . pull the cart . . . heart to heart . . . part . . . should . . . should you . . . no you better not . . . heart . . . cart . . . part my hair . . . hair there."

Data from Varcarolis EM: *Foundations of psychiatric mental health nursing*, ed 4, Philadelphia, 2002, WB Saunders.

Interpersonal Relationships

How satisfied are you with your interpersonal relationships? Are there people to whom you can talk about feelings and problems?

Achievement of satisfying interpersonal relationships is needed for mental health. Clients who have few to no interpersonal relationships may be depressed or out of touch with reality. Social support is important for interpersonal relationships.

Stressors

Have there been any recent changes in your life? How have these changes affected your stress level? What are the major stressors in your life now? How do you deal with stress? Are those methods of stress relief currently effective for you?

Inquire about stressors such as money, intimate relationships, death or illness of a family member or friend, and employment problems. One way to inquire further about stress is to

TABLE 7-2 Holmes Social Readjustment Rating Scale

EVENT	EVENT VALUE	EVENT	EVENT VALUE
1. Death of a spouse	100	22. Change in responsibilities at work	29
2. Divorce	73	23. Son or daughter leaving home	29
3. Marital separation	65	24. Trouble with in-laws	29
4. Jail term	63	25. Outstanding personal achievement	28
5. Death of a close family member	63	26. Spouse begins or stops work	26
6. Personal injury or illness	53	27. Begin or end school	26
7. Marriage	50	28. Change in living conditions	25
8. Fired at work	47	29. Revision of personal habits	24
9. Marital reconciliation	45	30. Trouble with boss	23
10. Retirement	45	31. Change in work hours or conditions	20
11. Change in health of family member	44	32. Change in residence	20
12. Pregnancy	40	33. Change in schools	20
13. Sex difficulties	39	34. Change in recreation	19
14. Gain of a new family member	39	35. Change in church activities	19
15. Business readjustment	39	36. Change in social activities	19
16. Change in financial state	38	37. Change in sleeping habits	16
17. Death of a close friend	37	38. Change in number of family get-togethers	15
18. Change to different line of work	36	39. Vacation	13
19. Change in number of arguments	35	40. Christmas	12
20. Mortgage or loan over $10,000	31	41. Minor violations of the law	11
21. Foreclosure of mortgage or loan	30	Total Points	

Directions for completion: Add up the point values for each of the events that you have experienced during the past 12 months.

Scoring

Below 150 points:
The amount of stress you are experiencing as a result of changes in your life is normal and manageable. There is only a 1 in 3 chance that you might develop a serious illness over the next 2 years based on stress alone. Consider practicing a daily relaxation technique to reduce your chance of illness even more.

150 to 300 points:
The amount of stress you are experiencing as a result of changes in your life is moderate. Based on stress alone, you have a 50/50 chance of developing a serious illness over the next 2 years. You can reduce these odds by practicing stress management and relaxation techniques on a daily basis.

Over 300 points:
The amount of stress you are experiencing as a result of changes in your life is high. Based on stress alone, your chances of developing a serious illness during the next 2 years approaches 90%, unless you are already practicing good coping skills and regular relaxation techniques. You can reduce the chance of illness by practicing coping strategies and relaxation techniques daily.

Reprinted from *Journal of Psychosomatic Research,* volume 11, Holmes T, Rahe RJ: Social readjustment rating scale, pp. 213-218, copyright 1967 with permission from Elsevier Science.

administer the Holmes Social Readjustment Rating Scale (Table 7-2). Coping with the stress of daily life is essential to maintain mental health. Answers to these questions help identify the client's stressors and how well they are being managed.

Anger

Have you been feeling angry? Do you feel angry now? How do you react when you are angry? Verbally, physically, or do you keep your anger inside? Can you talk about what has caused this anger?
Knowing how clients react to anger can help them find acceptable ways to express their feelings (e.g., hit a pillow instead of a person, verbally express anger in an empty room or elevator). Talking about the cause of the anger can be therapeutic and provides an opportunity for the nurse to make referrals for help.

Alcohol Use

How often do you drink alcohol, including beer, wine, or liquor?
Every adult and adolescent should be asked about alcohol consumption to determine if it is a health problem.

Recreational Drug Use

Do you ever use recreational drugs? If yes, tell me about your drug use.
Every adult and adolescent should be asked about recreational drug use to determine if it is a health problem.

Past Medical History

In the past, have you experienced any behaviors that could indicate a mental health problem? If yes, describe your experience. How have you coped in the

past with this disorder? Are those coping strategies still working for you?

Identifying the client's previous problems with mental health provides a baseline for interviewing, knowing that the client has had experience with mental health disorders. If previous coping strategies are working, they should be used again. If they have not been successful, other strategies may be suggested.

Family History

Do you have any blood relatives who have behaviors that could indicate a mental health problem? If so, can you describe the behavior they experience?

Some mental illnesses such as anxiety, depression, and schizophrenia have genetic links. Having a family member with a mental illness may be associated with the client's behavior.

PROBLEM-BASED HISTORY

Commonly reported problems related to mental health and mental status include depression, anxiety, alcohol abuse, drug abuse, and altered mental status. Although a symptom analysis is used when assessing physical manifestations, it is not as useful when asking questions about the client's behavior and feelings. When interviewing a client with mental health concerns, ask these questions over time so that the client does not become overwhelmed.

Depression

Risk factors for depression are listed in the box on p. 67.

During the past month, have you often been bothered by feeling down, depressed or hopeless? During the past month, have you often been bothered by having little interest or pleasure in doing things?

These two questions are used to screen for major depression. An affirmative answer to either question warrants a follow-up clinical interview (Bernstein, 2006).

Are you able to fall asleep and stay asleep without difficulty? Have you noticed any marked changes in your eating habits? Have you recently gained or lost weight without trying to? Have you noticed a lack of energy? Do you have crying spells? Do you have difficulty concentrating or making decisions? Describe your mood. Have you noticed an increase in irritability? How often have you experienced these feelings, how long did the feelings last, and how many of them occurred together in a two-week period?

These questions help identify possible symptoms of depression. Some clients can recognize symptoms but do not realize that the group of symptoms may indicate depression. Experiencing five or more of these symptoms in a two-week

period may indicate a need for a referral to a mental health professional (American Psychiatric Association, 2000).

Do you have friends whom you can trust and who are available when you need them?

Friends may be a source of social support to listen to the client's feelings and demonstrate their caring for the client.

Have you had feelings like this before? What did you do about depressive feelings at that time?

Depression can be assessed by administering the Beck Depression Inventory (Fig. 7-2). Depression may be a recurring disorder. Treatment that was successful in the past may be useful again.

Have there been times when you wanted to escape? Have you ever thought about escaping by hurting yourself or ending your life? If yes, do you feel like hurting yourself now? Do you have a plan for hurting yourself? If yes, what will you do to end your life? Where will this occur? Have you told anyone else about your plan? What would happen if you were dead?

These questions screen for suicidal thoughts. A client who has a specific plan for suicide is at higher risk than one who has no plan. Steps must be taken to protect the person who has a plan to hurt himself or herself.

What has kept you from hurting yourself in the past?

Ambivalence often keeps clients from ending their lives.

FREQUENTLY ASKED QUESTIONS

When clients say that they want to end their life, the nurse is supposed to ask if they have thought about hurting themselves or if they have a plan for hurting themselves. Doesn't that suggest to them that they should hurt themselves? Aren't you putting ideas in their heads?

Asking clients about a plan to hurt themselves may seem like a suggestion, but it is not. The purpose for asking the question is to determine if they are depressed enough or serious enough to make a plan to end their life. If the nurse learns that clients have a plan, they need immediate referral to a mental health professional.

Anxiety

Risk factors for anxiety are listed in the box on p. 67.

Have you had difficulty concentrating or making decisions? Have you been preoccupied or forgetful? Are you able to fall asleep and stay asleep without difficulty? Have you noticed a change in the amount of energy you have (fatigue)? Have you been more irritable than usual? Do your muscles seem tense? Do you feel a tightening in your throat?

These are symptoms of anxiety. See the description of the four levels of anxiety under Common Problems and Conditions later in this chapter.

Beck Depression Inventory, Short Form

Instructions: This is a questionnaire. On the questionnaire are groups of statements. Please read the entire group of statements in each category. Then pick out the one statement in that group which best describes the way you feel today, that is, *right now!* Circle the number beside the statement you have chosen. If several statements in the group seem to apply equally well, circle each one.
Be sure to read all the statements in each group before making your choice.

A. (Sadness)
  3 I am so sad or unhappy that I can't stand it.
  2 I am blue or sad all the time and I can't snap out of it.
  1 I feel sad or blue.
  0 I do not feel sad.

B. (Pessimism)
  3 I feel that the future is hopeless and that things cannot improve.
  2 I feel I have nothing to look forward to.
  1 I feel discouraged about the future.
  0 I am not particularly pessimistic or discouraged about the future.

C. (Sense of failure)
  3 I feel I am a complete failure as a person (parent, husband, wife).
  2 As I look back on my life, all I can see is a lot of failures.
  1 I feel I have failed more than the average person.
  0 I do not feel like a failure.

D. (Dissatisfaction)
  3 I am dissatisfied with everything.
  2 I don't get satisfaction out of anything anymore.
  1 I don't enjoy things the way I used to.
  0 I am not particularly dissatisfied.

E. (Guilt)
  3 I feel as though I am very bad or worthless.
  2 I feel quite guilty.
  1 I feel bad or unworthy a good part of the time.
  0 I don't feel particularly guilty.

F. (Self-dislike)
  3 I hate myself.
  2 I am disgusted with myself.
  1 I am disappointed in myself.
  0 I don't feel disappointed in myself.

G. (Self-harm)
  3 I would kill myself if I had the chance.
  2 I have definite plans about committing suicide.
  1 I feel I would be better off dead.
  0 I don't have any thoughts about harming myself.

H. (Social withdrawal)
  3 I have lost all of my interest in other people and don't care about most of them at all.
  2 I have lost most of my interest in other people and have little feeling for them.
  1 I am less interested in other people than I used to be.
  0 I have not lost interest in other people.

I. (Indecisiveness)
  3 I can't make any decisions at all anymore.
  2 I have great difficulty in making decisions.
  1 I try to put off making decisions.
  0 I make decisions about as well as ever.

J. (Self-image change)
  3 I feel that I am ugly or repulsive-looking.
  2 I feel that there are permanent changes in my appearance and they make me look unattractive.
  1 I am worried that I am looking old or unattractive.
  0 I don't feel that I look any worse than I used to.

K. (Work difficulty)
  3 I can't do any work at all.
  2 I have to push myself very hard to do anything.
  1 It takes extra effort to get started at doing something.
  0 I can work about as well as before.

L. (Fatigability)
  3 I get too tired to do anything.
  2 I get tired from doing anything.
  1 I get tired more easily than I used to.
  0 I don't get any more tired than usual.

M. (Anorexia)
  3 I have no appetite at all anymore.
  2 My appetite is much worse now.
  1 My appetite is not as good as it used to be.
  0 My appetite is no worse than usual.

Scoring
  0-4   None or minimal depression
  5-7   Mild depression
  8-15 Moderate depression
  16+   Severe depression

Fig. 7-2 Beck Depression Inventory. *(From Beck and Beck, 1972.)*

Have you felt nauseated? Does your heart feel as though it is racing? Have you had to urinate more often than usual?

Nausea, urinary frequency, and palpitations may be physiologic responses to anxiety.

Have you noticed a change in your feelings? If yes, describe those feelings. What do you think initiated those feelings? How did you handle or cope with those feelings?

Feelings of anger, guilt, worthlessness, and anguish often accompany anxiety. The client may report feeling that he or she is going to die or having a sense of impending doom.

Alcohol Abuse

What is the maximum number of drinks you've had on any given occasion during the last month? On a typical day when you drink, how many drinks do you have?

On average, how many days per week do you drink alcohol?

Accurate information is difficult to obtain because clients are unwilling to disclose their actual consumption. The four CAGE questions can be used as a screening tool (Box 7-1). The CAGE questionnaire is the most popular screening tool for primary care. It is less sensitive for early problem drink-

---

BOX 7-1   **CAGE**   *Questions Used to Screen for Alcoholism*

The four CAGE questions are used as a screening tool. CAGE is an acronym for *C*ut down, *A*nnoyed, *G*uilty, *E*ye opener (Ewing, 1984):

1. Have you ever felt you should *cut down* on your drinking?
2. Have people *annoyed* you by criticizing your drinking?
3. Have you ever felt bad or *guilty* about your drinking?
4. Have you ever had a drink first thing in the morning *(eye opener)* to steady your nerves, get rid of a hangover, or get the day started?

TABLE 7-3   *AUDIT Structured Interview**

QUESTION	SCORE				
	0	**1**	**2**	**3**	**4**
How often do you have a drink containing alcohol?	Never	Monthly or less	2-4 times/mo	Monthly 2-3 times/wk	4 or more times/wk
How many drinks do you have on a typical day when you are drinking?	None	1 or 2	3 or 4	5 or 6	7-9†
How often do you have 6 or more drinks on one occasion?	Never	Less than monthly	Monthly	Weekly	Daily or almost daily
How often during the last year have you found that you were unable to stop drinking once you had started?	Never	Less than monthly	Monthly	Weekly	Daily or almost daily
How often last year have you failed to do what was normally expected from you because of drinking?	Never	Less than monthly	Monthly	Weekly	Daily or almost daily
How often during the last year have you needed a first drink in the morning to get yourself going after a heavy drinking session?	Never	Less than monthly	Monthly	Weekly	Daily or almost daily
How often during the last year have you had a feeling of guilt or remorse after drinking?	Never	Less than monthly	Monthly	Weekly	Daily or almost daily
How often during the last year have you been unable to remember what happened the night before because you had been drinking?	Never	Less than monthly	Monthly	Weekly	Daily or almost daily
Have you or someone else been injured as a result of your drinking?	Never	Yes, but not in last year (2 points)	Yes, during the last year (4 points)		
Has a relative, doctor, or other health worker been concerned about your drinking or suggested you cut down?	Never	Yes, but not in last year (2 points)	Yes, during the last year (4 points)		

From Report of the U.S. Preventive Services Task Force: *Guide to clinical preventive services,* ed 2, Baltimore, 1996, Williams & Wilkins.

*Score of greater than 8 (out of 41) is suggestive of problem drinking and indicates need for more in-depth assessment. Cut-off of 10 points is recommended by some to provide greater specificity.

†5 points if response is 10 or more drinks on a typical day.

AUDIT, Alcohol Use Disorders Identification Test.

ing or heavy drinking (Report of U.S. Preventive Task Force, 1996).

The Alcohol Use Disorders Identification Test (AUDIT) is another screening tool. It is a 10-item scale with a score from 0 to 4 on each item (Table 7-3) (Report of the U.S. Preventive Services Task Force, 1996). These 10 AUDIT questions ask about quantity and frequency of drinking, binging, and drinking consequences.

Clients who report moderate or binge drinking need further assessment. *Moderate drinking* is defined as an average of two drinks per day or less for men and one drink a day or less for women. Results of a study reported that 14.3% of U.S. adults reported at least one binge drinking episode. *Binge drinking* is defined as consuming five drinks or more in a single occasion in the past 30 days. During the study, men accounted for 81% of all binge drinking episodes and whites accounted for 78% of all episodes (Naimi et al, 2003).

Drug Abuse

Tell me about your recreational drug use. Which drugs were used? How often are you using these drugs? Have you had any problems because of the drug use?

Recreational drug use may include illegal drugs such as heroine, cocaine, and marijuana as well as abuse of prescription drugs including narcotic analgesics such as hydroco-

done. These questions help identify the pattern of drug use and screen for drug abuse, which can contribute to health problems. The CAGE and AUDIT screening tools can be adapted to ask questions about recreational drug use.

ETHNIC & CULTURAL VARIATIONS

Drugs that are considered illegal in one society may be considered legal and useful in another. For example, in the United States and parts of Western Europe, caffeine, alcohol, and nicotine are used widely and accepted. In the Middle East cannabis is considered a legal drug, whereas alcohol is forbidden. Some Native American tribes use peyote, a hallucinogen causing visual and auditory hallucinations, for religious services (McKenry and Salerno, 2003).

Altered Mental Status

Changes in mental status may become evident when there is change in the client's orientation to time, place or person, attention span, or memory. When a client's orientation becomes a concern while taking a history or talking with the client, the nurse asks questions to collect additional data. Long-term memory can be assessed during the history by asking clients where they were born or about their previous surgeries.

HEALTH PROMOTION   *Mental Illness and Suicide Prevention*

Approximately 20% of the U.S. population is affected by mental illness in a given year. Depression is a major cause of disability and is associated with more than 65% of suicides each year. In the United States, approximately 30,000 individuals take their own life each year, and another 650,000 receive emergency care after attempting to take their own life.

Goals and Objectives—*Healthy People 2010*

Mental health is one of the leading health indicators identified by *Healthy People 2010*. The *Healthy People 2010* goal for mental health and mental disorders is to improve mental health and ensure access to appropriate, quality mental health services. Nine specific objectives are associated with improvement in mental health status, including the following:

- Reduce suicide rates and rates of adolescent suicide attempts.
- Reduce the proportion of homeless adults with serious mental illness.
- Increase the proportion of individuals with serious mental illness who are employed.
- Reduce the incidence of relapse for those with eating disorders.
- Increase the proportion of children and adults with mental health disorders who receive treatment.
- Increase the proportion of persons with mental health and substance abuse problems who receive treatment for both.

Recommendations to Reduce Risk (Primary Prevention)
Institute of Medicine (IOM)

The IOM makes four recommendations to reduce suicide:

- Develop a national network of interdisciplinary research on suicide prevention across the life cycle.
- Improve national monitoring of suicide.
- Develop and disseminate tools for recognition and screening for use by primary care providers.
- Programs for suicide prevention should be developed, tested, expanded, and implemented through funding from appropriate agencies.

Screening Recommendations (Secondary Prevention)
U.S. Preventive Services Task Force

- Screen adults for depression in clinical practice. Many tools to screen for depression are available—little evidence exists to recommend one over another.
- Clinicians should be alert to signs of suicidal ideation in persons with established risk factors.
- It is unknown if routine screening of children or adolescents for depression is effective.
- It is unknown if routine screening by primary care clinicians for suicide risk in asymptomatic persons is effective.

From: Institute of Medicine: *Reducing suicide: A national imperative,* Washington DC, 2000, National Academy Press; US Department of Health and Human Services: *Healthy people, 2010: understanding and improving health,* Washington DC, 2000 (available at *www.healthypeople.gov*); US Preventive Services Task Force, *Guide to clinical preventive services.* Screening for suicide risk, 2004, and Screening for Depression, 2002 (available at *www.ahrq.gov*).

HEALTH PROMOTION *Substance Abuse*

Substance abuse is a major problem within our society. It is associated with many other serious problems, including injury (often from motor vehicle crashes), violence (including child and spousal abuse), sexually transmitted disease, unwanted pregnancy, financial problems, and homelessness. It is estimated that approximately 20% of adolescents use alcohol and 10% report use of illicit drugs. Approximately 17% of adults report binge drinking and 6% admit to use of illicit drugs. Of the estimated 13 to 16 million individuals needing treatment for substance abuse each year, only 3 million receive treatment.

Goals and Objectives—*Healthy People 2010*

Substance abuse is one of the 10 leading health indicators identified by *Healthy People 2010*. The *Healthy People 2010* goal for substance abuse is to reduce substance abuse to protect the health, safety, and quality of life for all, especially children.

Recommendations to Reduce Risk (Primary Prevention)
National Institute on Drug Abuse

Strategies for prevention of drug abuse focus on two primary principles:

- *Enhance protective factors:* Protective factors include strong, positive bonds within the family; parental monitoring; clear rules of conduct consistently enforced within the family; parent involvement in the lives of children; success in school performance; strong bonds with institutions such as church and school; and adoption of conventional norms regarding drug use.
- *Reduce risk factors:* Risk factors include a chaotic home environment (especially with parents who have substance abuse problems or mental illness); ineffective parenting; lack of mutual attachments; shy or aggressive behavior in the classroom; failure in school performance; poor social coping skills; association with deviant peer group; and adoption of attitude that approves of drug use.

Screening Recommendations (Secondary Prevention)
U.S. Preventive Services Task Force

- Clinicians should be alert to signs and symptoms of drug/alcohol abuse.
- Screen all adults and adolescents for problem drinking through a history of alcohol use or use of standardized screening tools such as CAGE or AUDIT.
- Screen all pregnant women for problem drinking (more than two drinks per day or binge drinking).
- Research has not been able to demonstrate if screening for drug abuse with questionnaires or laboratory tests is effective in reducing drug/alcohol abuse.
- Routine screening using biomarkers is not recommended.

Recommendations for Treatment (Tertiary Prevention)
Substance Abuse and Mental Health Administration

National treatment plan includes several areas of recommendations for substance abuse treatment. Important general recommendations include the following:

- Establish standard insurance benefits for abuse treatment providing full continuum of care.
- Appropriate assessment, referral, and treatment are required for all systems serving individuals with substance abuse problems.
- The delivery of substance abuse treatment follows evidence-based treatment protocols, including monitoring the quality of care.
- Conduct educational initiatives about substance abuse and treatments that promote dignity and reduce stigma and discrimination directed at individuals in recovery.

From National Institute on Drug Abuse: Risk and protective factors in drug abuse prevention, *NIDA Notes* 16(6), 2002 (available at *www.drugabuse.gov/NIDA_Notes*); Substance Abuse and Mental Health Services Administration: *Changing the conversation, improving substance abuse treatment: the national treatment plan initiative,* 2000, US Department of Health and Human Services (available at *www.samhsa.gov*); US Department of Health and Human Services: *Healthy People 2010: understanding and improving health,* ed 2, Washington, DC, 2000, US Government Printing Office (available at *www.healthypeople.gov*); US Preventive Services Task Force: *Guide to clinical preventive services,* ed 2, 1996 (available at *www.ahrq.gov*).

EXAMINATION

PROCEDURES AND TECHNIQUES WITH NORMAL FINDINGS

ABNORMAL FINDINGS

OBSERVE the client's posture and movements.

The posture should be erect and the body relaxed.

Tense muscles, fidgeting, or pacing may indicate anxiety; a slumped posture and slow movements may indicate depression.

OBSERVE for appropriate dress and hygiene.

Outlandish dress and makeup may be worn by a client in a manic phase of a bipolar disorder. Soiled clothing or lack of hygiene may indicate depression or organic brain syndrome.

PROCEDURES AND TECHNIQUES WITH NORMAL FINDINGS	ABNORMAL FINDINGS

OBSERVE for changes in voice tone, rate of speech, perspiration, and muscle tension or tremors.

Speech should be smooth and even and without effort. The conversation should be clear, spontaneous, understandable, and appropriate to the context of the discussion. There should be no visible perspiration, and the client should appear relaxed.

Physical signs of anxiety include changes in tone of voice and rate of speech, body tremors, increased muscle tension, perspiration, and sweaty palms.

ASSESS mental status by determining orientation, memory, calculation ability, communication skills, judgment, and abstraction.

Orientation

Ask the client what year it is, where he or she is, and his or her name. Date and time are the first orientation to disappear. Orientation to place is the second orientation to be lost, and again the client is expected to remember the place, town, and state after reorientation. Orientation to person is the last orientation to be lost.

Loss of orientation to time, place, or person is only an abnormality when the client does not remember the day and date after reorientation.

Memory

Ask clients to repeat three unrelated objects that are spoken slowly, such as "dog," "cloud," and "apple."

The client has difficulty with or cannot remember the three words.

Calculation ability

The calculation ability can be tested by asking clients about making change. For example, the nurse asks a client, "You buy fruit that costs $2.45 and you gave the cashier $3.00. How much change would you expect to receive?"

The client gives an incorrect answer or is unable to perform the calculation.

Communication skills (naming, repeating, writing, and copying)

Ask the client to *name* common objects, such as a watch or pencil. *Repetition* is tested by asking clients to repeat a phrase such as, "No ifs, ands, or buts." To test repetition *Reading* is tested by asking clients to read a phrase that is written on a piece of paper and to do what it says, such as, "Lift your right hand." When clients complete this task, the nurse knows that they can read, comprehend what they read, and follow instructions. *Writing* is tested by asking clients to write a sentence. Do not tell them what to write. The sentence must have a subject and a verb to be sensible, but correct punctuation and grammar are not assessed. *Copying* is assessed by asking clients to copy a drawing of two geometric figures that overlap, such as an intersecting pentagon about 1 inch on a side.

The client is unable to name objects or names them incorrectly, unable to repeat a phrase, unable to comprehend a written phrase, unable to write a sentence with a subject and a verb, and/or unable to copy a drawing.

Judgment and reasoning

Ask a question such as, "What would you do if a car was speeding toward you?"

The client is unable to give an answer or gives one that is not related to the question.

Abstract reasoning

Ask the meaning of a proverb, such as "A bird in the hand is worth two in the bush."

The client is unable to provide a meaning or gives one that is not related to the proverb.

MEASURE the blood pressure.

Blood pressure varies with sex, body weight, and time of day, but the upper limits for adults are <120 mm Hg systolic and <80 mm Hg diastolic.

Anxiety, especially severe anxiety or panic, may cause elevated blood pressure as a result of sympathetic stimulation.

= core examination skill

PROCEDURES AND TECHNIQUES WITH NORMAL FINDINGS	ABNORMAL FINDINGS

☞ PALPATE the radial pulse for rate.

(See Chapter 13 for descriptions of pulses.)
Rate: 60 to 100 beats/min

Pulse rates for clients with anxiety may be elevated as a result of sympathetic stimulation.

☞ OBSERVE and COUNT respirations for rate and breathing pattern.

Note the respiratory rate. Breathing should be smooth and even. In adults, breathing should occur at a rate of 12 to 20 breaths per minute. Evaluate the rhythm or pattern of breathing. The chest wall should symmetrically rise and expand and then relax. It should appear easy, without effort.

Respiratory rate may be increased during anxiety as a result of sympathetic stimulation. The client may appear to be dyspneic. Respiratory rate may be decreased during depression, and the breathing pattern may include frequent, deep sighs.

OBSERVE eye movements and MEASURE pupil size.

When you suspect the client has drug intoxication, complete the Rapid Eye Test in Box 7-2.

Table 7-4 describes clinical findings of acute drug intoxication. Table 7-5 describes common eye signs detected after abuse of selected drugs.

TABLE 7-4   *Clinical Findings of Acute Drug Intoxication*

DRUG(S) ABUSED	CLINICAL FINDINGS
Cannabis drugs	Tachycardia and postural hypotension, conjunctival vascular congestion, distortions of perception, dryness of mouth and throat, possible panic
Cocaine	Increased stimulation, euphoria, increased blood pressure and heart rate, anorexia, insomnia, agitation; in overdose, increased body temperature, hallucinations, seizures, death
Opiates	Depressed blood pressure and respiration; fixed, pinpoint pupils; depressed sensorium; coma; pulmonary edema
Barbiturates and other general CNS depressants	Depressed blood pressure and respirations; ataxia, slurred speech, confusion, depressed tendon reflexes, coma, shock
Amphetamines	Elevated blood pressure, tachycardia, other cardiac dysrhythmias, hyperactive tendon reflexes, pupils dilated and reactive to light, hyperpyrexia, perspiration, shallow respirations, circulatory collapse, clear or confused sensorium, possible hallucinations, paranoid feelings
Hallucinogenic agents	Elevated blood pressure, hyperactive tendon reflexes, piloerection, perspiration, pupils dilated and reactive to light, anxiety, distortion of body image and perception, delusions, hallucinations

Adapted from McKenry LM, Tessier E, Hogan M: *Mosby's pharmacology in nursing,* ed 22, St Louis, 2006, Mosby.

CNS, Central nervous system.

TABLE 7-5 *Common Eye Signs Detected after Abuse of Selected Drugs*

	MARIJUANA	HEROIN	ALCOHOL	COCAINE	PCP
Pupil size	Normal	Constricted	Normal	Dilated	Normal
Slow or no reaction of pupil to light	Yes		Yes	Yes	Yes
Nonconvergence	Yes				
Redness of sclera	Yes		Yes		
Glazing of cornea	Yes	Yes	Yes		
Nystagmus	Yes		Yes		Yes
Swollen eyelids	Yes	Yes			Yes
Watering eyes	Yes				
Ptosis		Yes			
Decreased corneal reflex		Yes		Yes	Yes

Data from Tennant F: Is your patient abusing? *Postgrad Med 84:*108-114, 1988.

BOX 7-2 **RAPID EYE TEST TO DETECT CURRENT DRUG INTOXICATION**

General Observation
Look for redness of sclera, ptosis, retracted upper lid (white sclera visible above iris, causing blank stare), glazing, excessive tearing of eyes, and swelling of eyelids.

Pupil Size
Dilated (>6.5 mm) or constricted (<3.0 mm).

Pupil Reaction to Light
Slow, sluggish, or absent response.

Nystagmus
Hold finger in vertical position and have the client follow finger as it moves to the side, in a circle, and up and down. Positive test is failure to hold gaze or jerkiness of eye movements.

Convergence
Inability to hold the cross-eyed position after an examining finger is moved 1 foot away from client's nose and held there for 5 seconds.

Corneal Reflex
Decreased rate of blinking after touching cornea with cotton.

AGE-RELATED VARIATIONS

Infants, Children & Adolescents

Variations for neonates and infants include asking about drug and alcohol use of the mother during the pregnancy. Children are asked about their experiences in school, how they like school, and if they get into trouble at school. Also children are asked about their fears about any aspect of their life.

Adolescents are asked about school experience as well. Additionally they are asked about drug and alcohol use and about feelings of depression or anxiety. Assessing the self-esteem of this age group is important. Chapter 20 presents further information regarding the mental health assessment of these age groups.

Indications of depression in an older adult may be misinterpreted as expected manifestations of aging. For example, decrease in appetite or fatigue may be explained as a decrease in metabolism or a loss of taste buds that occur with aging. When older adults report problems concentrating or sleeping, it may be interpreted as an expected change with advanced age. Many older adults think that depression will go away without intervention, they are too old to get help, or reporting sadness may be a sign of weakness. Chapter 22 presents further information regarding the mental health assessment of this age group.

COMMON PROBLEMS & CONDITIONS

ALTERATIONS OF MOOD AND AFFECT

Major Depression

Major depression is an abnormal mood state in which a person characteristically has a sense of sadness, hopelessness, helplessness, worthlessness, and despair resulting from some personal loss or tragedy. A person may experience a single episode or may have recurrent episodes of depression. Feeling depressed is not the same thing as the illness of depression. Symptoms of depression interfere with the client's ability to work, study, sleep, eat, and enjoy pleasurable activities. **Clinical Findings:** A person must have been in a depressed mood or have lost interest or pleasure for at least 2 weeks, accompanied by significant distress or impairment and at least four of the classic clinical manifestations, before a diagnosis of major depression is made. These clinical manifestations include persistent sad, anxious, or "empty" mood; feelings of hopelessness or pessimism; feelings of guilt, worthlessness, and helplessness; reduced appetite with weight loss or increased appetite with weight gain; insomnia; excessive fatigue; difficulty concentrating and making decisions; and suicidal thoughts (*www.nimh. nih.gov/health/publications/depression/complete-publication. shtml,* accessed March 2008).

Bipolar Disorder

Bipolar disorder is a type of depression characterized by episodes of mania, depression, or mixed moods. Sometimes the mood switches are dramatic and rapid, but most often they are gradual. **Clinical Findings:** Characteristics of the manic phase are excessive emotional displays, excitement, euphoria, hyperactivity accompanied by elation, boisterousness, impaired ability to concentrate, decreased need for sleep, and limitless energy, often accompanied by delusions of grandeur. In contrast, in the depressive phase there is marked apathy and feelings of profound sadness, loneliness, guilt, and lowered self-esteem.

Anxiety

Anxiety is a feeling of uneasiness or discomfort experienced in varying degrees, from mild anxiety to panic. Unlike fear, which is a response to an actual object or event, anxiety is a response to no specific source or actual object. The energy that anxiety provides may mobilize a person to take constructive action such as solving a major problem or filling an unmet need. When used destructively, it can immobilize a person (*www.nimh.nih.gov/health/publications/anxiety-disorders/complete-publication.shtml,* accessed March 2008). **Clinical Findings:** Four levels of anxiety have been described: mild, moderate, severe, and panic. A mildly anxious person has a broad perceptual field because the anxiety heightens awareness to sensory stimuli. The person sees more, hears more, and thinks more logically. Learning occurs during mild anxiety. The moderately anxious person has a more narrow field of perception and uses selective inattention to ignore stimuli in the environment to focus on a specific concern. The severely anxious person has reduced perception of stimuli and develops compulsive mechanisms to avoid the anxiety-provoking object or situation. During severe anxiety the person experiences impaired memory, attention, and concentration, has difficulty solving problems, and is unable to focus on events in the environment. The panic level of anxiety is characterized by complete disruption of the perceptual field. The person experiences intense terror and is unable to think logically or make decisions. Physical manifestations of anxiety represent sympathetic nervous system stimulation. The person experiences muscle tension, tachycardia, dyspnea, hypertension, increased respiration, and profuse perspiration.

Obsessive-Compulsive Disorder

Obsessive-compulsive disorder is classified as an anxiety disorder because of the anxiety symptoms that develop when the client tries to resist an obsession or compulsion. *Obsessions* are defined as unwanted, intrusive, persistent ideas, thoughts, impulses, or images that cause marked anxiety or distress. Compulsions are unwanted, repetitive behavior patterns or mental acts that are intended to reduce anxiety. The person recognizes that the behaviors are excessive or unreasonable but continues them because of the relief from the discomfort of anxiety that they provide. **Clinical Findings:** Common obsessions include repeated thoughts about contamination, repeated doubts, a need to have everything in a particular order, and sexual imagery. Examples of compulsive behavior are praying, counting, or repeating words silently to relieve anxiety (Townsend, 2003).

Psychotic Disorders

Schizophrenia (Dopamine Dysregulation Disorder)

Schizophrenia is any one of a large group of psychotic disorders characterized by gross distortion of reality, disturbances of language and communication, withdrawal from social interaction, and the disorganization and fragmentation of thought perception and emotion reaction (Townsend, 2003). **Clinical Findings:** Clinical manifestations include apathy and confusion; delusions and hallucinations; rambling or stylized patterns of speech, such as echolalia, incoherence, or evasiveness; withdrawn, regressive, and bizarre behavior; and emotional lability.

Substance Abuse Disorders

Alcohol Withdrawal Syndrome

Ethyl alcohol, or ethanol, is a central nervous system depressant found in alcoholic beverages. The blood alcohol level (BAL) is used to measure the amount of alcohol in blood. The legal intoxication level in most states is 100 mg/dl (0.10%), with some states using 0.08%.

There are two phases of alcohol withdrawal syndrome (AWS): alcohol withdrawal and alcohol withdrawal delirium, or delirium tremens (DT). **Clinical Findings:** Early manifestations of alcohol withdrawal include hand tremors, sweating, nausea and vomiting, anxiety, and agitation. These manifestations begin 6 to 24 hours after the client's last drink, peak in 24 to 36 hours, and end after 48 hours of abstinence. About 7% of these clients experience hallucinations. Between 5% and 10% develop seizures. Only about 5% progress to delirium tremens, in which the client experiences cardiac dysrhythmias, hypertension, increased respirations, profuse sweating, delusion, and hallucinations (Compton, 2002).

Drug Intoxication

Clinical findings of intoxication from commonly abused drugs (cannabis, cocaine, opiates, barbiturates, amphetamines, and hallucinogenic agents) are presented in Tables 7-4 and 7-5.

Delirium and Dementia

Delirium

Delirium is characterized by a disturbance of consciousness and a change in cognition that develops rapidly over a short period of time. Manifestations are of a short duration (e.g., 1 week, rarely more than 1 month) and are reversible with treatment. **Clinical Findings:** Manifestations include attention deficits, disorganized thinking, confusion, disorientation, restlessness, incoherence, anxiety, excitement, and at times illusions. Emotional instability may be evident as fear, anxiety, depression, irritability, anger, euphoria, or apathy. Autonomic nervous system signs of tachycardia, sweating, flushed face, dilated pupils, and elevated blood pressure are common (Townsend, 2003).

Dementia

Dementia is a syndrome of acquired, progressive, intellectual impairment that compromises function such as memory, language, visual-spatial skills, emotion, personality, and cognition. Dementia usually is not reversible, a characteristic that distinguishes it from delirium. **Clinical Findings:** Initially symptoms are not apparent. As the dementia progresses, the client loses things and forgets people's names. Loss of short-term memory is common and disorientation becomes apparent. Psychomotor symptoms include wandering, obsessive-compulsiveness, agitation, and aggression. In the later stages the client is unable to recognize family members and is confined to bed (Townsend, 2003).

CLINICAL APPLICATION & CLINICAL REASONING

See Appendix E for answers to exercises in this section.

REVIEW QUESTIONS

1 Which question is appropriate for a nurse to ask at the beginning of a mental health history?
   1 "Have you been feeling anxious or sad?"
   2 "How have you been feeling about yourself?"
   3 "Are you alone a lot or do you have friends to socialize with?"
   4 "How are you dealing with the stressors in your life?"
2 During a history, the client says she is so uncomfortable with her life that she wishes that it were over. Which is an appropriate follow-up question from the nurse?
   1 "Have you thought of hurting yourself?"
   2 "Oh, I have felt that way many times."

3 "That feeling will go away, just give it some time."
4 "In what ways has your life been uncomfortable?"

3 During a health history a client says, "Stressors? Oh, yeah, I have stressors. I got a promotion at work and with the extra income I am going to move into a new house, but that has been delayed because my mother is in the hospital and my son is going off to college. To get through this time I just keep exercising and meditate." The nurse notes that this client is exhibiting:
   1 Flight of ideas.
   2 Anxiety.
   3 Positive coping strategies.
   4 Rationalization and denial.

4 Difficulty sleeping, financial concerns, problems with personal or work relationships, difficulty making decisions, tense muscles, and fatigue are indicators of which disorder?
1 Depression.
2 Anxiety.
3 Delirium.
4 Alcohol withdrawal syndrome.

5 A client reports nausea and vomiting and the nurse observes hand tremors, agitation, and sweating. In view of these findings, what additional data would the nurse need to collect?
1 What fears or stressors the client has been experiencing.
2 When the client last took illegal drugs and which one was taken.
3 What kinds of obsessions or compulsions the client has been experiencing.
4 When the client last drank alcohol and how much was consumed.

CASE STUDY

Sarah comes to the student health clinic with complaints of fatigue. The following data are collected by the nurse practitioner from interview and examination.

Interview Data

Sarah tells the nurse that she has felt constantly tired, and all she wants to do is sleep. She says that she does not have time to be tired, because final examinations are approaching, and she is very concerned about her grades. She begins to cry. "I am so afraid I will not pass my classes. If I don't pass, my parents will not help me with school anymore." When asked to describe herself, Sarah replies, "Friendly, but not very smart." Sarah goes on to tell the nurse that she has a boyfriend but only sees him occasionally because he lives in another state. When asked about other friends, Sarah replies, "I know all of the people in my class."

Examination Data

- *General survey:* Well-nourished, overweight young woman appearing unkept, with slightly swollen red eyes from crying. Makes infrequent eye contact.

- *Vital signs:* Blood pressure, 128/84 mm Hg; pulse, 96 beats per minute; respirations, 18 per minute; temperature, 98.6° F (36.7° C). Height: 5 feet 3 inches (160 cm). Weight: 148 lb (67 kg).
- *Mental status:* Oriented to person, place, and time. Slow speech pattern with flat affect.
- All body system findings are within normal limits.

Clinical Reasoning

1. What data deviate from normal findings, suggesting to the nurse that Sarah may have a mental health issue?
2. What additional information should the nurse ask or assess for?
3. Based on these data, what risk factors for depression does this client have?
4. What nursing diagnoses and collaborative problems should be considered for this situation?

INTERACTIVE ACTIVITIES

Open the interactive student CD-ROM, click on Chapter 7, and choose from the following activities shown on the menu bar:

- **Multiple Choice Challenge.** Click on the best answer for each question. You will be given immediate feedback, rationale for incorrect answers, and a total score. Good luck!

- **Risk Factors.** Review this client's history and identify risk factors. Complete your assessment by deciding which risks are modifiable and which are nonmodifiable. You only get one shot, so choose carefully!

- **The Name Game.** Identify each of the anatomic parts of the figure shown. Watch out where you place your answer—it won't stick if it's in the wrong place!

- **Printable Lab Guide.** Locate the Lab Guide for Chapter 7, and print and use it (as many times as needed) to help you apply your assessment skills. These guides may also be filled in electronically and then saved and e-mailed to your instructor!

- **Quick Challenge.** Use this critical thinking exercise to assess your skills through case study-style questions, then compare with expert answers!

CHAPTER 8

Sleep Assessment

Sleep disorders and sleep deprivation are an unmet public health problem of major proportions according to the Institute of Medicine (IOM), which calls for greater recognition of the contribution of sleep to health and safety. Between 50 and 70 million Americans suffer from a chronic disorder of sleep and wakefulness, hindering daily functioning and adversely affecting their health. The cumulative effects of sleep loss and sleep disorders have been associated with health consequences such as hypertension, diabetes mellitus, obesity, depression, myocardial infarction and stroke. Almost 20% of all serious car crash injuries are associated with driver sleepiness (IOM, 2006).

ANATOMY & PHYSIOLOGY

Sleep is a state of reduced consciousness from which a person can be aroused through the use of sensory stimuli: sounds, touch, bright light, or smells. During sleep there is an increased rate of anabolism (synthesis of cell structures) and a decreased rate of catabolism (breakdown of cell structures). Likewise, there is a decrease in the cardiac workload, a 5% to 10% reduction in systemic blood pressure, diminished skeletal muscle activity, and decreased metabolism.

Sleep physiology is a complex process involving the activation of several neurotransmitters in various areas of the brain. Structures of the brain believed to be involved with sleep are the reticular activating system (RAS) in the upper brainstem, the bulbar synchronizing region (BSR) in the pons and forebrain, the hypothalamus and thalamus in the diencephalon, and the frontal lobe in the cerebral cortex. The RAS receives sensory input to maintain wakefulness (Fig. 8-1). Norepinephrine, dopamine, and acetylcholine are neurotransmitters that contribute to wakefulness. Gamma-aminobutyric acid (GABA) is an inhibitory neurotransmitter that facilitates sleep.

Sleep patterns may be disrupted by physical or psychologic illnesses, by environmental factors such as noise or room temperature, by maturational factors such as age, and by drugs such as alcohol, hypnotics, antidepressants, and narcotics. When people are deprived of sleep, they have difficulty coping with stress, their immune system becomes impaired, and they feel fatigued, with a decreased ability to concentrate. They may demonstrate perceptual difficulties such as confusion, paranoia, and hallucinations, with increased anxiety and short-term memory loss.

STAGES OF SLEEP

Sleep stages are documented using overnight polysomnography, which includes the following measures: central and occipital electroencephalogram (EEG) to monitor brain wave activity; bilateral electrooculogram (EOG) to detect eye movement characteristic of rapid eye movement sleep; submental and anterior tibialis electromyograms (EMGs) to detect muscle tension of the chin and leg, respectively; electrocardiogram (ECG) to monitor cardiac rhythm; thermistor to measure nasal/oral airflow temperature; chest and abdominal belts to detect respiratory effort; and pulse oximetry to detect

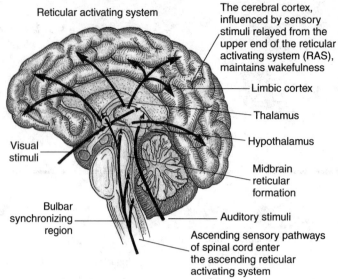

Reticular activating system

The cerebral cortex, influenced by sensory stimuli relayed from the upper end of the reticular activating system (RAS), maintains wakefulness

Limbic cortex

Thalamus

Hypothalamus

Midbrain reticular formation

Auditory stimuli

Ascending sensory pathways of spinal cord enter the ascending reticular activating system

Visual stimuli

Bulbar synchronizing region

Fig. 8-1   The RAS and BSR control sensory input, intermittently activating and suppressing the brain's higher centers to control sleep and wakefulness. *(From Potter and Perry, 2001.)*

TABLE 8-1 *Physiologic Changes during Sleep*	
STAGE OF SLEEP	**PHYSIOLOGIC CHANGES**
NREM	Basal metabolic rate decreases by 10 to 15%
	Temperature decreases 0.5° to 1° C (0.9° to 1.8° F)
	Heart rate decreases 10 to 30 beats per minute
	Blood pressure decreases
	Respirations decrease
	Muscle tone decreases
	Knee jerk reflexes are absent
	Pupils are constricted
REM	Bursts of rapid eye movement
	Loss of temperature regulation
	Alterations in heart rate, blood pressure, and respirations
	Lack of tone in antigravity muscles
	Penile erections in men
	Clitoral engorgement in women

From McCance K, Huether S: *Pathophysiology: The biologic basis for disease in adults and children*, ed 5, St. Louis, Mosby, 2006.

oxygen saturation. Data from these clinical parameters are used to identify two distinct phases of sleep: non–rapid eye movement (NREM) sleep followed by rapid eye movement (REM) sleep. Activities that occur during the four stages of NREM sleep are slow, regular respirations and low heart rate and blood pressure (Table 8-1). The subsequent phase—REM, or active, sleep—is characterized by irregular respiration, variable heart rate and blood pressure, rapid eye movement, and slight movement of the face and fingers. Dreaming is closely associated with REM sleep.

Sleep for an adult consists of three to five sleep cycles beginning with stage 1 NREM and progressing to REM sleep and then back to one of the stages of NREM sleep. An average sleep cycle lasts 90 minutes, but each cycle has varying amounts of NREM and REM sleep. Figure 8-2 illustrates the normal adult sleep cycle and stages of sleep. The first cycle usually follows an orderly progression from stage 1 to stage 4 of NREM sleep followed by the REM sleep phase. The subsequent cycles may omit stage 1 and proceed in a different order from stage 4 to stage 2 and then to REM sleep. During the first sleep cycle the NREM phase is longer than the REM phase. But as sleep continues, the time spent in NREM sleep decreases and REM sleep increases.

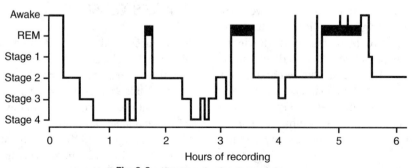

Fig. 8-2   Histogram showing stages of sleep.

A person's sleep patterns are highly individualized and change throughout life as the daily requirement for sleep gradually decreases. The National Sleep Foundation (NSF) reports 8 to 9 hours of sleep for adults as optimal. A 2005 NSF *Sleep in America* poll of adults revealed that women are more likely than men to have difficulty falling and staying asleep and to experience more daytime sleepiness at least a few times a week. Conditions unique to women, like the menstrual cycle, pregnancy and menopause, can affect how well a woman sleeps. This is because the changing levels of hormones that a woman experiences throughout the month and over her lifetime, like estrogen and progesterone, have an impact on sleep (National Sleep Foundation, 2007).

LINK TO CONCEPTS *Sleep*

The feature concept for this chapter is *Sleep*. This concept represents mechanisms that support or impair the pattern of natural periodic suspension of consciousness during which the body is restored.

Sleep is enhanced by good health; likewise, good health is impacted by adequate sleep. There are multiple factors that impair sleep, which include chronic illness, pain, medications, alcohol, nicotine, diet, environment, activity levels, and lifestyle. The relationships among concepts featured in this text with sleep are presented below.

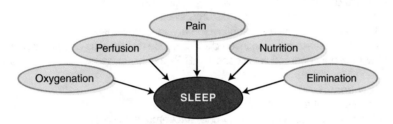

This model shows the interrelationship of concepts related to an individual's sleep patterns. As an example, an individual with heart failure potentially experiences sleep impairment. Familiarity with the concepts of perfusion, oxygenation, and elimination can help clarify why problems with sleep may arise. For example, reduced cardiac output (perfusion) can interfere with oxygen exchange (oxygenation) at night leading to orthopnea. Furthermore, it is not uncommon for the individual to awaken frequently at night with a need to urinate (elimination). Understanding the interrelationships among these concepts helps the nurse recognize risk factors and thus become more aware of issues to address when conducting a health assessment.

HEALTH HISTORY

RISK FACTORS　*Insomnia and Sleep Apnea*

As you conduct a health history related to sleep, it is important to consider common risk factors associated with insomnia and sleep apnea and follow up with additional questions should they exist.

INSOMNIA

- *Age:* People over 60 to 65 years are more likely to complain of insomnia because of bodily changes related to aging and because of chronic disorders that disturb sleep.
- *Chronic disease:*
  - Diabetes mellitus and kidney disease can cause frequent urination that can disturb sleep.
  - Chronic lung disease can cause frequent awakening due to decreased oxygen and feeling of air hunger.
  - Sleep apnea causes brief, often unnoticed, awakening and excessive daytime sleepiness.
  - Heart disease can cause difficulty breathing when lying down.
  - Arthritis disturbs sleep by causing joint pain and stiffness.
  - Fibromyalgia causes pain that disturbs sleep.
  - Restless leg syndrome causes involuntary limb movements during sleep.
  - Alzheimer disease and Parkinson disease cause restlessness and frequent awaking.
  - Gastroesophageal reflux disease (GERD) and hiatal hernia can cause heartburn when lying flat.
- *Medications:*
  - Decongestant and cold remedies
  - Corticosteroids for inflammatory and autoimmune disorders
  - Beta-adrenergic antagonists (beta-blockers) for hypertension
  - Theophylline for asthma
  - Phenytoin for seizure
- *Gender:* Insomnia occurs in women more than men. Pregnancy and hormonal shift can disturb sleep, as can premenstrual syndrome and menopause.
- *Psychological factors:* Stress, anxiety, depression, and bipolar disorders can disturb sleep.
- *Lifestyle:*
  - Smoking (M)
  - Drinking alcohol or beverages containing caffeine (M)
  - Exercising close to bedtime (M)
  - Night shift work when time of sleep varies with days off and days working
  - Poor sleep environment such as in a place that is too noisy, too hot, too cool, or too light (M)

SLEEP APNEA

Obstructive Sleep Apnea
- *Gender:* Male
- *Age:* Older than 65 years
- Family history of sleep apnea
- *Anatomic factors:* Anatomically narrowed airways, tonsillar hypertrophy, thick neck, enlarged tongue (e.g., people with Down syndrome)
- High blood pressure
- *Lifestyle:* Obesity, cigarette smoking, and use of alcohol, sedatives, and tranquilizers (M)

Central Sleep Apnea
- *Gender:* Male
- *Heart disorders:* Atrial fibrillation or heart failure
- *Neurologic disorders:* Stroke or brain tumor
- *Neuromuscular disorders:* Spinal cord injury, amyotrophic lateral sclerosis, or muscular dystrophy
- High altitude

From Swedish Medical Center, Seattle, Washington, *www.swedish.org/body,* May 2007, *Risk Factors for Insomnia.*
M = modifiable risk factor.

GENERAL HEALTH HISTORY

Present Health Status

Do you have any chronic problems that interfere with sleep, such as pain, difficulty breathing, anxiety, or needing to go to the bathroom during the night?
Chronic medical problems can interrupt sleep and sleep disorders are associated with chronic health problems. Correcting problems that interfere with sleep would be the goal of improving the client's sleep.

How many hours do you usually sleep per day?
Data are used to compare usual sleep patterns with the expected norms for the client's age. Adults sleep 7.5 to 8 hours.

BOX 8-1   DRUGS AND THEIR EFFECTS ON SLEEP

Hypnotics
Interfere with reaching deeper sleep stages
Provide only temporary (1 week) increase in quantity of sleep
Eventually cause "hangover" during day: excess drowsiness, confusion, decreased energy
May worsen sleep apnea in older adults

Diuretics
Nighttime awakenings nocturia

Antidepressants and Stimulants
Suppress REM sleep
Decrease total sleep time

Alcohol
Speeds onset of sleep
Reduces REM sleep
Awakens person during the night and causes difficulty in returning to sleep

Caffeine
Prevents person from falling asleep
May cause person to awaken during night
Interferes with REM sleep

Beta-Adrenergic Blockers
Cause nightmares
Cause insomnia
Cause awakening from sleep

Benzodiazepines
Alter REM sleep
Increase sleep time
Increase daytime drowsiness

Narcotics (Morphine/Demerol)
Suppress REM sleep
Cause increased daytime drowsiness

Anticonvulsants
Decrease REM sleep time
May cause daytime drowsiness

From Potter PA, Perry AG: *Fundamentals of nursing*, ed 6, St Louis, 2005, Mosby.

During what hours do you usually sleep? Are there variations in the time of day that you sleep?
Someone who rotates shifts at work, creating an inconsistent sleep-wake cycle, may develop altered sleep cycles.

Do you feel rested when you wake up from sleep?
This is a subjective indication of the quality of sleep time.

How often do you take naps? How long do you typically sleep?
The need for napping during the day may suggest inadequate length or quality of sleep at night. Long naps (longer than 1.5 to 2 hours) may disrupt nighttime sleep. In some cultures, however, an afternoon nap is the norm.

Do you ever fall asleep during the day when you do not want to fall asleep?
Falling asleep at inappropriate times may indicate excessive daytime sleepiness.

What is your usual bedtime routine (e.g., brushing teeth, bathing, reading, watching television, listening to music)?
Sleep may be disturbed when the usual ritual is changed.

What medication(s) do you take?
Side effects of many drugs may interfere with sleep (Box 8-1).

PROBLEM-BASED HISTORY

Commonly reported problems related to sleep are insomnia and sleep apnea. As with symptoms of all areas of health assessment, a symptom analysis is completed, which in the areas of sleep includes the chronology, setting, associated manifestations, and alleviating and aggravating factors (see Box 3-3 in Chapter 3).

Insomnia

How easily do you fall asleep? What helps you to fall asleep? How often do you wake up during sleep?
Difficulty falling asleep and staying asleep occurs with depression and insomnia.

What do you think is keeping you from sleeping? Examples are work-related issues, personal relationships, financial concerns, family concerns, stress, anxiety, depression, noise, environmental temperature, lights, discomfort, and thirst.
Responses help identify therapy for sleeplessness. Stress may cause tension that makes falling asleep difficult; stress causes release of adrenaline and corticosteroids that cause sleeplessness. As anxiety and depression increase, so does lack of sleep; lack of sleep, in turn, increases anxiety and depression.

Do you drink alcohol before bedtime?

Alcohol speeds onset of sleep, disrupts REM sleep, and causes difficulty in returning to sleep.

Do you eat or drink caffeine before bedtime?

Caffeine prevents clients from falling asleep and may cause awakening during the night.

Do you smoke? If so, how many packs per day?

Heavy smoking (more than one pack per day) causes difficulty falling asleep.

Does your need to urinate wake you from sleep?

Sleep Apnea

Do you snore loudly? Do you ever wake up because you cannot breathe? Has anyone ever told you that you often stop breathing for short periods during sleep?

(Spouse or bed partner/roommate may report this.) Waking frequently during the night, loud snoring, and not breathing for short periods may indicate sleep apnea.

Do you have difficulty staying awake during the day? Do you experience choking or gasping episodes during sleep? Have you had automobile or work-related accidents because of fatigue and sleepiness?

Positive responses may indicate obstructive sleep apnea.

Have you had cognitive changes such as difficulty concentrating, memory loss, irritability, or judgment problems because of fatigue?

These disorders may represent problems associated with obstructive sleep apnea.

Have you been diagnosed with hypertension, heart failure, coronary artery disease, or stroke since the sleeping difficulties began? Do you have to prop yourself on pillows to breathe while you sleep?

These disorders may represent adverse effects of central sleep apnea on the cardiovascular system.

EXAMINATION

PROCEDURES AND TECHNIQUES WITH NORMAL FINDINGS	ABNORMAL FINDINGS

 OBSERVE the client for mental status, thought patterns, and speech patterns.

The client should be alert and responsive. Responses should be easily understandable, spontaneous, and demonstrate clear thinking.

Slow or confused thought processes or slow or slurred speech may indicate sleep deprivation.

OBSERVE gross motor movements and posture.

The client's posture should be erect with smooth, coordinated, spontaneous muscle movement.

Slow, exaggerated movements or slumped posture may indicate sleep deprivation.

MEASURE blood pressure and weight.

Blood pressure should be within expected ranges and weight should be consistent with previous measurements for this client.

Hypertension and obesity are risk factors for sleep apnea.

INSPECT nasal septum for patency and deviation.

Nasal septum should be midline with unobstructed movement of air.

Deviated septum may obstruct nasal passages, contributing to airway obstruction that may contribute to sleep apnea.

INSPECT pharynx for tonsillar hypertrophy.

The tonsils should extend beyond the posterior pillars and should appear slightly pink with an irregular shape (see Chapter 11 for examination).

Large tonsils may obstruct airway during sleep.

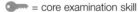 = core examination skill

AGE-RELATED VARIATIONS

Infants, Children, and Adolescents

During the first few weeks of life a neonate may sleep as much as 20 hours daily, with half the sleep time in the REM stage. Infants should be placed on their backs for sleep to prevent aspiration and sudden infant death syndrome (SIDS). Infants develop a nighttime pattern of sleep by 3 to 4 months of age. By age 2 years children usually sleep through the night and take a nap daily. Naps often cease by age 3. Sleep obtained by school-age children varies with their level of activity and state of health. Adolescents sleep 8 to 9 hours per day, of which a total of 2 hours is spent in REM sleep. Rapid growth and active lifestyle may contribute to fatigue. Chapter 20 presents further information regarding the sleep assessment for these age groups.

Older Adults

As adults age the time spent in nighttime sleep declines, with shortening of REM sleep and decrease in stages 3 and 4 of NREM sleep. The onset of sleep is delayed as adults age. Older adults frequently take a daily nap, but this does not necessarily indicate a sleeping problem at night. Chapter 22 presents further information regarding the sleep assessment for this age group.

COMMON PROBLEMS & CONDITIONS

INSOMNIA

Common factors contributing to insomnia are listed in the Risk Factors Box for Insomnia and Sleep Apnea. **Clinical Findings:** Clients may complain of difficulty getting to sleep or staying asleep, intermittent wakefulness during the night, early morning awakening, or combinations of any of these.

NARCOLEPSY

Narcolepsy is defined as a sudden onset of excessive daytime sleepiness that lasts from 10 to 30 minutes. It is accompanied by one or more of the following conditions: cataplexy, a transient loss of postural muscle tone; sleep paralysis, an awakening with transient inability to speak or move; hypnagogic hallucinations, dreamlike visual hallucinations occurring at the transitions from wakefulness to sleep; and disturbed nocturnal sleep, frequent, brief awakening during a night's sleep.

SLEEP APNEA

Sleep apnea is characterized by breathing abnormalities that vary from reduction of airflow (hypopnea) to complete cessation of airflow (apnea). There are three types of sleep apnea: central sleep apnea, obstructive sleep apnea, and mixed sleep apnea. Central sleep apnea is characterized by cessation of respiratory effort and thus no airflow. The breathing of clients with central sleep apnea has a gradual decline in respiratory effort followed by a gradual resumption of breathing effort. Obstructive sleep apnea is more common and is characterized by occlusion of upper airway with continued respiratory effort. The Risk Factors box lists different risk factors for obstructive and central sleep apnea (*www.mayoclinic.com*, 2006). The apnea ends when the clients awaken to reopen the airway. The frequent arousal interrupts the patterns of sleep. These clients experience sleepiness ranging from a subtle decrease in alertness to falling asleep in the middle of a conversation. Most data are collected from the bed partner because clients are unaware of their breathing pattern (Neubauer et al, 2002). **Clinical Findings:** Symptoms include reports of loud snoring and daytime sleepiness. Other clinical manifestations may include choking or gasping episodes at night and systemic and pulmonary hypertension.

CLINICAL APPLICATION & CLINICAL REASONING

See Appendix E for answers to exercises in this section.

REVIEW QUESTIONS

1 Nocturia and enuresis may be indicators of which sleep disorder?
1 Narcolepsy.
2 Sleep apnea.
3 Sleep terrors.
4 Insomnia.

2 What effect does drinking alcohol before sleep have on one's sleep patterns?
1 Nightmares.
2 Awakenings.
3 Awakening with difficulty returning to sleep.
4 Excessive drowsiness, confusion, and decreased energy.

3 Which are risk factors for obstructive sleep apnea?
1 Obesity, smoking, and thick neck circumference.
2 Heart disorders such as atrial fibrillation or heart failure.
3 Female, arid climate, and use of muscle relaxants.
4 Neuromuscular disorder such as spinal cord injury.

4 Which part of the brain maintains wakefulness?
1 The reticular activating system (RAS) in the upper brainstem.
2 The bulbar synchronizing region (BSR) in the pons and forebrain.
3 The hypothalamus and thalamus in the diencephalon.
4 The frontal lobe in the cerebral cortex.

5 What effect does heavy smoking (more than one pack per day) have on sleep?
1 Smoking interferes with REM dreaming.
2 Smoking causes nightmares.
3 Smoking enhances sleep by relaxation.
4 Smoking caused difficulty falling asleep.

SAMPLE DOCUMENTATION

Review the data obtained during an interview and examination by the nurse below.

D. H. is a 53-year-old black man who is accompanied by his wife to a follow-up appointment about his blood pressure. Vital signs recorded: temperature, 98.4° F (36.8° C); heart rate, 88 beats per minute; respiratory rate, 20 breaths per minute; blood pressure, 150/86 mm Hg. He says he is 6 feet 1 inch (185.42 cm) tall, and today he is weighed at 250 lb (113.6 kg). He is allergic to meperidine; it causes a rash. Mr. H. takes an aspirin daily as an anticoagulant and he also takes a multivitamin. He has been adhering to his low-fat diet and walking for 30 minutes three times a week with his wife to lose some weight. He quit smoking 2 years ago and does not drink alcohol for religious reasons. He has had a tonsillectomy, an appendectomy, and a right knee replacement. Mrs. H. mentions her husband's loud snoring and asks if anything can be done about it, because it has gotten worse during the past few months. Mr. H. sleeps 7 to 8 hours each night, but does not always feel rested when he wakes up. His bedtime routine is showering, brushing his teeth, and watching the nightly news. On days when he has difficulty staying awake, he takes a 1- to 2-hour nap in the afternoon. He has no difficulty going to sleep at night. Mrs. H. has noticed that his breathing sometimes stops at night, and other times he seems to be choking, so she wakes him up to make sure he is okay. Mr. H. reports some memory loss that he attributes to getting older. Mrs. H. says he seems to be more irritable and she thinks it is because he does not sleep well. Mr. H. is an alert and oriented obese black man with appropriate thought patterns. His speech is understandable and clear. His facial expressions and affect are appropriate. His nasal septum is aligned, symmetric, and open. He has a short, thick neck.

Below, note how the nurse recorded these same data in a documentation format and identified appropriate nursing diagnoses from the data.

53 y/o BM c̄ wife. CC: Follow up on treatment for HTN; wife c/o client snoring and choking. Medical Hx: tonsillectomy, appendectomy, TKA; Medications: ASA and MVI daily; Allergies: meperidine—rash.

SUBJECTIVE DATA
1800-calorie, low-fat diet, walking 30 min ×3 days per wk for wt loss, for HTN; quit smoking 2 yr ago, denies ETOH. Sleeps 7-8 hr/night c̄ 1-2 hr nap often; does not feel rested, difficulty staying awake often; c/o memory loss, irritable; periods of apnea during sleep—choking.

OBJECTIVE DATA
General survey: VS: T 98.4° F (36.8° C); HR 88, RR 20, BP 150/86; stated ht 6'1" (185.42 cm); measured wt 250 lb (113.6 kg).

General orientation: Alert, oriented obese black ♂ c̄ appropriate thought patterns. Speech is understandable, clear; facial expressions and affect appropriate.

Nose: Nasal septum is aligned, symmetric, and open.

Neck: Neck short, thick.

CASE STUDY

Brian is a 32-year-old man who comes to the clinic with a general complaint of feeling tired and not sleeping well. The following data are collected by the nurse from an interview and assessment.

Interview Data

Brian tells the nurse that he has not been sleeping well and wants something to help him sleep better. He states that lately he never feels rested. When asked about his sleep routine, he tells the nurse, "I go to bed about 11 PM each night and fall asleep quickly, but then I wake up around 2 AM and can't go back to sleep—I just end up tossing and turning." Brian tells the nurse that he does not have any specific routine before sleeping. "I just go to bed." When asked about stress in his life, Brian tells the nurse he is going through a divorce and may have to file bankruptcy. He states, "There has been so much stress lately that I have been having a couple of drinks every night to help me unwind."

Examination Data

- *Vital signs:* Blood pressure, 116/78 mm Hg; pulse rate, 92 beats/min; respirations, 20 breaths per minute; temperature, 98.6° F (37° C).
- *General survey:* Well-nourished adult male, ambulates slowly but smoothly. Hair matted. Slumped posture.
- *Mental status:* Oriented to person, place, and time. Speech slow with flat affect.
- All body system findings are within normal limits.

Clinical Reasoning

1. What data deviate from normal findings, suggesting to the nurse that Brian has a sleep pattern disturbance?
2. What additional information should the nurse ask or assess for?
3. Based on the data, what risk factors for insomnia does this client have?

INTERACTIVE ACTIVITIES

Open the interactive student CD-ROM, click on Chapter 8, and choose from the following activities on the menu bar:

- **Multiple Choice Challenge.** Click on the best answer for each question. You will be given immediate feedback, rationale for incorrect answers, and a total score. Good luck!

- **Crossword Wizard.** Complete the crossword puzzle using the clues associated with health assessment concepts. It's a whiz!

- **Marvelous Matches.** Drag each word or phrase to the appropriate place on the screen. Be careful where you place your answer—it won't stick if it's in the wrong place!

- **Printable Lab Guide.** Locate the Lab Guide for Chapter 8, and print and use it (as many times as needed) to help you apply your assessment skills. These guides may also be filled in electronically and then saved and e-mailed to your instructor!

- **Quick Challenge.** Use this critical thinking exercise to assess your skills through case study-style questions, then compare with expert answers!

CHAPTER 9

Nutritional Assessment

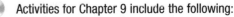
Because food and fluid are basic biologic needs, a nutritional assessment of the client is an integral part of the total health assessment. Nutritional assessment is not typically done in isolation: the collection of data specifically related to nutritional status and identifying risk factors for nutritional problems is usually part of a general examination. In addition to collecting a general health history, nurses explore questions detailing dietary intake and perceived nutrition-related problems. The nutritional examination includes anthropometric measurements, biochemical tests, and nutrition-focused examination. Although data collection varies with age groups and various stages in the life cycle (such as pregnancy), the general approach is consistent for clients of all ages.

ANATOMY & PHYSIOLOGY

Nutrients are necessary to provide the body calories for energy, to build and maintain body tissues, and to regulate body processes. The base energy requirement is called the *basal metabolic rate* (BMR), which is influenced by several factors. Activity levels, illness, injury, infection, ingestion of food, and starvation can all affect the BMR. When caloric intake meets energy needs, no weight change occurs. When energy needs exceed caloric intake, weight loss occurs. When caloric intake exceeds energy needs, weight gain occurs. Nutrients are classified into one of three groups: macronutrients, micronutrients, and water.

MACRONUTRIENTS

Carbohydrates, proteins, and fats are considered *macronutrients,* meaning nutrients needed in large amounts.

Carbohydrate is the main source of energy and fiber in the diet. Each gram of carbohydrate produces 4 kcal of energy. Fiber passes through the digestive tract partially undigested, providing bulk that stimulates peristalsis. The two main sources of carbohydrates are plant foods (fruits, vegetables, and grains) and lactose (from milk). Although a small amount of carbohydrate is stored in the liver and muscle in the form of glycogen (to serve as energy reserves between meals), moderate amounts of carbohydrates must be ingested at regular intervals to meet the energy demands. If more carbohydrate is ingested than needed, the excess is stored as adipose tissue. The recommended daily allowance (RDA) for carbohydrate intake is 130 g/day for children and adults but increases to 175 g/day during pregnancy and 210 g/day for lactating women (Institute of Medicine [IOM], 2002). Carbohydrates should account for 55% to 60% of total calories.

Protein plays an essential role in facilitating growth and repair of body tissues. Protein can also be a source of energy. The simplest form of protein is an amino acid. There are 20 different amino acids, and these combine in a number of different ways to form proteins. Ten of the amino acids are considered essential in the diet because they are not synthesized by the body. A complete-protein food contains all of the essential amino acids; complete proteins are also referred to as high–biologic-value proteins. Foods containing complete proteins include meat, fish, poultry, milk, and eggs. Foods that contain incomplete proteins include cereals, legumes, and some vegetables. Combinations of incomplete-protein foods can provide all the essential amino acids. If more protein is ingested than needed, the extra is used to supply energy or is stored as fat. Each gram of protein provides 4 kcal of energy. The RDA for protein intake in the adult diet is 0.8 g/kilogram of body weight, or an average of 56 g/day for adult males, and 46 g/day for adult females; 71 g/day for pregnant or lactating females (IOM, 2002). Ideally, protein should account for 12% to 20% of total kilocalories.

Fat is the main source of fatty acids, which are essential for normal growth and development. Other functions of fat include synthesis and regulation of certain hormones, tissue structure, nerve impulse transmission, energy, insulation,

and protection of vital organs. There are two essential fatty acids for metabolic processes: linoleic (or omega 3) and linolenic (or omega 6) acids. Fat is the body's major form of stored energy. One gram of fat yields 9 kcal of energy. If energy needs exceed carbohydrate intake, fat can be converted to glucose by a process known as gluconeogenesis. If more fat is ingested than needed, it is stored in adipose tissues. There is not an established RDA for total fat intake. The recommended percent of total calories from saturated fatty acids is less than 10% of total caloric intake; it is recommended that total fat intake should be between 25% to 30% of total caloric intake with most coming from polyunsaturated or monounsaturated fats (USDHH & USDA, 2005). It is estimated, however, that in the typical diet of Americans, 37% of caloric intake is derived from fats. When fats provide less than 10% of total calories, nutritional deficiencies may occur (Williams & Schlenker, 2003). Basic macronutrient calculations are shown in Box 9-1 and Box 9-2.

MICRONUTRIENTS

Micronutrients are nutrients required in small quantities. The two groups of micronutrients, vitamins and minerals, are essential for growth, development, and metabolic processes that occur continuously throughout the body.

Vitamins are classified as water soluble or fat soluble (Table 9-1). Water-soluble vitamins cannot be stored in the body, thus they must be ingested in the diet daily. Fat-soluble vitamins can be stored in the body, and vitamin toxicity can result if they are taken in large quantity. Deficiencies or toxicities in micronutrients result in nutritionally based diseases; when these deficiencies are clinically observed, it is usually a late sign of depletion.

Minerals are grouped into two categories: major minerals and trace minerals (Table 9-2). Major minerals are present in the body in large amounts with a required intake over 100 mg/day. Trace minerals are present in the body in smaller amounts; 10 of these are considered essential and have a required intake under 100 mg/day. The role of the remaining eight is unclear.

BOX 9-1 CALCULATING GRAMS OF A MACRONUTRIENT

To calculate the recommended number of grams of carbohydrate, proteins, and fats based on the number of calories in a diet, multiply the total calories by the recommended percent, and then divide by the number of kcals per gram.

(total kcals × recommended %) / kcals/gram

Example: Grams of carbohydrate, protein, and fat in a 1500 kcals diet.

Carbohydrates	1500 kcals × 55% carbohydrate = 825 calories/4 kcals = 206 grams
Protein	1500 kcals ×20% protein = 300 calories/4 kcals = 75 grams
Fat	1500 kcals × 25% fat = 375/9 kcal = 42 grams

BOX 9-2 CALCULATING THE PERCENT OF CALORIES FROM MACRONUTRIENTS

To calculate the percent of calories from carbohydrates, protein, and fat in a given food source, multiple the total grams by the kcal/gram and divide by the total number of calories.

(grams × kcal/gram) / total kcals

Example: Percent of kcals from carbohydrate, protein and fat in 8 oz of 2% milk. According to the label, 8 oz of milk has 125 kcals comprised of 12 grams of carbohydrate, 8 grams of protein, and 5 grams of fat.

Carbohydrates	12 grams of carbohydrates × 4 kcals/gram = 48 kcals/125 kcals = .38 or 38% carbohydrates
Protein	8 grams of protein × 4 kcals/gram = 32 kcals/125 kcals = .26 or 26% protein.
Fat	5 grams of fat × 9 kcals/gram = 45 kcals/125 kcals = .36 or 36% fat.

TABLE 9-1 *Vitamins*

Fat-Soluble Vitamins	Water-Soluble Vitamins
Vitamin A	Vitamin C
Vitamin D	B vitamins
Vitamin E	Thiamin
Vitamin K	Riboflavin
	Niacin
	Pyridoxine (B_6)
	Pantothenic acid
	Biotin
	Folate
	Cobalamin (B_{12})

TABLE 9-2 *Minerals*

MAJOR MINERALS	TRACE MINERALS	
	ESSENTIAL	UNCLEAR ROLE
Calcium	Iron	Silicon
Phosphorus	Iodine	Vanadium
Magnesium	Zinc	Nickel
Sodium	Copper	Tin
Potassium	Manganese	Cadmium
Chloride	Chromium	Arsenic
Sulfur	Cobalt	Aluminum
	Selenium	Boron
	Molybdenum	
	Fluoride	

WATER

Water composes 60% to 70% of total body weight, making it a critical component of the body. Cellular function depends on a well-hydrated environment. Because water is continually lost from the body, water replacement is required on a continual basis. Without water, an individual can survive for only a few days. The average adult metabolizes 2.5 to 3 L of water every day in the form of both foods and fluids. Fluid needs are increased in certain situations, especially fever, infection, gastrointestinal (GI) losses, and respiratory illness.

HEALTH HISTORY

RISK FACTORS *Nutrition*

As you conduct a health history related to nutrition, it is important to consider common risk factors associated with obesity, malnutrition, and eating disorders, and follow up with additional questions if such risk factors exist.

Obesity
- Sedentary lifestyle (M)
- High-fat diet (M)
- Genetics
- Ethnicity/Race
- Female

Protein Calorie Malnutrition (Undernutrition)
- Age
- Acute or chronic illness
- Side effects from medications or treatments
- Hospitalization or resident of long-term care facility
- Low socioeconomic status (M)

Eating Disorders
- Preoccupation with weight (M)
- Perfectionist (M)
- Poor self-esteem (M)
- Self-image disturbances (M)
- Peer pressure (M)
- Athlete—drive to excel (M)
- Compulsive or binge eating (M)

M = modifiable risk factor.

A nutritional history is a component of the health history discussed in Chapter 3. The nurse asks questions to elicit information about current health status, past medical history, family history, and risk factors. Specific questions are asked to assess the client's actual or potential nutritional needs and to assess for nutrition-related problems. Data gained from the history are used to evaluate the adequacy of the diet and to identify areas needed for client education.

GENERAL HEALTH HISTORY

Present Health Status

Do you have any chronic illnesses? If so, describe.
Many chronic illnesses are associated with nutritional problems or require special dietary measures and referral to a reg-

istered dietitian (e.g., diabetes, cystic fibrosis, phenylketonuria, celiac disease, heart failure, renal failure, and cancer).

What medications do you take? How often do you take them? Can you recall the dose?
Many medications can affect nutritional status. Some medications affect appetite; others may cause GI discomfort such as nausea, fullness, constipation, or diarrhea. Some medications are affected by foods ingested; thus food restrictions may be necessary.

Have you noticed any unexplained changes in your weight in the last 6 months? If so, describe.
Weight should remain fairly stable over time. Significant or rapid changes in weight require further evaluation.

Do you have any food intolerances or allergies? If so, describe.

Many persons have intolerance to foods such as lactose or are allergic to foods such as nuts or shellfish.

ETHNIC & CULTURAL VARIATIONS

Lactose intolerance affects a larger percentage of some ethnic groups than others. Approximately 50 million people in the United States have partial to complete lactose intolerance. This intolerance affects the following percentages of various groups:

- Native Americans: 95%
- Asian Americans: 90%
- Black Americans: 70%
- Jewish Americans: 60%
- Hispanic Americans: 50%
- White Americans: less than 25%

From McQuaid K: Alimentary tract. In Tierney LM, McPhee SJ, Papadakis MA, editors: *Current medical diagnosis and treatment,* New York, 2003, Lange Medical/McGraw-Hill.

Do you have any problems obtaining, preparing, or eating foods? If so describe.

Obtaining adequate nutrition may be a problem for low-income groups or those with disabilities. Many individuals with physical deficits or illness may have difficulty with food procurement and preparation. If this is an issue, assess support systems (someone willing to purchase and prepare food) or assess for community resources (e.g., meals on wheels).

Do you use street drugs or drink alcohol? If so, describe.

The use of drugs or alcohol can contribute to nutritional deficiencies. Alcohol is a source of "empty" calories, that is, calories that supply no nutrients, which in turn suppresses the appetite. Alcohol also impairs the absorption of nutrients. Additionally, money spent on drugs and alcohol may replace money available for the purchase of food. Alcohol consumption is often underreported by clients with alcoholic histories.

Past Medical History and Family History

What concerns have you had in the past regarding your weight or problems eating? What measures did you take in attempts to correct the problems (diet modification, exercise, medications, surgery, etc.)? Were these measures effective?

A personal history of excessive weight gain (such as during a pregnancy) or weight loss with an illness is important to note. Most individuals who have experienced weight gain attempt to reduce weight. Determine what measures they have used or attempted in the past, and if they were effective.

Have you or has anyone in your family ever had nutrition-related problems such as obesity or diabetes?

Obesity in one or both parents makes an individual at higher risk for excessive weight, which is partly genetic and partly from learned patterns of behavior regarding eating. Obesity is

the prime risk factor for type 2 diabetes. Individuals with a family history of diabetes are at risk of developing the disease.

Have you or has anyone in your family suffered from an eating disorder such as compulsive eating disorders, bulimia, or anorexia nervosa?

Eating disorders most commonly occur during adolescence and may cause lingering deficiency-related or psychologic-related problems in adulthood.

PROBLEM-BASED HISTORY

The most commonly reported problems related to nutrition include weight loss, weight gain, difficulty chewing and swallowing, and loss of appetite or nausea. As with symptoms in all areas of health assessment, a symptom analysis is completed, which includes the location, quality, quantity, chronology, setting, associated manifestations, alleviating factors, and aggravating factors (see Box 3-3 in Chapter 3).

Weight Loss

When did the weight loss start? What is your normal weight? What is your weight now? How many pounds have you lost in the last 6 months?

Determine onset and extent of weight loss. It is also important to determine if weight loss has been sudden or gradual.

What do you attribute the weight loss to? Was the weight loss desired or undesired? If desired, what measures did you take to lose the weight? If undesired, what do you think is causing you to lose weight?

Desired weight loss may be due to a change in eating habits or an increase in exercise. Strict calorie intake, fasting, bulimia, laxative abuse, and excessive exercise are indications of a preoccupation with body weight or a possible eating disorder (see Risk Factors: Nutrition box). Undesired weight loss may be caused by loss of appetite, vomiting, illness, stress, or medications. Individuals are usually able to explain what they think is causing the weight loss.

Have you had any symptoms associated with the loss of weight, such as fatigue, headaches, bruising, constipation, hair loss, or cracks in corners of the mouth?

Excessive weight loss may cause a number of symptoms because of inadequate energy and protein and deficiency in vitamins and minerals.

Weight Gain

When did you start gaining weight? What do you consider your normal weight? What is your weight now? How many pounds have you gained in the last 6 months?

Establish the total weight gained and the time frame over which it occurred, whether sudden or gradual.

To what do you attribute your weight gain? Has it been intentional? Unintentional?

Desired weight gain usually occurs from an intentional increase in caloric intake or use of dietary supplements (or both). Undesired weight gain may result from a decrease in activity levels, change in eating habits, increased appetite, or smoking cessation. It may also be associated with fluid retention as a result of certain medical conditions (e.g., heart failure) or as a side effect of certain medications (e.g., corticosteroids).

Difficulty Chewing or Swallowing

Tell me about the problems you are experiencing with chewing or swallowing (or both). When did this start?

Ask the client about the nature of the problem. Determine the time frame over which the chewing or swallowing difficulties have occurred. Choking and coughing are common symptoms associated with impaired swallowing.

What types of foods cause you the most problems eating?

Thin liquids and foods requiring forceful chewing (such as meat) may not be tolerated well.

What types of foods are you able to consume without difficulty?

Foods that are soft and highly viscous are most easily chewed and swallowed.

Has your weight changed since this problem developed?

Weight loss, particularly if undesired, may be an indication that food intake is hampered by chewing or swallowing difficulties.

Loss of Appetite or Nausea

Tell me about the problems you are experiencing with appetite or nausea (or both). When did you first notice this? Is the problem constant or does it come and go?

Establish the onset of the problem—this may provide clues as to the cause and potential nutritional deficiencies. Appetite may fluctuate from time to time. A reduction in appetite over an extended period of time may result in nutritional deficiencies.

To what do you attribute the loss of appetite or nausea (medications, illness, pregnancy, depression, etc.)?

The client often has an idea of what is causing a change in appetite or nausea. Medications, pregnancy, certain chronic illnesses, and depression can all contribute to changes in appetite or nausea.

What types of foods are the most offensive or most intolerable? What types of foods are you able to consume without difficulty?

In some cases, an individual may avoid an entire food group and eat from another. It is important to determine what nutrients the client is consuming and identify possible deficiencies in the diet.

Have you had a change of weight since this problem developed?

A significant change in weight indicates a problem and may suggest nutritional deficiencies as well.

ASSESSMENT OF DIETARY INTAKE

To complete an individual nutritional assessment, information regarding the client's dietary intake is collected. Obtaining accurate information on total dietary intake is a challenge because of the high incidence of underreporting, the wide variation in the day-to-day intake, and variations in serving portions. Thus a "snapshot" of nutrient intake over 1 day, or even over a course of several days, may not be an accurate reflection of intake over a long period of time. Nutrient intakes are estimated using a variety of instruments and techniques (Table 9-3). In addition to determining nutrient intakes, ask clients about their appetite, food preferences, food dislikes, and food intolerances. Also specifically ask clients about special diets they may be following and the use of dietary supplements or herbs. Diets may be followed for weight loss, weight gain, or disease control (e.g., low-salt diet), or as part of cultural/religious practice.

ETHNIC & CULTURAL VARIATIONS

Jewish Dietary Laws
Some people of the Jewish culture adhere to kosher standards. Laws that dictate which foods are permissible under religious law are found in Leviticus and Deuteronomy. The term *kosher* means "fit to eat"; it is not a method of food preparation. Because life is sacred and animal cruelty is forbidden, the kosher slaughter of animals is performed in a way so that the animals die instantaneously. All blood is drained from the animal before eating it.

Milk and meat may not be mixed together in cooking, serving, or eating. To avoid mixing foods, utensils used to prepare food and plates used to serve them are separated. Jewish people who follow these dietary laws have one set of dishes, pots, and utensils for milk products and one set for meat products. Because glass is nonabsorbent, it can be used for either meat or milk products.

From Purnell LD, Paulanka BJ: *Transcultural health care: a culturally competent approach*, ed 2, Philadelphia, 2003, FA Davis.

TABLE 9-3   *Techniques to Assess Dietary Intake*

Technique	Description	Comments
24-hour recall	Client recalls what he or she has eaten in the last 24 hours.	Very easy to use; does not need a trained interviewer Useful as a quick screening tool May not be reflective of typical daily intake
Typical food intake	Client describes what types of food he or she typically eats at specified times—breakfast, lunch, dinner, snacks.	Does not require trained interviewer Can be directed at specific nutrients (e.g., protein or fats) May not be accurate reflection of actual intake
Food diary	Client is asked to record all food eaten for a specified length of time (e.g., 3 days or 1 week).	Provides detailed information Not convenient—requires follow-up visit May not accurately reflect actual intake over time Analysis of data gained is time consuming
Food frequency questionnaires	Client indicates frequency of intake of certain foods over a period of time (e.g., number of servings and types of fruit eaten in a typical week).	Easy to use Client recalls types of foods typically eaten as opposed to actual foods eaten Does not assess intakes of all available foods—foods listed are usually those that are considered major contributors to the nutrients under study
Comprehensive diet history	An in-depth interview that provides detailed information regarding food intake.	May provide more accurate reflection of nutrient intake Is time consuming to acquire Requires a trained/skilled dietary interviewer

HEALTH PROMOTION   *Overweight and Obesity*

Obesity is one of the most serious health care problems in the United States not only because of the significant incidence found in all age groups, but also because obesity contributes to many other diseases, including hypertension, hyperlipidemia, type 2 diabetes, cardiovascular disease, gallbladder disease, sleep disturbances, respiratory disease, degenerative joint disease, and certain types of cancer. Over half the adults in the United States are overweight or obese, with the greatest prevalence among low socioeconomic groups and certain ethnic groups (African American and Mexican American). In children, obesity significantly increases the probability of developing type 2 diabetes.

Goals and Objectives—*Healthy People 2010*
Overweight and obesity is one of the leading health indicators identified by *Healthy People 2010*. The *Healthy People 2010* goal for nutrition and overweight is to promote health and reduce chronic disease associated with diet and weight. Three specific objectives address overweight and obesity:
- Increase the proportion of adults who are at a healthy weight.
- Reduce the proportion of adults who are obese.
- Reduce the proportion of children and adolescents who are overweight or obese.

Recommendations to Reduce Risk (Primary Prevention)
U.S. Preventive Services Task Force
- Intensive dietary counseling for adult patients with hyperlipidemia and other known risk factors for diet-related chronic disease is recommended.
- There is fair to good evidence that high-intensity counseling (for diet, exercise, or both) and behavioral interventions produce modest, sustained weight loss in adults who are obese.
- It is unknown if behavioral counseling in primary care settings to promote physical activity is effective; unable to determine if counseling leads to sustained increases in physical activity among adult patients.

Screening Recommendations (Secondary Prevention)
U.S. Preventive Services Task Force
- BMI assessment is reliable and valid for identifying adults at risk of morbidity and mortality due to overweight or obesity. For this reason, calculating BMI is recommended for all individuals on a periodic basis; the frequency of measurements is a matter of clinical discretion.
- Infants and children: height and weight should be compared to averages for weight, height, and gender to determine need for further evaluation.
- Adolescents: a body mass index (BMI) exceeding 85th percentile for age and gender may be used as a basis for further evaluation.
- Adults: BMI may be used as basis for evaluation of height and weight; insufficient evidence to recommend for or against using waist-to-hip ratio as routine screening test for obesity.

Recommendations for Treatment/Referral (Tertiary Prevention)
U.S. Preventive Services Task Force
- The evidence is insufficient to recommend for or against weight reduction counseling or behavioral interventions to promote sustained weight loss among overweight or obese individuals.

From: US Department of Health and Human Services: *Healthy People 2010: understanding and improving health,* ed 2, Washington, DC, 2000, US Government Printing Office (available at *www.healthypeople.gov*); US Preventive Services Task Force: Counseling for a healthy diet and *Screening and interventions to prevent obesity in adults.* In *Guide to clinical preventive services* (available at *www.ahrq.gov*).

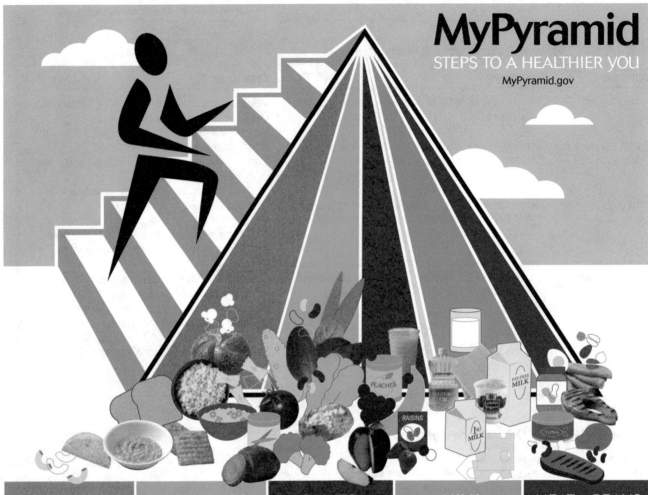

MyPyramid
STEPS TO A HEALTHIER YOU
MyPyramid.gov

GRAINS	VEGETABLES	FRUITS	MILK	MEAT & BEANS
Make half your grains whole	Vary your veggies	Focus on fruits	Get your calcium-rich foods	Go lean with protein
Eat at least 3 oz. of whole-grain cereals, breads, crackers, rice, or pasta every day 1 oz. is about 1 slice of bread, about 1 cup of breakfast cereal, or ½ cup of cooked rice, cereal, or pasta	Eat more dark-green veggies like broccoli, spinach, and other dark leafy greens Eat more orange vegetables like carrots and sweetpotatoes Eat more dry beans and peas like pinto beans, kidney beans, and lentils	Eat a variety of fruit Choose fresh, frozen, canned, or dried fruit Go easy on fruit juices	Go low-fat or fat-free when you choose milk, yogurt, and other milk products If you don't or can't consume milk, choose lactose-free products or other calcium sources such as fortified foods and beverages	Choose low-fat or lean meats and poultry Bake it, broil it, or grill it Vary your protein routine — choose more fish, beans, peas, nuts, and seeds

For a 2,000-calorie diet, you need the amounts below from each food group. To find the amounts that are right for you, go to MyPyramid.gov.

Eat 6 oz. every day	Eat 2½ cups every day	Eat 2 cups every day	Get 3 cups every day; for kids aged 2 to 8, it's 2	Eat 5½ oz. every day

Find your balance between food and physical activity
- Be sure to stay within your daily calorie needs.
- Be physically active for at least 30 minutes most days of the week.
- About 60 minutes a day of physical activity may be needed to prevent weight gain.
- For sustaining weight loss, at least 60 to 90 minutes a day of physical activity may be required.
- Children and teenagers should be physically active for 60 minutes every day, or most days.

Know the limits on fats, sugars, and salt (sodium)
- Make most of your fat sources from fish, nuts, and vegetable oils.
- Limit solid fats like butter, stick margarine, shortening, and lard, as well as foods that contain these.
- Check the Nutrition Facts label to keep saturated fats, *trans* fats, and sodium low.
- Choose food and beverages low in added sugars. Added sugars contribute calories with few, if any, nutrients.

MyPyramid.gov
STEPS TO A HEALTHIER YOU

U.S. Department of Agriculture
Center for Nutrition Policy and Promotion
April 2005
CNPP-15

USDA

Fig. 9-1 MyPyramid Food Guide. *(From the U.S. Department of Agriculture, Center for Nutrition Policy and Promotion. Available online at www.MyPyramid.gov.)*

HEALTH PROMOTION *Diabetes Mellitus*

The incidence of diabetes, particularly type 2 diabetes, is steadily increasing, making it a significant concern for the health and well-being of Americans. It is estimated that 800,000 new cases are diagnosed in the United States each year. Diabetes is most common in individuals over age 60 and has greatest incidence among Hispanics, American Indians, and African Americans. Long-term consequences of diabetes include blindness, end-stage renal disease, lower extremity amputations, increased risk for heart disease, and stroke. Diabetes is the seventh leading cause of death in the United States, primarily from diabetes-associated cardiovascular disease. Evidence exists that type 2 diabetes can be prevented or delayed.

Goals and Objectives—*Healthy People 2010*

The overall *Healthy People 2010* goals related to diabetes are to reduce the disease and economic burden of diabetes and improve the quality of life for all persons who have or are at risk for diabetes through prevention programs. Seventeen specific objectives have been identified, including the following: prevent diabetes/reduce the rate of new cases; reduce diabetes-related deaths; decrease the proportion of pregnant women with gestational diabetes; reduce the frequency of foot ulcers; reduce the rate of lower extremity amputations; increase the proportion of diabetics who have an annual urinary microalbumin test, glycosylated hemoglobin measurement, dilated eye examination, foot examination, and dental examination; increase the proportion of diabetics who take aspirin at least 15 days per month; and increase the proportion of diabetics who perform self-monitoring of glucose at least once daily.

Recommendations to Reduce Risk (Primary Prevention)
American Diabetes Association

- Encourage lifestyle modification in all overweight or sedentary individuals; modest weight loss (5% to 10% of body weight) and modest physical activity (30 minutes daily) are the recommended goals. Such recommendations should be made at every opportunity.

- There is insufficient evidence to support the use of drug therapy as a substitute for, or routinely used in addition to, lifestyle modification to prevent diabetes.

Screening Recommendations (Secondary Prevention)
American Diabetes Association

- Screen adults at 3-year intervals beginning at age 45, particularly in those with BMI > 25; consider screening at younger age or more frequently in individuals with several risk factors.
- The suggested screening test for diabetes is the fasting plasma glucose (FPG). The oral glucose tolerance test (OGTT) is also suitable; however, the FPG test is preferred because it is easier and faster to perform, more convenient and acceptable to patients, and less expensive. An FPG of 126 mg/dl (7.0 mmol/L) indicates a need for retesting; the test should be repeated on a different day to confirm a diagnosis.
- Screen children and adults with a substantial risk for development of type 2 diabetes. Those at substantial risk have two or more of the following risk factors: family history of type 2 diabetes; signs of insulin resistance; racial/ethnic group Native American, African American, or Hispanic American.
- Children who are overweight (BMI > 85th percentile) and have two risk factors listed previously should be tested every 2 years starting at age 10.
- It is unknown if community screening is a cost-effective approach to reduce the morbidity and mortality rates associated with diabetes in presumably healthy individuals.

Recommendations for Treatment (Tertiary Prevention)
American Diabetes Association

Individuals with diabetes should receive the following ongoing care to prevent progression of diabetic complications: annual foot examination, annual eye examination, annual renal evaluation; ongoing blood pressure management, lipid management, aspirin therapy.

From American Diabetes Association: *Standards of Medical Care in Diabetes, 2007* (available at *www.diabetes.org*); US Department of Health and Human Services: *Healthy people 2010: understanding and improving health,* ed 2, Washington, DC, 2000, US Government Printing Office (available at *www.healthypeople.gov*).

Once the client's dietary intake is obtained, the adequacy of the diet is evaluated. Several methods can be used to determine adequacy of dietary intake. Comparing diet intake to the food guide pyramid is the simplest approach to dietary assessment. Determine the number of servings per day for each of the six groups, and compare food intake with the recommended number of servings. The food guide pyramid (Fig. 9-1) indicates the recommended daily servings for each of the food groups. A web-based interactive program and additional information for consumers and health care professionals are easily located on the web at www.mypyramid.gov.

A more accurate approach is to compare the client's intake with the dietary reference intakes (DRIs), published by the Institute of Medicine. The DRIs are used to assess and plan diets of individuals or groups of individuals. DRIs comprise four nutrient-based reference values including estimated average requirement (EAR), recommended daily allowance (RDA), adequate intake (AI), and tolerable upper intake level (UI). Evaluating adequacy of dietary intake with DRIs is time consuming—because one needs to know an individual's requirement (based on DRI values) and the individual's long-term usual intake of nutrients—and requires expertise. For these reasons, this approach is not completed as part of a routine nursing assessment and is beyond the scope of this chapter. DRI tables are available on the United States Department of Agriculture website at *www.usda.gov.*

EXAMINATION

Many nutritional deficiencies become apparent through routine examination. Table 9-4 summarizes common findings associated with nutritional deficiencies. Some findings, however, may not be nutritionally related. For example, multiple bruises could be associated with nutritional deficiency, but they could also be related to trauma to the tissue. For this reason, findings must be considered in association with a detailed history.

TABLE 9-4 *Clinical Signs and Symptoms of Various Nutrient Deficiencies*

AREA OF EXAMINATION	SIGN/SYMPTOM	POTENTIAL NUTRIENT DEFICIENCY
Hair	Alopecia	Zinc, essential fatty acids
	Easy pluckability	Protein, essential fatty acids
	Lackluster	Protein, zinc
	"Corkscrew" hair	Vitamin C, vitamin A
	Decreased pigmentation	Protein, copper
Eyes	Xerosis of conjunctiva	Vitamin A
	Corneal vascularization	Riboflavin
	Keratomalacia	Vitamin A
	Bitot's spots	Vitamin A
Gastrointestinal tract	Nausea, vomiting	Pyridoxine
	Diarrhea	Zinc, niacin
	Stomatitis	Pyridoxine, riboflavin, iron
	Cheilosis	Pyridoxine, iron
	Glossitis	Pyridoxine, zinc, niacin, folate, vitamin B_{12}
	Magenta tongue	Riboflavin
	Swollen, bleeding gums	Vitamin C
	Fissured tongue	Niacin
	Hepatomegaly	Protein
Skin	Dry and scaling	Vitamin A, essential fatty acids, zinc
	Petechiae/ecchymoses	Vitamin C, vitamin K
	Follicular hyperkeratosis	Vitamin A, essential fatty acids
	Nasolabial seborrhea	Niacin, pyridoxine, riboflavin
	Bilateral dermatitis	Niacin, zinc
Extremities	Subcutaneous fat loss	Kcalories
	Muscle wastage	Kcalories, protein
	Edema	Protein
	Osteomalacia, bone pain, rickets	Vitamin D
	Arthralgia	Vitamin C
Neurologic	Disorientation	Niacin, thiamin
	Confabulation	Thiamin
	Neuropathy	Thiamin, pyridoxine, chromium
	Paresthesia	Thiamin, pyridoxine, vitamin B_{12}
Cardiovascular	Congestive heart failure, cardiomegaly, tachycardia	Thiamin
	Cardiomyopathy	Selenium

Data from Ross Products Division, Abbott Laboratories Inc. In Seidel HM et al: *Mosby's guide to physical examination,* ed 6, St Louis, 2006, Mosby.

ROUTINE TECHNIQUES	SPECIAL CIRCUMSTANCES OR ADVANCED PRACTICE
• MEASURE height and weight for body mass index. • ASSESS general appearance and level of orientation. • INSPECT skin for surface characteristics, hydration, and lesions. • INSPECT hair and nails for appearance and texture. • INSPECT eyes for surface characteristics. • INSPECT the oral cavity for dentition and mucous membranes. • INSPECT and PALPATE the extremities for shape, size, coordinated movement, and sensation.	• CALCULATE desirable body weight. • CALCULATE percent change in weight. • CALCULATE the waist-to-hip ratio. • ESTIMATE body fat by measuring triceps skinfold. ★ • ASSESS nutritional status by reviewing laboratory tests (if available).

EQUIPMENT NEEDED
Weight and height scale • Calculator • Tape measure • Skinfold calipers

★ = advanced practice

ROUTINE TECHNIQUES: NUTRITION

PROCEDURES AND TECHNIQUES WITH NORMAL FINDINGS

ABNORMAL FINDINGS

MEASURE height and weight for body mass index (BMI).

Body mass index (BMI) is a weight-to-height ratio that is significantly correlated with total body fat. It is an alternative to the traditional height-weight tables for assessing nutritional status. BMI can be estimated using a BMI table (Table 9-5) or a nomogram (Fig. 9-2), or it can be specifically calculated using the formula in Box 9-3.

The normal range for BMI is 18.5 to 24.9.

Clients increase their risk of developing nutrition-related problems the further their weight varies from the normal range.

BMI <18.5: underweight
BMI 25-29.9: overweight
BMI 30-34.9: obesity class I
BMI 35-39.9: obesity class II
BMI >40: obesity class III (extreme obesity)

ETHNIC & CULTURAL VARIATIONS

Prevalence of obesity (BMI > 30) differs among various racial groups.
• The highest prevalence of obesity is among African Americans (39.9%) followed by Hispanics (34.4%); the prevalence of obesity among Whites is 28.7%.
• Among women, African Americans have the highest prevalence of being obese (50.8%) followed by Hispanics (40.1%). The prevalence of obesity among white women is 30.6%
• Among men, the prevalence of obesity based on racial group is less significant. Hispanics, 29.4%; African Americans, 28.8%; Whites, 27.7.

From the CDC, National Center for Health Statistics, *National Health and Nutrition Examination Survey, 2002.*

ASSESS general appearance and level of orientation.

A well-nourished individual is alert and has a body that is well proportioned and within an acceptable weight range.

Poor nutritional status may be recognized from general observation. Excessive obesity or generalized edema is an obvious indicator of poor nutritional status. Prominent cheek and clavicle bones or wasted-appearing limbs (cachexia) suggest malnutrition. A client with insufficient caloric intake may be irritable or have a flat affect. Disorientation can be caused by niacin deficiency.

TABLE 9-5 *Body Mass Index Chart**

BMI HEIGHT (INCHES)	19	20	21	22	23	24	25	26	27	28	29	30	31	32	33	34	35
							BODY WEIGHT (POUNDS)										
58	91	96	100	105	110	115	119	124	129	134	138	143	148	153	158	162	167
59	94	99	104	109	114	119	124	128	133	138	143	148	153	158	163	168	173
60	97	102	107	112	118	123	128	133	138	143	148	153	158	163	168	174	179
61	100	106	111	116	122	127	132	137	143	148	153	158	164	169	174	180	185
62	104	109	115	120	126	131	136	142	147	153	158	164	169	175	180	186	191
63	107	113	118	124	130	135	141	146	152	158	163	169	175	180	186	191	197
64	110	116	122	128	134	140	145	151	157	163	169	174	180	186	192	197	204
65	114	120	126	132	138	144	150	156	162	168	174	180	186	192	198	204	210
66	118	124	130	136	142	148	155	161	167	173	179	186	192	198	204	210	216
67	121	127	134	140	146	153	159	166	172	178	185	191	198	204	211	217	223
68	125	131	138	144	151	158	164	171	177	184	190	197	203	210	216	223	230
69	128	135	142	149	155	162	169	176	182	189	196	203	209	216	223	230	236
70	132	139	146	153	160	167	174	181	188	195	202	209	216	222	229	236	243
71	136	143	150	157	165	172	179	186	193	200	208	215	222	229	236	243	250
72	140	147	154	162	169	177	184	191	199	206	213	221	228	235	242	250	258
73	144	151	159	166	174	182	189	197	204	212	219	227	235	242	250	257	265
74	148	155	163	171	179	186	194	202	210	218	225	233	241	249	256	264	272
75	152	160	168	176	184	192	200	208	216	224	232	240	248	256	264	272	279
76	156	164	172	180	189	197	205	213	221	230	238	246	254	263	271	279	287

From National Institutes of Health/National Heart, Lung, and Blood Institute: Clinical guidelines on the identification, evaluation, and treatment of overweight and obesity in adults: the evidence report, June 1998.

*To use the table, find the appropriate height in the left-hand column. Move across to a given weight. The number at the top of the column is the BMI at that height and weight. Pounds have been rounded off.

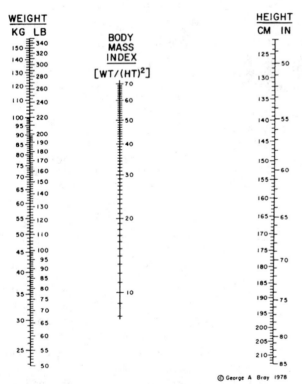

NOMOGRAM FOR BODY MASS INDEX

Fig. 9-2 **Nomogram to estimate body mass index.** Measure height to the nearest inch and weight to the nearest pound; mark on the two corresponding scales. Use a straight-edge ruler to connect the two points and circle the spot where the straight line crosses the center line. *(Reprinted with permission of the Nutrition Screening Initiative, a project of the American Academy of Family Physicians, the American Dietetic Association, and the National Council on Aging, Inc.)*

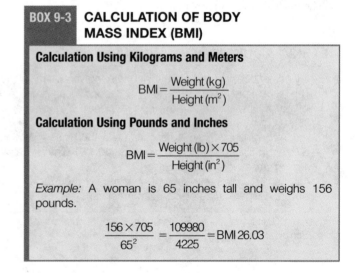

BOX 9-3 **CALCULATION OF BODY MASS INDEX (BMI)**

Calculation Using Kilograms and Meters

$$BMI = \frac{Weight\,(kg)}{Height\,(m^2)}$$

Calculation Using Pounds and Inches

$$BMI = \frac{Weight\,(lb) \times 705}{Height\,(in^2)}$$

Example: A woman is 65 inches tall and weighs 156 pounds.

$$\frac{156 \times 705}{65^2} = \frac{109980}{4225} = BMI\,26.03$$

PROCEDURES AND TECHNIQUES WITH NORMAL FINDINGS

INSPECT the skin for surface characteristics, hydration, and lesions.

The skin should be smooth, elastic, and without lesions, cracks, or bruising.

INSPECT the hair and nails for appearance and texture.

In well-nourished individuals, hair appears shiny, smooth, and firm. Nails should be pink, smooth, intact, and firm.

INSPECT the eyes for surface characteristics.

Mucous membranes (conjunctivae) around the eyes should be pink and free of lesions or drainage. The corneas should be clear and shiny.

ABNORMAL FINDINGS

Many nutritional deficiencies and fluid imbalance can be recognized by changes to the skin. The presence of edema indicates fluid retention (which may reflect protein depletion), whereas dry skin and decreased skin turgor may reflect dehydration. Multiple bruises are associated with vitamin C and K deficiencies; essential fatty acid deficiencies lead to dry flaking skin and eczema. Follicular hyperkeratosis is associated with vitamin A deficiency (Fig. 9-3).

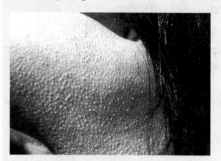

Fig. 9-3 Follicular hyperkeratosis. *(From McLaren, 1992.)*

Hair that is dull and falls out easily or observable hair loss indicates protein and fatty acid deficiencies. Spoon-shaped nails may be associated with iron deficiency.

Conjunctivae that are pale may be a sign of anemia. Excessively red conjunctivae may indicate riboflavin deficiency. Foamy-looking areas on the eyes (known as Bitot's spots) or excessively dry eyes are caused by vitamin A deficiency; with further deficiency the cornea becomes dry and hard, a condition known as xerophthalmia (Fig. 9-4).

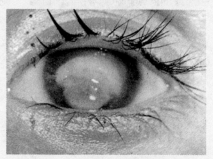

Fig. 9-4 Xerophthalmia. *(From McLaren, 1992.)*

PROCEDURES AND TECHNIQUES WITH NORMAL FINDINGS

INSPECT the oral cavity for dentition and intact mucous membranes.

The teeth should be present, clean, and intact; dentures, if present, should be assessed for fit. The mucous membranes and gums should be moist, pink, and free of lesions. The tongue and lips should be pinkish red, smooth, and without lesions.

INSPECT and PALPATE the extremities for shape, size, coordinated movement, and sensation.

Well-developed muscles should be observed, and these should be bilaterally equal. The client should have muscle strength and coordinated muscle movement, and full sensation to the extremities.

SPECIAL CIRCUMSTANCES OR ADVANCED PRACTICE: NUTRITION

CALCULATE desirable body weight (DBW).

Calculate the client's DBW and compare this to the actual body weight. These calculations allow you to express the current weight as a percentage of the DBW. The calculated weight can be increased or decreased by 10% to account for bone structure and amount of muscle or fat tissue. DBW is calculated using the formula in Box 9-4. Ideally, the client will fall between 90% and 110% of DBW.

BOX 9-4	CALCULATION OF DESIRABLE BODY WEIGHT (DBW)

Females: 100 lb (45.5 kg) for the first 5 feet (60 in); 5 lb (2.27 kg) for each inch greater than 5 feet; + or − 10%
Males: 106 lb (48 kg) for the first 5 feet (60 in); 6 lb (2.7 kg) for each inch greater than 5 feet; = or − 10%
Express the weight as a percentage of DBW by dividing the current weight by the DBW and multiplying by 100.

$$\text{Current weight}/\text{DBW} \times 100 = \% \text{ DBW}$$

Example:

$$\text{Current weight } 150 \text{ lb}/\text{DBW } 160 \text{ lb} = 0.9375 \times 100 = 93.8\% \text{ of DBW}$$

ABNORMAL FINDINGS

Poor dentition and painful oral lesions can negatively affect food intake. Dry mucous membranes may indicate dehydration. Bleeding gums may be a sign of vitamin C or vitamin K deficiency; vitamin B complex deficiency can cause cracks in the corners of the mouth or on the lips or an excessively red tongue. A reddish-purple tongue can be caused by riboflavin deficiency.

Muscle weakness and muscle wasting are signs of inadequate protein intake or excessive protein wasting. Uncoordinated muscle movements may interfere with the ability to feed self. Vitamin D deficiency can cause skeletal malformation. Thiamin deficiency can cause peripheral neuropathy and paresthesia.

Clients increase their risk of developing nutrition-related problems the further their weight varies from 100% DBW.

Severely underweight: 70% or less of DBW
Moderately underweight: 70% to 80% or less of DBW
Mild obesity: 20% to 40% above DBW
Moderate obesity: 40% to 100% above DBW
Morbid obesity: over 100% above DBW or over 45 kg higher than DBW.

PROCEDURES AND TECHNIQUES WITH NORMAL FINDINGS

ABNORMAL FINDINGS

CALCULATE percent change in weight.

Documentation of the amount of weight loss over a period of time may be helpful in determining the severity of weight loss. To determine the rate of weight loss, calculate the percentage change of weight by dividing current body weight by the usual body weight and multiplying by 100.

Current body weight/Usual body weight × 100 = % UBW

Moderate weight loss: 1% to 2% weight change over 1 week
Severe weight loss: >2% weight change over 1 week
Moderate weight loss: 5% weight loss over 1 month
Severe weight loss: >5% weight loss over 1 month, >7.5% weight loss over 3 months, or >10% weight loss over 6 months (Grodner et al., 2004).

CALCULATE the waist-to-hip ratio.

Waist-to-hip ratio is an indication of the risk of unhealthy fat distribution. To obtain the waist-to-hip ratio, measure the waist at the narrowest point, then measure the hips at the widest point. Calculate the waist-to-hip ratio using the following formula:

Waist (cm)/Hips (cm)
For example, if a man has a 44-inch waist (112 cm) and 40-inch hips (101 cm), the calculation would be as follows:
112 cm/101 cm = 1.1 waist-to-hip ratio
The desired waist-to-hip ratio for women is 0.8 or less and for men is 1.0 or less.

A ratio that exceeds the desired ratio is indicative of upper body obesity. This increases the risk of developing health problems related to obesity (e.g., diabetes, hypertension, coronary artery disease, gallbladder disease, osteoarthritis, and sleep apnea). Women typically collect fat in their hips, giving their bodies a pear (gynecoid) shape. Men, however, build up fat around their waists, giving them an apple (android) shape (Fig. 9-5).

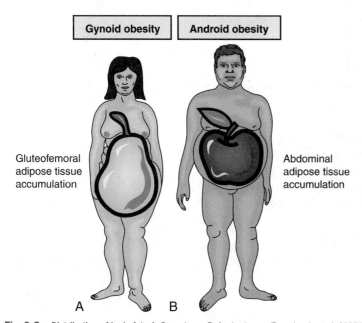

Gynoid obesity   Android obesity

Gluteofemoral adipose tissue accumulation

Abdominal adipose tissue accumulation

A   B

Fig. 9-5 **Distribution of body fat. A,** Pear shape. **B,** Apple shape. *(From Lewis et al, 2007.)*

PROCEDURES AND TECHNIQUES WITH NORMAL FINDINGS	ABNORMAL FINDINGS

★ **ESTIMATE body fat by measuring triceps skinfold.**

Skinfold measurements provide an estimate of total body fat (Fig. 9-6). Triceps skinfold measurements are made with skinfold calipers. The nurse uses the thumb and index finger to grasp and lift a fold of skin and fat about ½ inch (1.27 cm) on the posterior aspect of the client's arm halfway between the olecranon process (tip of the elbow) and acromial process on the lateral aspect of the scapula. Opened caliper jaws are placed horizontally to the raised skinfold; then the nurse releases the lever of the calipers to make the measurement to the nearest millimeter.

Values significantly higher than normal can indicate increased fat mass. Values significantly lower than normal can indicate decreased fat mass secondary to either an increase in lean mass or depleted fat stores.

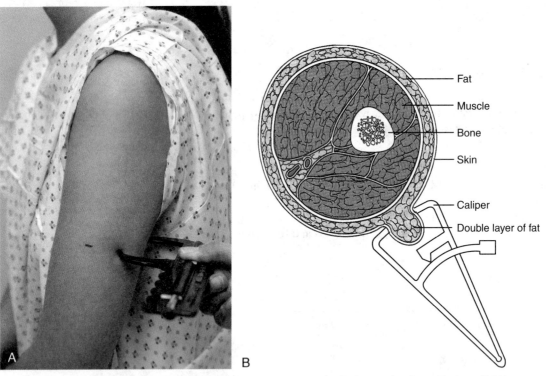

Fig. 9-6 **A,** Placement of calipers for triceps skinfold thickness measurement. **B,** Cross section of arm with triceps skinfold measurement. (**B,** From Barkauskus et al, 2002.)

Two or three measurements at the same site should be taken and the results averaged. Normal ranges for triceps skinfold fat measurements for men and women are included in Table 9-6. The desired skinfold measurement falls at or near the 50th percentile. Accuracy of this measurement is related to the skill of the nurse taking the measurements. Also, these measurements are not useful in clients who are acutely ill because of shifts in fluid.

★ = advanced practice

PROCEDURES AND TECHNIQUES WITH NORMAL FINDINGS

ABNORMAL FINDINGS

ASSESS nutritional status by reviewing laboratory tests.

Many laboratory tests are helpful in assessment of nutritional status. Not all of these tests are indicated for all situations.

Table 9-7 summarizes the tests, normal ranges, and abnormal findings for adults.

TABLE 9-6 *Percentiles for Triceps Skinfold Measurements (Adults)*

GENDER	TRICEPS SKINFOLD		
	5th	50th	95th
Males			
18-19	4	9	24
19-25	4	10	22
25-34	5	12	24
35-45	5	12	23
45-54	6	12	25
55-64	5	11	22
65-74	4	11	22
Females			
18-19	10	18	30
19-25	10	18	34
25-34	10	21	37
35-45	12	23	38
45-54	12	25	40
55-64	12	25	38
65-74	12	24	36

Data from Frisancho AR: New norms of upper limb fat and muscle areas for assessment of nutritional status, *Am J Clin Nutr* 34:2540-2545, 1981.

FREQUENTLY ASKED QUESTIONS

Why is body mass index (BMI) now used as opposed to the height and weight tables?
BMI still takes into account height and weight, but the difference is that a mathematical formula is applied to these data so that the same range is used for all individuals. A person with a BMI between 18.5 and 25 is within the normal range regardless of whether he or she is 5 feet 2 inches or 6 feet 7 inches tall.

FREQUENTLY ASKED QUESTIONS

What is the difference between serum albumin and pre-albumin?
Serum albumin simply measures circulating protein. Albumin can be affected by a number of factors, including fluid status, blood loss, liver function, and stress. Fluctuation of albumin levels occurs over 3 to 4 weeks. Prealbumin is a reflection of protein and calorie intake over the previous 2 to 3 days.

TABLE 9-7   *Laboratory Tests Used for Nutritional Assessment*

Test and Normal Value*	Purpose	Significance of Abnormal Findings
Serum albumin 3.5-5.0 g/dl or 35-50 g/L (SI units)	Measures circulating protein; levels can be affected by fluid status, blood loss, liver function, trauma, and surgery. Fluctuations in albumin levels occur over a 3- to 4-week period.	Low albumin levels suggest protein-calorie malnutrition. Levels between 2.8 and 3.5 g/dl are consistent with moderate protein deficiency; levels below 2.5 g/dl represent severe protein depletion. Rapid changes in albumin are most likely due to factors other than nutrition.
Prealbumin 15-36 mg/dl or 150-360 mg/L (SI units)	Prealbumin is a reflection of protein and calorie intake for the previous 2 to 3 days.	A deficiency of either calories or protein can cause prealbumin to decline. A malnourished individual undergoing refeeding therapy can produce rises in prealbumin levels.
Hemoglobin (Hgb) and hematocrit (Hct) Male: Hgb 14-18 g/dl or 8.7-11.2 mmol/L (SI units); Hct 42%-52% or 0.42-0.52 volume fraction (SI units) Female: Hgb 12-16 g/dl or 7.4-9.9 mmol/L (SI units); Hct 37%-47% or 0.37-0.47 volume fraction (SI units) Pregnancy: Hgb >11 g/dl; Hct >33%	Provides information regarding erythrocytes. These are clinically useful to screen for anemia caused by dietary deficiency such as iron, folate, and vitamin B_{12}. Hematocrit is also useful in evaluation of hydration.	Low hemoglobin and hematocrit levels suggest anemia. Causes of anemia are numerous, but dietary deficiencies of iron, vitamin B_{12}, or folate are a few possible causes. Elevated hemoglobin and hematocrit levels may occur in dehydration, chronic anoxia, and polycythemia. Elevated hematocrit levels suggest dehydration.
Blood glucose 70-105 mg/dl or 3.9-5.8 mmol/L (SI units)	Reflects carbohydrate metabolism. A fasting glucose level is used to screen for the presence of diabetes mellitus or glucose intolerance.	Hypoglycemia (blood glucose level less than 70 mg/dl) may indicate inadequate caloric intake. Hyperglycemia (blood glucose level over 126 mg/dl) may be an indication of diabetes mellitus.
Lipid profile *Serum cholesterol* <200 mg/dl or 5.20 mmol/L (SI units) *Serum triglyceride* Male: 40-160 mg/dl or 0.45-1.81 mmol/L Female: 35-135 mg/dl or 0.40-1.52 mmol/L *High-density lipoproteins (HDLs)* Male: >45 mg/dl or >0.75 mmol/L Female: >55 mg/dl or >0.91 mmol/L *Low-density lipoproteins (LDLs)* Male and female: 60-180 mg/dl or <3.37 mmol/L *Cholesterol to HDL* Male: 5.0 Female: 4.4	Lipid profile includes several tests that are indicators of lipid metabolism and are important determinants of risk factors for cardiovascular disease. A lipid profile includes total cholesterol and triglyceride levels, HDL level, LDL level, and cholesterol/high-density lipoprotein ratio. The cholesterol-to-HDL ratio is calculated by dividing the total cholesterol value by the HDL value.	Values equal to or greater than 200 mg/dl for total cholesterol and triglyceride levels indicate that the client is at increased risk for vascular disease. Elevations of LDL are associated with increased risk for developing coronary heart disease; elevated HDL levels reduce the risk.
BUN/creatinine ratio Up to 20:1.0	Blood test is used as an indication of hydration.	Levels 21:1-24:1 are associated with impending dehydration; levels >25:1 indicate dehydration.
Urine specific gravity	Urine test is used as an indication of hydration	Levels >1.029 are associated with dehydration.

From Pagana DK, Pagana TJ: *Mosby's diagnostic and laboratory test reference,* ed 8, St Louis, 2007, Mosby.

*Values for adults only; refer to a laboratory reference for other age groups.

BUN, Blood urea nitrogen.

AGE-RELATED VARIATIONS

INFANTS AND CHILDREN

The pediatric nutritional assessment includes many of the same components described for the adult, although some specific differences exist including assessing feeding patterns, assessment of body weight, plotting weight, length, and head circumference on a growth chart, observing for the presence of rooting reflex and effective suck effort and swallowing in infants, and observing for presence of tooth decay in children. Chapter 20 presents further information regarding the nutritional assessment from this age group.

OLDER ADULTS

The nutritional assessment for an older adult essentially is the same as previously described for adults with a few exceptions including ability to acquire and prepare food, social interactions, and general functional assessment. Chapter 22 presents further information regarding the nutritional assessment of older adults.

COMMON PROBLEMS & CONDITIONS

OBESITY

Obesity occurs when there is greater energy intake than energy expenditure. This condition is caused by genetics, overeating, and inactivity. In the United States, 65% of individuals are classified as overweight or obese (NCHS, 2005). **Clinical Findings:** Obesity is characterized by excessive adipose tissue to the face and neck, trunk, and extremities

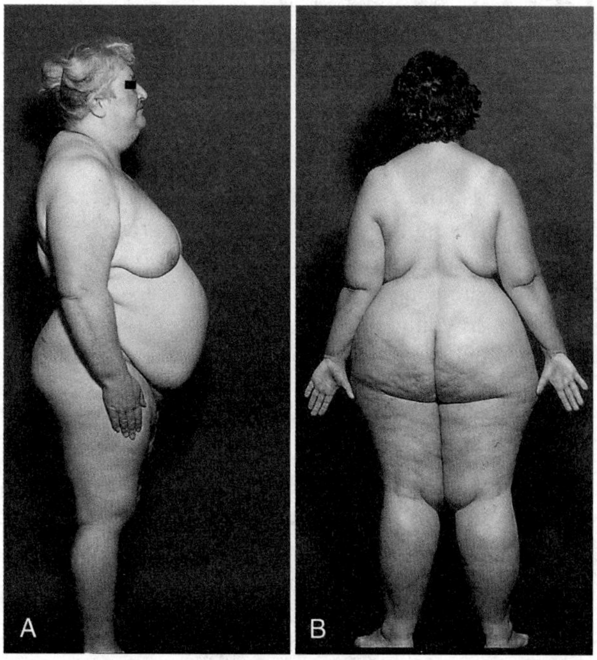

Fig. 9-7   Obesity. *(From Lewis et al, 2007).*

(Fig. 9-7). Overweight and obesity are clinically defined as a BMI greater than 25 and 30, respectively.

HYPERLIPIDEMIA

Hyperlipidemia is a condition associated with elevated serum lipids that can include cholesterol, triglycerides, and phospholipids. Causes include excessive dietary fat and genetics. Over 105 million American adults have total blood cholesterol values of 200 mg/dL and higher; 36.6 million American adults have levels of 240 mg/dL or above. **Clinical Findings:** Hyperlipidemia is not associated with any clinical symptoms until a significant cardiovascular event occurs. Biochemical indications include elevations in serum lipids. In adults, total cholesterol levels from 200 to 239 mg/dL are considered borderline-high; levels of 240 mg/dL or higher are considered high.

PROTEIN CALORIE MALNUTRITION (PCM)

Protein Calorie Malnutrition refers to the state of inadequate protein and calorie intake. PCM is the most common form of undernutrition and can result from poor or limited food intake, wasting disease (such as cancer), malabsorption syndromes, endocrine imbalances, and poor living conditions. **Clinical Findings:** The malnourished individual often appears thin with muscle wasting and a loss of subcutaneous fat (Fig. 9-8), and other protein deficiency findings presented in Table 9-4. One is considered underweight with a BMI of less than 18.5 or if more than 10% below DBW. Biochemical indications such as low serum levels of albumin or protein may exist.

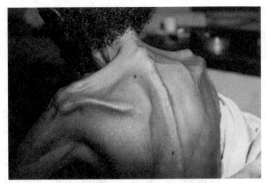

Fig. 9-8   Loss of subcutaneous fat and muscle wasting in patient with protein calorie malnutrition. *(From Swartz, 2006.)*

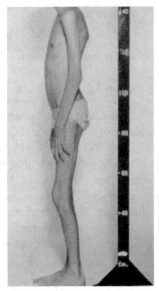

Fig. 9-9   Anorexia nervosa. *(From McCance, 2005.)*

EATING DISORDERS

Eating disorders refer to a group of psychiatric conditions resulting in altered food consumption. Three prevalent eating disorders are anorexia nervosa, bulimia nervosa, and binge eating disorder. It is estimated that 7% to 8% of females experience anorexia nervosa or bullemia nervosa during their lifetime (American Psychiatric Association, 2000). **Clinical Findings:** Clinical findings depend on type of eating disorder. **Anorexia Nervosa**: refusing to eat, extreme thinness, along with other symptoms of protein calorie malnutrition (Fig. 9-9). **Bullemia Nervosa:** recurrent binge-and-purge eating cycles, electrolyte imbalances, chronic irritation or erosion of the pharynx, esophagus, and teeth (from exposure to hydrochloric acid). **Binge Eating Disorder:** consumption of large quantities of food until uncomfortably full. Frequently the individual experiences feelings of being out of control during the binge episodes.

CLINICAL APPLICATION & CLINICAL REASONING

See Appendix E for answers to exercise in this section.

REVIEW QUESTIONS

1 The nurse is teaching a client how to evaluate the percentage of fat in a serving of food. She explains that if the label on a package of a toaster pastry states that there are 6 grams of fat and 210 calories per serving, the percentage of fat per serving is:
   1 26%.
   2 35%.
   3 54%.
   4 72%.

2 A man weighs 265 pounds and is 6 feet 4 inches tall. Based on these data, the nurse classifies his weight condition as:
   1 Overweight.
   2 Class I obesity.
   3 Class II obesity.
   4 Class III obesity.

3 An elderly woman is 5 feet 2 inches tall and weighs 100 pounds. To best understand her dietary intake, which of the following questions is most appropriate?
   1 "Who prepares your meals?"
   2 "What are your favorite foods?"
   3 "How do you get to the grocery store?"
   4 "Could you describe what you eat on a typical day?"

4 The nurse asks a client what medications he takes as part of a nutritional assessment for which of the following reasons?
   1 Medications must be taken with food to avoid irritation to the gastrointestinal system.
   2 Many drugs affect nutritional intake requirements; thus adjustments to the diet must be made.
   3 The absorption and bioavailability of some medications are affected by food.
   4 Some medications taste bad.

5 A client states that he has experienced "a lot" of unintentional weight loss over the past 4 months. The nurse measures his height and weight (5 feet 11 inches, 170 pounds) and determines that his BMI is 22.7. Which of the following is the most appropriate action to better evaluate his recent weight loss?

1 Calculate his desirable body weight.
2 Ask, "What is your usual body weight?"
3 Record what he ate in the last 24 hours.
4 Determine his hip-to-waist ratio.

SAMPLE DOCUMENTATION

Review the data obtained during an interview and examination by the nurse below.

Evelyn Dodson is a 73-year-old white woman new to the community who is seeking a health care professional to treat her hypertension and weight management. She states that she has had high blood pressure for about 15 years. She describes her overall health as good. Her current medication is a diuretic (furosemide, 40 mg daily) taken for blood pressure control. She has no illness other than hypertension. She states that she has had an ongoing weight problem for years, although she has had no weight change for several years. Her appetite is described as "good"; she eats three meals per day and admits to snacking a lot during the day. Her food preferences include fried foods and sweets such as cookies and cakes. She likes nearly all foods and does not have any food intolerances or food allergies. Ms. Dodson was advised to eat a low-salt diet in the past by her former physician, but admits she does not know what that means. She drinks five to six glasses of water per day, and she also drinks five to six cups of coffee per day. She does not drink any alcoholic beverages. She does not exercise—she says she is "too old and fat." Her activity is primarily housework and watching TV. Ms. Dodson says she thinks she is at risk for "heart problems" and would like assistance in reducing her risk. Vital signs recorded: Temperature, 98.3° F (36.8° C); heart rate, 82 beats/min; respiratory rate, 18; blood pressure, 142/100 mm Hg; measured height, 5 feet 3 inches (160 cm); measured weight, 172 lb (78 kg); body mass index, 30.5; desirable body weight, 115 lb. Serum cholesterol, 220 mg/dl; HDL, 55 mg/dl; LDL, 258 mg/dl. She is alert and oriented, and she is moderately obese in general appearance. She walks slowly but without difficulty, and her gait is smooth. Her skin is pink and somewhat dry, with loose turgor. She does not have any visible skin lesions. Her hair color is gray, and her hair is thick and full. Inside her mouth her gums are pink and moist without lesions or cracks. Her teeth are in good condition. Ms. Dodson wears glasses. Her eyes are clear, without any discharge or noticeable lesions, and the conjunctivae are pink. Her arms and legs appear similar in size on right and left sides; she has 5/5 muscle strength in arms and legs.

To the right, note how the nurse recorded these same data in a documentation format and identified appropriate nursing diagnoses and collaborative problems from the data.

E. D.; 73 y/o W F. Reason for seeking health care: HTN management and wt control.

SUBJECTIVE DATA

New to community; seeking health care professional for wt control and HTN mgt. HTN × 15 yr. Is concerned about risk for "heart problems"; requests assistance to reduce risk. Describes health as "good."

Current meds: Furosemide 40 mg daily for BP control (× 8 years).

Appetite: Described as "good."

Intake patterns: 3 full meals/day plus snacks; preference for fried foods and sweets; no food intolerances or allergies.

Dietary limitations: Previously advised to eat low-salt diet; admits to not understanding this.

Fluid intake: 5-6 glasses of water per day; 5-6 cups of coffee.

Activity: No exercise; sedentary lifestyle.

OBJECTIVE DATA

Vital signs and measurements: T 98.3° F (36.8° C); HR 82/min; RR 18/min; BP 142/100. Height 5 feet 3 inches (160 cm); weight 172 lb (78 kg); BMI 30.5; DBW 115 lb; 49% over DBW.

Labs: Serum cholesterol, 220 mg/dl; HDL, 55 mg/dl; LDL, 258 mg/dl.

General survey: Alert, moderate obesity; walks slowly and smoothly without difficulty.

Skin: Pink, even skin tone; dryness noted; no lesions or edema; loose skin turgor.

Hair: Gray; thick, full.

Oral cavity: Mucous membranes pink, moist, without lesions or cracks; teeth intact, good condition.

Eyes: Wears glasses; conjunctivae pink, no lesions or discharge.

Extremities: Upper and lower bilaterally equal; muscle strength 5/5.

CASE STUDY

Marian is a 45-year-old woman who is brought to the hospital after an episode of fainting.

Interview Data

Marian states that she has been very tired lately and gets short of breath and fatigues very easily. She also complains of cracks in the corners of her mouth that won't heal. When asked about her diet, she tells the nurse she is a "new vegetarian." She states that she started a vegetarian diet about 4 months ago "to prevent diseases and because animals are unclean." She acknowledges weight loss since starting the diet but states, "I am healthy because of what I eat and because I am thin." She refuses foods that contain meat or animal products. Her diet is described as "healthy," typically eating beans, rice, breads, and salad. She is not specific about portions, stating, "I eat the amount I am hungry for." Her fluid intake consists of coffee, tea, and water. She does not use drugs or alcohol. She also tells the nurse that her financial resources are very limited.

Examination Data

Vital signs and other measurements: Blood pressure, 118/76 mm Hg; pulse rate, 92 beats/min; respirations, 20; temperature, 98.2° F (36.8° C); height, 5 feet 4 inches (162 cm); weight, 110 lb (50 kg).

General observation: Very thin, protruding bony prominence to cheeks and clavicles.

Skin: Warm, very dry with scaling—especially on arms and legs.

Hair: Brown, thin, dull, easily plucked.

Oral cavity: Pink, moist mucous membranes without lesions. Teeth present, in good repair. Cracks noted in corners of mouth.

Eyes: Conjunctivae pale; no drainage or lesions.

Extremities: Bilaterally equal; extremities thin; small amount of muscle mass noted; muscle strength 4/5.

Clinical Reasoning

1. What data deviate from normal findings, suggesting a need for further investigation?

2. What additional information should the nurse ask or assess for?

3. What risk factors for nutritional problems can be identified?

4. What nursing diagnosis and collaborative problems should be considered for this situation?

INTERACTIVE ACTIVITIES

Open the interactive student CD-ROM, click on Chapter 9, and choose from the following activities on the menu bar:

- **Multiple Choice Challenge.** Click on the best answer for each question. You will be given immediate feedback, rationale for incorrect answers, and a total score. Good luck!

- **Printable Lab Guide.** Locate the Lab Guide for Chapter 9, and print and use it (as many times as needed) to help you apply your assessment skills. These guides may also be filled in electronically and then saved and e-mailed to your instructor!

- **Quick Challenge.** Use this critical thinking exercise to assess your skills through case study-style questions, then compare with expert answers!

CHAPTER 10

Skin, Hair, and Nails

ANATOMY & PHYSIOLOGY

The skin and the accessory structures—hair, nails, sweat glands, and sebaceous glands—form what is referred to as the *integumentary system.* The skin is an elastic, self-regenerating cover for the entire body. Because they are composed of several tissues that perform specialized tasks, the skin and related structures are considered a body organ. The skin has several important functions. The primary function is protection: the skin protects the body from microbial and foreign-substance invasion and protects internal body structures from minor physical trauma. The skin also helps retain body fluid and electrolytes—without skin, an individual would suffer tremendous water loss. The skin provides the body with its primary contact with the outside world, providing sensory input about the environment. Its sensitive surface detects and reports, via nerve endings and specialized receptors, comfort factors such as temperature and surface textures, enabling the body to adapt through either temperature regulation or position changes. This regulation of body temperature is accomplished continuously through radiation, conduction, convection, and evaporation. Other functions of the skin include production of vitamin D; excretion of sweat, urea, and lactic acid; expression of emotion (e.g., blushing); and even repair of its own surface wounds by exaggerating the normal process of cell replacement. The skin and appendages often mirror systemic disease and thus may provide valuable clues to an internal disorder.

SKIN

The skin is composed of three layers that are functionally related: the epidermis, the dermis, and the subcutaneous layer, also known as the hypodermis. The main components of each of these layers and their functional and spatial relationships are shown in Fig. 10-1.

Epidermis

The epidermis is the thin, outermost layer of the skin and is composed of stratified squamous epithelium. This layer of skin is *avascular,* meaning it has no direct blood supply. The deepest aspect of the epidermis is the stratum germinativum. This layer lies adjacent to the dermis, close to a rich supply of blood. Within this deepest layer of epidermis, active cell generation takes place. As cells are produced, they push up the older cells toward the skin surface. As the cells move toward the surface, they begin to die (because they move away from their nutritional source) and they undergo a process known as *keratinization,* in which keratin (a protein) is deposited, causing the cells to become flat, hard, and waterproof. The outermost aspect of the epidermis, the stratum corneum, is composed of 30 layers of these dead, flattened, keratinized cells. This exposed layer serves as the protective barrier and regulates water loss. The dead cells are continuously sloughed off and replaced by new cells moving up

111

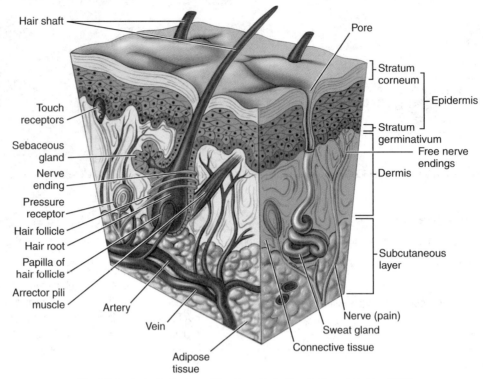

Fig. 10-1   Anatomic structures of the skin and hair. *(From Herlihy and Maebius, 2000.)*

from the underlying epidermal layers. The entire process takes about 30 days.

In addition to the generation of skin cells, the underlying epidermal layers contain hair roots, apocrine sweat glands, eccrine sweat glands, and sebaceous glands. Hair and nails arise from these underlying layers and are composed primarily of keratin. Melanocytes, located in the basal cell layer of the epidermis, secrete melanin, which provides pigment for the skin and hair and serves as a shield against ultraviolet radiation.

Dermis

The dermis is made up of highly vascular connective tissue. The blood vessels dilate and constrict in response to external heat and cold and to internal stimuli such as anxiety or hemorrhage, resulting in the regulation of body temperature and blood pressure. The dermal blood nourishes the epidermis, and the dermal connective tissue provides support for the outer layer. The dermis also contains sensory nerve fibers that react to touch, pain, and temperature. The arrangement of connective tissue enables the dermis to stretch and contract with body movement. Dermal thickness varies from 1 to 4 mm in different parts of the body.

Subcutaneous Layer

The subcutaneous tissue (hypodermis) is not actually skin tissue, but is a support structure for the dermis and epidermis—literally acting as an anchor for these upper layers. This layer is composed primarily of loose connective tissue interspersed with subcutaneous fat. These fatty cells help to retain heat, provide a protective cushion, and provide calories.

APPENDAGES

Hair, nails, and glands (the eccrine sweat glands, the apocrine sweat glands, and the sebaceous glands) are considered appendages. These structures are formed at the junction of the epidermis and the dermis.

Hair

Epidermal cells in the dermis form hair. Each hair consists of a root, a shaft, and a follicle (the root and its covering). At the base of the follicle is the papilla, a capillary loop that supplies nourishment for growth. Melanocytes within the hair shaft provide color. Variations in hair color, density, and pattern of distribution vary considerably as a result of age, gender, race, and hereditary factors. Structures of the hair follicle are shown in Fig. 10-1.

Nails

Nails are really epidermal cells converted to hard plates of keratin. The nails assist in grasping small objects and protect the fingertips from trauma. The nail is composed of a free edge, the nail plate, and the nail root—the site of nail growth. The white crescent-shaped area at the base, the lunula, represents new nail growth (Fig. 10-2). Skin tissue adjacent to the nail is referred to as paronychium; the cuticle is epidermal tissue (stratum corneum) that grows on the nail plate at the nail base. Tissue directly under the nail plate is highly vascular, providing clues to oxygenation status and blood perfusion.

Eccrine Sweat Glands

Eccrine sweat glands regulate body temperature by water secretion through the skin's surface. They are the most numerous and widespread sweat glands on the body. They are distributed almost everywhere throughout the skin's surface, found in greatest numbers on the palms of the hands, the soles of the feet, and the forehead.

Apocrine Sweat Glands

These structures are much larger and deeper than the eccrine glands; they are found only in the axillae, nipples, areolae, anogenital area, eyelids, and external ears. In response to emotional stimuli, the glands secrete an odorless fluid containing protein, carbohydrates, and other substances. Decomposition of apocrine sweat produces what we associate with body odor.

Sebaceous Glands

These glands secrete a lipid-rich substance, sebum, which keeps the skin and hair from drying out. The greatest distribution of sebaceous glands is found on the face and scalp, although they are found in all areas of the body with the exception of the palms and soles. Sebum secretion, stimulated by sex hormone activity, varies throughout the life span.

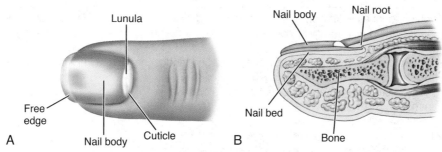

Fig. 10-2   Structures of the nail. *(From Herlihy and Maebius, 2000.)*

LINK TO CONCEPTS   *Tissue Integrity*

The feature concept for this chapter is *Tissue Integrity.* This concept represents the structural intactness and physiologic function of tissues and conditions that affect integrity. Several concepts featured in this textbook have an interrelationship with this concept including perfusion, oxygenation, motion, tactile sensory perception, elimination, nutrition, and pain. The maintenance of tissue integrity requires adequate perfusion of oxygenated blood; interference with this process results in tissue injury or necrosis. Adequate nutrition is also required maintain and sustain tissues. Sustained pressure over tissue may occur if an individual has limited mobility and or if the individual has limited tactile sensory perception. Urinary or bowel incontinence can also contribute to impairment of tissue integrity. Finally, a loss of tissue integrity often results in pain. These interrelationships are depicted in the model below.

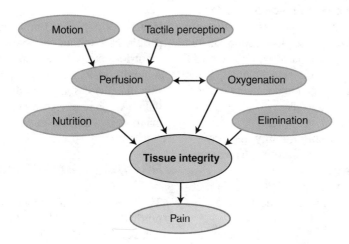

This model shows the interrelationship of concepts impacting adequate tissue integrity. As an example, an individual who has a spinal cord injury has reduced motion and tactile sensation, which can lead to sustained pressure, contributing to breakdown of skin over bony prominences. Understanding the interrelationship of these concepts helps the nurse recognize risk factors and thus increases awareness when conducting a health assessment.

ETHNIC & CULTURAL VARIATIONS

Native Americans, Alaskan Natives, Pacific Islanders, and Asian Americans have fewer apocrine glands than whites. They perspire less and produce less body odor. In Alaskan Natives, most eccrine sweat glands are located in the face. Chloride concentrations in sweat decrease as skin color darkens.

HEALTH HISTORY

RISK FACTORS *Skin, Hair, and Nails*

As you conduct a health history, it is important to consider common risk factors for problems associated with the skin, hair, and nails, and follow up with appropriate questions should they exist.
- Systemic disease (such as liver, kidney, collagen, endocrine, or autoimmune disease)
- Infection (viral, bacterial, or fungal)
- Family history of skin cancer or autoimmune disease
- Immobility
- Excessive sun exposure (M)
- Exposure to chemicals or allergens (M)
- Medications (allergic outbreaks, photosensitive response) (M)

M = modifiable risk factor.

GENERAL HEALTH HISTORY

Present Health Status

Do you have any chronic illnesses? If so, describe.
Some chronic illnesses (such as liver failure, renal failure, and autoimmune disease) cause changes to the skin such as pruritus, excessive dryness, and skin lesions.

Do you take any medications? If so, what do you take and how often? What are the medications for?
Medications can cause a number of side effects that are manifested in the skin, including allergic reactions in the form of hives or rashes, lesions associated with photosensitivity, or other systemic effects such as acne, thinning of the skin, and stretch marks. The nurse should document medications that are used to treat skin problems.

What do you do to keep your skin healthy (e.g., hygiene measures, use of lotions, protection from sun exposure, use of sunscreen)?
Health care practices may be clues for underlying skin problems, as well as areas for education. Specifically determine products and frequency used.

Have you noticed any changes in the way your skin and hair looks or feels? Any changes in the sensation of your skin? If so, where? Describe.
Ask clients if they have noticed changes as opposed to asking them if they have any problems. Clients may have a pathologic skin condition yet may not be aware of it or may not consider it a problem. This information helps identify clients at risk for injury to their skin or development of skin ulcers.

Past Medical History and Family History

Have you ever had problems with your skin such as skin disease, infections involving the skin or nails, or trauma involving the skin? If so, describe.
Past skin injuries and conditions may provide clues to current skin lesions or findings.

Has anyone in your family ever had skin-related problems such as skin cancer or autoimmune-related disorders such as systemic lupus erythematosus?
A family history helps determine predisposition to certain skin disorders. Some skin disorders have familial or genetic links. Autoimmune disorders tend to be familial and may manifest in a number of ways, including rash and alopecia.

PROBLEM-BASED HISTORY

The most commonly reported symptom of skin disease is pruritis (Etter and Myers, 2002). Other common problems related to the skin include rashes, pain/discomfort, lesions, wounds, and changes in skin color or texture, hair, or nails. As with symptoms in all areas of health assessment, a symptom analysis is completed, which includes the onset, location, duration, characteristics, aggravating and alleviating factors, related symptoms, and treatment (see Box 3-3 in Chapter 3).

Skin

Pruritis

When did the itching first start? Did it start suddenly or over time? Where did it start? Has it spread?

Understanding the onset and location of the itching may provide clues to the cause.

Does anything make the itching worse? Is there anything that relieves it? What have you done to treat yourself?

Document characteristics and aggravating and alleviating factors of the itching; these data may provide clues to the cause.

What were the circumstances when you first noticed the itching? Taking medications? Contact with possible allergens such as animals, foods, drugs, plants?

Pruritus may be caused by an allergic response (hives) or may occur secondary to an infestation of scabies, lice, or insect bites. Systemic diseases such as biliary cirrhosis and some types of cancer such as lymphoma may also cause pruritus (Etter and Myers, 2002).

Do you have dry or sensitive skin?

Dry or sensitive skin may make an individual more prone to itching.

Rash

When did the rash start? Where did you first notice the rash? Describe what the rash looked like initially: Flat? Raised? How long has the rash been present?

Determining onset, location, and duration of the rash may provide clues to the cause.

Does the rash itch or burn? What makes it better? Worse? What have you done to treat it? Have you noticed any other symptoms associated with this rash, such as joint pains, fatigue, or fever?

Document aggravating and alleviating factors, related symptoms, and measures of self-treatment to better understand the cause.

Do you have any known allergies to foods, plants, skin/hair products, laundry detergent, chemicals, or animals? Does anyone else in your family have a similar rash? Have you been exposed to others with a similar rash?

A rash is not generally a disease in itself, but rather a symptom of an allergic response, skin disorder, or systemic illness. Some of these questions help differentiate the cause of the rash.

Pain/Discomfort of Skin

Describe the pain or discomfort you are experiencing. When did the pain start? Describe the location of the pain. Does the pain or discomfort extend from where it started? Does it spread anywhere? Does the pain stay on the skin surface, or does it go deep inside?

There are multiple causes of pain; onset and location are important factors in determining the cause (Box 10-1).

BOX 10-1   FOCUS ON PAIN   *Skin, Hair, and Nails*

When a client complains of pain or discomfort associated with the skin, hair, and nails, the nurse should conduct a focused symptom analysis. Pain and discomfort are associated with a number of skin and nail disorders ranging from mild discomfort (such as pruritus associated with dry skin) to intense, severe pain (such as pain associated with a large abscess or herpes zoster). The degree of pain one experiences is highly individualized and may vary by the severity or stage of the disorder. Additionally, the effect of a lesion on body image can have a tremendous impact on the pain perceived by an individual.

Describe the pain or discomfort—sharp, dull, achy, burning, itching. How bad is your pain on a scale of 0 to 10? Is the pain constant, or does it come and go? If constant, does the pain vary? If pain comes and goes, how long does the pain last?

Document characteristics of the pain or discomfort to better understand the cause.

What triggers the pain? Are there things that make the pain worse? Better?

Document aggravating and relieving factors for the discomfort. (Box 10-1 focuses on pain associated with the skin, hair, and nails.)

Lesion or Changes in Mole

Describe the lesion you are concerned with. Where is the lesion? When did you first notice it? Do you have any symptoms associated with the lesion such as pain, discomfort, pruritis, or drainage? If so, describe.

Lesions may result from acne, trauma, infections, exposure to chemicals or other irritants, tumors, or other systemic disease.

Describe the changes you have noticed in the mole (color, shape, texture, tenderness, bleeding, or itching).

A changing or irregular mole may be a sign of a malignant lesion.

Change in Skin Color

Has there been any generalized change in your skin color, such as a yellowish tone or paleness?

Changes in overall skin color may have a number of causes, including medications, anemia, or an internal systemic disease such as liver disease causing jaundice.

Have there been any localized changes in your skin color, such as redness, discoloration of one or both feet, or areas of bruises or patches?

Localized changes may be associated with changes in tissue perfusion, causing a discoloration to the affected area, cyanosis, bruising (may be a sign of a hematologic condition, abuse, frequent falls), or vitiligo—a loss of pigmentation in the skin.

Skin Texture

In what way has the texture of your skin changed (e.g., skin thinning, fragile, excessive dryness)?

Changes in the skin texture may be normal (e.g., associated with aging) or may indicate a metabolic or nutritional problem.

Do you have excessively dry (xerosis) or oily (seborrhea) skin? If so, is it seasonal, intermittent, or continuous? What do you do to treat it?

A history of dry skin may provide information about an existing system disease (e.g., thyroid disease), or it may be related to an environmental condition such as low humidity. Dry skin may also be associated with poor skin lubrication.

Wounds

Where is your wound located? How long have you had the wound? Do you have any associated symptoms such as pain or drainage? If so, describe.

The location of a wound and how long it has been there are important to document. These may provide clues as to the cause of the wound. Chronic wounds on the lower legs, for example, suggest problems with peripheral perfusion.

What have you done to treat the wound?

Self-treatment of a wound may provide insight to the appearance of a wound, particularly if the client reports problems associated with wound healing.

Do you typically have problems with wound healing?

A history of problems associated with wound healing can point to nutritional or metabolic problems, infection, or poor circulation.

Hair

What changes or problems with your hair are you experiencing? When did you notice the changes? Did the changes occur suddenly?

Establish the type of problem, the onset, and the nature of the changes with the hair. Common problems associated with hair include excessive dryness, brittleness, hair loss, and pain/dryness to the scalp.

Can you think of any contributory factors associated with the problems or changes? Have you recently experienced stress? Fever? Other illness? Itching? What kinds of hair products have been used on your hair recently?

Reports of changes in the hair such as excessive dryness or brittle hair may indicate stress or systemic disease. Exposure to hair care products may account for changes in texture or condition of hair.

Has there been a change in your diet in the last few months?

Nutritional deficiencies may be observed by changes in hair appearance or texture. For example, dullness and hair that is easily plucked could be caused by a protein deficiency.

HEALTH PROMOTION   *Skin Cancer*

Skin cancer is the most common cancer, accounting for almost half of all cancers. Nonmelanoma (basal and squamous cell) skin cancers are the most common, with more than 1 million cases diagnosed per year. Melanoma accounts for 55,000 new cases of skin cancer per year. The estimated number of skin cancer–related deaths in 2007 was 10,250, of which 7900 were related to melanoma. In the elderly, melanoma tends to be diagnosed at a later stage and is more likely to be lethal.

Goals and Objectives—*Healthy People 2010*

The overall *Healthy People 2010* goal related to cancer is to reduce the number of new cancer cases and reduce illness, disability, and death caused by cancer. Two specific objectives relate to skin cancer:

- Reduce the rate of melanoma cancer deaths.
- Increase the proportion of persons who use at least one measure that may reduce risk (avoid sun exposure between 10 AM and 4 PM; wear sun-protective clothing when exposed to sunlight; use sunscreen with a sun-protective factor of 15 or higher; avoid artificial sources of ultraviolet light).

Recommendations to Reduce Risk (Primary Prevention)
American Cancer Society (ACS)

- Avoid sun exposure, especially between 10 AM and 4 PM. Seek shade whenever possible. Special care should be taken when the ultraviolet (UV) index levels are moderate or higher (between 5 and 10).
- Avoid artificial sources of UV light (sunlamps and tanning booths).
- Wear protective clothing (including a wide-brimmed hat) when out in the sun.
- Wear sunglasses with 99% to 100% UV absorption to provide optimal protection for the eyes and the surrounding skin.
- Apply sunscreen with a sun protection factor of 15 or higher to sun-exposed skin; reapply every 2 hours. Use sunscreen even on hazy or overcast days.

Screening Recommendations (Secondary Prevention)
American Cancer Society

Screening: Skin examination as part of a cancer-related checkup is recommended every 3 years for people age 20 to 40 and on a yearly basis for anyone older than 40.

Self-examination: Monthly self-examination of skin starting at age 20 is recommended. Use the ABCDEF mnemonic for evaluating lesions (see Box 10-2).

From American Cancer Society: *Cancer facts and figures,* Atlanta, 2007, American Cancer Society; US Department of Health and Human Services: *Cancer.* In *Healthy People 2010: understanding and improving health,* ed 2, Washington, DC, 2000, US Government Printing Office (available at *www.healthypeople.gov*).

Have you noticed any changes in the distribution of hair growth on your arms or legs?

A decrease in hair growth on an extremity, particularly the lower extremity, may indicate problems with arterial circulation. Increases in hair growth may be caused by an ovarian or adrenal tumor.

Nails

What kind of problem or changes are you experiencing with your nails? When did you first notice the changes?

The health and consistency of the fingernails and toenails may be an important sign about the client's general health. Establish onset of the changes or problem.

Have you been exposed to or do you handle any chemicals at home or work?

Exposure to chemicals can cause the nails to change in appearance or consistency.

Are your nails brittle? Have you noticed a pitting type of pattern to your nail?

Pitting, brittle nails, crumbling, and changes in color can be caused by nutritional deficiencies, systemic diseases, or localized fungal infections.

Do you chew your nails? Do you now have, or have you ever had, an infection of the nail or around the nail bed? If so, describe.

Clients who have a habit of nail biting may use the biting as an unconscious way to handle stress. The nails may show signs of local infection such as fungal infection.

Do you have difficulty keeping your nails clean? Do your nails appear dirty?

Hyperthyroidism may cause the nail to separate from the nail bed and make the nail appear "dirty."

EXAMINATION

ROUTINE TECHNIQUES

- INSPECT the skin for general color and localized ⚷ variations in skin color.
- PALPATE the skin for texture, temperature, moisture, mobility, turgor, and thickness.
- INSPECT and PALPATE the scalp and hair for surface characteristics, hair distribution, texture, quantity and color.
- INSPECT facial and body hair for distribution, color, quantity, and hygiene.
- INSPECT and PALPATE the nails for shape, contour, consistency, color, thickness, and cleanliness.

SPECIAL CIRCUMSTANCES OR ADVANCED PRACTICE

- INSPECT and PALPATE skin lesions. ⚷
- INSPECT lesions using a Wood's lamp. ★

EQUIPMENT NEEDED

Light source (e.g., overhead light, penlight) • Centimeter ruler • Magnifying lens if needed • Gloves (if open lesions present) • Wood's lamp

⚷ = core examination skill   ★ = advanced practice

PROCEDURES AND TECHNIQUES WITH NORMAL FINDINGS

ROUTINE TECHNIQUES

Start with a general survey, noting the color of the skin, general pigmentation, vascularity or bruising, and lesions or discoloration. Note any unusual odors. Next, inspect and palpate the skin more closely, moving systematically from the head and neck to the trunk, arms, legs, and back. In a head-to-toe assessment, the skin can be examined in conjunction with other body systems. Before you begin, be sure to have adequate lighting so that subtle changes will not be missed.

ABNORMAL FINDINGS

PROCEDURES AND TECHNIQUES WITH NORMAL FINDINGS

ABNORMAL FINDINGS

 INSPECT the skin for general color.

Inspect the skin for general color and uniformity of color. The skin color should be consistent over the body surface, with the exception of vascular areas (such as the cheeks, upper chest, and genitalia), which may appear pink or have a reddish purple tone. The normal range of skin color varies from whitish pink, to olive tones, to deep brown. Table 10-1 compares clinical findings between clients with light and dark skin. Sun-exposed areas may show evidence of slightly darker pigmentation.

Abnormal skin color may be evidence of local or systemic disease. Common abnormal findings of particular importance include *cyanosis, pallor,* and *jaundice* (see Table 10-1). Less common findings include:

- *Hypopigmentation,* also known as *albinism* (a complete absence of pigmentation; pale white skin tone is noted over the entire body surface).
- *Hyperpigmentation* (increased melanin deposition) may be an indication of an endocrine disorder (such as Addison's disease) or liver disease.

TABLE 10-1 *Comparison of Skin-Related Findings in Clients with Light Skin and Clients with Dark Skin*

CLINICAL SIGN	LIGHT SKIN	DARK SKIN
Cyanosis	Grayish blue tone, especially in nail beds, earlobes, lips, mucous membranes, palms, and soles of feet.	Ashen-gray color most easily seen in the conjunctiva of the eye, oral mucous membranes, and nail beds.
Ecchymosis (bruise)	Dark red, purple, yellow, or green color, depending on age of bruise.	Deeper bluish or black tone, difficult to see unless it occurs in an area of light pigmentation.
Erythema	Reddish tone with evidence of increased skin temperature secondary to inflammation.	Deeper brown or purple skin tone with evidence of increased skin temperature secondary to inflammation.
Jaundice	Yellowish color of skin, sclera of eyes, fingernails, palms of hands, and oral mucosa.	Yellowish green color most obviously seen in sclera of eye (do not confuse with yellow eye pigmentation, which may be evident in dark-skinned clients), palms of hands, and soles of feet.
Pallor	Pale skin color that may appear white.	Skin tone will appear lighter than normal. Light-skinned African Americans may have yellowish brown skin; dark-skinned African Americans may appear ashen. Specifically evident is a loss of the underlying healthy red tones of the skin.
Petechiae	Lesions appear as small, reddish purple pinpoints.	Difficult to see; may be evident in the buccal mucosa of the mouth or sclera of the eye.
Rash	May be visualized as well as felt with light palpation.	Not easily visualized but may be felt with light palpation.
Scar	Narrow scar line.	Frequently has keloid development, resulting in a thickened, raised scar.

 = core examination skill

PROCEDURES AND TECHNIQUES WITH NORMAL FINDINGS

ABNORMAL FINDINGS

➤ **INSPECT the skin for localized variations in skin color.**

Almost all healthy individuals have natural variations in skin pigmentation. A common intentional localized variation in skin color is a tattoo. If a tattoo is present, its location and the characteristics of the surrounding areas should be examined and documented. Normal localized variations of the skin pigmentation include the following:

- *Pigmented nevi (moles):* Moles are considered a normal finding—most adults have between 10 and 40 moles scattered over the body. They are most commonly located above the waist on sun-exposed body surfaces (chest, back, arms, legs, and face). Moles tend to be uniformly tan to dark brown, are typically less than 5 mm in size, and may be raised or flat. The expected shape of a mole is round or oval with a clearly defined border (see Table 10-2 later in this chapter).
- *Freckles:* Small, flat hyperpigmented macules that may appear anywhere on the body, particularly on sun-exposed areas of the skin. The most common locations are on the face, arms, and back.
- *Patch:* An area of darker skin pigmentation that is usually brown or tan and typically is present at birth (birthmarks). Some of these patches fade, but many do not change over time.
- *Striae:* Silver or pink "stretch marks" secondary to weight gain or pregnancy (see Table 10-3 later in this chapter).

- *Melanoma.* The nurse should be familiar with abnormal characteristics of pigmented moles that might point to melanoma (Box 10-2). Moles located below the waist or on the scalp or breast are rarely "normal" moles.
- *Vitiligo* is an acquired condition associated with the development of unpigmented patch or patches; it is more common in dark-skinned races and thought to be an autoimmune disorder (see Table 10-2 later in this chapter).
- Localized areas of hyperpigmentation may be associated with endocrine disorders (pituitary, adrenal) and autoimmune disorders (systemic lupus erythematosus).

ETHNIC & CULTURAL VARIATIONS

- "Coining" is a treatment practiced by Cambodians and Vietnamese. The body is rubbed vigorously with a coin while exerting pressure until red marks appear over the bony prominence of the rib cage on the back and chest. Marks created by this treatment frequently have been mistaken as signs of abuse or mistreatment.
- "Cupping" is a treatment for arthritis, stomachaches, bruises, and paralysis. A cup is heated and placed on the skin. As a result of the heat, the cup adheres to the skin and may leave a reddened area or mark. This is practiced by Latin American and Russian cultures (Monteleone, 1996).

BOX 10-2	**EARLY SIGNS OF MELANOMA**

To help you remember the early signs of melanoma, use the mnemonic ABCDEF:
A—Asymmetry (not round or oval)
B—Border (poorly defined or irregular border)
C—Color (uneven, variegated)
D—Diameter (usually greater than 6 mm)
E—Elevation (recent change from flat to raised lesion)
F—Feeling (sensation of itching, tingling, or stinging within the lesion)

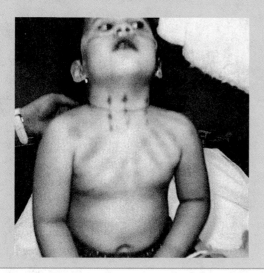

➤ = core examination skill

PROCEDURES AND TECHNIQUES WITH NORMAL FINDINGS

ABNORMAL FINDINGS

PALPATE the skin for texture, temperature, moisture, mobility, turgor, and thickness.

Texture

The skin should be smooth, soft, and intact, with an even surface. Normal variations include calluses over the hands, feet, elbows, and knees.

Excessive dryness, flaking, cracking, or scaling of the skin may occur secondary to environmental conditions or may be signs of systemic disease or nutritional deficiency. Look for areas of maceration, discoloration, or rashes under skin folds (Fig. 10-3).

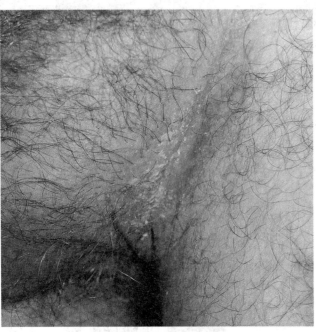

Fig. 10-3   Maceration in a skin fold. *(From Habif, 2004.)*

Temperature

The skin temperature is best evaluated using the dorsal aspect of your hands. The skin should be warm. The skin temperature should be consistent for the entire body with the exception of the hands and feet, which may be cooler, particularly in a cool environment.

Cool Skin. Generalized cool or cold skin is an abnormal finding and may be associated with shock or hypothermia. Localization of cold skin, particularly in the extremities, may be an indication of poor peripheral perfusion.

Hot Skin. Generalized hot skin is a reflection of hyperthermia. This may be associated with a fever, increased metabolic rate (e.g., hyperthyroidism), or exercise. Localized areas of skin that are hot may reflect an infection, traumatic injury, or thermal injury such as a sunburn.

Moisture

The skin is normally dry. There should be minimal perspiration or oiliness, although increased perspiration may be a normal finding associated with increased environmental temperatures, strenuous activity, or anxiety.

Diaphoresis (excessive sweating) is an abnormal finding in the absence of strenuous activity. This may be a reflection of hyperthermia, extreme anxiety, pain, or shock. Excessively moist skin may often be seen with metabolic conditions such as hyperthyroidism (Leonhardt and Heymann, 2002).

PROCEDURES AND TECHNIQUES WITH NORMAL FINDINGS

Mobility and Turgor

Skin mobility and turgor are assessed by picking up and slightly pinching the skin on the forearm or under the clavicle. The skin should move easily when lifted and should return to place immediately when released. The technique and expected findings for skin turgor are shown in Fig.10-4.

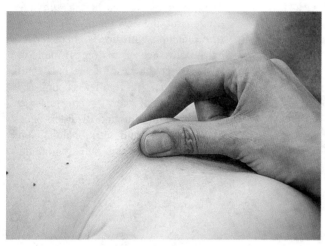

Fig. 10-4 Elastic skin turgor.

Thickness

Skin thickness varies based on age and area of the body. Typically skin thickens until adulthood, and then decreases in thickness after age 20. The skin is thickest over the palms of hands and soles of feet, and thinnest over the eyelids. A callus is an area of excessive thickening of skin that is a normal variation associated with friction or pressure over a particular surface area. A callus is commonly found on the hands or feet (Fig. 10-6).

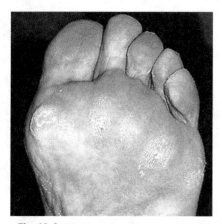

Fig. 10-6 Callus. *(From White and Cox, 2000.)*

ABNORMAL FINDINGS

Edema, excessive scarring to the skin, or some connective tissue disorders (such as scleroderma) reduce skin mobility. Poor skin turgor is noted if "tenting" is observed, or the skin slowly recedes back into place. Decreased turgor may result from dehydration or may be a finding in an individual who has experienced significant weight loss (Fig. 10-5).

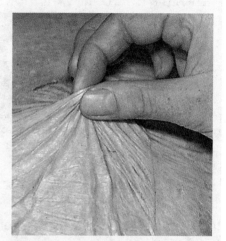

Fig. 10-5 Poor skin turgor. *(From Kamal and Brocklehurst, 1991.)*

An increase in skin thickness is seen in diabetic clients and is thought to be caused by abnormal collagen caused by hyperglycemia (Ferringer and Miller, 2002). Excessively thin skin may take on a shiny or transparent appearance and is seen in hyperthyroidism, arterial insufficiency, and aging.

PROCEDURES AND TECHNIQUES WITH NORMAL FINDINGS

ABNORMAL FINDINGS

INSPECT and PALPATE the scalp and hair for surface characteristics, hair distribution, texture, quantity, and color.

The scalp should be smooth to palpation and should show no evidence of flaking, scaling, redness, or open lesions. The hair should be shiny and soft. The texture of the hair may be fine or coarse. Note the quantity and distribution of the hair for balding patterns and isolated areas of hair loss. If there are areas of isolated hair loss, note whether the hair shaft is broken off or whether it is absent completely. Men may show a gradual, symmetric hair loss on the scalp due to genetic disposition and elevated androgen levels.

ETHNIC & CULTURAL VARIATIONS

Hair texture varies widely across races:
- Fine, thick, and very curly or kinky hair may be characteristic of African Americans.
- Curly facial hair that some African American males have tends to ingrow, producing a condition known as "razor bumps."
- Coarse, straight hair may be characteristic of Asian Americans, Pacific Islanders, Native Americans, and Alaskan Natives.
- Body hair and facial hair is sparse or absent in many Native Americans, Alaskan Natives, and Asian Americans.
- Balding patterns are frequently seen in Native American women, but balding is rare in Native American men.

INSPECT facial and body hair for distribution, quantity, and texture.

Examine the quantity and distribution of facial and body hair. Men generally have noticeable hair present on the lower face, neck, nares, ears, chest, axilla, back, shoulders, arms, legs, and pubic region. The noticeable hair distribution in women is most commonly limited to the arms, legs, axillae, pubic region, and around the nipples. Women may also have fine or light-colored hair on the back, face, and shoulders. The women in some cultural groups may also have facial or chin hair. Fine vellus hair covers the body, whereas coarser hair is found on the eyebrows and lashes, pubic region, axillary area, male beards, and to some extent on the arms and legs. The male pubic hair configuration is an upright triangle, with the hair commonly extending midline to the umbilicus. The female pubic hair configuration forms an inverse triangle; the hair may also extend midline to the umbilicus.

Dull, coarse, and brittle hair is seen with nutritional deficiencies, hypothyroidism, and exposure to chemicals in some hair products and bleach. Hyperthyroidism makes the hair texture fine (Leonhardt and Heymann, 2002). *Parasitic infection* with lice is characterized by the presence of nits (eggs) found on the scalp at the base of the hair shaft. *Alopecia* (hair loss) often occurs as a manifestation of many systemic diseases (including autoimmune disorders, anemic conditions, and nutritional deficiencies) or treatment with radiation or antineoplastic agents.

Hair loss on the legs may indicate poor peripheral perfusion. Thinning of the eyebrows is a prominent finding in hypothyroidism (Sperling, 2002). *Hirsutism* (hair growth in women with an increase of hair on the face, body, and pubic area) may be a sign of an underlying endocrine disorder. Pubic hair distribution that deviates from typical gender patterns may indicate a hormonal imbalance.

| **PROCEDURES AND TECHNIQUES WITH NORMAL FINDINGS** | **ABNORMAL FINDINGS** |

INSPECT and PALPATE the nails for shape, contour, consistency, color, thickness, and cleanliness.

Inspect the edges of the nails to determine if they are smooth and rounded. The nail surface should be flat in the center and slightly curved downward at the edges. The skin adjacent to the nail should be intact and not inflamed.

- Inflammation characterized by edema and erythema of the folds of the finger tissue may indicate infection.
- *Koilonychia* (spoon nail) presents as a thin, depressed nail with the lateral edges turned upward (Fig. 10-7). This is associated with anemia or may be congenital.

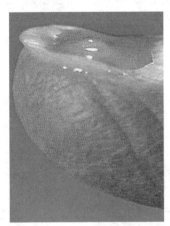

Fig. 10-7   Severe spooning with thinning of the nail. *(From Beaven and Brooks, 1994.)*

In light-skinned individuals, nails are pink and blanch with pressure. Individuals with darker-pigmented skin typically have nails that are yellow or brown, and vertical banded lines may appear (Fig. 10-8).

- *Leukonychia* appears as white spots on the nail plate (Fig. 10-9). This is usually caused by minor trauma or manipulation of the cuticle.

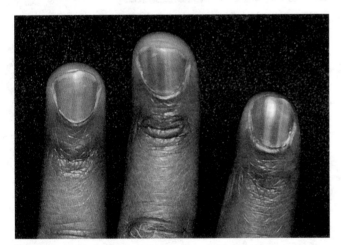

Fig. 10-8   Nail bed color of a dark-skinned person (pigmented bands occur as a normal finding in over 90% of African Americans). *(From Habif, 1990.)*

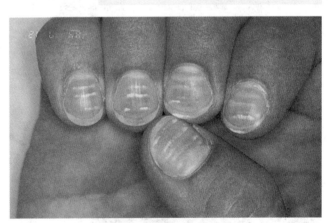

Fig. 10-9   Leukonychia punctata. Transverse white bands result from repeated minor trauma to the nail matrix. *(From Baran et al, 1991.)*

PROCEDURES AND TECHNIQUES WITH NORMAL FINDINGS

ABNORMAL FINDINGS

Inspect the nail base angle—that is, the angle of the proximal nail fold and the nail plate. The expected angle of the nail base is 160 degrees.

- Clubbing is present when the angle of the nail base exceeds 180 degrees (Fig. 10-10). It is caused by proliferation of the connective tissue resulting in an enlargement of the distal fingers. It is most commonly associated with chronic respiratory or cardiovascular disease.

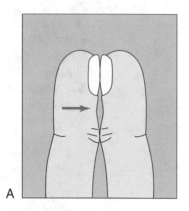
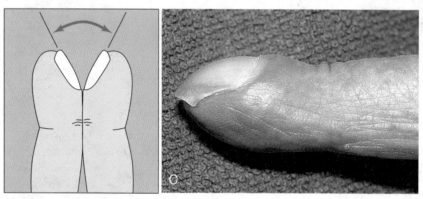

Fig. 10-10 **Assessment of finger clubbing. A,** Normally when opposing fingers are placed together, a small space is visible between the fingers and the nail beds meet. **B,** With finger clubbing, no space is observed between the fingers, and the nail beds angle away from one another. **C,** With finger clubbing, the base if the nail is enlarged and curved. *(A, and B, From Seidel, 2006; C, From White and Cox, 2000.)*

Inspect the nail surface itself to determine its smoothness. Note grooves, depressions, pitting, and ridges.

- *Beau's lines* manifest as a groove or transverse depression running across the nail (Fig. 10-11). It results from a stressor that temporarily impairs nail formation (such as trauma). The groove first appears at the base of the nail by the cuticle and moves forward as the nail grows out.

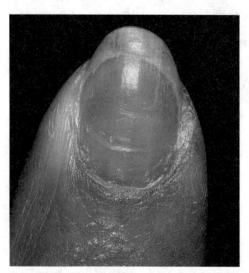

Fig. 10-11 Beau's lines. *(From Habif, Campbell, Chapman et al, 2005.)*

PROCEDURES AND TECHNIQUES WITH NORMAL FINDINGS

ABNORMAL FINDINGS

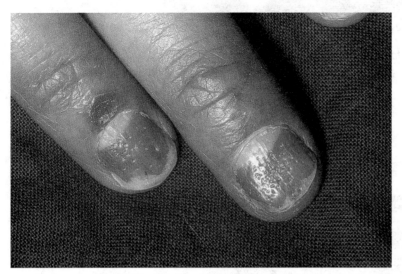

Fig. 10-12 Nail pitting. *(From White and Cox, 2000.)*

Examine the thickness of the nail itself. The nail should be smooth and have a uniform thickness. Finally, palpate the nail to ensure that the nail base feels firm and adheres to the nail bed.

SPECIAL CIRCUMSTANCES OR ADVANCED PRACTICE

INSPECT and PALPATE the skin for lesions.

An in-depth examination of lesions is not routinely performed during every health assessment. However, when the client has a new lesion, or when a lesion has changed (such as a change in appearance or has become painful), the lesion should be examined. A strong light source is helpful to determine the exact color, elevation, and borders. A centimeter ruler to measure the size of lesions may also be helpful. The lesion is documented based on its characteristics, including location, distribution, color, pattern, edges, depth, and size (Box 10-3 and Fig. 10-13). Lesions are classified as primary, secondary, or vascular.

- Pitting of the nail is commonly associated with psoriasis. Minor pitting may also be seen in persons with no health care problems (Fig. 10-12).

- Thinning or brittleness of the nail may be secondary to poor peripheral circulation or inadequate nutrition.

BOX 10-3 | **LESION CHARACTERISTIC TO BE NOTED DURING EXAMINATION**

- Note the **location and distribution** of the lesion. Is the lesion generalized over the entire body or section of the body, or is it localized to a specific area such as around the waist, under a piece of jewelry, or in the hair?
- Describe the **color** of the lesion and describe how this lesion may be different in color from other lesions noted on the body (e.g., a mole or freckle). Has the client noticed a change in the color of the lesion?
- What is the **pattern** of the lesion? Are the lesions clustered? Are they in a line? How does the client describe the development of the pattern of the lesion? (See Fig. 11-7.)
- What are the **edges** of the lesion like? Is the edge of the lesion regular or irregular? Has the client noticed a change in the shape of the lesion?

- Is the lesion flat, raised, or sunken?
- What is the current **size** of the lesion? Measure using a centimeter ruler. Has the client noticed a change in the size of the lesion?
- What are the **characteristics** of the lesion? Is it hard, soft, or fluid filled? If there is an exudate, what is the color of the drainage fluid? Does the exudate have an odor? Note both the color and odor if present. Has the client noticed a change in either the characteristics or drainage of the lesion? If so, how and when?

= core examination skill

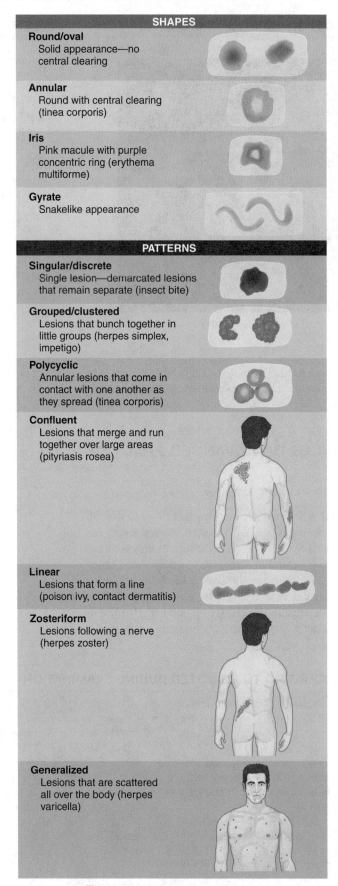

SHAPES

Round/oval
Solid appearance—no central clearing

Annular
Round with central clearing (tinea corporis)

Iris
Pink macule with purple concentric ring (erythema multiforme)

Gyrate
Snakelike appearance

PATTERNS

Singular/discrete
Single lesion—demarcated lesions that remain separate (insect bite)

Grouped/clustered
Lesions that bunch together in little groups (herpes simplex, impetigo)

Polycyclic
Annular lesions that come in contact with one another as they spread (tinea corporis)

Confluent
Lesions that merge and run together over large areas (pityriasis rosea)

Linear
Lesions that form a line (poison ivy, contact dermatitis)

Zosteriform
Lesions following a nerve (herpes zoster)

Generalized
Lesions that are scattered all over the body (herpes varicella)

Fig. 10-13 Shapes and patterns of lesions.

PROCEDURES AND TECHNIQUES WITH NORMAL FINDINGS

Primary Lesions

Many primary lesions are considered normal variations of the skin and include moles, freckles, and patches. These have been discussed in previous sections. (Table 10-2).

★ Use a Wood's lamp to identify fluorescing lesions, indicating fungal infection. Darken the room and shine the light on the area to be examined. If there is no fungal infection, the light tone on the skin will appear soft violet.

ABNORMAL FINDINGS

Many primary lesions are considered abnormal findings and are associated with a specific disease process or injury (Table 10-2).

A yellow-green or blue-green fluorescence indicates the presence of fungal infection.

TABLE 10-2 *Primary Skin Lesions*

SKIN LESIONS	EXAMPLES		
Macule A flat, circumscribed area that is a change in the color of the skin; less than 1 cm in diameter	Freckles, flat moles (nevi), petechiae, measles, scarlet fever	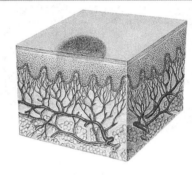	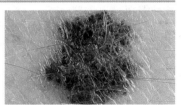 Flat nevi. *(From Habif, Campbell, Chapman et al, 2005.)*
Papule An elevated, firm, circumscribed area less than 1 cm in diameter	Wart (verruca), elevated moles, lichen planus, cherry angioma, skin tag	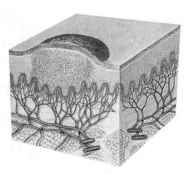	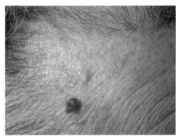 Cherry angioma. *(From Baran et al, 1991.)*
Patch A flat, nonpalpable, irregular-shaped macule more than 1 cm in diameter	Vitiligo, port wine stains, mongolian spots, café-au-lait spots	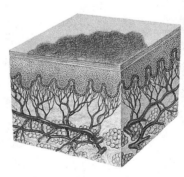	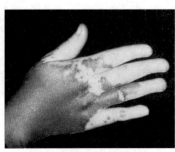 Vitiligo. *(Courtesy Medical College of Georgia, Division of Dermatology. From Goldstein and Goldstein, 1997.)*

Continued

★ = advanced practice

TABLE 10-2   *Primary Skin Lesions—cont'd*

SKIN LESIONS	EXAMPLES

Plaque
Elevated, firm, and rough lesion with flat top surface greater than 1 cm in diameter

Psoriasis, seborrheic and actinic keratoses, eczema

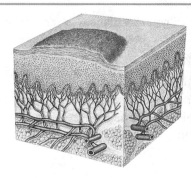
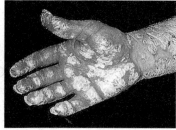

Plaque type of psorias. *(From Goldstein and Goldstein, 1997.)*

Wheal
Elevated irregular-shaped area of cutaneous edema; solid, transient; variable diameter

Insect bites, urticaria, allergic reaction, lupus erythematosus

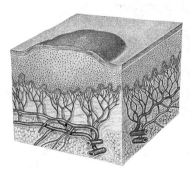
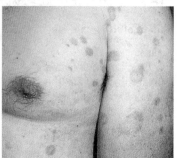

Wheals of urticaria. *(From Goldstein and Goldstein, 1997.)*

Nodule
Elevated, firm, circumscribed lesion; deeper in dermis than a papule; 1 to 2 cm in diameter

Dermatofibroma erythema nodosum, lipomas, melanoma, hemangioma, neurofibroma

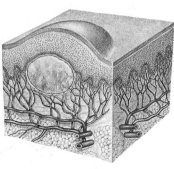
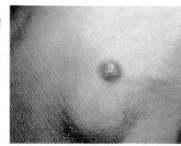

Dermatofibroma. *(From Goldstein and Goldstein, 1997.)*

Tumor
Elevated and solid lesion; may or may not be clearly demarcated; deeper in dermis; greater than 2 cm in diameter

Neoplasms, lipoma, hemangioma

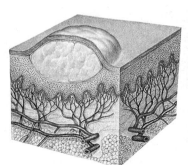
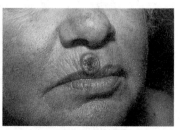

Tumor of upper lip. *(From Goldstein and Goldstein, 1997.)*

TABLE 10-2 *Primary Skin Lesions—cont'd*

SKIN LESIONS	EXAMPLES		

Vesicle
Elevated, circumscribed, superficial, not into dermis; filled with serous fluid; less than 1 cm in diameter

Varicella (chickenpox), herpes zoster (shingles), impetigo, acute eczema

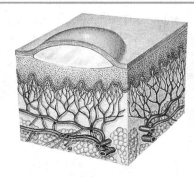

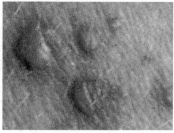

Vesicles. *(From Farrar et al, 1992.)*

Bulla
Vesicle greater than 1 cm in diameter

Blister, pemphigus vulgaris, lupus erythematosus, impetigo, drug reaction

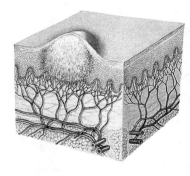

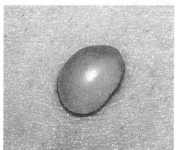

Blister. *(From White, 1994.)*

Pustule
Elevated, superficial lesion; similar to a vesicle but filled with purulent fluid

Impetigo, acne, folliculitis, herpes simplex

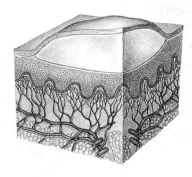

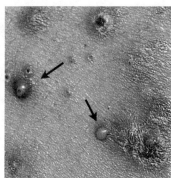

Acne. *(From Weston, Lane, and Morelli, 2002.)*

Cyst
Elevated, circumscribed, encapsulated lesion; in dermis or subcutaneous layer; filled with liquid or semisolid material

Sebaceous cyst, cystic acne

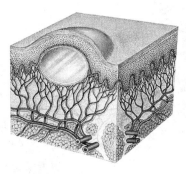

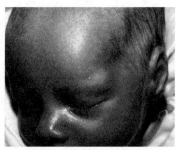

Sebaceous cyst. *(From Weston, Lane, and Morelli, 2002.)*

PROCEDURES AND TECHNIQUES WITH NORMAL FINDINGS

ABNORMAL FINDINGS

Secondary Lesions

Some secondary lesions are considered normal variations. A scar, for example, is a common variation seen on the skin, caused by past physical trauma to the skin. Scars often lack significance.

Abnormal secondary lesions result from changes from a primary lesion or trauma to a primary lesion (Table 10-3). Scars may be an indication of past physical abuse. Scarring caused by needle-track marks is generally indicative of intravenous drug use.

TABLE 10-3   *Secondary Skin Lesions*

SKIN LESIONS	EXAMPLES		
Scale Heaped-up keratinized cells; flaky skin; irregular; thick or thin; dry or oily; variation in size	Flaking of skin with seborrheic dermatitis following scarlet fever, or flaking of skin following a drug reaction; dry skin, pityriasis rosea, eczema, xerosis	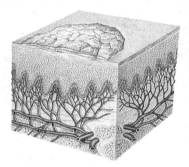	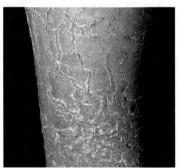Scaling. *(From Habif, 1996.)*
Lichenification Rough, thickened epidermis secondary to persistent rubbing, itching, or skin irritation; often involves flexor surface of extremity	Chronic dermatitis	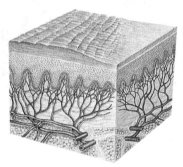	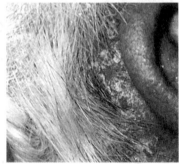Stasis dermatitis in an early stage. *(From Marks and DeLeo, 1992.)*
Keloid Irregular-shaped, elevated, progressively enlarging scar; grows beyond the boundaries of the wound	Keloid formation following surgery	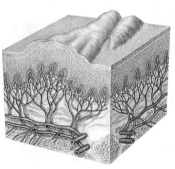	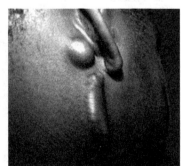Keloid. *(From Weston, Lane, and Morelli, 2002.)*

TABLE 10-3 *Secondary Skin Lesions—cont'd*

SKIN LESIONS	EXAMPLES		

Scar

Thin to thick fibrous tissue that replaces normal skin following injury or laceration to the dermis

Healed wound or surgical incision

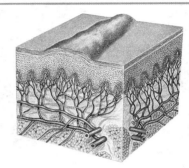

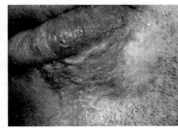

Hypertrophic scar. *(From Goldman and Fitzpatrack, 1994.)*

Excoriation

Loss of the epidermis; linear hollowed-out crusted area

Abrasion or scratch, scabies

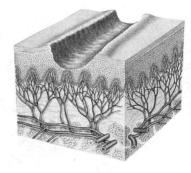

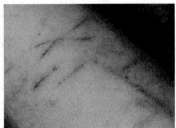

Excoriation. *(From Lemmi, 2000.)*

Fissure

Linear crack or break from the epidermis to the dermis; may be moist or dry

Athlete's foot, cracks at the corner of the mouth, chapped hands, eczema, intertrigo labialis

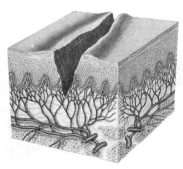

(From Seidel, 2003.)

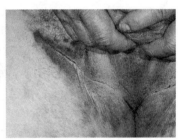

Fissure. *(From Habif, 1996.)*

Crust

Dried drainage or blood; slightly elevated; variable size; colors variable—red, black, tan, or mixed

Scab on abrasion, eczema

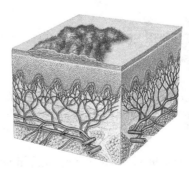

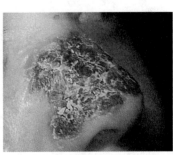

Scab. *(From Seidel, 2006.)*

Continued

TABLE 10-3 *Secondary Skin Lesions—cont'd*

SKIN LESIONS	EXAMPLES	

Erosion

Loss of part of the epidermis; depressed, moist, glistening; follows rupture of a vesicle or bulla

Varicella, variola after rupture, candidiasis, herpes simplex

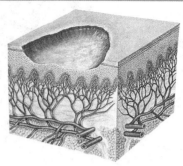 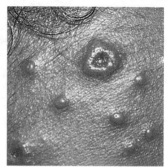

Erosion. *(From Cohen, 1993.)*

Ulcer

Loss of epidermis and dermis; concave; varies in size

Pressure ulcer, stasis ulcers, syphilis chancre

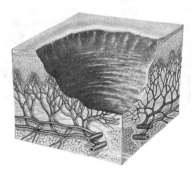 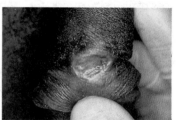

Ulcer caused by syphilis. *(From Goldstein and Goldstein, 1997.)*

Atrophy

Thinning of the skin surface and loss of skin markings; skin appears translucent and paper-like

Aged skin, striae, discoid lupus erythematosus

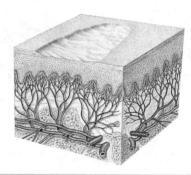 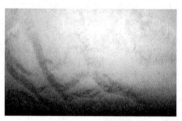

Striae. *(Courtesy Antoinette Hood, MD, Dept. of Dermatology, University of Indiana, Dept. of Medicine, Indianapolis. From Seidel, 2006.)*

PROCEDURES AND TECHNIQUES WITH NORMAL FINDINGS

Vascular Lesions

Many vascular lesions are considered common variations (Table 10-4). Ecchymosis (bruising) on a bony prominence is generally considered a common finding secondary to the activities of daily living. Other vascular lesions include the following:

- *Telangiectasia:* A fine, irregular red line caused by permanent dilation of a group of superficial blood vessels.
- *Cherry angioma:* A small, slightly raised, bright red area that typically appears on the face, neck, and trunk of the body. These increase in size and number with advanced age (Fig. 10-14).

ABNORMAL FINDINGS

Abnormal vascular lesions are presented in Table 10-4. A *hematoma* forms when there is a leakage of blood in a confined space caused by a break in a blood vessel. Bruising over soft tissue areas of the body in the absence of injury, or the presence of multiple bruises on the body in various stages of healing, is considered an abnormal finding warranting further investigation. Possible causes include physical abuse or a bleeding disorder.

TABLE 10-4 *Vascular Skin Lesions*

SKIN LESIONS	CAUSE/EXAMPLES

Petechiae

Tiny, flat, reddish purple, nonblanchable spots in the skin less than 0.5 cm in diameter; appears as tiny red spots pinpoint to pinhead in size

Cause: tiny hemorrhages within the dermal or submucosa—due to intravascular defects and infection

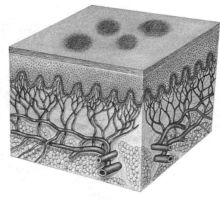

(From Seidel, 2006.)

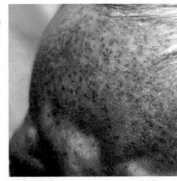

Petechiae. *(From Weston, Lane, and Morelli, 2002.)*

Purpura

Flat, reddish purple, nonblanchable discoloration in the skin greater than 0.5 cm in diameter

Cause: infection or bleeding disorders resulting in hemorrhage of blood into the skin

Examples: senile, actinic purpura, progressive pigmented purpura, vasculitis purpura, thrombocytopenic purpura

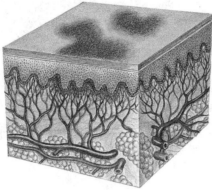

(From Seidel, 2006.)

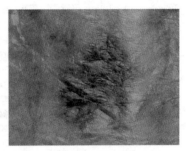

Senile purpura. *(From Lemmi, 2000.)*

Ecchymosis (Bruise)

A reddish purple, nonblanchable spot of variable size

Cause: trauma to the blood vessel resulting in bleeding under the tissue

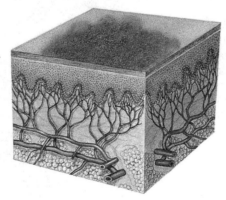

(From Seidel, 2006.)

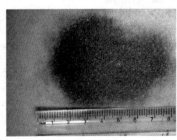

Ecchymosis. *(From Lemmi, 2000.)*

Angioma

Benign tumor consisting of a mass of small blood vessels; can vary in size from very small to large

Examples: cherry angioma, hemangioma, cavernous hemangioma, strawberry hemangioma

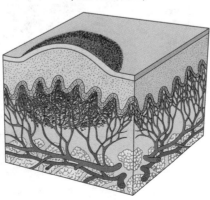

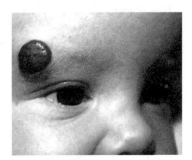

Strawberry hemangioma. *(From Habif, 2004.)*

Continued

TABLE 10-4 *Vascular Skin Lesions—cont'd*

SKIN LESIONS	CAUSE/EXAMPLES

Capillary Hemangioma (Nevus Flammeus)

A type of angioma that involves the capillaries within the skin producing an irregular macular patch that can vary from light red to dark red, to purple in color

Cause: congenital vascular malformation of capillaries
Example: port wine stain, stork bite

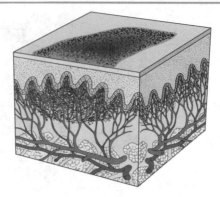

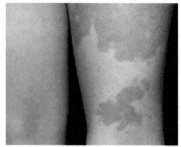

Port wine stain. *(From McCance and Huether, 2002.)*

Telangiectasia

Permanent dilation of preexisting small blood vessels (capillaries, arterioles, or venules) resulting in superficial, fine, irregular red lines within the skin

Causes: rosacea, collagen vascular disease; actinic damage, increased estrogen levels
Examples: essential telangiectasia, hereditary hemorrhagic telangiectasia, spider telangiectasia

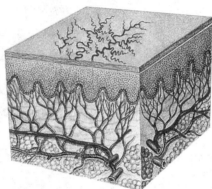

(From Seidel, 2006.)

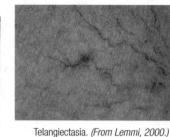

Telangiectasia. *(From Lemmi, 2000.)*

Vascular Spider (Spider Angioma)

A type of telangiectasia characterized by a small central red area with radiating spider-like legs; this lesion blanches with pressure

Causes: may occur in absence of disease, with pregnancy, in liver disease, or with vitamin B deficiency

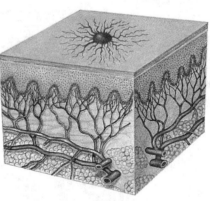

(From Seidel, 2006.)

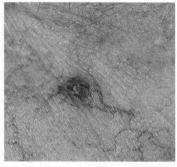

Vascular spider. *(From Habif, Campbell, Chapman et al, 2005.)*

Venous Star

A type of telangiectasia characterized by a nonpalpable bluish star-shaped lesion that may be linear or irregularly shaped

Cause: increased pressure in the superficial veins

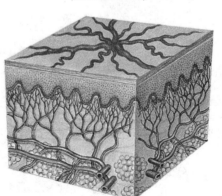

(From Seidel, 2006.)

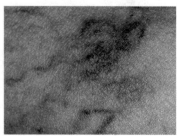

Venous star. *(From Lemmi, 2000.)*

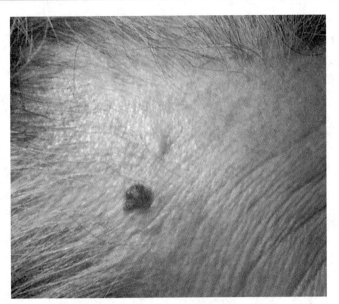

Fig. 10-14 Cherry angioma. *(From Baran et al, 1991.)*

FREQUENTLY ASKED QUESTIONS

What is the best way to memorize all the different types of skin lesions?

As a student, it is much more important that you learn to accurately describe a lesion than memorize the types of lesions themselves. As you become more proficient with descriptions, you will also begin to remember the names. When you describe a lesion, be sure to include the following information:

- Location, size, and color of the lesion
- Shape of the lesion (oval, round, irregular) and borders (regular or irregular)
- Elevation of the lesion (flat, raised, or sunken)
- Characteristics (hard, soft, fluid filled, etc.)
- Pattern (if more than one lesion)

FREQUENTLY ASKED QUESTIONS

How is a nurse supposed to be able to tell if a skin lesion is cancerous?

The only way to tell if a lesion is malignant or benign is through biopsy and pathologic examination of the tissue. The role of the nurse is not to diagnose skin cancer, but to recognize skin lesions that are suspicious (and make appropriate referrals) and to teach individuals measures to minimize the risk of skin cancers and to recognize warning signs of suspicious lesions.

Documenting Expected Findings

Skin Assessment: Adult Female

The skin is expected color for race: it is smooth, soft, warm, dry, and intact with an even surface and elastic turgor. Freckles are noted on face, back, arms, and legs. Hair on the scalp is red, shiny, soft, and fine. Facial and body hair are consistent with female distribution. Nails are clean, pink, smooth, and unpolished and blanche with pressure.

CLINICAL REASONING *Skin, Hair, and Nails*

A 74-year-old man with type 2 diabetes mellitus and peripheral vascular disease arrives at a medical clinic complaining of a painful area on his right lower leg near the ankle.

Noticing: The experienced nurse immediately has a perceptual grasp of the situation at hand. Extensive practical knowledge about what to expect with this age group and diagnoses allows the nurse to recognize risk factors given his situation. Age, diabetes mellitus, and peripheral vascular disease impact perfusion and immunity. This background knowledge sets up the possibility of noticing signs of a prevalent complication in an individual presenting with these data. The man indicates the pain started several days ago and has become progressively worse. The nurse observes a large area of redness swelling over the medial aspect of the lower left leg; the area is extremely painful to the touch and hot.

Interpreting: Early in the encounter, the nurse considers two possible causes of this client's leg pain: potential deep vein thrombosis or infection, both of which the client is at high

risk for. To determine whether either has any probability of being correct, the nurse gathers additional data.

Has there been a recent injury to the area, creating a mechanism for bacterial entrance into the skin? The only injury the client can recall is scratching his leg in that area the previous week while cutting weeds.

The experienced nurse not only recognizes inflammation and infection by the signs (erythema, heat, and edema) and symptoms (pain), but interprets this information in the context of an injury to an extremity of an individual with type 2 diabetes mellitus and peripheral artery disease. The nurse verifies medication allergies in anticipation for the need of antibiotics.

Responding: The nurse initiates appropriate initial interventions to reduce the inflammation and treat the infection, determine which type of health care provider may best assist the client, and ensure that the client receives appropriate immediate and follow-up care including instruction about how to prevent infections.

AGE-RELATED VARIATIONS

Infants & Children

The assessment of skin among infants and children follows the same general principals as previously described for the adult. Skin lesions common to infants and children include milia, erythema toxicum, diaper rash, and rashes associated with allergens. Chapter 20 presents further information regarding the assessment of skin, hair, and nails for these age groups.

Adolescents

The most common and concerning skin lesions among adolescents is acne because of the increase in sebaceous gland activity. Not only are these lesions painful, but they are concerning to the client because of personal appearances. Chapter 20 presents further information.

Older Adults

The skin and hair undergo significant changes with aging. Lesions are commonly found on older adults. Although many lesions are considered expected variations associated with the aging process, the incidence of skin cancer increases with age. Further information related to changes of the skin and lesions commonly found among older adults is presented in Chapter 22.

CLIENTS WITH SITUATIONAL VARIATIONS

CLIENTS WITH LIMITED MOBILITY (HEMIPLEGIA, PARAPLEGIA, QUADRIPLEGIA)

Clients with limited mobility are at risk for skin breakdown secondary to pressure and body fluid pooling because of an inability to feel pressure or a decreased ability to independently change position to relieve pressure. The nurse should examine the client's skin, especially over bony prominences. The nurse may need assistance to turn the client so that a complete skin assessment may be performed. In addition, clients who operate their own wheelchairs are at high risk for developing hand calluses. Therefore special care should be taken to examine the client's hands.

Expected and Abnormal Findings (Skin)

Assess all contact and skin pressure points for clients who have limited mobility (Fig. 10-15). When a red area of skin is noted, blanch the skin by applying gentle pressure over the red areas. If the skin becomes white (blanches) when pressure is applied and reddens again after pressure is relieved, the circulation to that area is sufficient and the redness will disappear. If the skin does not blanch when pressure is applied, a stage I pressure ulcer has developed. Pressure ulcers are staged as follows: stage I, prolonged redness with unbroken skin; stage II, partial-thickness skin loss appears as a superficial abrasion, blister, or excoriation; stage III, full-thickness skin loss with damage to the subcutaneous tissue (may note serosanguineous drainage); and stage IV, full-thickness skin loss with invasion of deeper tissue into the muscle or bone (or both). The wound appears as an open ulceration with purulent drainage and peripheral crusting (Table 10-5).

ETHNIC & CULTURAL VARIATIONS

Pressure areas in darker-skinned people often are harder to see in the early stages, because their skin does not become red or blanche under pressure. Applying manual pressure to a suspected pressure area produces a grayish or yellow-brown pallor that becomes purple. When the pressure is removed, the skin returns to normal color. An area that remains purple after pressure is released indicates tissue damage from a pressure ulcer.

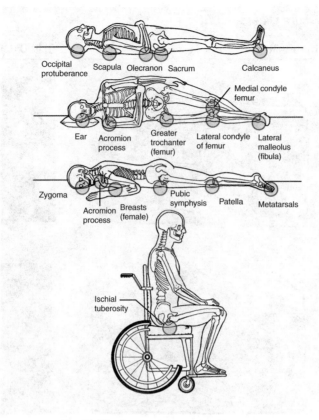

Fig. 10-15 Bony prominences vulnerable to pressure.

TABLE 10-5 *Staging of Pressure Ulcers*		
DESCRIPTION	**DIAGRAM**	**CLINICAL PRESENTATION**
Stage I A stage I pressure ulcer is an observable pressure–related alteration of intact skin whose indicators, as compared to an adjacent or opposite area of the body, may include changes in one or more of the following: Skin temperature (warmth or coolness) Tissue consistency (firm or boggy feel) Sensation (pain, itching) The ulcer appears as a defined area of persistent redness in lightly pigmented skin, whereas in darker skin tones, the ulcer may appear with persistent red, blue, or purple hues.	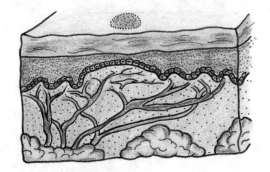	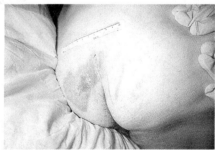

Continued

TABLE 10-5 *Staging of Pressure Ulcers—cont'd*

DESCRIPTION	DIAGRAM	CLINICAL PRESENTATION
Stage II Partial-thickness skin loss involving epidermis, dermis, or both. The ulcer is superficial and appears clinically as an abrasion, blister, or shallow crater.	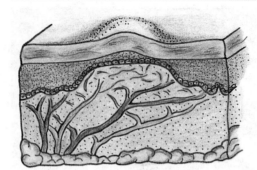	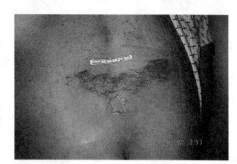
Stage III Full-thickness skin loss involving damage to or necrosis of subcutaneous tissue that may extend down to, but not through, underlying fascia. The ulcer manifests clinically as a deep crater with or without undermining of adjacent tissue.	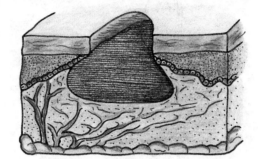	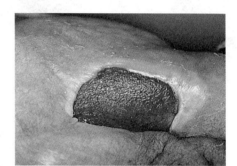
Stage IV Full-thickness skin loss with extensive destruction, tissue necrosis, or damage to muscle, bone, or supporting structures (e.g., tendon, joint capsule). Undermining and sinus tracts may also be associated with stage IV pressure ulcers.	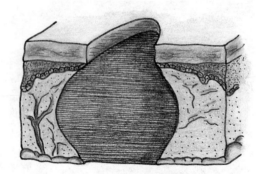	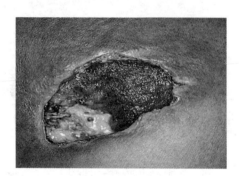

From Fifth National NPUAP Conference: Task Force on Darkly Pigmented Skin and Stage I Pressure Ulcers, approved Feb 1998, National Pressure Ulcer Advisory Panel. *Illustrations from Lewis, 2007.*

COMMON PROBLEMS & CONDITIONS

SKIN

Hyperkeratosis

Clavus (Corn)

A corn is a lesion that develops secondary to chronic pressure from a shoe over a bony prominence. **Clinical Findings:** The corn is a flat or slightly raised, painful lesion that generally has a smooth, hard surface (Fig. 10-16). A "soft" corn is a whitish thickening commonly found between the fourth and fifth toes. A "hard" corn is clearly demarcated and has a conical appearance.

Dermatitis

The term *dermatitis* is used to describe a variety of superficial inflammatory conditions of the skin that can be acute or chronic.

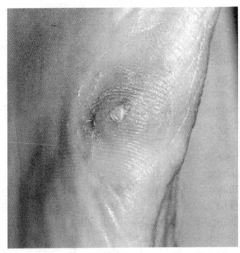

Fig. 10-16 Corn (clavus). *(From White, 1994.)*

Atopic Dermatitis

Atopic dermatitis is a chronic superficial inflammation of the skin with an unknown cause; however, it is commonly associated with hay fever and asthma and it is thought to be familial. It is seen in all age groups, although it is more common in infancy and childhood. **Clinical Findings:** During infancy and early childhood, red, weeping, crusted lesions appear on the face, scalp, extremities, and diaper area (Fig. 10-17). In older children and adults, lesion characteristics include erythema, scaling, and lichenification. The lesions are usually localized to the hands, feet, arms, and legs (particularly at the antecubital fossa and popliteal space) and are associated with intense pruritus.

Contact Dermatitis

Contact dermatitis is an inflammatory reaction of the skin in response to irritants or allergens such as metals, plants, chemicals, and detergent. This condition affects people of all ages and ethnic groups. **Clinical Findings:** Contact dermatitis appears as an area of localized erythema that may also include edema, wheals, scales, or vesicles that may weep, ooze, and become crusted. Pruritus is a common associated symptom of contact dermatitis (Fig. 10-18). The inflammatory response can vary from no reaction to extreme; thus it is highly individualized.

Seborrheic Dermatitis

Seborrheic dermatitis is a chronic inflammation of the skin of unknown cause affecting individuals throughout their entire life, often with periods of remission and exacerbation. (In infants, this condition is known as cradle cap.) **Clinical Findings:** The lesions appear as scaly, white, or yellowish plaques involving skin on the scalp, eyebrows, eyelids, nasolabial folds, ears, axillae, chest, and back. Lesions typically cause mild pruritus; lesions on the scalp cause dandruff (Fig. 10-19).

Stasis Dermatitis

Stasis dermatitis is an inflammation of the skin on the lower legs most commonly seen in the older adult. It is thought to be caused by venous stasis, chronic edema, and poor peripheral circulation. **Clinical Findings:** Initially this condition is characterized by an area or areas of erythema and pruritus followed by scaling, petechiae, and brown pigmentation

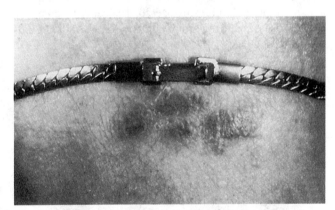

Fig. 10-18 **Contact dermatitis.** In this case, allergic reaction to nickel. *(From Cohen, 1993.)*

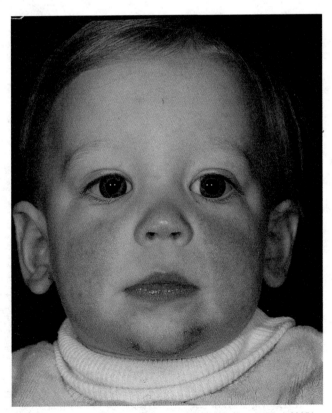

Fig. 10-17 Atopic dermatitis. *(From Habif, Campbell, Chapman et al, 2005.)*

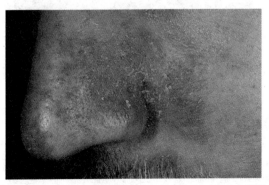

Fig. 10-19 Seborrheic dermatitis. *(From McCance and Huether, 2002.)*

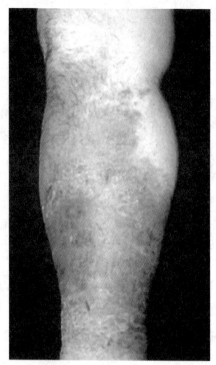

Fig. 10-20 Stasis dermatitis. *(From Marks and DeLeo, 1992.)*

(Fig. 10-20). Stasis dermatitis progresses to ulcerated lesions (known as stasis ulcers) if untreated.

Psoriasis

This is a common chronic skin disorder that can occur at any age, but usually develops by age 20. The cause is unknown, and the disease can range from mild to severe. **Clinical Find-**

ings: The lesions appear as well-circumscribed, slightly raised, erythematous plaques with silvery scales on the surface. The lesions appear most frequently on the elbows, knees, buttocks, lower back, and scalp. A specific characteristic of this condition is the observance of small bleeding points if the lesion is scratched. Associated symptoms include pruritus, burning, and bleeding of the lesions and pitting of the fingernails (Fig. 10-21).

Pityriasis Rosea

Pityriasis rosea is a common, acute, self-limiting inflammatory disease that usually occurs in young adults during the winter months. The cause is unknown, but might be associated with a virus. **Clinical Findings:** The initial manifestation is a lesion referred to as a "herald patch"—a single lesion, usually located on the trunk, resembling tinea corporis (Fig. 10-22, *A*). One to three weeks following the initial lesion, a generalized eruption of pale, erythematous, and macular lesions occurs on the trunk and extremities (Fig. 10-22, *B*); occasionally, they appear as vesicular lesions. The client generally feels well but may complain of mild itching.

Lesions Caused by Viral Infection

Warts (Verruca)

A wart is a small benign lesion caused by human papillomavirus (HPV). Because there are more than 60 different types of HPV, many different types of warts occur in many locations and in many sizes. Warts may appear at any age. **Clinical Findings:** Common warts (verrucae vulgaris) are round

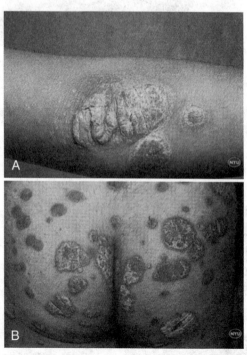

Fig. 10-21 **Psoriasis on elbow and buttocks.** *(Courtesy American Academy of Dermatology and Institute for Dermatologic Communication and Education, Schaumburg, Illinois.)*

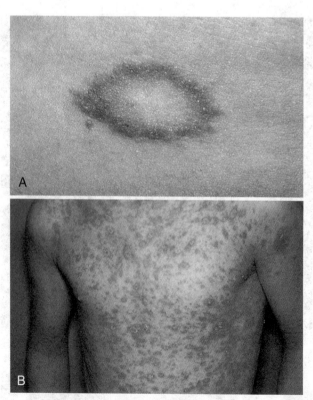

Fig. 10-22 **Pityriasis rosea. A,** Large herald patch on the chest. **B,** Many oval lesions on the chest. *(From Cohen, 1993.)*

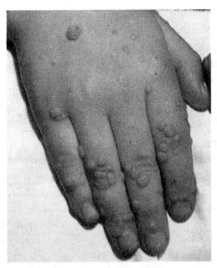

Fig. 10-23 Common warts on hand and fingers. *(Courtesy American Academy of Dermatology and Institute for Dermatologic Communication and Education, Schaumburg, Illinois.)*

or irregular-shaped papular lesions that are light gray, yellow, or brownish black. They commonly appear on hands, fingers, elbows, and knees (Fig. 10-23). Plantar warts are found on the sole of the foot and are typically tender to pressure.

Herpes Simplex

The term *herpes simplex* represents a group of eight DNA viruses. Herpes simplex virus (HSV) is a chronic, noncurable condition; between outbreaks, the virus is dormant. Outbreaks are triggered by a number of factors, including sun exposure, stress, and fever. **Clinical Findings:** Before the onset of lesions, many clients report a sensation of slight stinging and increased sensitivity. The classic manifestation of HSV is the development of grouped vesicles on an erythematous base. The lesions are very painful and highly contagious after direct contact with skin. Lesions caused by herpes simplex virus type 1 (HSV-1) often appear on the upper lip (often referred to as a cold sore), nose, around the mouth, or on the tongue (Fig. 10-24). Herpes simplex virus

type 2 (HSV-2) lesions usually appear on the genitalia. As the lesions erupt they move through maturational stages of vesicles, pustules, and finally crusting. The lesions typically last for approximately 2 weeks. (See Chapter 18 for further discussion of HSV-2.)

Herpes Varicella (Chickenpox)

This is a highly communicable viral infection, spread by droplets, that commonly occurs in children but can also infect adults who did not have the infection as children. **Clinical Findings:** The lesions first appear on the trunk and then spread to the extremities and the face. Initially the lesions are macules; they progress to papules, then vesicles, and finally the old vesicles become crusts. The lesions erupt in crops over a period of several days. For this reason, lesions in various stages are seen concurrently. The period of infectivity is from a few days before lesions appear until the final lesions have crusted, usually about 6 days after the first lesions erupt (Fig. 10-25).

Herpes Zoster (Shingles)

A dormant herpes varicella virus causes herpes zoster—which is an acute inflammation by reactivation of the virus. Herpes zoster follows varicella infection years later in some individuals. **Clinical Findings:** Linearly grouped vesicles

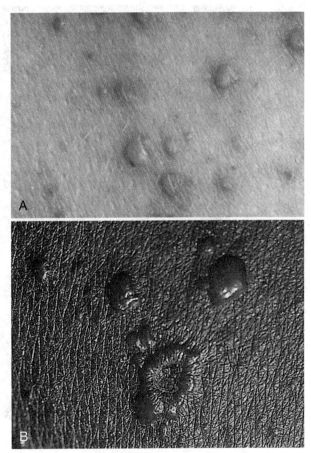

Fig. 10-25 **Herpes varicella (chickenpox).** Lesions in various stages of development, including red papules, vesicles, umbilicated vesicles, and crusts. **A,** Light-skinned person. **B,** Dark-skinned person. *(From Farrar et al, 1992.)*

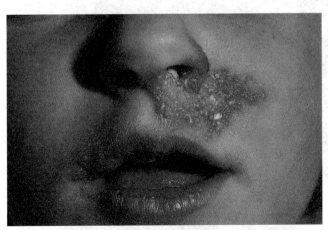

Fig. 10-24 **Herpes simplex.** Typical manifestation with vesicles appearing on the lips and extending onto the skin. *(From Habif, 2004.)*

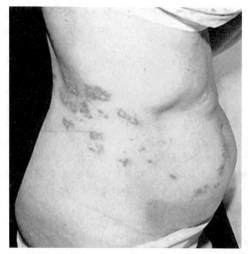

Fig. 10-26 Herpes zoster (shingles). *(From Raj, 1992.)*

appear along a cutaneous sensory nerve line (dermatome) (Fig. 10-26). As the disease progresses, the vesicles turn into pustules followed by crusts. This painful condition is generally unilateral and commonly appears on the trunk and face. Pain may precede lesion eruption by several days.

Lesions Caused by Fungal Infections

Tinea Infections

Tinea infections are caused by a number of dermophyte fungal infections involving the skin, hair, and nails that affect children and adults. **Clinical Findings:** *Tinea corporis* (ringworm) involves generalized skin areas (excluding scalp, face, hands, feet, and groin) and appears as circular, well-demarcated lesions that tend to have a clear center (Fig. 10-27, *A*). These lesions appear on nonhairy parts of the body. They are hyperpigmented in light-colored skin and hypopigmented in dark-skinned persons. *Tinea cruris* ("jock itch") affects the groin area and is characterized by small erythematous and scaling vesicular patches with a well-defined border spreading over the inner and upper surfaces of the thighs (Fig. 10-27, *B*). *Tinea capitis* involves the scalp, causing scaling and pruritis with balding areas due to hair that breaks easily (Fig. 10-27, *C*). *Tinea pedis* is a chronic infection involving the foot ("athlete's foot"). It initially appears as small weeping vesicles and painful macerated areas between the toes and sometimes on the sole of the foot. As the lesions develop, they may become scaly and hard and cause discomfort and itching (Fig. 10-27, *D*).

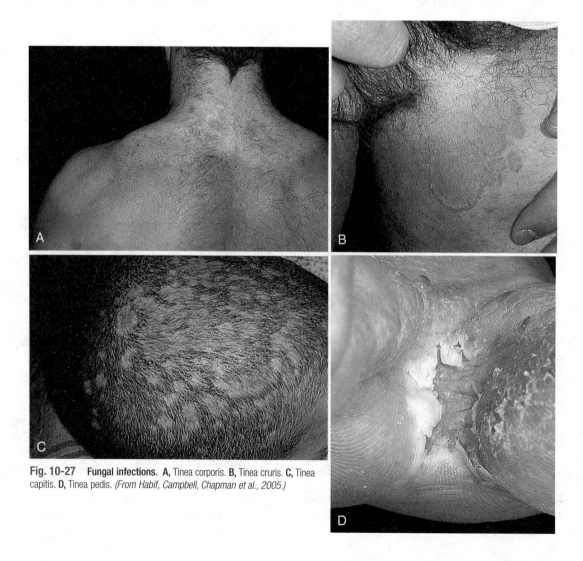

Fig. 10-27 **Fungal infections. A,** Tinea corporis. **B,** Tinea cruris. **C,** Tinea capitis. **D,** Tinea pedis. *(From Habif, Campbell, Chapman et al., 2005.)*

Candidiasis

This fungal infection is caused by *Candida albicans*. This fungus is normally found on the skin, mucous membranes, gastrointestinal tract, and vagina, but can cause an infection under certain conditions such as a favorable environment (warm, moist, or tissue maceration); disease states (diabetes, Cushing syndrome, debilitated states, immunosuppression); and systemic antibiotic administration. **Clinical Findings:** A *Candida* infection affects the superficial layers of skin and mucous membranes. It appears as a scaling red rash with sharply demarcated borders. The area is generally a large patch but may have some loose scales. Common areas for candidiasis involving the skin include the genitalia, the inguinal areas, and along gluteal folds (Fig. 10-28).

Lesions Caused by Bacterial Infections

Cellulitis

Cellulitis is an acute streptococcal or staphylococcal infection of the skin and subcutaneous tissue. Cellulitis can occur at any age and can involve any skin area on the body. **Clinical Findings:** The skin is red, warm to the touch, and tender, and appears to be indurated. There may be regional lymphangitic streaks and lymphadenopathy (Fig. 10-29).

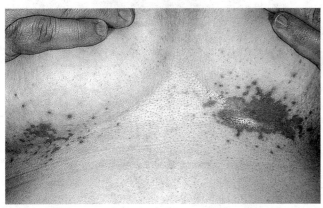

Fig. 10-28 Candidiasis. *(From Habif, Campbell, Chapman et al, 2005.)*

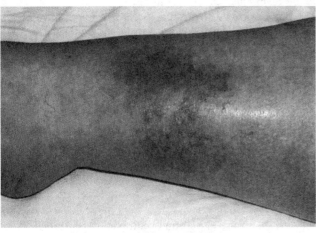

Fig. 10-29 Cellulitis to the lower leg.

Impetigo

This is a common and highly contagious bacterial infection caused by staphylococcal or streptococcal pathogens. It can occur in any age group; however, impetigo is most prevalent in children, especially among individuals living in crowded conditions with poor sanitation. It occurs most commonly in mid-to-late summer, with the highest incidence in hot, humid climates. **Clinical Findings:** This infection appears as an erythematous macule that becomes a vesicle or bulla and finally a honey-colored crust after the vesicles or bullae rupture (Fig. 10-30). The lesions commonly occur on the face around the nose and mouth, although other skin areas can be involved.

Folliculitis

This is an inflammation of hair follicles. **Clinical Findings:** An acute lesion appears as an area of erythema with a pustule surrounding the hair follicle (Fig. 10-31), most commonly on the scalp and extremities. A chronic condition occurs when deep hair follicles are infected (usually seen in bearded areas).

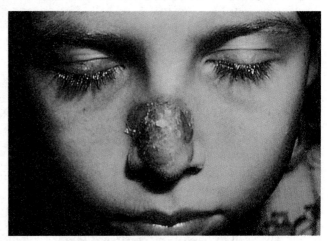

Fig. 10-30 Impetigo. *(From Goldstein and Goldstein, 1997. Courtesy Department of Dermatology, University of North Carolina at Chapel Hill.)*

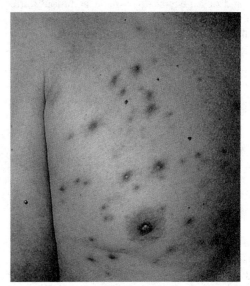

Fig. 10-31 Folliculitis. *(From Goldstein and Goldstein, 1997. Courtesy Beverly Sanders, MD.)*

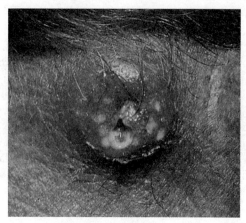

Fig. 10-32 Furuncle. *(From Thompson et al, 2002. Courtesy J. A. Tschen, MD, Baylor College of Medicine, Department of Dermatology, Houston, Texas.)*

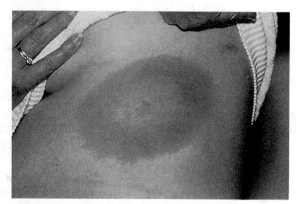

Fig. 10-33 **Lyme disease.** Note expanding erythematous lesion with central clearing on trunk. *(From Goldstein and Goldstein, 1997. Courtesy John Cook, MD.)*

Furuncle or Abscess (Boil)

A furuncle, also known as a boil, is a localized bacterial lesion caused by a staphylococcal pathogen. Furuncles often develop from folliculitis. **Clinical Findings:** Initially, a furuncle is a nodule surrounded by erythema and edema. As it progresses, it becomes a pustule; the center (or core) fills with a sanguineous purulent exudate. The skin around a furuncle is red, hot, and extremely tender (Fig. 10-32).

Lesions Associated with Arthropods

Scabies

Scabies is a highly contagious infestation associated with the mite *Sarcoptes scabiei*. The female mite burrows into the superficial layer of skin and lays eggs. Transmission usually occurs with direct skin-to-skin contact. **Clinical Findings:** Severe pruritus is the hallmark of scabies. The pruritus is caused by a hypersensitivity to the mite and its feces. The lesions are small papules, vesicles, and burrows that result from the mite entering the skin to lay eggs. The burrows appear as short irregular marks that look as if they were made by the end of a pencil. Areas most commonly affected include the hands, wrists, axillae, genitalia, and inner aspects of the thigh.

Lyme Disease

Lyme disease occurs after a bite from a tick infected with *Borrelia burgdorferi*. The large majority of Lyme disease cases in the United States occur in the Northeast states (CDC, 2005). **Clinical Findings:** The classic manifestation of Lyme disease is the development of an expanding erythemic rash with central clearing at the site of the tick bite (Fig. 10-33). This rash typically exceeds 5 cm and persists for several weeks. Most individuals also have flulike symptoms (such as fever, headache, muscle aches).

Spider Bites

The majority of bites that are of concern to humans are caused by two spiders—the black widow spider and the brown recluse spider. Black widow spiders are found throughout the United States; brown recluse spiders are

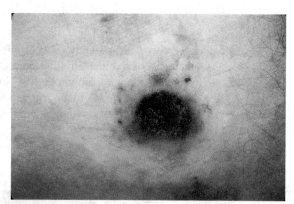

Fig. 10-34 **Brown recluse spider bite.** Note necrotic ulcer and erythema. *(From Goldstein and Goldstein, 1997. Courtesy Marshall Guill, MD.)*

found predominantly in the central and south central United States. **Clinical Findings:** The bite of the black widow and brown recluse spiders tends to cause minimal symptoms at the time of the bite. The initial lesion of a black widow spider bite appears as an area of erythema with two red puncta at the bite site. Within a few hours, symptoms of severe abdominal pain and fever typically develop. The bite of a brown recluse spider initially appears as a lesion with erythema and edema that evolves into a necrotic ulcer with erythema and purpura (Fig. 10-34). Other symptoms include fever, nausea, and vomiting.

Neoplasia

Basal Cell Carcinoma

Basal cell carcinoma is the most common form of skin cancer. It predominantly afflicts light-skinned individuals between ages 40 and 80. It is locally invasive and rarely metastasizes. The incidence increases with age and is more common in males than females (American Cancer Society [ACS], 2007). **Clinical Findings:** The lesion has different forms but usually appears as a nodular pigmented lesion with depressed centers and rolled borders. In some cases the center is ulcerated. It is usually found in areas that have had repeated exposure to the sun or ultraviolet light, such as the face (Fig. 10-35).

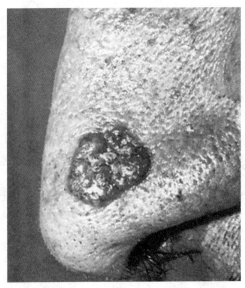

Fig. 10-35 Basal cell carcinoma. *(From Thompson et al, 1993. Courtesy Gary Monheit, MD, University of Alabama at Birmingham School of Medicine.)*

Squamous Cell Carcinoma

Squamous cell carcinoma is the second-most frequent form of skin cancer. It is an invasive skin cancer that typically appears on the head and neck and occurs as a result of excessive sun or ultraviolet light exposure. Those most commonly affected are individuals over age 50 who have blue eyes and childhood freckling (light pigmentation). Men are more commonly affected than women (ACS, 2007). **Clinical Findings:** Initially this cancer appears as a red, scaly patch that has a sharply demarcated border (Fig. 10-36). As the lesion develops further, it is soft, mobile, and slightly elevated. As the tumor matures, a central ulcer may form with surrounding redness.

Melanoma

Melanoma is the most serious form of skin cancer. It is a malignant proliferation of pigmented cells (melanocytes). These lesions typically arise from already present nevi. **Clinical Findings:** The mnemonic ABCDEF (see Box 10-2)

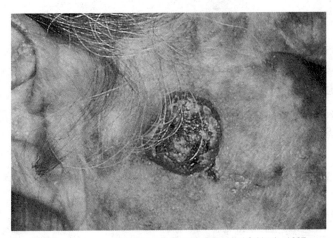

Fig. 10-36 Squamous cell carcinoma. *(From Goldstein and Goldstein, 1997. Courtesy Department of Dermatology, Medical College of Georgia.)*

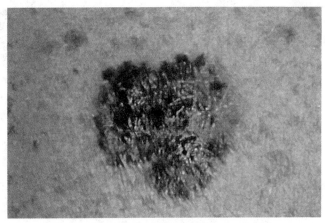

Fig. 10-37 Malignant melanoma. *(From Hill, 1994.)*

is used to remember the classic manifestations of melanoma: *A*symmetry, *B*order irregularity, *C*olor variation, *D*iameter greater than 6 mm, *E*levation (recent change from a flat to raised lesion), and *F*eeling (a reported sensation of itching, tingling, or stinging within the lesion). The lesion may have a flaking or scaly texture, and its color may vary from brown to pink to purple, or it may have mixed pigmentation (Fig. 10-37).

Kaposi's Sarcoma

Kaposi's sarcoma is a malignant neoplasm that develops in connective tissues such as cartilage, bone, fat, muscle, blood vessels, or fibrous tissues. It affects those with acquired immunodeficiency syndrome (AIDS) and those who have drug-induced immunosuppression. **Clinical Findings:** The initial lesions appear on the lower extremities and are characterized by dark blue-purple macules, papules, nodules, and plaques (Fig. 10-38). The lesions eventually spread all over the body, particularly the trunk, arms, neck, face, and oral mucosa. Associated symptoms are pain and pruritus to the lesions.

Skin Lesions Caused by Abuse

Injuries to the skin are among the most easily recognized signs of physical abuse. It is important to compare the type of injury or injuries to the history and to the developmental level (if it involves an infant or child). Injuries to the skin are generally recognized in three forms: bruises, bites, and burns.

Bruise (Ecchymosis)

A bruise is a discoloration of the skin or mucous membrane caused by blood seeping into the tissues as a result of a trauma to the area. It can indicate superficial injury or a deep injury such as injury to muscle or abdominal organs. Consider the location, appearance, and pattern of bruises and the type of mark made. **Clinical Findings:** A recent bruise (1 to 3 days old) is purple to deep black in appearance. A bruise that is 3 to 6 days old is green to brown in color, whereas an older bruise (6 to 15 days old) changes from green to tan to yellow and then fades. Look for a pattern in the bruise markings. Bruises associated with abuse may be caused by objects

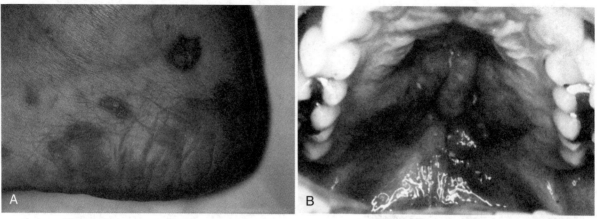

Fig. 10-38   **A,** Kaposi's sarcoma of the heel and lateral foot. **B,** Oral Kaposi's sarcoma. **(A,** *From Grimes et al, 1991.* **B,** *Courtesy Sol Silverman, Jr., DDS, University of California, San Francisco.)*

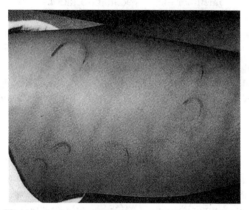

Fig. 10-39   Loop mark pattern of bruising caused by whipping with an electrical cord. *(From Monteleone, 1996.)*

that leave distinctive patterns, such as a loop pattern from being hit with a cord (Monteleone, 2003) (Fig. 10-39).

Bites

Bites are always intentional and are a common injury associated with abuse (Fig. 10-40). Bite marks are ovoid with tooth imprints that may or may not break the skin. They may have a suck mark (bruising) in the middle. The size of the bite mark is important to note to determine the age of the person who may have left the mark (i.e., child versus adult). Bite marks on infants and children are frequently located on the genitals or buttocks (Monteleone, 2003).

Burns

Burns are frequently associated with abuse. The most common type is an immersion burn. This is easily recognizable by a "glove" or "stocking" burn pattern (a line of demarcation) where the child is immersed into scalding hot water. Look for this pattern on hands and arms, feet and legs, and buttocks (Fig. 10-41). Another common type of burn associated with abuse is a *contact burn*—a burn caused by intentionally placing a hot object, such as a cigarette, light bulb, lighter, or hot iron, on the skin (Fig. 10-42). Intentional contact burns are easily recognizable because they literally leave a "branded pattern" on the skin. An accidental burn with an object typically leaves a glancing burn pattern with a nonuniform pattern (Giardino and Giardino, 2002).

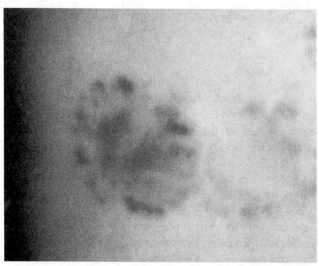

Fig. 10-40   Bite injury. *(From Monteleone, 1996.)*

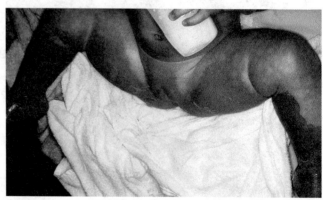

Fig. 10-41   Stocking burn patterns to perineum, thighs, legs, and feet. *(From Zitelli and Davis, 2002. Courtesy Dr. Thomas Layton, Mercy Hospital, Pittsburgh, Pennsylvania.)*

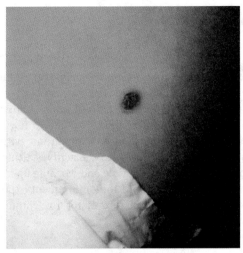

Fig. 10-42 Cigarette burn to a child's abdomen. *(From Zitelli and Davis, 2007.)*

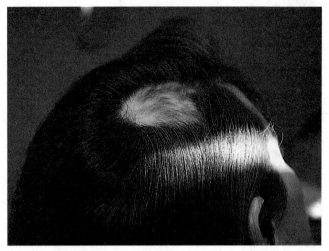

Fig. 10-44 **Alopecia areata.** Note areas of regrowth (fine, light-colored hairs). *(From Goldstein and Goldstein, 1997.)*

HAIR

Pediculosis (Lice)

Lice are parasites that invade the scalp, body, or pubic hair regions. Lice on the body are called pediculosis corporis, and pubic lice are called pediculosis pubis. **Clinical Findings:** The eggs (nits) are visible as small, white particles at the base of the hair shaft (Fig. 10-43). The skin underlying the infested area may appear red and excoriated.

Alopecia Areata

Alopecia areata is a chronic inflammatory disease of the hair follicles resulting in hair loss on the scalp. The cause is unknown, but is associated with autoimmune disorders, metabolic disease, and stressful events. **Clinical Findings:** Hair loss is observed in multiple round patch areas of the scalp (Fig. 10-44). The affected areas are either completely smooth or have short shafts of hair. The poorly developed and fragile hair shafts break and will generally grow back within 3 to 4 months, although some individuals suffer total scalp hair loss.

Hirsutism

This is a condition associated with an increase in the growth of facial, body, or pubic hair in women. This condition has familial tendency and can be associated with endocrine disorders, menopause, and side effects of medications, especially corticosteroid or androgenic steroid therapy. **Clinical Findings:** An increase of body or facial hair is seen; the amount of hair is variable (Fig. 10-45). This condition is more pronounced among individuals

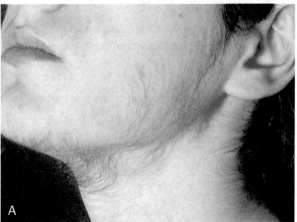
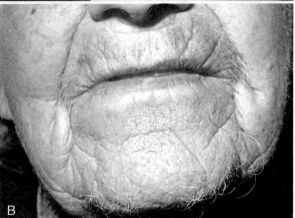

Fig. 10-45 **Facial hirsutism. A,** Hair growth on the jaw line and neck of a young woman. **B,** Hair growth on the chin of a postmenopausal woman. *(From Baran et al, 1991.)*

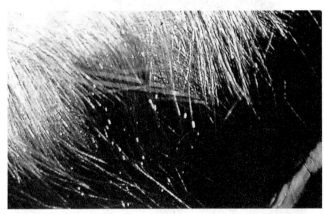

Fig. 10-43 **Pediculosis (lice).** The eggs, or nits, are visible attached to hair shafts. *(From Farrar et al, 1992. Courtesy Dr. E. Sahn.)*

with dark-pigmented hair. Increased hair growth may or may not be associated with other signs of virilization.

NAILS

Onychomycosis

This is a fungal infection of the nail plate caused by tinea unguium. Although the prevalence is variable, it occurs in up to 18% of the population in given areas. **Clinical Findings:** The nail plate turns yellow or white as hyperkeratotic debris accumulates. As the problem progresses, the nail separates from the nail bed, and the nail plate crumbles (Fig. 10-46).

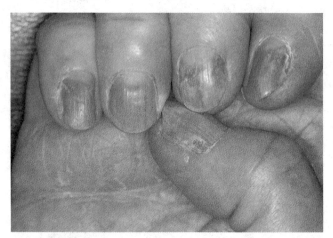

Fig. 10-46 Onychomycosis (fungal infection of the fingernail). *(From Baran et al, 1991.)*

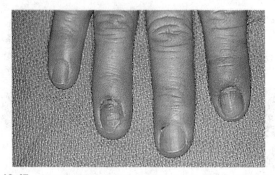

Fig. 10-47 Chronic paronychia with swollen posterior nail folds and nail dystrophy. *(From Goldstein and Goldstein, 1997. Courtesy Department of Dermatology, University of North Carolina at Chapel Hill.)*

Paronychia

Paronychia involves an acute or chronic infection of the cuticle. The infection is usually caused by staphylococci and streptococci, although *Candida* may also be the causative organism. **Clinical Findings:** Acute infection involves the rapid onset of very painful inflammation at the base of the nail, often after minor trauma to the area. In some cases an abscess may form. With chronic paronychia the inflammation develops slowly, usually starting at the base of the nail within the cuticle and working up along the sides of the nails (lateral nail folds). Frequent exposure of the hands to moisture is a risk factor for chronic paronychia (Fig. 10-47).

Ingrown Toenail

An ingrown toenail occurs when the nail grows through the lateral nail and into the skin. This condition usually involves the great toe. **Clinical Findings:** The individual experiences pain, redness, and edema. An acute infection may occur, resulting in purulent drainage (Fig. 10-48). Common risk factors for an ingrown toenail include trauma, poorly fitting shoes, and excessive trimming of the lateral nail plate.

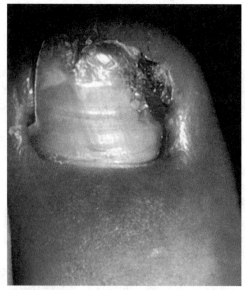

Fig. 10-48 Ingrown toenail. *(From Baden, 1987).*

CLINICAL APPLICATION & CRITICAL THINKING

See Appendix E for answers to exercises in this section.

REVIEW QUESTIONS

1 A client has edema and redness of the skin surrounding the nail on his right index finger. Which of the following data elicited from his history best explains this condition?
1 He has a family history of liver disease.
2 There has been a scabies outbreak among his family members.
3 He has a new full-time position as a dishwasher at a local restaurant.
4 He had several warts removed from his hands 2 years ago.

2 When examining a 16-year-old male client, the nurse notes multiple pustules and comedones on the face. The nurse recognizes this is due to increased activity of the:
1 Epidermal cells.
2 Eccrine glands.
3 Apocrine glands.
4 Sebaceous glands.

3 A client with darkly pigmented skin has been admitted to the hospital with hepatitis. To assess for jaundice in this patient, the nurse knows that:
1 Jaundice is best seen in the sclera.
2 In dark-skinned persons, jaundice results in a darkening of genitalia.
3 Jaundice is best determined by blanching the fingernails.
4 It is not possible to assess for jaundice in clients with darkly pigmented skin.

4 A client has multiple solid, red, raised lesions on her legs and groin that she describes as "itchy insect bites." The nurse documents these lesions as:
1 Wheals.
2 Bullae.
3 Tumors.
4 Plaques.

5 The nurse observes multiple red circular lesions with central clearing that are scattered all over the abdomen and thorax. The nurse documents the shape and pattern of the lesions as:
1 Gyrate and linear.
2 Annular and generalized.
3 Iris and discrete.
4 Oval and clustered.

6 Which of the following is an example of a vascular lesion?
1 Dermatofibroma.
2 Vitiligo.
3 Sebaceous cyst.
4 Port wine stain.

7 A 60-year-old male client states he has a sore above his lip that has not healed and is getting bigger. The nurse observes a red scaly patch with an ulcerated center and sharp margins. The nurse recognizes that these features are commonly associated with:
1 Kaposi's sarcoma.
2 Malignant melanoma.
3 Basal cell carcinoma.
4 Squamous cell carcinoma.

8 A 48-year-old woman asks the nurse how to best protect herself from excessive sun exposure while at the beach. Which response would be most appropriate?
1 "Limit your time in the sun to 5 minutes every hour."
2 "Wear a wet suit that covers your arms and legs."
3 "Apply a waterproof sunscreen (SPF 15 or higher) to exposed skin surfaces—reapply at least every 2 hours."
4 "Apply sunscreen with a minimum SPF 50 to all skin surfaces before leaving for the beach; this will provide all-day coverage."

SAMPLE DOCUMENTATION

Review the data obtained during an interview and examination by the nurse below.

Darren Muller is an 18-year-old college freshman who lives in the dormitory with four roommates. He presents to the college health center clinic with a chief complaint of "bad rash." He states that he has no medical problems, takes no medications, and has no allergies. Vital signs: temperature, 99.2° F (37.3° C); pulse rate, 104; respirations, 24. The rash was first noticed by Darren 2 days ago. He states that he does not know what is causing it but thinks it is getting worse. At first he noticed the rash under his nose and just assumed it was red from a runny nose. Today Darren states the rash is "wet, sticky, and drains a lot." When Darren was asked about other symptoms he stated, "It is really itchy, but it only hurts a little." He also reports that he has not had a very good appetite lately and he has not been drinking very much either. When asked if anything makes the rash better or worse, he stated nothing. He applied A & D ointment to the rash, but it did not help. Darren is up-to-date on immunizations. The overall skin appearance is dry with olive skin color. There are several lesions grouped together on the face around the mouth, the left side of the nose, and under the left eye. The lesions appear as raised vesicles and pustules with erythematous bases. A clear yellow exudate is seen draining from the lesions. Some of the exudate has dried into a crust. Lesions range in size from 1 to 2 cm. The hair on the scalp appears normal. There is normal body hair distribution, texture, and quality. No lesions are seen on the scalp. The fingernails appear intact without evidence of lesions. There is dirt under the nails.

Below, note how the nurse recorded these same data in a documentation format and identified appropriate nursing diagnoses from the data.

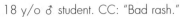

18 y/o ♂ student. CC: "Bad rash."

Medical history: none. Medications: none. Allergies: NKDA. Immunizations: up to date. Lives on campus in dormitory with 4 roommates.

SUBJECTIVE DATA

Rash first noticed under nose 2 days ago; rash is getting worse; Rash described as "wet, sticky, itchy, and drains a lot." Other symptoms: ↓ appetite and fluid intake. No specific aggravating or alleviating factors. Home tx: A and D ointment applied to rash over last 24 hours; no improvement.

OBJECTIVE DATA

Vitals: T 99.2° F (37.3° C); HR 104; RR 24

Skin: Overall skin appearance is dry/olive tone. Grouped lesions noted on face around mouth, L side of nose, and under L eye. Lesions—raised vesicles and pustules c̄ erythematous base; clear yellow, sticky exudates and crust noted. Lesion size from 1 to 2 cm.

Hair: Hair distribution, texture, quality WNL; no scalp lesions.

Nails: Fingernails intact; no lesions; dirt under nails observed.

CASE STUDY

Don Hillerman is a 38-year-old male paraplegic admitted to the hospital for unexplained weakness and depression. The following data are collected by the nurse during an interview and assessment.

Interview Data

Don states that he became a paraplegic 2 years ago after a motorcycle accident. He claims he is fully independent and needs no assistance. However, the past month or so he has felt weak and has had a loss of appetite. Normally he is able to transfer himself in and out of a wheelchair but admits that the last few weeks he has engaged in very little activity. His mother and father keep telling him he is depressed, and this makes him feel very angry. He has no other medical problems, and he has no allergies to medications.

Examination Data

- *General survey:* Alert, very thin male with flat affect lying in a supine position. Height, 6 feet 2 inches (188 cm); weight, 153 lb (69.5 kg). Slight foul-smelling odor noted.
- *Skin:* Skin color is pale. No evidence of bruising, no skin discoloration. Presence of skin breakdown over the left greater trochanter and over the sacrum.
- *Hair:* Full hair distribution on head with soft texture.
- *Abdomen:* Active bowel sounds. Abdomen soft, nondistended, nontender.
- *Musculoskeletal:* Paralysis, atrophy to both lower extremities; upper extremities fully functional.

Clinical Reasoning

1. What data deviate from normal findings, suggesting a need for further investigation?
2. What additional information should the nurse ask or assess for?
3. Based on the data, what risk factors for pressure ulcers does this client have?
4. Based on the data, what recommendations for health promotion would you make for this client?
5. What nursing diagnosis and collaborative problems should be considered for this situation?

INTERACTIVE ACTIVITIES

Open the interactive student CD-ROM, click on Chapter 10, and choose from the following activities on the menu bar:

- **Multiple Choice Challenge.** Click on the best answer for each question. You will be given immediate feedback, rationale for incorrect answers, and a total score. Good luck!

- **Marvelous Matches.** Drag each word or phrase to the appropriate place on the screen. Test your ability to match a lesion description to the lesion category.

- **A Day in the Clinic.** Complete an examination by choosing a technique and an examination area on this patient. You'll be able to collect data, document, and compare your answers with those of the experts. All that you need for a successful assessment is at your fingertips!

- **Printable Lab Guide.** Locate the Lab Guide for Chapter 10, and print and use it (as many times as needed) to help you apply your assessment skills. These guides may also be filled in electronically and then saved and e-mailed to your instructor!

- **Quick Challenge.** Use this critical thinking exercise to assess your skills through case study-style questions, then compare with expert answers!

- **Core Examination Skills Checklists.** Make sure you've got frequently-used exam skills down pat! Use these checklists to help cover all the bases for your examination.

CHAPTER 11

Head, Eyes, Ears, Nose, and Throat

ANATOMY & PHYSIOLOGY

The head and neck regions contain multiple structures that make examination of these areas complex. The skull encloses the brain; facial structures include the eyes, ears, nose, and mouth. Structures of the neck include the upper portion of the spine, the esophagus, the trachea, the thyroid gland, arteries, veins, and lymph nodes. Because of the regional relationship, all these structures are presented in this chapter.

THE HEAD

The skull is a bony structure that protects the brain and upper spinal cord (Fig. 11-1). The special senses of vision, hearing, smell, and taste are also contained within the skull. Six bones form the skull (one frontal bone, two parietal bones, two temporal bones, and one occipital bone) and are fused together at sutures. The skull is covered by scalp tissue, which is typically covered with hair.

The face consists of 14 bones that protect facial structures including the eyes, ears, nose, and mouth; these structures are generally symmetric. Like the skull, these bones are immobile and are fused at sutures, with the exception of the mandible. The mandible articulates with the temporal bone of the skull at the temporomandibular joint, allowing for movement up, down, in, out, and from side to side. The facial muscles are innervated by cranial nerves V (trigeminal) and VII (facial).

THE EYES

External Ocular Structures

The external eye is composed of the eyebrows, upper and lower eyelids, eyelashes, conjunctivae, and lacrimal glands (Fig. 11-2). The opening between the eyelids is termed the *palpebral fissure*. The eyelashes curve outward from the lid margins, filtering out dirt. Two thin, transparent mucous membranes termed *conjunctivae* lie between the eyelids and the eyeball. The bulbar conjunctiva covers the scleral surface of the eyeballs. The palpebral conjunctiva lines the eyelids and contains blood vessels, nerves, hair follicles, and sebaceous glands. One of the sebaceous glands, the meibomian gland, secretes an oily substance that lubricates the lids, prevents excessive evaporation of tears, and provides an airtight seal when the lids are closed. Tears, formed by the lacrimal glands, combine with sebaceous secretions to maintain a constant film over the cornea. In the inner (or medial) canthus, small openings termed the *lacrimal puncta* drain tears from the eyeball surface through the lacrimal sac into the nasolacrimal ducts.

Ocular Structures

The globe of the eye, also known as the "eyeball," is surrounded by three separate layers: the sclera, uvea, and retina (Fig. 11-3). The *sclera* is a tough, fibrous outer layer com-

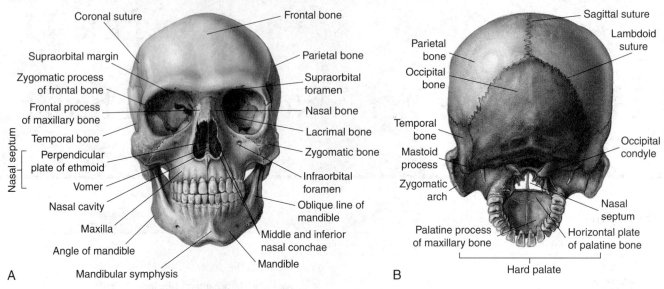

Fig. 11-1 **Bones of the skull and face. A,** Anterior view. **B,** Posterior view. *(From Seeley, Stephens, and Tate, 1995. The McGraw Hill Companies, Inc.)*

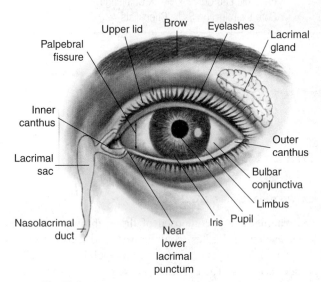

Fig. 11-2 External ocular structures. *(From Thompson, 2002.)*

monly referred to as the "white" of the eye. The sclera merges with the cornea in front of the globe at a junction termed the *limbus.* The cornea covers the iris and the pupil. It is transparent, avascular, and richly innervated with sensory nerves via the ophthalmic branch of the trigeminal nerve (cranial nerve V). The constant wash of tears provides the cornea with its oxygen supply and protects its surface from drying. An important corneal function is to allow light transmission through the lens to the retina.

The middle layer, termed the *uvea,* consists of the choroid posteriorly and the ciliary body and iris anteriorly. The choroid layer is highly vascular and supplies the retina with blood. The iris is a circular, muscular membrane that regulates pupil dilation and constriction via the oculomotor nerve (cranial nerve III). The central opening of the iris, the pupil, allows light transmission to the retina through the transparent lens. The ciliary body has two functions: It adjusts the shape

of the lens to accommodate vision at varying distances, and it produces transparent aqueous humor—a fluid that helps maintain the intraocular pressure and metabolism of the lens and posterior cornea. Aqueous humor fills the anterior chamber between the cornea and lens and flows between the lens and the iris.

The inner layer of the eye, the *retina,* is an extension of the central nervous system. This transparent layer has photoreceptor cells, termed *rods* and *cones,* scattered throughout its surface. As the term *photoreceptor* suggests, these cells perceive images and colors in response to varying light stimuli. Rods respond to low levels of light and cones to higher levels of light. These rods and cones, although scattered throughout the retina, are not evenly distributed. The macula lutea, a pigmented area about 4.5 mm in diameter, is densely packed peripherally with rods. The fovea centralis, a small depression in the center of the macula lutea on the posterior wall of the retina, contains no rods.

Perforating the retina is the optic disc, which is the head of the optic nerve (cranial nerve II). It contains no rods or cones, causing a small blind spot located about 15 degrees laterally from the center of vision. The central retinal artery and central vein bifurcate at the optic disc and feed into smaller branches throughout the retinal surface as shown in Fig. 11-3. (Also see Fig. 11-27 later in this chapter.)

Ocular Function

Vision, the primary function of the eyes, occurs when rods and cones in the retina perceive images and colors in response to varying light stimuli. The lenses are constantly adjusting to stimuli at different distances through accommodation. When the lenses bring an image into focus, nerve impulses transmit the information from the retina along the optic nerve and optic tract, reaching the visual cortex (located in the occipital lobe of each cerebral hemisphere) for cognitive interpretation (Fig. 11-4).

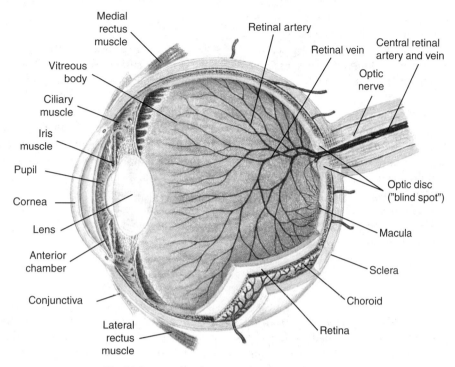

Fig. 11-3   Anatomy of the human eye. *(From Seidel et al, 2006).*

Six extraocular muscles and three cranial nerves allow for eye movement in six directions. The medial, inferior, and superior rectus muscles, as well as the inferior oblique muscles, guided by the oculomotor nerve (cranial nerve III), control upward outer, lower outer, upward inner, and medial eye movements. The superior oblique muscle controls lower medial movement, innervated by the trochlear nerve (cranial nerve IV). The lateral rectus muscle controls lateral eye movement, innervated by the abducens nerve (cranial nerve VI).

THE EAR

External Ear

The external ear is made up of the auricle (pinna) and the external auditory ear canal. The auricle is composed of cartilage and skin. The helix is the prominent outer rim; the concha is the deep cavity in front of the external auditory meatus (Fig. 11-5). The bottom portion of the ear is referred to as the lobule. The auricle is attached to the head by skin, extension cartilage to the external auditory canal

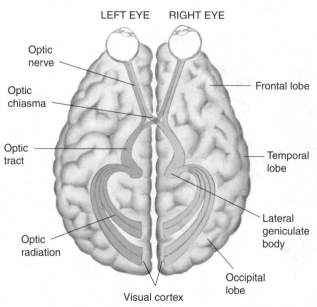

Fig. 11-4   Visual pathway. *(From Thompson, 2002).*

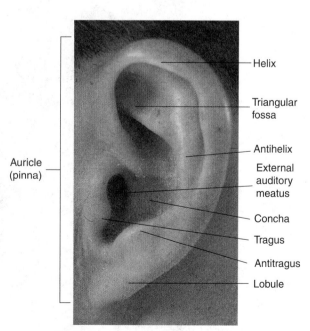

Fig. 11-5   Anatomic structure of the auricle (pinna).

cartilage, ligaments, and muscles (the anterior, superior, and posterior auricular muscles). The auricle serves three main functions: collection and focus of sound waves, location of sound (by turning the head until the sound is loudest), and protection of the external ear canal from water and dirt.

The adult's external ear canal is an S-shaped pathway leading from the outer ear to the tympanic membrane (TM)—commonly known as the eardrum (Fig. 11-6). The lateral one third of the ear canal has a cartilaginous framework; the medial two thirds of the canal is surrounded by bone. The skin covering the cartilaginous portion of the auditory canal has hair follicles surrounded by sebaceous glands that secrete cerumen (earwax). The hair follicles and cerumen protect the middle and inner ear from particles and infection.

Middle Ear

The middle ear is an air-filled cavity separated from the external ear canal by the TM. The TM is made of layers of skin, fibrous tissue, and mucous membrane that is shiny and pearl-gray. It is translucent, permitting limited visualization of the middle ear cavity. The middle ear contains three tiny bones—the malleus, incus, and stapes that are collectively known as ossicles (see Fig. 11-6). Lying between the nasopharynx and the middle ear is the eustachian tube. It opens briefly during yawning, swallowing, or sneezing to equalize the pressure of the middle ear to the atmosphere.

The function of the middle ear is amplification of sound. Sound waves cause the TM to vibrate; this vibration is transmitted through the ossicles to the inner ear. The amplification results from the ossicles and from the size (area) difference between the TM and the oval window.

Inner Ear

The inner ear is encased in a bony labyrinth that contains three primary structures: the vestibule, the semicircular canals, and the cochlea (Fig.11-6). The vestibule and the semicircular canals contain receptors responsible for balance and equilibrium. The coiled snail-shaped cochlea contains the organ of Corti, the structure that is responsible for hearing. Specialized hair cells on the organ of Corti act as sound receptors. Sound waves that reach the cochlea cause movement of the hair cells, which in turn transmit the impulses along the cochlear nerve branch of the acoustic nerve (cranial nerve VIII) and then to the temporal lobe of the brain, where interpretation of sound occurs.

THE NOSE

The nose serves as a passageway for inspired and expired air. It humidifies, filters, and warms air before it enters the lungs, and conserves heat and moisture during exhalation. Other functions of the nose include identifying odors and giving resonance to laryngeal sounds.

The upper third of the nose is encased in bone and the lower two thirds of the nose is composed of cartilage. The floor of the nasal cavity is the hard palate. The septal cartilage maintains the shape of the nose and separates the nares (nostrils), which maintain an open passage for air. The nasal cavity is lined with highly vascular mucous membranes containing cilia (nasal hairs) that trap airborne particles and prevent them from reaching the lungs. Three turbinates (inferior, middle, and superior) line the lateral walls of the nasal cavity, providing a large surface area of nasal mucosa for heat and water exchange as air passes through the nose. The middle meatus is an outlet for drainage from the frontal, maxillary,

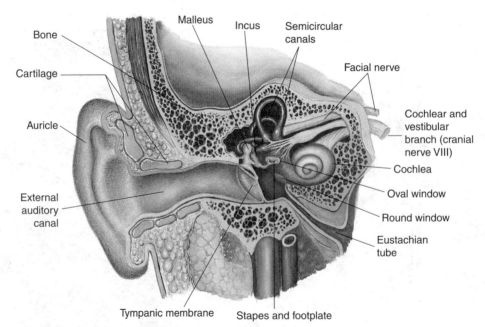

Fig. 11-6 Anatomy of the ear showing the outer ear, external auditory canal, tympanic membrane, and structures of the middle and inner ear. *(From Seidel et al, 2006.)*

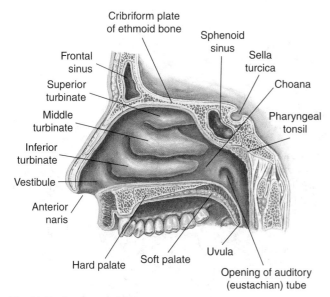

Cribriform plate
of ethmoid bone

Sphenoid
sinus

Frontal
sinus

Sella
turcica

Superior
turbinate

Choana

Middle
turbinate

Pharyngeal
tonsil

Inferior
turbinate

Vestibule

Anterior
naris

Hard palate   Soft palate   Uvula

Opening of auditory
(eustachian) tube

Fig. 11-7 Cross-sectional view of the structures of the nose and nasopharynx. *(From Seidel et al, 2006.)*

and anterior ethmoid sinuses. The nasolacrimal duct drains into the inferior meatus and the posterior ethmoid sinus drains into the middle and superior meatus (Fig. 11-7).

Paranasal sinuses extend out of the nasal cavities through narrow openings into the skull bones to form four bilateral (paired), air-filled cavities that make the skull lighter (sphenoid, frontal, ethmoid, and maxillary) (Fig. 11-8). They are lined with mucous membranes and cilia that move secretions along excretory pathways.

THE MOUTH AND OROPHARYNX

Within the mouth are several structures, including the lips, tongue, teeth, gums, and salivary glands (Fig. 11-9). The roof of the mouth consists of the hard palate, near the front portion of the oral cavity, and the soft palate, toward the back of the pharynx. The tongue has hundreds of taste buds (papillae) on its dorsal surface. The taste buds distinguish sweet, sour, bitter, and salty tastes. The ventral (bottom) surface of the tongue is smooth and highly vascular.

Humans have two sets of teeth: deciduous teeth (baby teeth) and permanent teeth. There are 32 permanent teeth: 12 incisors, 8 premolars, and 12 molars. Teeth are tightly encased in mucous membrane–covered, fibrous gum tissue and rooted in the alveolar ridges of the maxilla and mandible.

Three pair of salivary glands (the parotid, submandibular, and sublingual) release saliva through small openings (ducts) in response to the presence of food (Fig. 11-9). The parotid glands lie anterior to the ears, immediately above the mandibular angle, and drain into the oral cavity through Stensen's ducts (parotid gland openings). These are visible adjacent to the upper second molars. The submandibular glands are tucked under the mandible and lie approximately midway between the chin and the posterior mandibular angle. Wharton's ducts, the openings for the submandibular glands, are visible on either side of the lingual frenulum under the tongue. The sublingual glands, the smallest salivary glands, lie on the floor of the mouth and drain through 10 to 12 tiny ducts that cannot be seen with the naked eye.

Oropharynx

The oropharynx includes the structures at the back of the mouth that are visible on examination: the uvula, the anterior and posterior pillars, the tonsils, and the posterior pharyngeal wall (see Fig. 11-9). The uvula is suspended, midline, from the soft palate, which extends out to either side to form the anterior pillar. The tonsils are masses of lymphoid tissue that are tucked between the anterior and posterior pillars. These may be atrophied in adults to the point of being barely visible. The posterior pharyngeal

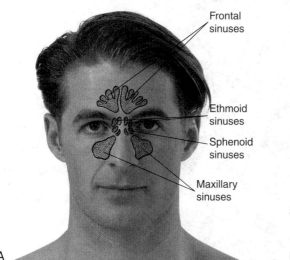

Frontal
sinuses

Ethmoid
sinuses

Sphenoid
sinuses

Maxillary
sinuses

A

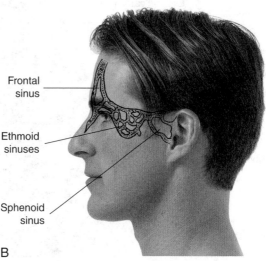

Frontal
sinus

Ethmoid
sinuses

Sphenoid
sinus

B

Fig. 11-8 Paranasal Sinuses. **A,** Front view. **B,** Side view.

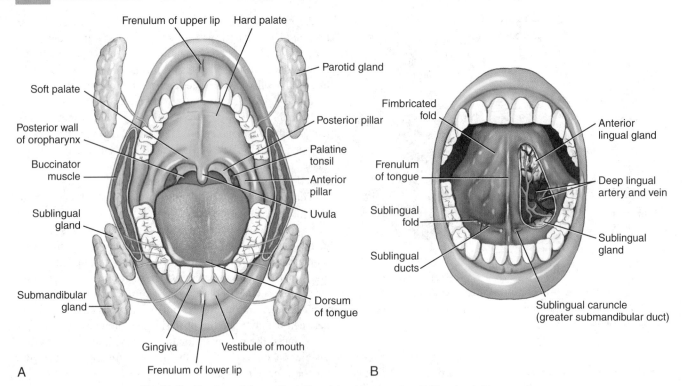

Fig. 11-9   Structures of the mouth. **A,** View of dorsal tongue surface. **B,** View of ventral tongue surface.

wall is visible when the tongue is extended and depressed. This wall is highly vascular and may show color variations of red and pink because of the presence of small vessels and lymphoid tissue. The epiglottis, a cartilaginous structure that protects the laryngeal opening, sometimes projects into the pharyngeal area and is visible as the tongue is depressed.

NECK

Structures within the neck include the cervical spine, sternocleidomastoid muscle, hyoid bone, larynx, trachea, esophagus, thyroid gland, lymph nodes, carotid arteries, and jugular veins (Fig. 11-10). The neck is formed by the bones within the upper spine (cervical vertebrae), which are supported by

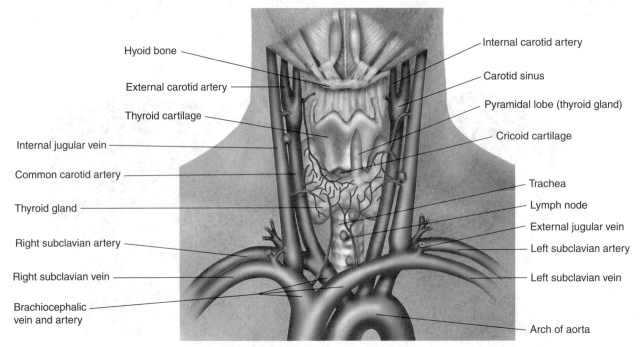

Fig. 11-10   Underlying structures of the neck. *(From Seidel et al, 2006.)*

ligaments and by the sternocleidomastoid and trapezius muscles. These structures allow for the extensive movement within the neck. The relationship of neck muscles to each other and to adjacent bones creates anatomic landmarks called triangles (Fig. 11-11). The medial borders of sternocleidomastoid muscles and the mandible form the anterior triangle. Inside this triangle lie the hyoid bone, thyroid and cricoid cartilage, larynx, trachea, esophagus, and anterior cervical lymph nodes. The hyoid bone is a U-shaped bone at the base of the mandible that anchors the tongue. It is the only bone in the body that does not articulate with another bone. The posterior triangle is formed by the trapezius and sternocleidomastoid muscles and the clavicle; it contains the posterior cervical lymph nodes.

Larynx

The larynx (also known as the voice box) lies just below the pharynx and just above the trachea. The larynx acts as a passageway for air (into the trachea) and allows for vocalization with the vocal cords. The largest component of the larynx is the thyroid cartilage (also known as the "Adam's apple"), located in the anterior portion of the neck (see Fig. 11-10). The thyroid cartilage is a tough, shield-shaped structure with a notch in the center of its upper border that protrudes in the front of the neck protecting the other structures within the larynx (epiglottis, vocal cords, and upper aspect of the trachea).

Thyroid Gland

The thyroid gland, the largest endocrine gland in the body, produces two hormones, thyroxine (T_4) and triiodothyro-

nine (T_3), that regulate cellular metabolism. Mental and physical growth and development depend on thyroid hormones. The thyroid gland is positioned in the anterior portion of the neck, just below the larynx, situated on the front and sides of the trachea (see Fig. 11-10). The right and left lobes of the thyroid gland are butterfly shaped, joined in the middle by the isthmus. The isthmus lies across the trachea under the cricoid cartilage (the uppermost ring of the tracheal cartilages) and tucks behind the sternocleidomastoid muscle.

Cardiovascular Structures

The carotid arteries and internal jugular vein lie deep and parallel to the anterior aspect of the sternocleidomastoid muscle (see Fig. 11-10). These large vessels provide important information regarding a client's cardiovascular status. See Chapter 13 for further information about these vessels.

LYMPH NODES

Lymph nodes are tiny oval clumps of lymphatic tissue, usually located in groups along blood vessels. Nodes located in subcutaneous connective tissue are called superficial nodes; those beneath the fascia of muscles or within various body cavities are called deep nodes. Deep nodes are not accessible to inspection or palpation. However, superficial nodes are accessible and become enlarged and tender, providing early signs of inflammation.

In the head, lymph nodes are categorized as preauricular, postauricular, occipital, parotid, retropharyngeal (tonsillar), submandibular, submental, and sublingual. In the neck, lymph nodes are found in chains and are named according to their relation to the sternocleidomastoid muscle and the neck's anterior and posterior triangles. Lymph nodes in the neck include the anterior and posterior cervical chains, sternomastoid nodes, and the supraclavicular nodes (Fig. 11-12).

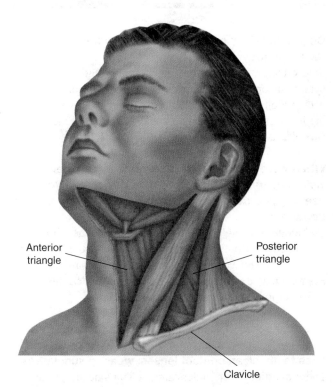

Fig. 11-11 Anterior and posterior triangles of the neck. *(From Seidel et al, 2006.)*

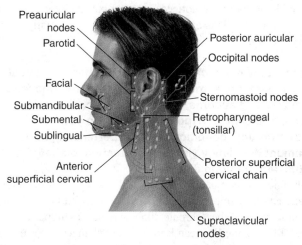

Fig. 11-12 Lymph nodes of the head and neck. *(Modified from Seidel et al, 2006.)*

LINK TO CONCEPTS   *Sensory Perception*

The feature concept for this chapter is *Sensory Perception.* The concept of sensory perception refers to the ability to understand and interact with the environment through senses (sight, hearing, smell, taste, and touch) and conditions that negatively affect these perceptions. Sensory perception occurs through a variety of body systems and a complex interaction between sensory structures and neurologic function.

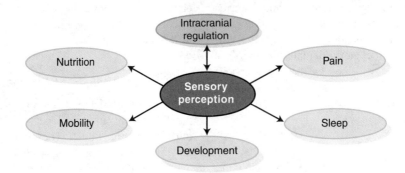

This model shows the interrelationship of concepts that are impacted by sensory perception, and the relationship sensory perception has to neurologic function. As an example, a child with chronic ear infections may be impacted by pain, interrupted sleep, and developmental delay. An individual with a visual disturbance may experience changes in mobility. Having an understanding of the interrelationship of these concepts helps the nurse recognize potential risk factors and thus increases awareness when conducting a health assessment. This is an important step associated with clinical judgment.

HEALTH HISTORY

GENERAL HEALTH HISTORY

Present Health Status

Have you noticed any changes in your overall health, or changes to your eyes, ears, nose, or mouth?
The client may have noticed a change but may not consider it a "problem." This question allows you to potentially identify problems.

Do you have any chronic conditions that affect your eyes, ears, nose, mouth, head, or neck regions (e.g., cataracts, glaucoma, migraine headaches, hearing loss, oral cancer, hypothyroidism)? Do you have other chronic conditions (e.g., hypertension, human immunodeficiency virus [HIV] infection, diabetes mellitus, autoimmune disorders)?
Chronic diseases can impact clinical findings. For example, cataracts may impact visual acuity and may be visible upon examination. Other chronic illnesses such as hypertension and diabetes mellitus can lead to visual changes; HIV infection and immunodeficiency disorders can lead to mouth lesions.

Do you take any medications? If so, what do you take and how often?
Side effects of medications are common and may explain symptoms or clinical findings associated with the head and neck regions. Headaches, dizziness, changes in vision, ringing in the ears, and dry mouth are all examples of medication side effects.

When were your last routine examinations (dental, vision, hearing)? What corrective devices do you use (e.g., contact lenses, glasses, hearing aids, dentures)?
These questions help to understand a client's health promotion practices. Routine dental examinations and examination of the eyes and ears are recommended. The frequency of examinations depends on the client's age, underlying medical conditions, and use of corrective devices.

Describe some of your daily practices to maintain the health of your eyes, ears, and mouth (e.g., brush and floss teeth; clean contact lenses; wearing sunglasses).
These questions help understand a client's health promotion practices and potential risks.

RISK FACTORS *Vision, Hearing, Mouth Cancer*

As you conduct a health history, consider common risk factors associated with hearing and vision loss and mouth cancers. Follow up with additional questions should they exist.

Hearing Loss
- Age: increased incidence after age 50
- Environmental noise (repeated exposure to loud noise >80 dB) (M)
- Ototoxic medications (aminoglycosides, salicylates, furosemide) (M)
- Family history (sensorineural hearing loss)
- Autoimmune disorders (sensorineural hearing loss)
- History of congenital hearing loss

Cataracts
- Age: Between 65 and 74 years, 70% of adults had opaque areas and 18% had cataracts; between 75 and 84 years, 90% of adults had opaque areas and about 50% had cataracts.
- Gender: Women have a higher risk than men.
- Ethnicity: African Americans have highest risk.
- Smokers: Those who smoke 20 or more cigarettes daily have twice the risk. (M)
- Alcohol: Chronic drinkers of alcohol have increased risk. (M)
- Light Exposure: Exposure to low-level ultraviolet B (UVB) radiation increases risk. Occupational exposure such as arc welding increases risk. (M)
- Medication: People who take corticosteroids may have increased risk. (M)
- Chronic disease: Diabetes mellitus increases risk.

Glaucoma
- Age: Risk increases each year over age 50.
- Family history: Those with a history of glaucoma in a first-degree relative have three times the risk.
- Ethnicity: African Americans are more likely to develop open-angle glaucoma than Caucasians. Asians and Eskimos have an increased risk for closed-angle glaucoma.
- Medication: People who take corticosteroids (including inhaled steroids) on a regular, long-term basis have increased risk. (M)
- Chronic disease: Diabetes mellitus and hypertension significantly increase risk.

Macular Degeneration
- Age: Macular degeneration exists in 25% of those between ages 65 and 74 years and 33% of those above age 75 years.
- Smoking: Cigarette smokers have twice the risk. (M)
- Chronic disease: Hypertension is associated with increased risk.
- Diet: High intake of monosaturated, polyunsaturated, and vegetable fats (M)

Oropharyngeal Cancer
- Age (increased incidence after age 40 with peak incidence between ages 64 and 74)
- Gender (2:1 male-to-female incidence)
- Race (African Americans have highest incidence)
- Tobacco: 90% of individuals who develop oral cancer are tobacco users. (M)
- Alcohol: 75% to 80% of individuals who develop oral cancer consume excessive amounts of alcohol. (M)
- Exposure to sunlight: 30% of those who have cancer on the lip have an outdoor occupation with prolonged exposure to the sun. (M)
- History of previously diagnosed cancer
- Immunosuppression

M = modifiable risk factor.
National Eye Institute, *www.nei.nih.gov/health/*
American Cancer Society, *www.cancer.org*
National Institute on Deafness and Communication Disorders, *www.nidcd.nih.gov/*

Do you know of any occupational or recreational risks for injury to your eyes, ears, or mouth?

Assessment of environmental risk factors that can contribute to vision or hearing loss is an important component of a health history. Clients should be encouraged to take protective action to minimize injury such as avoiding loud sounds, wearing ear plugs, wearing goggles, wearing eye and/or mouth protection when engaging in contact sports. Regulatory agencies such as the Occupational Safety and Health Administration (OSHA) have guidelines and regulations to reduce injuries in the work environment.

Do you use nicotine products or drink alcohol? If so, how much?

These questions help understand a client's potential risks for problems involving the head, eyes, ears, and mouth. Chronic alcohol intake and smoking are risk factors for many problems including cataracts, glaucoma, and cancers of the oropharynx.

Past Medical History

Have you ever had an injury to your eyes, ears, mouth, or neck? If so, describe when and what happened. Do you continue to have any problems related to the injury?

Injuries, either recent or past, may provide information relevant to a client's clinical findings. Although not common, some individuals have lost an eye due to disease or injury and have an eye prosthesis.

Have you had surgery involving your eyes, nose, ears, mouth, or neck? If so, what was the purpose of the surgery?

Knowledge of past surgeries may provide information that may be applied to symptoms or clinical findings. Teeth extraction and removal of tonsils are common surgical procedures that affect findings within the mouth. Common surgical procedures on the eyes include cataract and surgery for corrective vision. Myringotomy is a common surgical procedure of the ears among children.

In the past, have you had chronic infections affecting your eyes, ears, sinuses, or throat? If so, did this occur during childhood? Adulthood? How was the problem treated?

Establish baseline information for persons with a history of chronic infections—even if they don't currently have problems. These data may shed light on other findings.

Family History

Is there a history of cancer in your family? If so, which family member(s)? What kind of cancer was diagnosed?

The client could have a genetic predisposition to cancer.

Does anyone in your family have conditions impacting hearing, vision, or thyroid?

Cataracts, glaucoma, sensorineural hearing loss, Ménière's disease, and hyperthyroidism are examples of conditions that have familial tendencies, and may increase a client's risk.

PROBLEM-BASED HISTORY

The most commonly reported problems related to the head and related structures (eyes, ears, nose, throat, and neck) include headache, dizziness, difficulty with vision, hearing loss, ringing in the ears, earache, nasal discharge, sore throat, and mouth lesions. As with symptoms in all areas of health assessment, a symptom analysis is completed, which includes the location, quality, quantity, chronology, setting, associated manifestations, alleviating factors, and aggravating factors (see Box 3-3 in Chapter 3).

Headache

How long have you been having headaches? How often do you have a headache? How long does the headache last? Does it follow a pattern?

Many times a headache may be a sign of stress. At other times, headaches may be a sign of chemical imbalance in the body or even a sign of a more serious pathologic condition. Identification of headache patterns may help determine aggravating factors and causes. Cluster headaches occur more than once a day and last for less than an hour to about 2 hours. They may follow this pattern for a couple of months and then disappear for months or years. Migraine headaches may occur at periodic intervals and may last from a few hours to 1 to 3 days.

Where do the headaches occur? Is the pain in one area, or is it generalized? What does the pain feel like? How intense is the pain on a scale of 0 to 10?

Sinus headaches may cause tenderness over frontal or maxillary sinuses. Tension headaches tend to be located in the front or back of the head, and migraine and cluster headaches are usually unilateral. Cluster headaches produce pain over the eye, temple, forehead, and cheek. Tension headaches are described as viselike, migraine headaches produce throbbing pain, and cluster headaches cause a burning or stabbing feeling behind one eye.

What other symptoms do you experience with the headaches?

Migraines may be accompanied by visual disturbances, nausea, and vomiting. Cluster headaches may occur with nasal stuffiness or discharge, red teary eyes, or drooping eyelids.

Can you think of any factors that trigger headaches? If so, describe.

Possible triggers include stress, fatigue, exercise, food, and alcohol. Box 11-1 lists foods that trigger headaches for some individuals. Conditions that can precipitate headaches include hypertension, hypothyroidism, and vasculitis. Migraines are frequently associated with menstrual periods.

HEADACHE-TRIGGERING FOODS

Alcohol: sulfites	Meats, processed: bologna,
Avocado	salami, pepperoni
Bacon: nitrites	Monosodium glutamate
Bananas	(Chinese food)
Canned figs	Nuts
Chicken livers	Onions
Chocolate	Sunflower seeds
Citrus fruits: lemon, lime,	Tea and coffee (caffeinated
orange, grapefruit	or decaffeinated)
Herring	Yogurt
Hot dogs	

From Smith L, Schumann L: Differential diagnosis of headache, *J Am Acad Nurse Pract* 10(11):519, 1998.

What do you usually do to treat the headache? If medication, what kind? Is the medication effective in relieving the pain? How often do you take the medication?

Knowing what brings relief may help in determining the cause of the headache. Rest can help relieve migraine headaches, whereas movement helps relieve cluster headaches.

Dizziness and Vertigo

Describe the sensation of dizziness that you are experiencing. When did it first begin? How often does it occur? How long does the dizziness last?

Ask the client to define what he or she means when reporting a history of dizziness. Dizziness is a feeling of faintness experienced within the client. By contrast, vertigo is a sensation that the environment is whirling around external to the client. The perception of movement distinguishes dizziness from vertigo (Box 11-2). Nearly all clients who self-report a sensation of motion have vertigo (Sandhaus, 2002).

DIFFERENTIATING DIZZINESS

Dizziness is a symptom used by many clients to describe a wide range of sensations, including faintness or inability to maintain normal balance in a standing or seated position. Based on the description and findings, a generalized symptom of dizziness can be more specifically classified as presyncope, disequilibrium, vertigo, or light-headedness.

Presyncope: feeling of faintness and impending loss of consciousness—often a cardiovascular symptom.

Disequilibrium: feeling of falling—often a locomotor problem.

Vertigo: sensation of movement, usually rotational motion such as whirling or spinning. Subjective vertigo is the sensation that one's body is rotating in space; objective vertigo is the sensation that objects are spinning around the body. Vertigo is the cardinal symptom of vestibular dysfunction.

Light-headedness: vague description of dizziness that does not fit any of the other classifications—usually idiopathic or psychogenic.

Does the dizziness interfere with your normal daily activities? Do you experience these symptoms when driving a car or operating machinery? Have you ever fallen as a result of the dizziness?

Knowing the effect on activities of daily living (ADLs) helps determine the extent to which the dizziness is interfering with the client's life and the frequency of the problem. It is also important to assess if the client is at risk for injury during periods of dizziness. If the client describes symptoms consistent with vertigo, he or she should be advised about the potential hazard of driving or operating machinery.

What have you done to treat the dizziness? Has this been effective?

It is important to note any attempts at self-treatment by the client.

Difficulty with Vision

What type of difficulty are you having with vision? When did it begin? Did it begin suddenly or gradually? Does the problem affect one eye or both? Is it constant, or does it come and go?

The client's description is essential in determining the cause of the visual difficulty. A sudden onset of visual symptoms may indicate a detached retina and requires an emergency referral. Involvement of both eyes tends to indicate a systemic problem, whereas involvement of one eye is a local problem.

What other symptoms are you experiencing?

Headaches, dizziness, and nausea are symptoms commonly associated with visual difficulty.

What makes your vision worse? What makes your vision better? What treatment have you tried for the vision difficulty? How effective was the treatment?

Determining what therapies have been used successfully or unsuccessfully helps in understanding the problem and guiding current treatment strategies.

Has your vision problem interfered with your daily life? If so, describe how.

Determine the impact this visual difficulty has had on the client's quality of life and evaluate the adjustments the client has made to lifestyle and routines.

Hearing Loss

How long have you had trouble hearing? What tones or sounds are difficult for you to hear?

Establish onset of problem (sudden or gradual onset over time). A sudden hearing loss in one or both ears that is not associated with an ear infection or upper respiratory infection requires further evaluation. Hearing loss associated with aging (presbycusis) occurs gradually and increases with advancing age, particularly with high frequencies.

Have you noticed other symptoms associated with the hearing loss?

Explore other symptoms such as fevers, headaches, or visual changes.

To what degree does your hearing loss bother you? Does it interfere with your daily routine or create problems on the job or social interactions?

Hearing loss may cause individuals to withdraw or become isolated because they cannot hear or because they are embarrassed. This may lead to reduced interpersonal communication, depression, and exacerbation of coexisting psychiatric conditions.

Ringing in the Ears (Tinnitus)

Describe the noise that you are hearing. Is it ringing, hissing, crackling, or buzzing? When did it first begin?

Ringing of the ears (tinnitus) is a sensation or sound heard only by the affected individual. It can manifest differently with a variety of sounds or sensations.

Does the sound occur all of the time, or does it come and go? If it comes and goes, does it occur with certain activities or at the same time of day?

Establish the pattern of the symptom; this may provide clues to determine the cause of the problem.

Earache

How long have you had an earache? Do you know what might be causing the pain?

Determine the onset of pain. Ear pain can be related to an infection in the mouth, sinuses, or throat (Box 11-3).

Describe the location of the pain. Is the pain constant, or does it come and go? If it comes and goes, how often does it occur, and how long does it last?

Determine the location of the pain. Ear pain can be unilateral or bilateral; it can be internal or external. Also determine the duration of the pain. If the pain is intermittent, explore possible triggering mechanisms.

What does the pain feel like? On a scale of 0 to 10, how would you rate the intensity of your ear pain? Does it hurt when you pull on or touch your ear? Does the pain change when you change your position, such as lying down?

Description of the pain may help determine the cause. Pain caused by an ear infection involving the external ear or ear canal increases with movement of the ear; pain caused by otitis media does not change with manipulation of the ear.

Is there any discharge from the ear? If so, what does it look like? Does the discharge have an odor?

BOX 11-3 | **FOCUS ON PAIN** *Earache*

The medical term for ear pain or earache is *otalgia*. Otalgia can be primary (pain caused by a disorder within the ear) or referred (pain caused by a disorder outside of the ear). Clues regarding the cause of the pain can be gained from taking a history—specifically ask the client what events may have triggered the pain. A recent history considered significant that may explain the onset of ear pain includes the following:

Infection to the upper respiratory tract (viral or bacterial)

Injury or trauma to the head

Exposure to a loud noise

Stress (which leads to grinding teeth)

Airplane travel

Data from Black JM, Matassarin-Jacobs E: *Medical-surgical nursing: clinical management for continuity of care,* ed 5, Philadelphia, 1997, WB Saunders.

A description of ear discharge might help determine the cause of the symptoms.

Nasal Discharge / Nose Bleed

When did the nasal discharge / nose bleed begin? How would you describe the discharge (color, consistency, odor)? Is it on one side of your nose or both?

A thick or purulent green-yellow, malodorous discharge usually results from a bacterial infection. A foul-smelling discharge, especially unilateral discharge, is associated with a foreign body or chronic sinusitis. Profuse watery discharge is typically seen with allergies. Bloody discharge may result from a neoplasm, trauma, or an opportunistic infection such as a fungal disease. A nose bleed (epistaxis) may occur secondary to trauma, chronic sinusitis, malignancy, or a bleeding disorder; it may also result from cocaine abuse.

What other symptoms do you have?

Associated symptoms consistent with allergic rhinitis include itching, swelling, discharge from the eyes, postnasal drip, and cough (Silvers, 2003). Fatigue, fever, and pain may be associated symptoms for individuals with infections.

What do you do to treat the discharge/bleeding? How effective is the treatment?

Determining what has been used successfully in the past may guide current treatment strategies and provide an opportunity for teaching. If the client uses nasal spray other than normal saline, alert him or her that it should be used for only 3 to 5 days to avoid causing rebound congestion.

Sore Throat

How long have you had a sore throat? Describe what it feels like—a lump, burning, scratchy? Does it hurt

to swallow? Is your sore throat associated with fever, cough, fatigue, painful lymph nodes?

A sore throat may have many causes, from nasal congestion or sinus drainage to an infection or allergy. Often, edema and pain associated with throat infections make it difficult to swallow. Common associated symptoms include fever, fatigue, and pain when swallowing. Nasal congestion that requires mouth breathing during the night may cause a sore throat in the morning.

Are others in your home ill or have they just recovered from a sore throat or cold? Do you inhale dust or fumes at work? Is the air in your home or office dry?

These questions explore possible environmental factors that contribute to sore throat and whether the sore throat may be communicable.

How have you been treating your sore throat? How effective was the treatment?

Determining what has been used successfully in the past may guide current treatment strategies.

Mouth Lesions

Where is the mouth sore? How long has it been present?

Mouth lesions can be caused by many things including trauma, infection, nutritional deficits, immunologic problem, or cancer.

What other symptoms have you noticed? Does the sore bother you when eating or talking?

Bleeding, lumps, thickened areas in the mouth are possible symptoms of oral cancer. Enlarged lymph nodes might be associated with cancer or an infection. Painful ulcerations may impair adequate nutritional intake.

Are there any other sores anywhere else on your body, such as in the vagina? In the urethra? On the penis? In the anus?

Sexually transmitted diseases such as herpes may be transmitted through oral sex.

HEALTH PROMOTION *Hearing*

It is estimated that some 28 million people in the United States have a hearing impairment. Hearing impairment is caused by a number of factors, including genetics (congenital), exposure to excessive noise (noise-induced hearing loss), trauma, infections (especially otitis media), and certain drugs. Hearing is a necessary component for child development; therefore identification of hearing impairment at an early age is critical. Newborn hearing screening is required by law in many states.

Goals and Objectives—*Healthy People 2010*
The *Healthy People 2010* goal for vision and hearing is to improve the visual and hearing health of the nation through prevention, early detection, treatment, and rehabilitation. Eight specific objectives relate to hearing: increase the number of newborns screened for hearing loss by 1 month; reduce the incidence of otitis media in children and adolescents; increase access to hearing rehabilitation services and adaptive devices; increase the proportion of persons who have had a hearing examination; increase the number of persons referred for hearing evaluation and treatment; increase the use of ear protection devices; reduce noise-induced hearing loss in children and adolescents; and reduce adult hearing loss.

Recommendations to Reduce Risk (Primary Prevention)
American Speech-Language Hearing Association (ASLHA)
Wear hearing protection when exposed to loud or potentially damaging noise at work, in the community, or at home.
Limit periods of exposure to noise.
Reduce volume when using stereo headsets or listening to amplified music in a confined place such as a car.
Be aware of and minimize noise in personal environment. Consider noise rating when purchasing recreational equipment, children's toys, household appliances, and power tools; look for those items with lower noise ratings.

Screening Recommendations (Secondary Prevention)
Healthy People 2010
Screen newborns for hearing loss by age 1 month; if loss is identified, perform audiologic evaluation by age 3 months, and enroll in appropriate intervention services by age 6 months as needed.
Screen adults every decade between ages 18 and 50; more frequent monitoring after age 50 years.

Intervention Recommendations (Tertiary Prevention)
CDC
Infants identified with a hearing loss should be enrolled in an intervention program by 6 months of age.

From: American Speech-Language-Hearing Association website (available at *www.asha.org*); Centers for Disease Control and Prevention: *Hearing detection and intervention program* (available at *www.cdc.gov*); US Department of Health and Human Services: Vision and hearing. In *Healthy People 2010: understanding and improving health,* ed 2, Washington, DC, 2000, US Government Printing Office (available at *www.healthypeople.gov*).

EXAMINATION

ROUTINE TECHNIQUES

HEAD
- INSPECT the head:
  - Skull
  - Facial structures 🔑

EYES
- TEST visual acuity.
- INSPECT the external ocular structures: 🔑
  - Eyebrows, eyelids, eyelashes
  - Conjunctiva
- INSPECT the ocular structures: 🔑
  - Eyes for position
  - Corneal light reflex
  - Sclera
  - Cornea transparency and surface characteristics
  - Iris
  - Pupils

EARS
- ASSESS hearing based on response from conversation. 🔑
- INSPECT the external ears:
  - Alignment and position
  - Size, shape, symmetry, skin color, and skin intactness
  - External auditory meatus

NOSE
- INSPECT the nose.

MOUTH
- INSPECT the mouth and oropharynx: 🔑
  - Lips
  - Teeth and gums
  - Tongue
  - Buccal mucosa and anterior and posterior pillars
  - Palate, uvula, posterior pharynx and tonsils

NECK
- INSPECT the neck for:
  - Appearance
  - Position
  - Skin characteristics

SPECIAL CIRCUMSTANCES OR ADVANCED PRACTICE

HEAD
- PALPATE structures of the head:
  - Skull
  - Bony structures of the face and jaw
  - Temporal arteries

EYES
- ASSESS visual fields for peripheral vision.
- ASSESS eye movement:
  - Six Cardinal Fields of Gaze
  - Cover-uncover test
- PALPATE the eye, eye lids, and lacrimal puncta.
- TEST the corneal reflex.
- INSPECT anterior chamber.
- INSPECT intraocular structures: ★
  - Red reflex
  - Optic disc
  - Retinal vessels
  - Retinal background
  - Macula

EARS
- PALPATE the external ears and mastoid areas.
- INSPECT the internal ear structures: ★
  - External ear canal
  - Tympanic membrane
- TEST auditory function.

NOSE
- PALPATE and ASSESS the nose.
- INSPECT the internal nasal cavity.
- PALPATE the paranasal sinuses.
- TRANSILLUMINATE the sinuses. ★

MOUTH
- PALPATE structures of the mouth:
  - Teeth, inner lips, and gums
  - Tongue

NECK
- INSPECT the neck for range of motion.
- PALPATE the neck for:
  - Anatomic structures
  - Tenderness
  - Muscle strength
  - Thyroid gland ★

LYMPH NODES
- PALPATE regional lymph nodes.

EQUIPMENT NEEDED

Ophthalmoscope • Otoscope • Stethoscope • Penlight • Snellen's chart or Snellen's "E" chart • Handheld vision screener (Rosenbaum or Jaeger) • Cover card (opaque) • Tuning fork • Audiometer • Nasal speculum • Examination gloves • Tongue blade • 4 × 4 gauze

---

🔑 = core examination skill   ★ = advanced practice

PROCEDURES AND TECHNIQUES WITH NORMAL FINDINGS	ABNORMAL FINDINGS

ROUTINE TECHNIQUES: HEAD

INSPECT the head.

Head for size, shape, skin characteristics.
Look at the head in relation to the neck and shoulders for size and shape. *Normocephalic* is the term designating that the skull is symmetric and is appropriately proportioned for the size of the body. The head should be held upright in a straight position. To inspect the scalp, part the hair in various locations. The scalp should be intact, without lesions, redness, or flakes.

Microcephaly is an abnormally small head. *Macrocephaly* is an abnormally large head.

Facial structures for size, symmetry, movement, intactness, skin characteristics, and facial expression.
The facial features (eyes and eyebrows, palpebral fissures, nasolabial folds, and sides of the mouth) should appear symmetric with a calm facial expression (Fig. 11-13). Facial bones should be symmetric and appear proportional to the size of the head.

Note abnormal skin color, uneven skin pigmentation, skin lesions, coarse facial hair (in women), asymmetry, edema, or abnormal facial movements (tics) (Fig. 11-14).

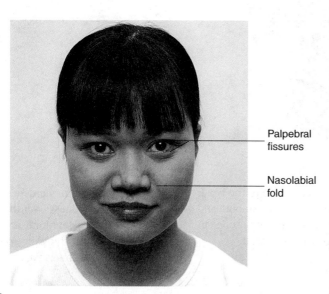

Palpebral fissures

Nasolabial fold

Fig. 11-13 Symmetry of facial features (the eyebrows, palpebral fissures, nasolabial folds, and corners of the mouth) is a normal finding.

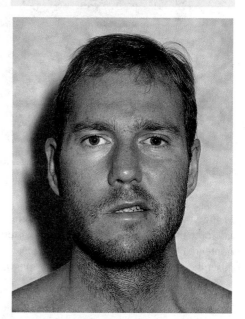

Fig. 11-14 Right facial palsy causing asymmetry of facial features. *(From Swartz, 2006.)*

SPECIAL CIRCUMSTANCES OR ADVANCED PRACTICE: HEAD

PALPATE the structures of the head.

Skull for contour, tenderness, and intactness.
Palpate the skull from front to back using a gentle rotary motion. The skull should be symmetric and should feel firm without tenderness. The frontal, parietal, and bilateral occipital prominences may be felt. Examination gloves should be worn if the client has scalp lesions, injury, or poor hygiene.

Lumps, marked protrusions, or tenderness should be differentiated to determine if they are on the scalp or actually part of the skull. Depressions or unevenness of the skull may occur secondary to skull injury.

= core examination skill

| **PROCEDURES AND TECHNIQUES WITH NORMAL FINDINGS** | **ABNORMAL FINDINGS** |

Bony structures of the face and jaw noting size, intactness, and tenderness, and jaw movement.

To palpate jaw movement, place two fingers in front of each ear and ask the client to slowly open and close the mouth and then move the lower jaw from side to side. The jaw should move smoothly and without pain (Fig. 11-15).

Pain associated with palpation of facial structures should be explored further. Limited movement, pain with movement, and a jaw that clicks or catches with movement may indicate TMJ disease (Okeson, 2003).

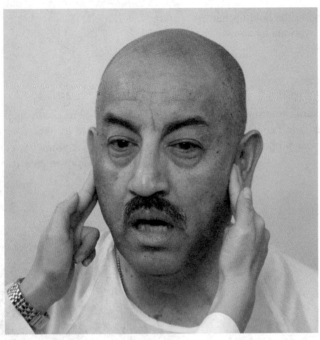

Fig. 11-15   Position fingers in front of each ear to palpate the temporomandibular joint (TMJ).

Temporal arteries.

Using your fingertips, palpate over the temporal bone on each side of the head, lateral to each eyebrow for the temporal artery. The artery should be smooth and nontender, with pulsation noted. If indicated, use the bell of your stethoscope to auscultate the temporal arteries. A normal finding is absence of a bruit.

Tender, edematous, or hardened temporal arteries with redness over the temporal region suggest temporal arteritis. A bruit (a low-pitched blowing sound) indicates a vascular abnormality.

ROUTINE TECHNIQUES: EYES

TEST visual acuity (distance vision).

Procedure: Place Snellen's chart on the wall in a well-lighted room. The client may sit or stand 20 feet (6 m) from the chart. If the client wears contact lenses or glasses, he or she should leave them in place.

- Have the client cover one eye with an opaque card and read the line of smallest letters that it is possible for the client to read. Test the other eye and then test both eyes using the same procedure.
- Document the line read completely by the client, using the fraction printed at the end of the line; also indicate if the client was wearing glasses or contacts.
- Next, to assess perception ask the client to use both eyes to distinguish which of the two horizontal lines is longer. Finally, ask the client to name the colors of the two horizontal lines to document red and green color perception.

PROCEDURES AND TECHNIQUES WITH NORMAL FINDINGS

ABNORMAL FINDINGS

NOTE: Use the "E" chart for clients who cannot read letters. This can be a very sensitive area for adults who do not know how to read. The client is asked to indicate the direction in which the "E" points (see Fig. 4-12, *B,* in Chapter 4).

Findings: The reading pattern should be smooth and without hesitation. A finding of 20/30 means the client can read at 20 feet what a person with normal vision can read at 30 feet. If the client can read all the letters in the 20/30 line and two letters in the 20/20 line, document the finding as 20/30 + 2.

Note any hesitancy, squinting, leaning forward, blinking or facial expressions indicating that the client is struggling to see. Note that the larger the denominator, the poorer the vision. If vision is poorer than 20/30, or the client is unable to distinguish colors or line length, refer to an ophthalmologist or optometrist. A person is considered legally blind when the best corrected visual acuity is 20/200.

TEST visual acuity (near vision).

Assess near vision for people over 40 years of age or for those who feel they have difficulty reading. Ask the client to cover one eye and hold a Jaeger or Rosenbaum card or a newspaper at about 14 inches and to read the smallest line possible (see Fig. 4-13 in Chapter 4). Repeat the assessment, covering the other eye. Document the line read completely using the fraction at the end of the line. The findings are the same as those for the Snellen's chart.

With age, there is a loss of elasticity of the lens of the eye; this finding is termed *presbyopia.* As a result, the client needs to move the card farther away to see it clearly.

INSPECT the external ocular structures.

Eyebrows, eyelashes, and eyelids for symmetry, hair distribution, skin characteristics, and discharge.

Skin should be intact and eyebrows symmetric. Note whether the eyebrow extends over the eye. Eyelashes should be equally distributed and curled slightly outward. Palpebral fissures should be bilaterally equal. The color of the eyelids should correspond to skin color. The eyelid margins should be pale pink and fit flush against the eyeball surfaces; the upper lid should cover part of the iris but not the pupil while the lower lid generally covers to just below the limbus (see Fig. 11-13). Lid closure should be complete, with smooth, easy motion. Blinking is typically frequent, bilateral, involuntary movements, averaging 15 to 20 blinks per minute. No draining or discharge should be present.

Flakiness, loss of hair, scaling, and unequal alignment of movement are abnormal as are asymmetrical palpebral fissures. The lid of either eye covering part of the pupil is known as ptosis (Fig. 11-16). Sclera is visible between the upper lid and iris in hyperthyroid exophthalmos (Fig. 11-17). Closure of the lid that is incomplete or accomplished only with pain or difficulty may occur with infections. Edema of the lid may occur with trauma or infection. The presence of lesions, nodules, erythema, flaking, crusting, excessive tearing, or discharge should be documented. Note inward deformity of the lid and lashes. This is a finding seen in enophthalmos (Fig. 11-18).

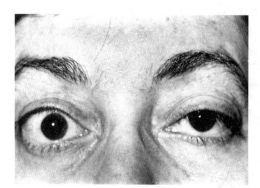

Fig. 11-16 **Ptosis.** Client with left ptosis and right upper lid retraction. *(From Nesi et al, 1998.)*

⟜ = core examination skill

PROCEDURES AND TECHNIQUES WITH NORMAL FINDINGS	**ABNORMAL FINDINGS**

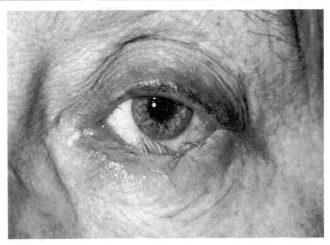

Fig. 11-18 **Enophthalmos.** The eyelid and lashes are rolled in. *(From Bedford, 1986.)*

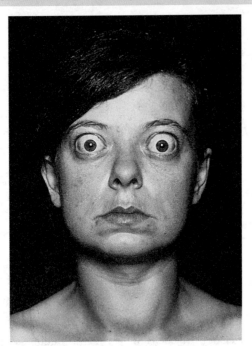

Fig. 11-17 Exophthalmos. *(From Seidel et al, 1999.)*

ETHNIC & CULTURAL VARIATIONS

The palpebral fissures are horizontal in non-Asians, whereas Asians normally have an upward slant to the palpebral fissures (see Fig. 11-13).

ETHNIC & CULTURAL VARIATIONS

For white clients, the eyeball does not protrude beyond the supraorbital ridge of the frontal bone. For African American clients, the eyeball may protrude slightly beyond the supraorbital ridge.

Conjunctiva for color, moisture, drainage, lesions.
Procedure: Ask the client to look up. Gently separate the lids widely with the thumb and index finger, exerting pressure over the bony orbit surrounding the eye. Have the client look up, down, and to each side. Next, pull down and evert the lower lid; ask the client to look up (Fig. 11-19).

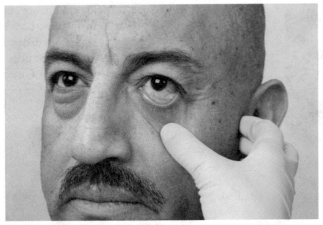

Fig. 11-19 To inspect the palpebral conjunctiva, gently pull down and evert the lower eyelid.

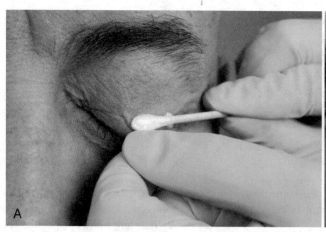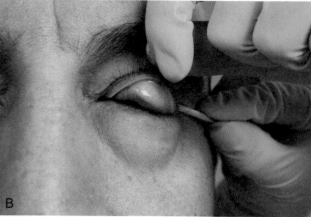

Fig. 11-20 Everting upper eyelid.

PROCEDURES AND TECHNIQUES WITH NORMAL FINDINGS

Occasionally eversion of the upper eyelid is necessary when you must inspect the conjunctiva of the upper lid (such as when clients complain of eye pain or a foreign body is suspected). Wearing gloves, gently grasp the upper eyelashes and pull gently downward while the client is looking down with the eyes slightly open. Place a cotton-tipped applicator stick about 1 cm above the upper lid margin and push gently down with the applicator while still holding the lashes to evert the lid (Fig. 11-20, *A*). Hold the lashes of the everted lid against the upper ridge of the bony orbit, just below the eyebrow, and examine the lid (Fig. 11-20, *B*). Return the lid to its normal position by moving the lashes slightly forward and asking the client to look up and then blink.

Findings: The bulbar conjunctiva should be pink and clear; tiny red vessels are often noted.

ABNORMAL FINDINGS

Red and congested conjunctiva may indicate conjunctivitis (see Fig. 11-54 later in this chapter). A sharply defined area of blood adjacent to normal-appearing conjunctiva may indicate subconjunctival hemorrhage. Lesions, nodules, or foreign bodies are abnormal findings.

⚷ INSPECT the ocular structures.

Corneal light reflex for symmetry (Hirschberg's test).

Ask the client to stare straight ahead with both eyes open. Shine a penlight toward the bridge of the nose at a distance of 12 to 15 inches (30 to 38 cm). Light reflections should appear symmetrically in both corneas (Fig. 11-21). *NOTE: When an imbalance is found in the corneal light reflex, perform the cover-uncover test (discussed in sections that follow).*

If light reflections appear at different spots in each eye (asymmetrically), this may indicate weak extraocular muscles.

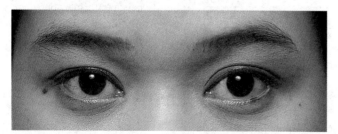

Fig. 11-21 **Normal position of eyes and eyelids.** The symmetric light reflection in both corneas is a normal finding.

Sclera for color, surface characteristics.

Sclera should be white and clear, although slight yellowing may be seen in darkly pigmented individuals.

Yellow sclera may indicate jaundice caused by liver disease or obstruction of

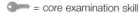 = core examination skill

PROCEDURES AND TECHNIQUES WITH NORMAL FINDINGS

ETHNIC & CULTURAL VARIATIONS

The sclera appears white except in darker-skinned clients, in whom it is normally a darker shade. Tiny black dots of pigmentation may be present near the limbus in dark-skinned individuals. In light-skinned individuals, there may be a slight yellow cast.

Cornea for transparency and surface characteristics.
Use oblique lighting and slowly move the light reflection over the corneal surface. Observe for transparent quality and a smooth surface that is clear and shiny.

Iris for shape and color.
The iris should be round with consistent coloration. Some people may have a normal variation in color in which each iris is a different color. This is due to genetic factors.

Pupils for size, shape, reaction to light, accommodation, and consensual reaction.
Procedure: To determine the pupil size, use a pupil gauge like the one found at the bottom of a Rosenbaum Pocket Vision Screener (see Fig. 4-13 in Chapter 4). To assess reaction to light, dim the room lights if possible. Ask the client to hold the eyes open and fix his or her gaze on an object across the room. Approach with a penlight beam from the side and shine it directly on the pupil. Repeat with the other eye. To test accommodation, ask the client to fix his or her gaze on a distant object across the room. Then ask the client to shift his or her gaze to your finger, placed about 6 inches from the client's nose.
Findings: The pupil diameter is normally between 2 and 6 mm. Pupils should be round and equal in size. The illuminated pupil should constrict (direct response); the other pupil should constrict simultaneously (consensual response). The pupils should dilate when visualizing a distant object and constrict when focusing on a near object. Box 11-4 provides tips used to document normal findings of pupils.

BOX 11-4 DOCUMENTATION TIPS FOR EYES

PERRLA
Pupils are
Equal,
Round and
React to
Light and
Accommodation

Remembering C's and D's for Expected Findings for Accommodation
Pupils **C**onstrict when focusing on a **C**lose object
Pupils **D**ilate when focusing on a **D**istant object
Even the name helps you remember the expected findings. The **C** in a**C**commodation is close to the beginning of the word, whereas the **D** in accommo**D**ation is distant from the beginning of the word.

ABNORMAL FINDINGS

the common bile duct with gallstones. Redness within the sclera is suggestive of inflammation or hemorrhage. A blue tone to the sclera may be due to osteogenesis imperfecta.

Note opacities, irregularities in light reflections, lesions, abrasions, or foreign bodies. Especially note any white opaque ring encircling the limbus, termed *corneal arcus,* seen in many clients over 60 years old and in individuals with hyperlipidemia.

Clients who have had an iridectomy to correct glaucoma will have a section of the iris missing. Coloboma is a congenital defect of the iris. Blunt trauma to the eye can cause an iridodialysis, a circumferential tearing of the iris from the sclera.

Pupillary abnormalities are described in Table 11-1. Failure of either one or both eyes to constrict to light in speed or magnitude indicates dysfunction of the oculomotor nerve (cranial nerve III). *Mydriasis* is pupil size greater than 6 mm that fails to constrict. *Miosis* is constriction to less than 2 mm. Unequal pupils may be normal, but it may occur as a result of past eye surgery, trauma, or congenital anomalies.

TABLE 11-1 *Pupil Abnormalities*

ABNORMALITY	CONTRIBUTING FACTORS	APPEARANCE
Miosis (pupillary constriction; usually less than 2 mm in diameter)	Miotic eyedrops (such as pilocarpine given for glaucoma)	
Mydriasis (pupillary dilation; usually more than 6 mm in diameter)	Mydriatic or cycloplegic drops (such as atropine); midbrain (reflex arc) lesions or hypoxia; oculomotor (CN III) damage; acute-angle glaucoma (slight dilation)	
Oval pupil	Sometimes occurs with head injury or intracranial hemorrhage; transitional stage between normal pupil and dilated, fixed pupil with increased intracranial pressure (ICP); in most instances returns to normal when ICP is returned to normal	
Anisocoria (unequal size of pupils)	Congenital (approximately 20% of normal people have minor or noticeable differences in pupil size, but reflexes are normal) or caused by local eye medications (constrictors or dilators), amblyopia, or unilateral sympathetic or parasympathetic pupillary pathway destruction (NOTE: Nurse should test whether pupils react equally to light; if response is unequal, nurse should note whether larger or smaller pupil reacts more slowly [or not at all], since either pupil could be abnormal size)	
Iridectomy	Surgical excision of portion of iris usually done in superior area so upper lid will cover additional exposure	

From Thompson JM et al: *Mosby's clinical nursing*, ed 5, St. Louis, 2002, Mosby.

PROCEDURES AND TECHNIQUES WITH NORMAL FINDINGS

ABNORMAL FINDINGS

SPECIAL CIRCUMSTANCES OR ADVANCED PRACTICE: EYE

ASSESS visual fields for peripheral vision (confrontation test).

Procedure: Face the client, standing or sitting at a distance of 2 to 3 feet (60 to 90 cm). Ask the client to cover one eye with an opaque card and look directly at you as you cover your own eye directly opposite the client's covered eye.
- Hold a pencil or use your finger and extend it to the farthest periphery and gradually bring the object close to the midline (equal distance between you and the client). Ask the client to report when he or she first sees the object; you should see the object at the same time.

PROCEDURES AND TECHNIQUES WITH NORMAL FINDINGS

- Slowly move the object inward from the periphery in four directions. Move your fingers anteriorly (from above the head down into field of vision), inferiorly (from upper chest up toward field of vision), temporally (move in laterally from behind the client's ear into field of vision), and nasally (move medially into the field of vision) (Fig. 11-22).
- Estimate the angle between the anteroposterior axis of the eye and the peripheral axis when the pencil or finger is first seen.

(NOTE: This test assumes that the nurse has normal peripheral visual fields.)

Findings: Normal values are 50 degrees anteriorly, 70 degrees inferiorly, 90 degrees temporally, and 60 degrees nasally. The temporal value is greater than the nasal value because of the position of the opaque card covering one of the eyes.

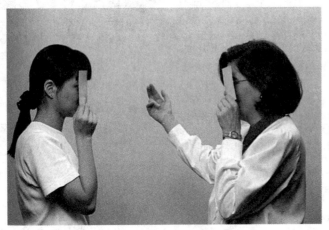

Fig. 11-22   Assessing a client's peripheral vision nasally by moving object medially into the field of vision.

ASSESS eye movement.

Six Cardinal Fields of Gaze (tests cranial nerves III, IV, and VI).
Procedure. While the client is looking at you, position your finger 10 to 12 inches from the client's nose. Ask the client to keep the head still and use the eyes only to follow your finger or an object in your hand (Fig. 11-23).

ABNORMAL FINDINGS

If the client cannot see the pencil or finger at the same time that you see it, peripheral field loss is suspected. A person whose visual field is 20 degrees or less is considered legally blind. Refer the client to an eye care specialist for more precise testing.

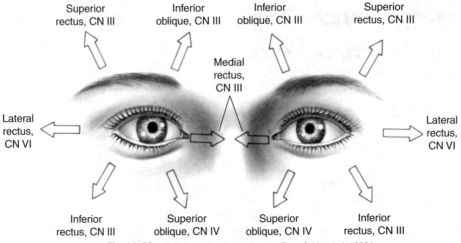

Superior rectus, CN III   Inferior oblique, CN III   Inferior oblique, CN III   Superior rectus, CN III

Medial rectus, CN III

Lateral rectus, CN VI   Lateral rectus, CN VI

Inferior rectus, CN III   Superior oblique, CN IV   Superior oblique, CN IV   Inferior rectus, CN III

Fig. 11-23   The six cardinal fields of gaze. *(From Seidel et al, 1999.)*

PROCEDURES AND TECHNIQUES WITH NORMAL FINDINGS

- Move the object from its center position to upper outer extreme, hold there, move back to center, to lower inner extreme, and hold there.
- Move the object to temporal-nasal extremes, holding there momentarily. Move the object to opposite upper outer extreme and back to opposite lower inner extreme.

An alternative method is to move your finger slowly in a circle to each of the six directions. Stop in each position so that the client can hold the gaze briefly before moving to the next position.

Findings: Normally there will be parallel tracking of the object with both eyes. Mild nystagmus at extreme lateral gaze is also normal.

Cover-Uncover Test

Perform this test if the corneal light reflex is asymmetric. Ask the client to stare straight ahead at your nose.

- Cover one of the client's eyes with the opaque card. Observe the uncovered eye for any deviation or movement from a steady, fixed gaze (Fig. 11-24, *A*).
- Remove the card from the covered eye; observe if this eye moves to try to focus. It should not move (Fig. 11-24, *B, C*).
- Repeat steps with the other eye.

ABNORMAL FINDINGS

Nystagmus is involuntary movement of the eyeball in a horizontal, vertical, rotary, or mixed direction. It may be congenital or acquired (from multiple causes).

If the uncovered eye moves to focus, it is the weaker eye and strabismus is present (see Fig. 11-55 later in this chapter).

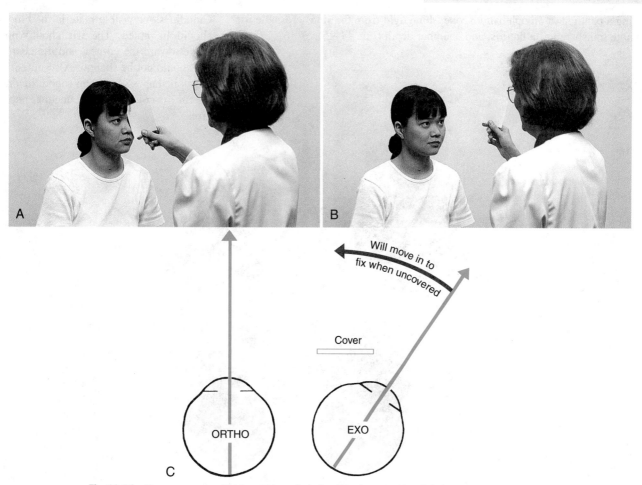

Fig. 11-24 The cover-uncover test is used to evaluate function of eye muscles. **A,** Left eye covered; observe right eye. **B,** Left eye uncovered; observe it for movement. **C,** Exophoria; the right eye shifted from right to center when the eye was uncovered. *(C, From Prior, Silberstein, and Stang, 1981.)*

PROCEDURES AND TECHNIQUES WITH NORMAL FINDINGS

ABNORMAL FINDINGS

PALPATE the eye, eyelids, and lacrimal puncta.

Ask the client to look down with lids closed so that you will not palpate the cornea. Gently palpate the eyeball; it should indent with slight pressure. Palpate the lower orbital rim near the inner canthus. This pressure slightly everts the lower lid. Puncta are seen as small elevations on the nasal side of the upper and lower lid margins. Mucosa should be pink and intact despite pressure. Eyes should be moist, without excessive tears. Gently palpate the upper and lower lids for tenderness or nodules; there should be no pain.

An eyeball that is very firm and resists palpation may occur in glaucoma. Lacrimal puncta that are clogged with mucus or dirt cause inflammation (dacryocystitis). Fluid or purulent material may be discharged from the puncta in response to pressure. Excessive tearing (epiphora) may be caused by blockage of the nasolacrimal duct. Tenderness, nodules, or irregularities indicate a problem.

TEST the corneal reflex.

Test the corneal reflex *only* in selected cases, such as unconscious clients. Lightly touch the cornea with cotton. The lids of both eyes blink when either cornea is touched. This reflex tests the sensory reception of the ophthalmic branch of the trigeminal nerve (cranial nerve V) and the motor branch of the facial nerve (cranial nerve VII), which creates a blink.

Edema of the brainstem might impair the function of cranial nerve V and cranial nerve VII and may occur after head injury or with cerebral hemorrhage or tumor.

INSPECT the anterior chamber for transparency, iris surface, and chamber depth.

Using a penlight or an ophthalmoscope, shine light from the side across the iris to note transparency, a flat iris, and chamber depth (Fig. 11-25).

Cloudiness or visible material or blood should be noted. The iris should not bulge toward the cornea, and the chamber should not be shallow. Also note iris or pupil shapes other than round, inconsistent iris coloration, and unequal pupil sizes.

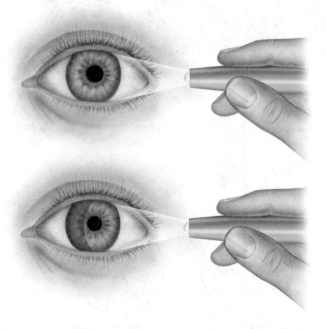

Fig. 11-25   Evaluation of depth of anterior chambers. **A,** Normal anterior chamber. **B,** Shallow anterior chamber. *(From Seidel et al, 2006.)*

PROCEDURES AND TECHNIQUES WITH NORMAL FINDINGS	ABNORMAL FINDINGS

★ INSPECT intraocular structures (ophthalmoscopic examination).

To use an ophthalmoscope, darken the room to help dilate the client's pupils. Have the client remove glasses; contact lenses may be left in. You may leave your glasses or contact lenses in place. Turn on the ophthalmoscope light and set the diopter wheel to 0.

To examine the client's right eye, hold the ophthalmoscope in your right hand and use your right eye. To examine the client's left eye, hold the ophthalmoscope in the left hand and use your left eye. Place your index finger on the diopter wheel so that you can change the focus as needed to visualize the internal structures. Red numbers (minus) compensate for myopia (nearsighted) and black numbers (positive) compensate for hyperopia (farsighted).

Direct the client to continuously gaze at a point across the room and slightly above your shoulder. Begin about 10 inches (25 mm) from client's eye at a 15-degree angle lateral to the client's line of vision. Shine the light of the ophthalmoscope on the pupil while looking through the viewing lens.

Inspect for a red reflex.

The red reflex is a red or orange glow over the client's pupil (Fig. 11-26, *A*) created by light illuminating the retina. Keep the red reflex in sight and move closer to the eye, adjusting the lens with the diopter wheel as needed to focus; there should be no interruption in the red reflex. Absence of the red reflex may be caused by movement of the light away from the pupil; correct by repositioning the light.

Decreased or irregular red reflex, dark spots, and opacities should be noted. Dark shadows or black dots may indicate opacities that occur with cataracts or may be due to hemorrhage in the vitreous humor.

Inspect the optic disc for discrete margin, shape, size, color, and physiologic cup.

Procedure: After seeing the red reflex, continue to move closer until you nearly touch foreheads with the client (Fig. 11-26, *B*). Placing your middle finger on the client's cheek stabilizes the ophthalmoscope. Focus varies depending on the refractive state of both the nurse and the client; adjust your focus with the diopter wheel. When you locate a blood vessel, follow it inward toward the nose until you see the optic disc.

Cataracts prevent inspection of the optic disc because the light cannot penetrate the opacity of the lens.

Findings: The margin should be regular and have a distinct, sharp outline. Scattered or dense pigment deposits may be seen at the border. A gray crescent may appear at the temporal border.

Blurred margin may indicate papilledema, which is caused by increased intracranial pressure relayed along the optic nerve.

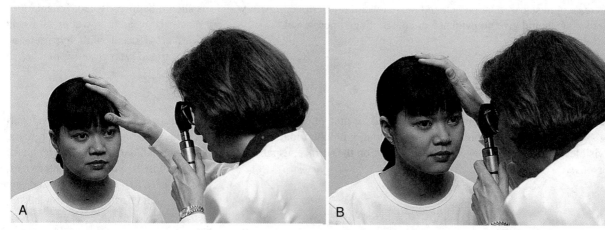

Fig. 11-26 **Examining the retina. A,** The red reflex is created by light illuminating the retina. **B,** Move close to the client until you nearly touch foreheads.

★ = advanced practice

PROCEDURES AND TECHNIQUES WITH NORMAL FINDINGS

The optic disc should be round or slightly vertically oval. Marked myopic refractive errors may make the disc appear larger, and hyperopic errors may make it appear smaller. The optic disc's color should be creamy yellow to pink, lighter than the retina, possibly with tiny blood vessels visible on the surface (Fig. 11-27).

The physiologic cup is a small depression just temporal to the disc center that does not extend to the border. It usually appears lighter than the rest of the disc and occupies less than one half of the disc's diameter. Vessels entering the disc may drop abruptly into the cup or appear to fade gradually.

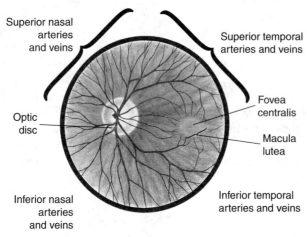

Superior nasal arteries and veins

Superior temporal arteries and veins

Fovea centralis

Optic disc

Macula lutea

Inferior nasal arteries and veins

Inferior temporal arteries and veins

Fig. 11-27   Retinal structures of the left eye. *(From Seidel et al, 2006.)*

Inspect the retinal vessels for color, arteriolar light reflex, artery-to-vein ratio, and arteriovenous crossing changes.

From the optic disc, follow each of the four sets of retinal vessels from the disc to the periphery. Arteries are on average one fourth narrower than veins; artery-to-vein width should be 2:3 to 4:5. Arteries are light red and may have a narrow band of light in the center. By contrast, veins are larger than arteries and have no light reflex. They are darker, and venous pulsations may be visible (see Fig. 11-27).

Overall, the caliber of both arteries and veins should be regular and uniformly decreasing in size as they branch and move toward the periphery. Artery and vein crossing should give no evidence of constricting either vessel.

Inspect the retinal background for color, presence of microaneurysms, hemorrhages, and exudates.

The color is uniform throughout and may be pink, red, or orange; it varies with skin color. The retinal surface should be finely granular, with choroidal vessels possibly visible. Movable light reflections may appear on the surface, usually in young persons.

ABNORMAL FINDINGS

Irregular disc or discs that differ in size or shape between the two eyes should be noted. Impaired blood flow may cause the disk to appear whiter than expected. Hyperemic discs with engorged or tortuous vessels on the surface are abnormal.

The depression of the physiologic cup should not extend to the border of the disc and should not occupy more than one half of the diameter of the disc. The appearance (size or placement) of the physiologic cup should not differ between eyes.

Extremely narrow arteries are abnormal. The width of the light reflex should not cover more than one third of the artery. Arteries should not be pale or opaque.

Irregularities of caliber, either dilation or constriction, should be noted. Compact areas of tortuous, narrow vessels should be investigated. Indentations or pinched appearances where veins and arteries cross occur with hypertension and are termed *arteriovenous nicking.*

Pale fundus, either in general or in localized areas, or hemorrhages (linear, flame shaped, round, dark red, large, or small) must be noted. Note microaneurysms, which appear as fine red dots, and any exudates (soft, hard, fuzzy, or well defined).

PROCEDURES AND TECHNIQUES WITH NORMAL FINDINGS

ABNORMAL FINDINGS

Inspect the macula for color and surface characteristics.

Ask the client to look directly into the ophthalmoscope light. The macula is about one disc diameter (DD) in size and lies about two DDs temporal to the optic disc. The macula and its center should be slightly darker than the rest of the retina. Tiny vessels may appear on the surface. Fine pigmentation and granular appearance may be visible. The macula may be difficult to see if the client's pupil has not been chemically dilated.

Drusen bodies are deposits that form within the layer under the retina and appear as small, discrete spots in the retina. They become yellow as the spots enlarge. When drusen bodies increase in size or number, they may contribute to macular degeneration.

ROUTINE TECHNIQUES: EARS

ASSESS hearing based on response from conversation.

As you conduct the history, note the client's ability to hear by observing communication patterns. A client's ability to engage in conversation is considered an expected finding. *NOTE: Perform further tests for hearing if findings suggest a hearing deficit (described in the following Special Circumstances section).*

Subtle indications of hearing loss includes the client who asks you to repeat yourself; repeatedly misunderstands questions you ask; has garbled speech sounds with word distortion; leans forward or tilts his or her head; watches your lips as you speak; or speaks in a loud monotone voice.

INSPECT the external ears.

Observe the alignment and position.

The pinna of the ear should align directly with the outer canthus of the eye and be angled no more than 10 degrees from a vertical position (Fig. 11-28).

Low-set ears (the pinna is located below the external corner of the eye) or ears that are misaligned (the ear is angled more than 10 degrees from a vertical position) should be considered abnormal. Low-set ears are seen in persons with congenital diseases such as Down syndrome.

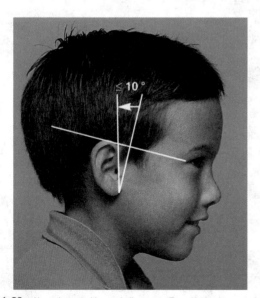

Fig. 11-28   Normal ear position and alignment. *(From Hockenberry et al, 2003.)*

PROCEDURES AND TECHNIQUES WITH NORMAL FINDINGS

Inspect for size, shape, symmetry, skin color, and skin intactness.
The ears should be between 4 and 10 cm in length and appear the same bilaterally. If the ears are pierced, note the skin around the piercing for skin intactness, edema, or discharge. The skin should be an even skin tone, with color about the same skin tone as that noted on the face. The skin should be intact and without lesions. A small, painless nodule, called a Darwin tubercle, is a normal deviation and may be noted at the helix of the ear (Fig. 11-29).

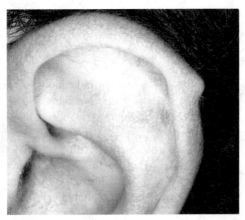

Fig. 11-29   A darwinian tubercle. *(From Bingham, Hawke, and Kwok, 1992.)*

ABNORMAL FINDINGS

If the ears are smaller than 4 cm in length, they are referred to as *microtia* ears. If the ears are larger than 10 cm in length, they are referred to as *macrotia* ears.

Other abnormal findings include lesions or deformities, such as nodules, tophi sebaceous cysts, cauliflower ear, hematoma, or edema (Table 11-2).

TABLE 11-2   Abnormal Findings of the External Ear

Cauliflower Ear
A thickened, disfigured auricle resulting from repeated episodes of minor or major blunt trauma. When observed in infants and young children, child abuse should be suspected.

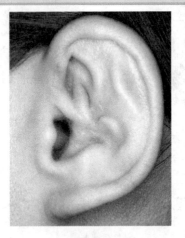

Hematoma
Most commonly caused by direct trauma, usually from a contact sport (e.g., football, rugby, wrestling) or a blow to the side of the head (e.g., trauma from a motor vehicle accident, assault). When observed in infants and young children, child abuse should be suspected.

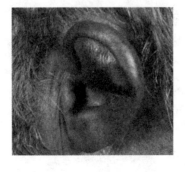

Tophi
Small, hard, whitish yellow, nontender nodules in or near the helix of the ear. They contain uric acid crystals and are a sign of gout.

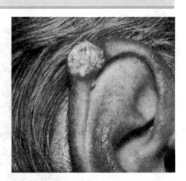

Sebaceous Cyst
Manifests as a nodule usually found behind the earlobe in the postauricular fold. This is very painful if it becomes infected.

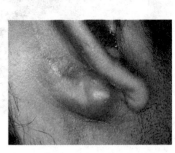

PROCEDURES AND TECHNIQUES WITH NORMAL FINDINGS

Inspect the external auditory meatus for discharge or lesions.
There should be no lesions or discharge.

SPECIAL CIRCUMSTANCES OR ADVANCED PRACTICE: EARS

PALPATE the external ears and mastoid areas for tenderness, edema, and nodules.

The upper part of the ear should be firm and flexible; the earlobe should be soft. All areas should be without tenderness or edema. Gently pull on the helix of the ear to determine if there is any discomfort or pain. There should be none.

★ INSPECT the internal ear structures.

Procedure. This procedure requires the use of an otoscope. If you have a choice of speculum size, always choose the largest speculum that will comfortably fit into the external auditory meatus.

Proper technique using the otoscope is necessary to optimize visualization and prevent discomfort or injury.

- When examining the client's right ear, grasp the pinna with the left hand and gently pull the helix upward and slightly toward the back of the head (Fig. 11-30, *A*). This straightens the S-shaped curve of the auditory canal. (When examining the client's left ear, pull back on the client's ear with the right hand, and hold the scope in the left hand.)

ABNORMAL FINDINGS

Discharge from the ear should be considered abnormal. A bloody or clear discharge from the ear accompanied by a history of head injury should lead to suspicion of possible skull fracture. A purulent or crusty discharge usually indicates infection or the presence of a foreign body.

Tenderness of the mastoid area may indicate mastoiditis. Pain when the helix of the ear is pulled may indicate an inflammation within the auditory canal.

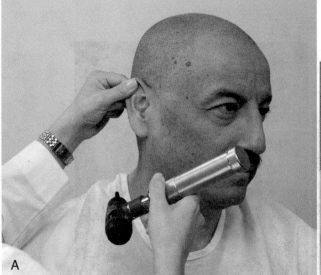

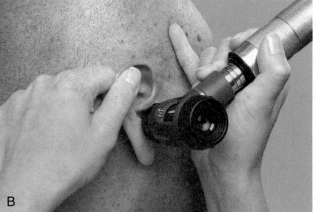

Fig. 11-30 **Use of an otoscope. A,** Pull the client's helix upward and slightly toward the back of the head. **B,** Holding the otoscope "upside down," rest the back of your hand against the client's temple area to steady the otoscope.

★ = advanced practice

PROCEDURES AND TECHNIQUES WITH NORMAL FINDINGS

- Holding the otoscope upside down in the right hand, insert the lighted speculum of the otoscope 1.0 to 1.5 cm into the client's external auditory canal. Rest the back of the right hand against the client's temple area to steady the positioning of the otoscope (Fig. 11-30, *B*). Be careful not to insert the otoscope speculum into the canal too far because the bony section of the ear canal is very sensitive.

Inspect the external ear canal for cerumen, edema, erythema, discharge, and foreign bodies.

Once the otoscope is properly positioned, look through the lens of the otoscope to visualize the walls of the canal. Cerumen is almost always in the canal (Fig. 11-31, *A*). Note the characteristics of the cerumen. The color may be black, brown, dark red, creamy, or brown-gray. The texture ranges from moist, to dry and flaky, to hard. There should be no odor.

ETHNIC & CULTURAL VARIATIONS

White and dark-skinned races have cerumen that is moist, sticky, and dark. Asians, Native Americans, and Alaskan Natives have cerumen that is generally sparse, dry, flaky, and lighter.

BOX 11-5   REMOVING CERUMEN FROM THE AUDITORY CANAL

To remove cerumen from the auditory canal, the nurse may first fill the canal with a cerumen-softening agent. Block the opening of the canal with a cotton ball and wait 5 to 10 minutes. The cerumen may then be easily removed from the canal by irrigating the canal with warm water. Some nurses prefer to remove the cerumen with a cerumen spoon. This technique requires skill so as not to scrape the walls of the canal or injure the tympanic membrane.

CAUTION: Do not use water irrigation of the canal if any of the following are suspected: otitis externa, tympanic membrane perforation, or myringotomy tubes in place.

ABNORMAL FINDINGS

Erythema and edema of the auditory canal may be an indication of otitis externa. The infection may cause the canal to become swollen and completely closed.

Purulent discharge may occur secondary to otitis externa or with rupture of the TM associated with acute otitis media. Clear fluid or frank bloody drainage following a head injury may indicate a basilar skull fracture. Other abnormal findings in the auditory canal include the presence of foreign bodies, excessive cerumen, or a polyp. If an excessive amount of cerumen is present in the ear, it may occlude the entire ear canal (Fig. 11-31, *B*). If this has occurred, the cerumen must be removed before the examination can continue (Box 11-5).

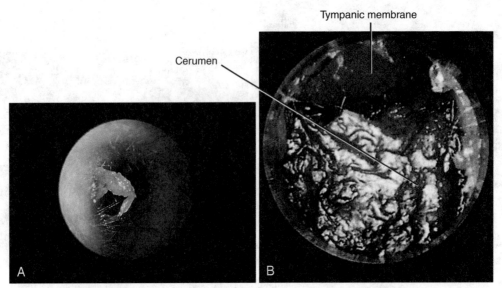

Tympanic membrane

Cerumen

Fig. 11-31   A, Normal piece of cerumen (earwax) in the external meatus. **B,** Excessive earwax in the external auditory canal. *(**A,** From Bingham, Hawke, and Kwok, 1992. **B,** Courtesy Dr. Richard A. Buckingham, Abraham Lincoln School of Medicine, University of Illinois, Chicago. From Barkauskas et al, 2002).*

PROCEDURES AND TECHNIQUES WITH NORMAL FINDINGS

Inspect the tympanic membrane for landmarks, color, contour, translucence, and fluctuation.

Locate all landmarks of the tympanic membrane (TM). Most of the TM is taut and is known as the pars tensa; a smaller, less taut part is the pars flaccida, and the dense fibrous ring around the membrane is the annulus. The cone of light may be seen downward and anteriorly. Part of the malleus and incus may be visualized through the TM (Fig. 11-32). Note the color and contour. It should be a translucent, pearly gray color.

Mobility of the TM is evaluated by attaching a pneumatic bulb to the otoscope. To perform this procedure, make sure that the speculum is fully inserted into the canal and that the speculum is large enough to completely occlude the canal. Gently squeeze the bulb so that puffs of air are transmitted to the TM. A normal response is that the TM slightly fluctuates with the puffs of air. This procedure can be performed with any age group, but is most commonly done when examining infants and young children because they are unable to provide a history regarding the pain they are experiencing.

ABNORMAL FINDINGS

Absence or distortion of the landmarks on the TM should be considered abnormal. A hole in the TM is referred to as a perforation (Fig. 11-33), which occurs with untreated acute otitis media, a blow to the head, or penetration by a foreign body. Variations in the color and characteristics of the TM indicating an abnormality are presented in Box 11-6.

Bulging of the TM with no mobility indicates pus or fluid behind the TM. Retraction of the TM with no mobility of the TM with negative pressure indicates obstruction of the eustachian tube.

Increased mobility of only one part of the TM (as determined with the pneumatic bulb) indicates an area of healed TM perforation.

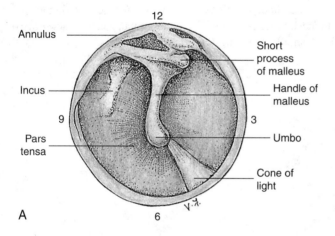

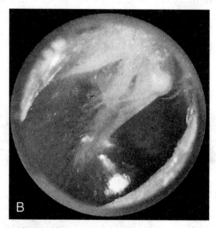

Fig. 11-32   The tympanic membrane. A, Landmarks of tympanic membrane with "clock" superimposed (right ear). **B,** Photograph of a normal-appearing tympanic membrane. *(A, From Potter and Perry, 1991. B, Courtesy Dr. Richard A. Buckingham, Clinical Professor, Otolaryngology, Abraham Lincoln School of Medicine, University of Illinois, Chicago. From Barkauskas et al, 2002.)*

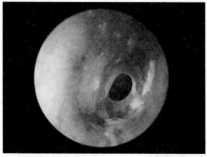

Fig. 11-33   Perforated tympanic membrane. *(From Bingham, Hawke, and Kwok, 1992.)*

BOX 11-6	ABNORMAL COLOR CHARACTERISTICS OF THE TM AND POSSIBLE CAUSES

- *Yellow/amber:* serous fluid in the middle ear, which may indicate otitis media with effusion
- *Redness:* infection in the middle ear, such as acute purulent otitis media
- *Chalky white:* infection in the middle ear, such as otitis media
- *Blue or deep red:* blood behind the TM, which may have occurred secondary to injury
- *Red streaks:* injected/increased vascularization may be due to allergy
- *Dullness:* fibrosis or scarring of the TM secondary to repeated infections
- *White flecks/plaques:* healed inflammation of the TM

PROCEDURES AND TECHNIQUES WITH NORMAL FINDINGS

ABNORMAL FINDINGS

TEST the acoustic cranial nerve (VIII) to evaluate auditory function.

Whispered Voice Test

Stand 1 to 2 feet in front of or to the side of the client. Instruct the client to cover one ear with his or her hand so that one ear may be tested at a time. Shield your mouth so that the client cannot read your lips. Softly whisper several monosyllabic (e.g., ball, chair, cat) and disyllabic (e.g., streetcar, baseball, highchair) words and ask the client to repeat what is heard. The client should be able to hear and repeat at least 50% of all words whispered. Repeat the procedure with the other ear. Although this test is simple, standardization of the results is difficult because of variance of the loudness of whispers among nurses.

It should be considered abnormal if the client cannot repeat at least 50% of the spoken words. Consider each ear separately.

Finger-Rubbing Test

Another simple hearing screening test may be done by holding your hand 3 to 4 inches from the client's ear and briskly rubbing your index finger against your thumb. The client should be able to hear the noise generated by rubbing the fingers together. Repeat the technique with the other ear.

Clients with a high-frequency hearing loss may not be able to hear the noise generated by your fingers.

Weber's Test

This test uses a tuning fork to assess hearing. Activate the tuning fork by holding it by the base stem and striking the forked section against the base of the palm. Immediately place the base of the fork on the midline of the client's skull. Ask the client to indicate which ear the sound is heard loudest. Because sound is transmitted along the skull to the inner ear, the client should hear the tone equally in both ears (Fig. 11-34).

If the sound lateralizes to one side (the client hears the tone better in one ear than the other) the test should be considered abnormal. Lateralization of sound to the affected ear suggests conductive hearing loss (Fig. 11-35, *A*). Lateralization of sound to the unaffected ear suggests sensorineural hearing loss (Fig. 11-35, *B*).

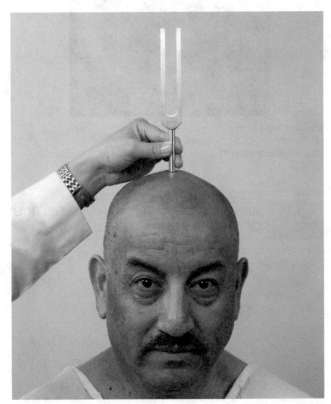

Fig. 11-34   Weber's test. The tuning fork is placed on the midline of the skull.

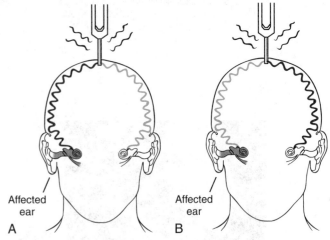

Affected ear

A

Affected ear

B

Fig. 11-35   A, Client with conduction loss; sound lateralizes to the defective ear because the sound transmits through the bone rather than air. **B,** Client with sensorineural loss; sound lateralizes to the unaffected ear.

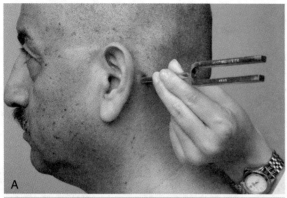

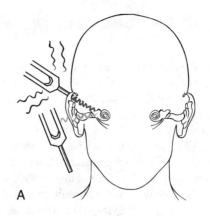

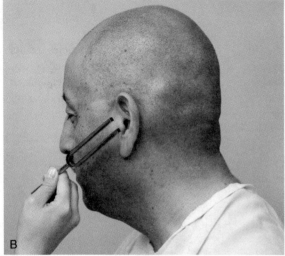

Fig. 11-36 **Rinne test. A,** The tuning fork is placed on the mastoid bone for bone conduction. **B,** The tuning fork is placed in front of the ear for air conduction.

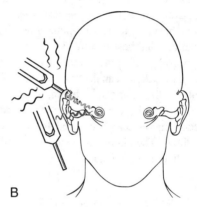

Fig. 11-37 **A,** Client with conduction loss will hear bone conduction longer than air conduction (BC greater than AC). **B,** Client with sensorineural loss will hear air conduction longer than bone conduction (AC greater than BC).

PROCEDURES AND TECHNIQUES WITH NORMAL FINDINGS

Rinne Test

The Rinne test also uses a tuning fork to assess hearing by comparing air conduction (AC) of sound to bone conduction (BC) of sound. The AC route through the ear canal is a more sensitive route.

Procedure: Explain the procedure and ask the client to indicate when the sound is no longer heard when the tuning fork is placed on the bone and when it is placed in the front of the ear.

- Activate the tuning fork by holding it by the base stem and striking the forked section against the base of the palm of your hand. Immediately place the base of the tuning fork directly on the client's mastoid process (Fig. 11-36, *A*).
- Begin timing by counting the seconds. The client should be able to hear the tone. Instruct the client to tell you when the tone can no longer be heard.

ABNORMAL FINDINGS

Consider the test abnormal when the sound is heard longer by bone conduction than air conduction (BC > AC). Clients with conductive hearing loss will have bone conduction longer than air conduction in the affected ear (Fig. 11-37, *A*). Clients with sensorineural hearing loss will have air conduction longer than bone conduction (AC > BC) in the affected ear, but it will be less than 2:1 ratio (Fig. 11-37, *B*).

- When the client indicates the tone can no longer be heard, note the number of seconds counted; and quickly remove the fork from the mastoid process, invert the fork, and hold the vibrating section of the tuning fork in front of the client's ear (Fig. 11-36, *B*).
- Begin timing again. The client should be able to hear the tone again. Instruct the client to tell you when the vibration is no longer heard.
- When the client no longer hears the tone, note the time.

Findings: The tone heard in front of the ear should last twice as long as the tone heard when the fork was on the mastoid process (AC greater than BC by 2:1). This is the normal (positive) response. Repeat the test with the other ear.

Audioscope

Each of the screening tests listed previously may identify an individual with decreased hearing, but none of these tests measures the degree of hearing loss. An audioscope provides a measurement of hearing (see Fig. 4-25 in Chapter 4). Select a speculum that best fits the ear canal (a snug fit is desired to screen out surrounding noise). Attach the speculum to the probe, and insert in the ear sealing the external auditory canal. As tones are delivered at each frequency, the client indicates if the tone can be heard, thus providing objective measurement of hearing. Because of the high degree of accuracy, and ease of use, the audioscope is becoming increasingly used for hearing screening in primary care (Yueh et al, 2003). The client who hears well will be able to hear all tones at all frequencies delivered by the audioscope.

A 20-dB loss in high frequencies results in difficulty hearing high-pitched consonants. A 40-dB loss in all frequencies causes moderate difficulty in hearing normal speech.

ROUTINE TECHNIQUES: NOSE

INSPECT the nose for general appearance, symmetry, discharge, and tenderness.

The skin should be smooth and intact, with the color matching the rest of the face. The nose should appear symmetric and midline. The nostrils should be symmetric, not flaring or narrowed. There should be no nasal discharge present.

Lesions, erythema, and discoloration are abnormal and may be signs of a systemic illness. Marked asymmetry of the nose may be the result of current or past injury.

Edema, nasal discharge, and crusting are possible signs of infection, allergy, or injury. Watery, unilateral nasal discharge following a history of head injury may indicate skull fracture. Unilateral, purulent, thick nasal drainage may indicate a foreign body. Hypertrophy of the sebaceous glands and soft tissue of the nose is a condition known as rhinophyma (see Fig. 11-61 later in this chapter).

SPECIAL CIRCUMSTANCES OR ADVANCED PRACTICE: NOSE

PALPATE the nose for tenderness and to assess patency.

Apply pressure to occlude one nostril; ask the client to close his or her mouth and sniff through the opposite nostril; repeat on the other side. There should be noiseless, free exchange of air on each side. The nose should not be tender with palpation.

Narrowing of the nostrils when the client inhales may be associated with chronic obstruction that may necessitate mouth breathing. Noisy or obstructed breathing may occur secondary to nasal congestion, trauma to the nasal passage, polyps, or allergies. Instability or tenderness from trauma or inflammation may be noted on palpation.

INSPECT the internal nasal cavity.

Procedure: The internal nasal cavity is inspected using a nasal speculum and a light source. Hold the speculum in the palm of the hand and use your index finger to stabilize the speculum against the side of the nose. Insert the speculum slowly and cautiously; open the speculum on a slightly oblique axis (not horizontally) because direct pressure on the septum is painful (Woodson, 2001). Use your other hand to hold the light source. Alternatively, an otoscope with a nasal speculum attached may be used for the examination (Fig. 11-38).

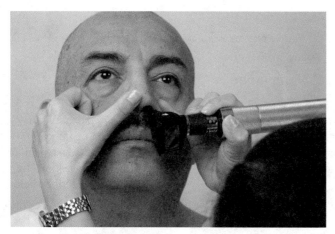

Fig. 11-38   Inspect the nasal cavity with a light source.

PROCEDURES AND TECHNIQUES WITH NORMAL FINDINGS

Findings: With the client's head erect, note the floor of the nose, inferior turbinate, nasal hairs, and mucosa, which should be slightly darker red than the oral mucosa. The client's nasal septum should be straight, intact, and midline. With the client's head back, inspect the middle meatus and middle turbinate (Fig. 11-39). Turbinates should be a deep pink color, similar to the color of the surrounding tissue.

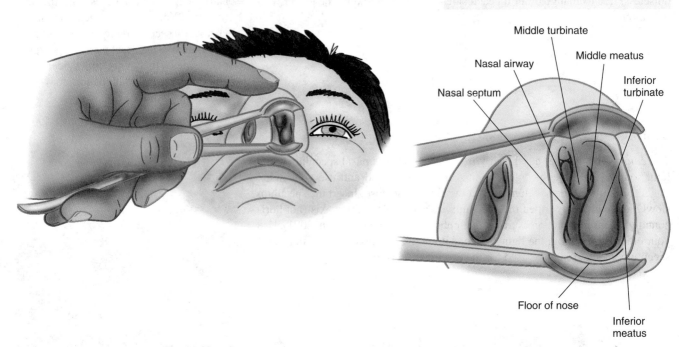

Fig. 11-39   View of the nasal mucosa through the nasal speculum. *(From Seidel et al, 2006.)*

PALPATE the frontal and maxillary paranasal sinus areas for tenderness.

To palpate the frontal sinuses, press upward on the frontal sinuses with your thumbs on the supraorbital ridge just below the eyebrows. Be careful not to press directly over the eyeballs. To palpate the maxillary sinuses, press over the sinus area above the cheekbones (Fig. 11-40). There should be no tenderness or pain with palpation over the sinuses.

★ TRANSILLUMINATE the sinus area.

If the client complains of sinus pain or shows signs of sinus congestion, transilluminate the sinuses using a transilluminator or bright penlight. After darkening the room, place the source of light lateral to the nose, just beneath the medial aspect of the eye. Look through the client's open mouth for illumination of the hard palate. Transilluminate the frontal sinuses by placing the light source against the medial aspect of each supraorbital rim. Look for a dim red glow as light is transmitted above the eyebrows.

ABNORMAL FINDINGS

There should be no perforations, bleeding, or crusting. A deviated nasal septum with a decrease in airflow is abnormal. Increased redness may occur secondary to infection, whereas localized erythema and edema in the vestibule may indicate a furuncle or localized infection.

Tenderness on palpation may indicate sinus congestion or infection. If the client complains of sinus pain or shows signs of sinus congestion, transilluminate the sinuses (described below).

An absence of a glow during transillumination of the sinuses may indicate that the sinus is congested and is filled with secretions, or that the sinus never developed.

★ = advanced practice

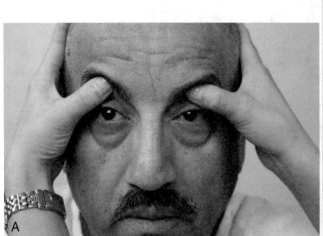
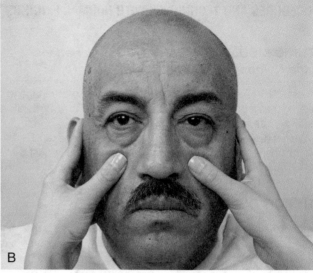

Fig. 11-40   Palpation of the sinuses. A, Frontal. **B,** Maxillary.

| PROCEDURES AND TECHNIQUES WITH NORMAL FINDINGS | ABNORMAL FINDINGS |

ROUTINE TECHNIQUES: MOUTH

🔑 **INSPECT the mouth and oropharynx.**

Lips for color, symmetry, moisture, and texture.

Lips should appear pink and symmetric both vertically and laterally. The lips should be smooth and moist and have slight vertical linear markings. There should be a distinct border between the lips and the facial skin (vermillion border).

Pale lips may indicate anemia or shock. Cyanotic (bluish) lips and circumoral cyanosis may indicate hypoxemia or hypothermia. Dry, flaking, or cracked lips may be caused by dehydration, exposure to dry air or wind. Cracks and erythema in the corners of the mouth may be caused by vitamin B deficiencies (Williams & Schlenker, 2003). Lesions, plaques, vesicles, nodules, or ulcerations may be signs of infection, irritation (such as lip biting), or skin cancer. Lips may be edematous due to an allergic reaction.

Teeth and gums for condition, color, surface characteristics, stability, and alignment.

The teeth should be white, yellow, or gray, with smooth edges. Inspect the condition of the teeth, making note of caries, and broken and missing teeth.

Observe alignment by asking the client to clench the teeth and smile. The upper back teeth should rest directly on the lower back teeth, with the upper incisors slightly overriding the lower ones. The teeth should be evenly spaced and firmly anchored. The gingiva around the base of the teeth should have a pink, moist appearance with a clearly defined margin at each tooth. For clients who wear dentures, observe the gum line beneath the dentures.

Missing teeth may occur secondary to tooth extraction or trauma. Darkened or stained teeth may occur secondary to coffee, medications, poor dental care, or frequent vomiting. Brown spots in the crevices or between the teeth may indicate caries.

Excessively exposed tooth neck with receding gums may occur secondary to aging or gingival disease.

Protrusion of the upper or lower incisors or upper incisors that do not overlap

🔑 = core examination skill

PROCEDURES AND TECHNIQUES WITH NORMAL FINDINGS

ETHNIC & CULTURAL VARIATIONS *Variations in the Number and Size of Teeth*

About 30% of Asian Americans, 15% of Native Americans, and 10% of whites have agenesis of the third molar and thus have only 28 teeth as adults. This pattern is rare in African Americans.

Whites have the smallest teeth; African Americans tend to have larger teeth than whites; Asians and Native Americans have the largest teeth.

ETHNIC & CULTURAL VARIATIONS

Darker-skinned persons often have darker oral pigmentation and may have a patchy brown pigmentation of the gums. There may also be a dark melanotic line along the gingival margin.

Tongue for movement, color, and surface characteristics.

Ask the client to stick out his or her tongue. (This maneuver also tests cranial nerve XII—the hypoglossal nerve.) The forward thrust should be smooth and symmetric, and the tongue itself should appear symmetric. The tongue should be pink and moist with a glistening surface dorsally and laterally. The surface may appear slightly rough because of the papillae on the dorsal surface of the tongue. Also, note any edema or variation in size, color, coating, or ulceration.

Buccal mucosa and anterior and posterior pillars for color and surface characteristics.

Ask the client to open the mouth widely to allow you to inspect the buccal mucosa using a penlight and tongue blade. Inspect the anterior and posterior pillars. Note the color of the mucosa and the symmetry of the pillars. The color of the tissue should be pale coral or pink with slight vascularity. Using a tongue blade, gently pull the buccal mucosa away from the molars. The buccal mucosa should be smooth, with a transverse occlusion line appearing adjacent to where teeth meet. Clear saliva should cover the surface. The parotid gland duct opening (also known as Stensen's duct) is on the buccal mucosa adjacent to the upper second molar. It appears as a slightly elevated pinpoint red mark. Also, note the odor of the breath. The mouth should have a slightly sweet odor or no odor at all.

ABNORMAL FINDINGS

the lower ones on closure are indications of malocclusion (Fig. 11-41).

Presence of debris usually occurs because of poor dental habits. Redness, edema, and bleeding of the gums may occur secondary to gingivitis, systemic disease, hormonal changes, and drug therapy (see Fig. 11-63 later in this chapter).

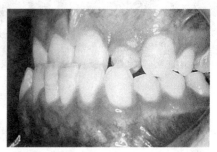

Fig. 11-41   Malocclusion of the teeth.

Atrophy of the tongue on one side or deviation of the tongue may be a sign of a neurologic disorder. A smooth or beefy-red colored, edematous tongue with a slick appearance may indicate B vitamin deficiency (Williams and Schlenker, 2003). A hairy tongue with yellow-brown to black elongated papillae may occur secondary to antibiotic therapy, superinfection, or pipe smoking. An enlarged tongue may be seen in clients with mental retardation or hypothyroidism. Lesions and sores are always considered abnormal.

Aphthous ulcers on the buccal mucosa appear as white, round, or oval ulcerative lesions with a red halo (see Fig. 11-66 later in this chapter). *Leukoplakia* is a white patch or plaque found on the oral mucosa that cannot be scraped off (Fig. 11-42). *Erythroplakia* is a red patch found on the oral mucosa. An excessively dry mouth or excessive salivation may indicate salivary gland blockage or may occur secondary to medications, dehydration, or stress.

An acetone odor on the breath may indicate diabetic ketoacidosis. A fetid

PROCEDURES AND TECHNIQUES WITH NORMAL FINDINGS

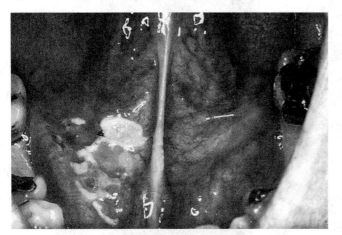

Fig. 11-42 Leukoplakia. *(From Dunlap and Barker, 1991.)*

Palate, uvula, posterior pharynx, and tonsils for texture, color, surface characteristics, and movement.

Instruct the client to tilt his or her head back so that the palate and uvula may be inspected. The hard palate should be smooth, pale, and immovable with irregular transverse rugae. The soft palate and uvula should be smooth and pink, with the uvula in a midline position. Instruct the client to say "ah." (If necessary, depress the tongue with a tongue depressor.) Observe if the soft palate rises symmetrically with the uvula remaining in the midline position. (This tests cranial nerves IX and X—the glossopharyngeal and vagus nerves.)

Using a tongue depressor to hold the tongue down, examine the posterior wall of the pharynx (Fig. 11-43). The tissue should be smooth and have a glistening pink coloration. The tonsils extend beyond the posterior pillars. The tonsils should appear slightly pink with an irregular surface.

ETHNIC & CULTURAL VARIATIONS

A split uvula occurs in up to 10% of Asians and 18% of some Native American groups (Giger and Davidhizar, 2008).

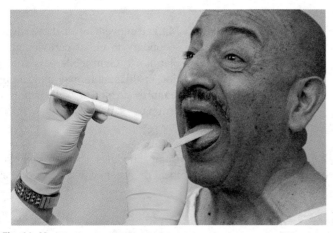

Fig. 11-43 Displace the tongue with a tongue depressor for inspection of the pharynx.

ABNORMAL FINDINGS

odor may occur secondary to gum disease, caries, poor dental care, or sinusitis.

Nodules observed on the palate that are not at the midline may indicate a tumor. Lesions associated with Kaposi's sarcoma may be present on both the hard and soft palates. Opportunistic infections may occur when an individual has been on antibiotics or is immunosuppressed. Failure of the soft palate to rise bilaterally, as well as uvula deviation during vocalization, may indicate a neurologic problem.

Exudate or mucoid film on the posterior pharynx may be present secondary to postnasal drip or infection. A grayish tinge to the membrane may occur with allergies or diphtheria. Edematous, erythematous tonsils with or without exudate may indicate infection. Tonsil enlargement is graded from 1+ to 4+ (Fig. 11-44).

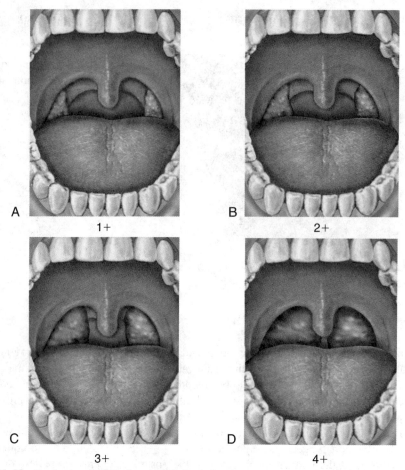

Fig. 11-44 **Tonsil enlargement. A,** 1+, visible; **B,** 2+, halfway between tonsilar pillars and uvula; **C,** 3+, nearly touching the uvula; **D,** 4+, touching each other. *(From Seidel et al, 2006.)*

PROCEDURES AND TECHNIQUES WITH NORMAL FINDINGS	ABNORMAL FINDINGS

SPECIAL CIRCUMSTANCES OR ADVANCED PRACTICE: MOUTH

PALPATE structures of the mouth.

Teeth, inner lips, and gums for condition and tenderness.
Wearing gloves, palpate the teeth and inner aspects of the lips and upper and lower gingivobuccal fornices and gingivae (gums). The teeth should be firmly anchored.

Marked movement of the teeth may be secondary to either periodontal disease or trauma. Gum tenderness with palpation or thickening may indicate that the dentures do not fit well or presence of lesions.

Tongue for texture
Wearing examination gloves, grasp the tongue with a 4×4 inch gauze pad, and palpate all sides (Fig. 11-45). The tongue should feel relatively smooth and even. Papillae create slight roughness on the dorsum of the tongue. During palpation, note any lumps, nodules, or areas of thickening.

Lumps, nodules, or masses may indicate local or systemic disease or oral cancer.

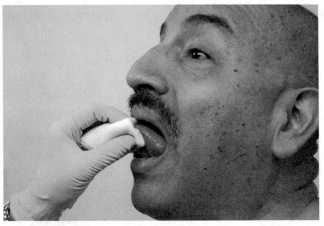

Fig. 11-45 Grasp the tongue with a 4 × 4 inch gauze pad.

PROCEDURES AND TECHNIQUES WITH NORMAL FINDINGS	ABNORMAL FINDINGS

ROUTINE TECHNIQUES: NECK

INSPECT the neck.

Position in relation to the head and trachea.
The neck should be centered, and the trapezius and sternocleidomastoid muscles should be bilaterally symmetric (Fig. 11-46). The trachea should be midline.

Note rhythmic movements or tremor of the neck and head. Observe also for tics or spasms. Tracheal deviation suggests displacement by a mass in the chest.

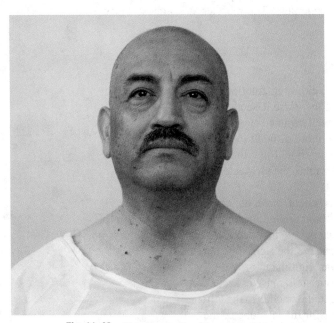

Fig. 11-46 Bilateral symmetry of the neck muscles.

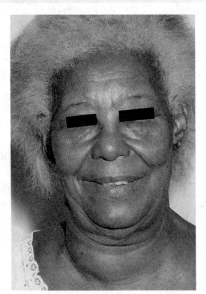

Fig. 11-47 **Goiter.** Note visible enlargement over the anterior neck. *(From Bingham, Hawke, and Kwok, 1992.)*

Skin characteristics, presence of lumps, masses.
The skin color should match other skin areas. In some individuals (particularly in thin men) the thyroid cartilage may protrude enough to be visible. The thyroid gland is usually not clearly visualized.

Lesions or masses on the neck are not normal. A goiter (enlarged thyroid) may be seen as a fullness in the neck (Fig. 11-47).

| PROCEDURES AND TECHNIQUES WITH NORMAL FINDINGS | ABNORMAL FINDINGS |

SPECIAL CIRCUMSTANCES OR ADVANCED PRACTICE: NECK

INSPECT the neck for range of motion.

Ask the client move the neck forward (chin to chest, 45 degrees), backward (toward ceiling, 55 degrees), and side to side (ear to shoulder, 40 degrees). The shoulders should remain stationary during assessment. Next, ask the client to rotate the head laterally to the right and left (70 degrees in both directions). All movements should be controlled, smooth, and painless.

Limited ROM or pain during movement may indicate either a systemic infection with meningeal irritation, a musculo-skeletal problem such as muscle spasm, or degenerative vertebral disks. Note weakness of muscles or tremors. Note if the client complains of pain throughout the movement or at particular points.

PALPATE the neck.

Positioning of anatomic structures and trachea.

Palpate the neck and trachea just above the suprasternal notch. Palpate for the tracheal rings, cricoid cartilage, and thyroid cartilage. All structures should be midline and nontender.

Assess sternocleidomastoid muscle strength by asking the client to turn his or her head from side to side against the resistance of your hand. Assess trapezius muscle strength by asking the client to shrug the shoulders against the resistance of your hands pressing down on the client's shoulders. By doing this, you are also assessing the spinal accessory nerve (cranial nerve XI). Palpation of the neck muscles helps assess for areas of muscle tenderness. The muscles should be firm and nontender with palpation.

Abnormalities include tenderness or masses on palpation or location of the structures away from the midline posi-tion.

Unilateral or bilateral muscle weak-ness is an abnormal finding.

Tenderness, muscle spasms, and edema are abnormal findings and may suggest injury.

★ *Thyroid gland for size, shape consistency, tenderness, and presence of nodules.*

Procedure: Palpation of the thyroid may be done using either an anterior or a posterior approach. The technique used is the choice of the nurse. Use a gentle touch to palpate the thyroid. Your fingernails should be well trimmed at or below the fingertips. Nodules and asymmetric position will be more difficult to detect if the pressure is too hard. In either technique, the client should flex the neck slightly forward and toward the side being examined to relax the sternocleido-mastoid muscle.

Posterior approach (Fig. 11-48, *A*): Stand behind the client. Have the client sit straight with the head slightly flexed. Reach from behind around the client's neck and place your fingers on either side of the trachea below the cricoid car-tilage. Use two fingers of the left hand to push the trachea to the right. Instruct the client to swallow while using the finger pads of your right hand to feel for the right lobe of the thyroid gland, the right sternocleidomastoid muscle, and the trachea. Repeat the technique using the right hand to push the trachea to the left. Instruct the client to swallow while your left hand feels for the left lobe of the thyroid.

Anterior approach (Fig. 11-48, *B*): You should be standing in front of the client. Ask the client to sit up straight, then bend the head slightly forward and to the right. Push the client's trachea to the right with your left thumb. Palpate the thyroid gland below the cricoid process. Instruct the client to swallow; the client's displaced right thyroid lobe may be palpated between the sternocleido-mastoid muscle and the trachea by the finger pads of your left index and middle fingers. Use the same examination techniques with reversed hand position to examine the left thyroid lobe.

★ = advanced practice

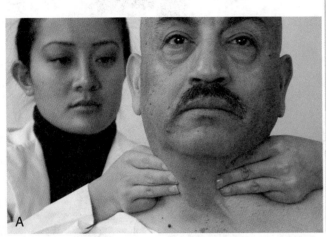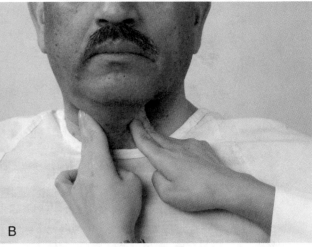

Fig. 11-48 Palpation of the thyroid gland. **A,** Posterior approach. **B,** Anterior approach.

PROCEDURES AND TECHNIQUES WITH NORMAL FINDINGS

Findings: The thyroid gland is a little larger than the size of your thumb pad. The thyroid gland often is not detected, and this is considered a normal finding. If the thyroid is felt, it should feel small, smooth, and soft, and the gland should move freely during swallowing. The thyroid should be nontender.

Findings: Lymph nodes may or may not be palpable. If they are palpable, they should be soft, mobile, and nontender and bilaterally equal.

SPECIAL CIRCUMSTANCES OR ADVANCED PRACTICE: LYMPH NODES

PALPATE lymph nodes for size, consistency, mobility, boarders, tenderness, and warmth.

Regional lymph nodes include occipital nodes (at base of skull), preauricular nodes (in front of the ear), postauricular nodes (behind the ear), anterior and posterior cervical chain nodes (within the neck), parotid nodes (along the angle of the jaw), submental and submandibular nodes (under the mandible), and supraclavicular nodes (under the clavicle).

Procedure: Palpate the nodes using your fingertips. You may want to use both hands, one on each side of the head and neck, to compare the findings. However, the submental nodes are easier to palpate with one hand.

Begin with the preauricular nodes and palpate them (Fig. 11-49), followed by the parotid, postauricular, occipital, retropharyngeal, submandibular, and submental nodes. Next, examine the anterior and posterior cervical chain by tipping the client's head toward the side being examined (Fig. 11-50); palpate the anterior chain on either side of the sternocleidomastoid muscle and the deep

ABNORMAL FINDINGS

A bruit indicates an abnormally large volume of blood flow and suggests a goiter. A thyroid that is easily palpable before swallowing is enlarged—a common finding in hyperthyroidism. If the thyroid gland is enlarged, use the bell of the stethoscope to auscultate the thyroid for vascular sounds. Lumps, nodules, or tenderness are abnormal findings.

Lymph nodes that are enlarged, tender, and firm but freely movable may suggest an infection of the head or throat. Malignancy may be suspected when nodes are unilateral, hard, asymmetric, fixed, and nontender.

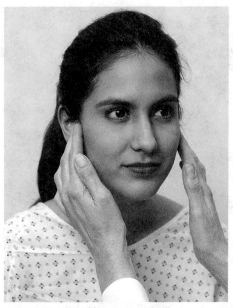

Fig. 11-49   Palpation of the preauricular nodes.

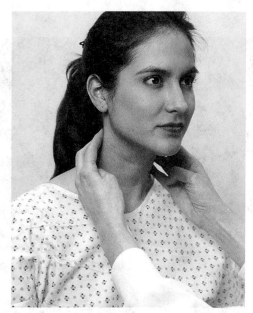

Fig. 11-50   Palpation of the posterior superficial cervical chain nodes.

PROCEDURES AND TECHNIQUES WITH NORMAL FINDINGS

ABNORMAL FINDINGS

posterior cervical nodes at the anterior border of the trapezius muscle. Palpate the supraclavicular nodes by having the client hunch the shoulders forward and flex the chin toward the side being examined. Place your fingers into the medial supraclavicular fossa. Ask the client to take a deep breath while you press deeply behind the clavicles to detect nodes.

Documenting Expected Findings

Head, Ears, Eyes, Nose, and Throat in an Adult Male

Head. The head symmetric and proportioned for the body size. Scalp clean, intact with male-patterned balding. Face and jaw symmetric and proportional. TMJ moves smoothly. Temporal arteries palpable bilaterally with a regular rate and rhythm, grade 2.

Eyes: Distance and near vision are 20/20 OU with contact lens. Horizontal and color perceptions intact. Eyebrows symmetric with eyelashes evenly distributed and curled upward. Palpebral fissures equal bilaterally and the eyelid color appropriate for race. Eyelid margins pale pink and cover the top of the brown iris. Lid closure complete with frequent, bilateral and involuntary blinking. Bulbar conjunctiva pink and clear. Corneal light reflex symmetric. Sclera white, clear, and moist; corneas are transparent. PERRLA. Peripheral vision present. EOM intact. Eyeballs indent with slight pressure, no tenderness of eyelids. The irises are clear, with no shadow noted. *Ophthalmic examination:* Red reflex present, disc margins distinct, round, yellow, physiologic cup temporal to disc center; artery-to-vein ratio 2:3, retina red uniformly; macula and fovea slightly darker.

Ears: Hearing present with conversation. Pinna aligned with outer canthus of eyes. The upper part of ear firm, flexible, and soft without discomfort; aligned with eyes; ears symmetric. Cerumen in auditory canal; TM pearly gray, cone of light reflex present. Whispered words repeated correctly, tone heard bilaterally in Weber Test, AC:BC 2:1.

Nose: Skin, smooth, intact and oily. Nasal passages patent, turbinates pink without exudate, septum midline, sinuses nontender.

Mouth, Throat and Neck: Breath without odor. Lips symmetric, moist, smooth; 32 white, smooth, aligned teeth. Tongue symmetric, pink, moist, and movable. Gingiva pink and moist, symmetric pillars, clear saliva. Hard palate smooth, pale, soft palate smooth, pink and rises as expected, uvula midline; posterior pharynx pink, smooth tonsils pink with irregular surface. Trachea is midline; thyroid smooth, soft, moves freely with swallow. Neck is centered with full ROM, no palpable lymph nodes.

CLINICAL REASONING *HEENT*

A 17-year-old Native American woman brings her 5-month-old son to a medical clinic reporting that he is fussy and his skin is very hot. She also reports the baby has low energy and is not sleeping or eating well.

Noticing: Extensive practical knowledge about what to expect with infants allows the experienced nurse to recognize that these are common findings associated with fever. This background knowledge sets up the possibility of noticing when there are signs of a prevalent complication (such as respiratory compromise and dehydration) in an infant presenting with fever and considering possible causes of fever. The nurse observes an infant who is crying with adequate air exchange and appears well hydrated; the nurse confirms the infant has a fever when the temperature is measured at 100.7° F. His respiratory rate is 40.

Interpreting: Early in the encounter, the nurse knows the two most common causes of fever in an infant this age are a respiratory or ear infection. In order to determine if either has any probability of being correct, the nurse gathers additional data.

- Are there signs of respiratory involvement? No evidence of nasal flaring or discharge, cough, stridor, grunting, retractions are observed; lung sounds are clear; the left tympanic membrane is red.
- Has the infant had a recent cough or nasal drainage? Has the infant been pulling at his ear? The mother denies cough or nasal drainage, but reports ear rubbing. The experienced nurse not only recognizes infection by the clinical signs (red tympanic membrane, fever) and symptoms (fussy, poor sleeping, eating, rubbing the ear), but interprets this information in the context of his age.

Responding: The experienced nurse initiates appropriate initial interventions, determines the type of health care provider for the baby, and ensures that the infant receives appropriate immediate and follow-up care, including family teaching about otitis media and fever management.

AGE-RELATED VARIATIONS

INFANTS AND CHILDREN

There are several important differences to be aware of when conducting an assessment of the head, eyes, ears, nose, and throat of infants and young children. These differences include interview questions to ask, anatomical differences, examination procedures, and findings. Refer to Chapter 20 for a detailed discussion related to assessment for this age group.

OLDER ADULTS

Multiple changes occur as a consequence of advancing age; many of these age-related changes impact assessment findings presented within this chapter. See Chapter 22 for further information about the differences of assessment for this age group.

COMMON PROBLEMS & CONDITIONS

HEAD & NECK

Headaches

Headaches are one of the most common medical complaints of humans. Most recurrent headaches are symptoms of a chronic primary headache disorder, but they can also be associated with other problems such as ophthalmologic problems, dental problems, sinusitis, infections, side effects from medications, cerebral hemorrhage, or tumors. The pain associated with headaches can be mild or severe.

Typically, headaches can be classified based on the symptoms and history.

Migraine Headache

Migraine headache is the second most common headache syndrome in the United States. These headaches can occur in childhood, adolescence, or early adult life; young women are most susceptible. **Clinical Findings:** The headache generally starts with an aura caused by a vasospasm of intracranial arteries and is described as a throbbing unilateral distribution of the headache pain. Accompanying signs may include feelings of depression, restlessness or irritability, photophobia, and nausea or vomiting. The headache may last up to 72 hours.

Cluster Headache

A cluster headache is considered to be the most painful of primary headaches. Cluster headaches are most common from adolescence to middle age. **Clinical Findings:** This type of headache is characterized by intense episodes of excruciating unilateral pain. A cluster headache may last from 30 minutes to 1 hour but may repeat daily for weeks at a time (hence the term *cluster*) followed by periods of remission during which the person is completely free from the attacks. On average, a cluster period lasts from 6 to 12 weeks and remissions last for an average of 12 months, although remissions may last for years (Dodick and Campbell, 2001). The pain is described as "burning," "boring," or "stabbing" pain behind one eye and may be accompanied by unilateral ptosis, ipsilateral lacrimation, and nasal stuffiness and drainage. Generally the headaches occur without warning, although some report a vague premonitory warning such as slight nausea.

Tension Headache

A tension headache is the most common type of headache experienced by adults between 20 and 40 years of age. **Clinical Findings:** It is usually bilateral and may be diffuse or confined to the frontal, temporal, parietal, or occipital area. The onset may be very gradual and may last for several days. The headache may be accompanied by contraction of the skeletal muscles of the face, jaw, and neck. Clients frequently describe this headache as feeling as if a tight band was around their head.

Posttraumatic Headache

This is a headache that occurs secondary to a head injury or concussion. The most common cause of head injury is motor vehicle accidents. **Clinical Findings:** A posttraumatic headache is characterized by a dull, generalized head pain. Accompanying symptoms may be a lack of ability to concentrate, giddiness, or dizziness.

Hydrocephalus

Hydrocephalus is abnormal accumulation of cerebrospinal fluid (CSF) that may develop from infancy to adulthood. In infants, hydrocephalus is usually a result of an obstruction of the drainage of CSF in the head. In adults, it may be caused by obstruction, as well as increased production or impaired absorption of CSF. **Clinical Findings:** In infants, a gradual increase in intracranial pressure occurs leading to an actual enlargement of the head (Fig. 11-51). As the head enlarges, the facial features appear small in proportion to the cranium; fontanels may bulge, and the scalp veins dilate. In adults the signs of increased intracranial pressure (decreased mental status, headache) are noted because the skull is unable to expand.

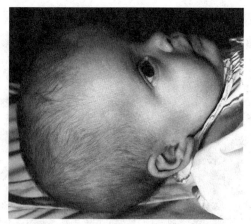

Fig. 11-51 Three-month-old infant with hydrocephalus. *(From McCullough, 1989.)*

EYES

External Eye

Chalazion

A chalazion is a nodule of the meibomian gland in the eyelid. It may be tender if infected and often follows hordeolum or chronic inflammation such as conjunctivitis, blepharitis, or meibomian cyst (Fig. 11-52). **Clinical Findings:** A firm, nontender nodule is observed in the eyelid.

Hordeolum (Sty)

An acute infection originating in the sebaceous gland of the eyelid is termed a *hordeolum*. It is usually caused by *Staphylococcus aureus* (Fig. 11-53). **Clinical Findings:** The affected area usually is painful, red, and edematous.

Conjunctivitis

An inflammation of the palpebral or bulbar conjunctiva is termed *conjunctivitis*. It is caused by local infection of bacteria or virus, as well as by an allergic reaction, systemic in-

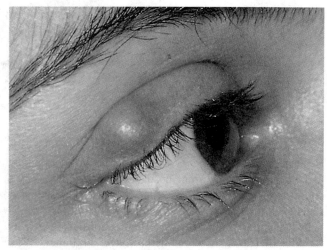

Fig. 11-52 Chalazion (right upper eyelid). *(From Newell, 1992.)*

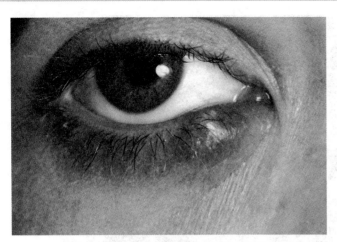

Fig. 11-53 Hordeolum (sty). *(From Bedford, 1986.)*

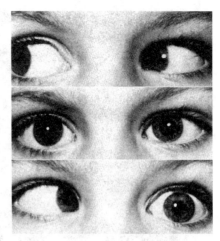

Fig. 11-55 Paralytic strabismus involving left lateral rectus muscle innervated by cranial nerve VI (abducens nerve). *(From von Noorden, 1990.)*

fection, or chemical irritation (Fig. 11-54). **Clinical Findings:** The eye appears red, with thick, sticky discharge on the eyelids in the morning.

Corneal Abrasion or Ulcer

Disruptions of the corneal epithelium and stroma create a corneal abrasion or ulcer. It is caused by fungal, viral, or bacterial infections or desiccation (dryness) because of incomplete lid closure or poor lacrimal gland function. It can also be caused by scratches, foreign bodies, or contact lenses that are poorly fitted or overworn. **Clinical Findings:** The client feels intense pain, has a foreign body sensation, and reports photophobia. Tearing and redness are observed.

Strabismus

An abnormal ocular alignment in which the visual axes do not meet at the desired point is termed *strabismus* (Fig. 11-55). Nonparalytic strabismus is due to muscle weakness, focusing difficulties, unilateral refractive error, or anatomic

differences in eyes. Paralytic strabismus is a motor imbalance caused by paresis or paralysis of an extraocular muscle. **Clinical Findings:** Two of the most common types of strabismus are esotropia and exotropia. Esotropia is an inward-turning eye and is the most common type of strabismus in infants. Exotropia is an outward-turning eye.

Internal Eye

Cataract

A cataract is an opacity of the crystalline lens. It most commonly occurs from denaturation of lens protein caused by aging, but can also be congenital or caused by trauma (Fig. 11-56). **Clinical Findings:** Clients report cloudy or blurred vision; glare from headlights, lamps, or sunlight; and diplopia. They also report poor night vision and frequent changes in their glasses prescriptions. A cloudy lens can be observed on inspection. The red reflex is absent and examination because the light cannot penetrate the opacity of the lens.

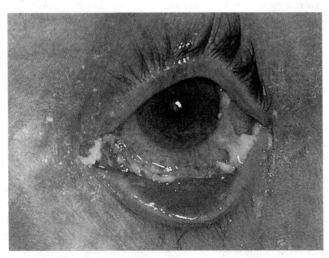

Fig. 11-54 Acute conjunctivitis. *(From Newell, 1996.)*

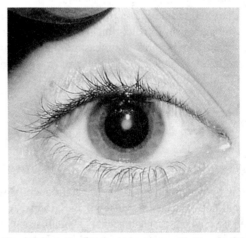

Fig. 11-56 **Cataract.** Note cloudy white spot over pupil. *(From Zitelli and Davis, 2007.)*

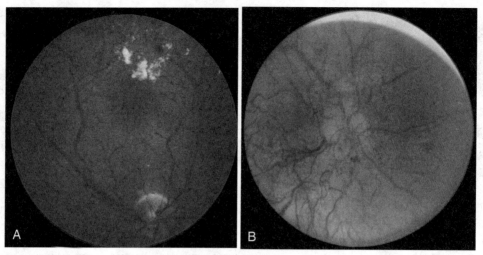

Fig. 11-57 **Diabetic retinopathy. A,** Nonproliferative. **B,** Proliferative. *(A, From Bedford, 1986. B, Courtesy John W. Payne, MD, The Wilmer Ophthalmological Institute, The Johns Hopkins University and Hospital, Baltimore, MD. From Seidel et al, 2006.)*

Diabetic Retinopathy

Visual alteration caused by diabetes mellitus is termed *diabetic retinopathy*. It is caused by changes in the retinal capillaries and is the leading cause of blindness in working Americans (Gallichan, 2006). Diabetic retinopathy is classified as background and proliferative. **Clinical Findings:** Clients report decrease in vision. In background diabetic retinopathy, microaneurysms and hemorrhages are seen. Exudates may also be seen around the macula (Fig. 11-57, *A*). Clients with proliferative diabetic retinopathy may report an image of a curtain coming down over their eye from a detached retina. On examination, a network of new blood vessels is seen along the retinal surface (Fig. 11-57, *B*).

Glaucoma

Glaucoma is a group of diseases characterized by an increase in the intraocular pressure. Untreated, it causes damage to the optic nerve and leads to blindness (Kanner and Tsai, 2006). Types of glaucoma include open angle (most common), closed angle, congenital glaucoma, and secondary glaucoma. **Clinical Findings:** There are no specific symptoms of open-angle glaucoma. Clients may report gradual and painless loss of peripheral vision and the eye may be very firm to palpation. The most reliable indicator is an intraocular pressure measurement. Clients with closed-angle glaucoma complain of sharp eye pain and seeing a halo around lights.

EARS

Foreign Body

A foreign body within the ear is most frequently seen in children, although it may occur in all age groups. A foreign body can be any small object such as a small stone, a small part of a toy, or even an insect. **Clinical Findings:** The client feels a sense of fullness in the ear and experiences decreased hearing. If the foreign body is a live insect, the client may report hearing movement of the insect and often experiences severe pain. In this case, symptoms may include ear pain and fever. Inspection of the auditory canal reveals the foreign body (Fig. 11-58).

Infection

Acute Otitis Media

Acute otitis media (AOM) is an infection of the middle ear. It can occur at any age, but is one of the most common of all childhood infections (Rovers et al, 2007). **Clinical Findings:** The major symptom associated with AOM is ear pain (otalgia). Infants unable to verbally communicate pain may demonstrate irritability, fussiness, crying, lethargy, and pulling at the affected ear. Associated manifestations include fever, vomiting (infants), and decreased hearing (older children and adults). On inspection in the early stages, the TM appears inflamed—it is red and may be bulging and immobile (Fig. 11-59). Later stages may reveal discoloration (white or yellow drainage) and opacification to the TM. Purulent drainage from the ear canal with a sudden relief of pain suggests perforation.

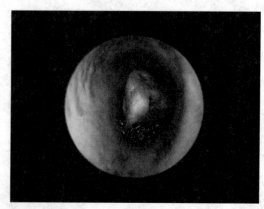

Fig. 11-58 Client inserted a small stone into the deep part of the external ear canal. It is lying against the tympanic membrane. *(From Bingham, Hawke, and Kwok, 1992.)*

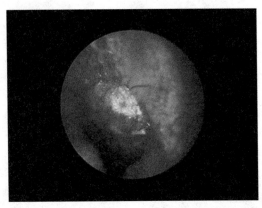

Fig. 11-59   Acute otitis media with redness and edematous swelling of the pars flaccida, shown in the central part of the illustration (left ear). *(From Bingham, Hawke, and Kwok, 1992.)*

Otitis Media with Effusion

Otitis media with effusion (OME) is an inflammation of the middle ear space resulting in accumulation of serous fluid in the middle ear. **Clinical Findings:** Common symptoms include a clogged sensation in the ears, problems with hearing and balance. Some report clicking or popping sounds within the ear. Because OME is not associated with acute inflammation, fever and ear pain are absent. On examination, the TM is often retracted and is yellow or gray with limited mobility (Fig. 11-60).

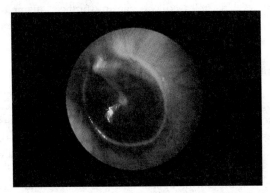

Fig. 11-60   Otitis media with effusion. *(From Bingham, Hawke, and Kwok, 1992.)*

Hearing Loss

Conductive Hearing Loss

Conductive hearing loss is caused by the interference of air conduction to the middle ear. This can result from blockage of the external auditory canal (such as a cerumen impaction), problems with the tympanic membrane (perforations, retraction pockets, or tympanosclerosis), or problems within the middle ear (otitis media with effusion, otosclerosis, trauma, or cholesteatoma) (Zadeh and Selesnick, 2001). **Clinical Findings:** Typically the chief complaint is a decreased ability to hear and the report of muffled tones. Other findings are dependent on the cause; obstructions within the auditory canal or problems with the TM may be visible with otoscopic examination, whereas problems within the middle ear may not be visible.

Sensorineural Hearing Loss

Sensorineural hearing loss (SNHL) is caused by structural changes, disorders of the inner ear, or problems with the auditory nerve. SNHL accounts for over 90% of hearing loss cases (Yueh et al, 2003). Presbycusis, the most common cause of SNHL, is caused by atrophy and deterioration of the cells in the cochlea or atrophy, degeneration, and stiffening of cochlear motion. **Clinical Findings:** Presbycusis usually manifests as a gradual and progressive bilateral deafness with a loss of high-pitched tones. Clients with presbycusis have difficulty filtering background noise, making listening difficult.

NOSE

Epistaxis

The term *epistaxis* means bleeding from the nose. Epistaxis is recognized as one of the most common problems of the nose, estimated to occur in 60% of individuals (Kucik & Klenny, 2005). Common causes of nosebleeds include forceful sneezing or coughing, trauma, picking the nose, or heavy exertion. Some nosebleeds occur spontaneously without an obvious causative event. **Clinical Findings:** The primary sign and symptom is bleeding from the nose. Bleeding can be mild or heavy. Because of the high vascularity, most nosebleeds occur from Kiesselbach's area, which is located in the anterior aspect of the septum; however, bleeds from the posterior septum may also occur and tend to be more severe.

Inflammation

Allergic Rhinitis

The term *rhinitis* refers to inflammation of the nasal mucosa. Chronic rhinitis affects millions of individuals and is usually caused by an inhalant allergy—this may be a seasonal allergy or a year-round sensitivity to dust and molds. There is a strong family history associated with allergic rhinitis. **Clinical Findings:** After exposure to the allergen the individual experiences sneezing, nasal congestion, and nasal drainage. Other symptoms can include itchy eyes, cough, and fatigue (Silvers, 2003). Turbinates are often enlarged and may appear pale or darker red.

Rhinophyma

Rhinophyma is a hypertrophy of the nose caused by rosacea, a chronic inflammatory disorder of the skin. It most commonly affects middle-age and older adults with fair complexion. The cause is unknown. **Clinical Findings:** Initial findings are pronounced flushing reactions, especially in response to heat, emotional stimuli, alcohol, hot drinks, or spicy foods. With advanced disease, papules, pustules, telangiectasia, and tissue hypertrophy of the nose are common findings (Fig. 11-61).

Acute Sinusitis

This is an infection of the sinuses that typically occurs as a result of pooling of secretions within the sinuses, which often occurs after an upper respiratory infection. These

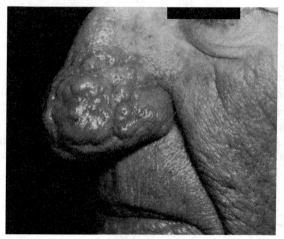

Fig. 11-61 Rhinophyma associated with rosacea. *(From Callen et al, 1993.)*

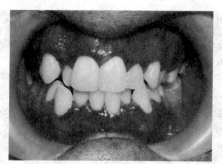

Fig. 11-63 Gingivitis. Note enlargement of the gums. *(From Bingham, Hawke, and Kwok, 1992.)*

pooled secretions provide a medium for bacterial growth. **Clinical Findings:** The most common symptom is throbbing pain within the affected sinus. The sinus is tender to palpation. The client may also have fever, thick purulent nasal discharge, and edematous, erythematous nasal mucosa. If transillumination is performed, absence of a red glow is noted in the affected sinus (Ivker, 2003).

MOUTH

Inflammation/Infection

Herpes Simplex Type 1 (Cold Sore)

A cold sore is a highly contagious, common viral infection caused by the herpes simplex type 1 virus. It is spread by direct contact. Recurrent infections occur following a stimulus of sun exposure, cold temperature, fever, or allergy. **Clinical Findings:** The client typically has a prodromal burning, tingling, or pain sensation before the outbreak of the lesions (Marx and Stern, 2002). The lesions usually appear on the lip-skin junc-

tion as groups of vesicular lesions with an erythematous base. Like other herpes infections, the lesions progress from vesicles, to pustules, and finally to crusts (Fig. 11-62).

Gingivitis

A common condition among adults, gingivitis is an inflammation of the gingivae (gums). Gingivitis can be acute, chronic, or recurrent. The most common cause is poor dental hygiene leading to the formation of bacterial plaque on the tooth surface at the gumline resulting in inflammation. **Clinical Findings:** Hyperplasia of the gums, erythema, and bleeding with manipulation are the most common signs (Fig. 11-63). Edema of the gum tissue deepens the crevice between the gingivae and teeth, allowing for the formation of gingival pockets where food particles collect, causing further inflammation. Periodontitis occurs when the inflammatory process causes erosion of the gum tissue and loosening of the teeth.

Tonsillitis

Tonsillitis is infection of the tonsils. Common bacterial pathogens include beta-hemolytic and other streptococci. **Clinical Findings:** The classic presentation of tonsillitis includes sore throat, pain with swallowing (odynophagia), fever, chills, and tender cervical lymph nodes. Some clients may also complain of ear pain (Johnson and Aijaz, 2003). On inspection, the tonsils appear enlarged and red and may be covered with white or yellow exudates (Fig. 11-64).

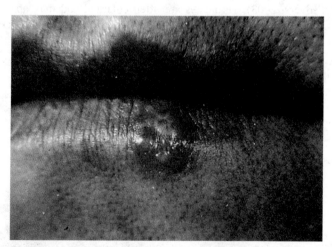

Fig. 11-62 Herpes simplex lesion (cold sore) of the lower lip. *(From Grimes, 1991.)*

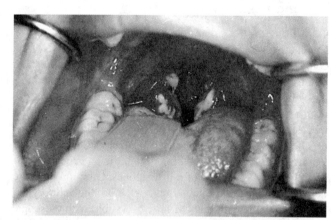

Fig. 11-64 Tonsillitis and pharyngitis. *(Courtesy Dr. Edward L. Applebaum, Head, Department of Otolaryngology, University of Illinois Medical Center.)*

Candidiasis (Thrush)

Candidiasis is an opportunistic oral infection typically caused by *Candida albicans*. Thrush is commonly seen among individuals who are chronically debilitated, in clients who are immunosuppressed, or as a result of antibiotic therapy. **Clinical Findings:** Oral candidiasis appears as soft white plaques on the tongue, buccal mucosa, or posterior pharynx (Fig. 11-65). If the membrane is peeled off, a raw, bleeding, erythematous, eroded or ulcerated surface results.

Lesions

Aphthous Ulcer (Canker Sore)

A canker sore is a common oral lesion with an unknown etiology that affects up to 30% of adults and 37% of school-age children (Zunt, 2003). **Clinical Findings:** These lesions are very painful and appear on the buccal mucosa, the lips, the tongue, or the palate as round or oval ulcerative lesions with a yellow-white center and with an erythematous halo (Fig. 11-66). The ulcers may last up to 2 weeks.

Oral Cancer

Oral cancers can occur on the lip or within the oral cavity and oropharynx. **Clinical Findings:** Oral cancer lesions are often subtle and asymptomatic in early stages; premalignant changes of the oral mucosa such as red or white patches (leukoplakia and erythroplakia) may be seen. These lesions progress to painless, nonhealing ulcers (Fig. 11-67). Later-stage signs and symptoms include enlarged, hard, nontender cervical chain or submental lymph nodes; noticeable mass, bleeding, loosening of teeth, difficulty wearing dentures, and difficulty swallowing.

Oral Kaposi's Sarcoma

This malignancy is seen in persons with acquired immunodeficiency syndrome (AIDS). **Clinical Findings:** Oral Kaposi's sarcoma appears as incompletely formed blood vessels in the mouth (Fig. 11-68). These vessels form lesions of various shades and sizes as the blood escapes into tissues in response to the malignant tumor of the mucous membranes.

NECK

Thyroid Disorders

Hyperthyroidism

Hyperthyroidism is a condition associated with excessive production and secretion of thyroid hormone. Of the several diseases that can cause hyperthyroidism, Graves' disease, a familial autoimmune disorder, is the most common cause (Weeks,

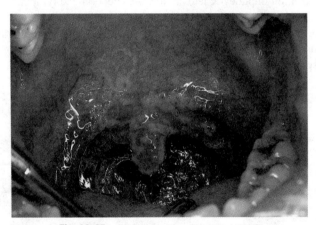

Fig. 11-65   Candidiasis. *(From Regezi et al, 2003.)*

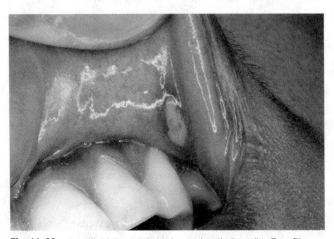

Fig. 11-66   A small aphthous ulcer (canker sore) on the lower lip. *(From Bingham, Hawke, and Kwok, 1992.)*

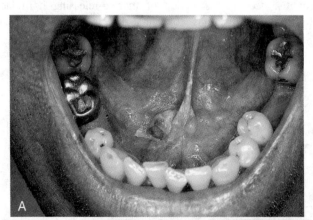

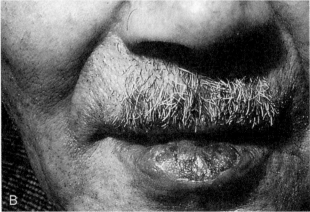

Fig. 11-67   **A,** Early squamous cell carcinoma on the floor of the mouth. **B,** Squamous cell carcinoma on the lip. *(**A,** From Regezi et al, 2003. **B,** From Hill, 1994.)*

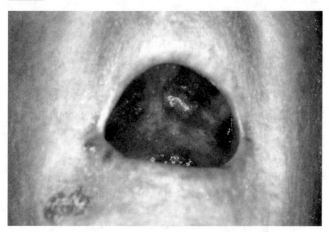

Fig. 11-68   The bluish raised lesion seen on the palate of this client who has AIDS is Kaposi's sarcoma. *(From Bingham, Hawke, and Kwok, 1992.)*

2005). **Clinical Findings:** Because thyroid hormone affects all body tissue, most body systems are affected. The signs and symptoms reflect increased metabolism and may include enlargement of the thyroid gland and exophthalmos (see Fig. 11-17). Auscultation of the goiter may reveal a bruit.

Hypothyroidism

Hypothyroidism, the most common problem associated with thyroid function, is characterized by a decreased production of thyroid hormone by the thyroid gland. Several etiologies have been linked to hypothyroidism, including autoimmune thyroiditis, decreased secretion of thyroid-releasing hormone from the hypothalamus, congenital defects, a result of treat-ment for hyperthyroidism (antithyroid drugs or surgical resection of thyroid tissue), atrophy of the thyroid gland, and iodine deficiency (Braverman and Utiger, 2005). **Clinical Findings:** Clinical findings reflect an overall decreased metabolism; clients seem to be in "slow motion," with a depressed affect. Goiter may be seen with hypothyroidism because of increases in thyroid-stimulating hormone (see Fig. 11-47).

Thyroid cancer

Thyroid cancer is the most common type of endocrine malignancy. **Clinical Findings:** Thyroid cancer frequently does not cause symptoms. Typically, thyroid cancer is first discovered as a small nodule on the thyroid gland. As the tumor grows, changes in the voice and problems with swallowing or breathing may be experienced because of invasion of the tumor into the larynx, esophagus, and trachea, respectively.

Lymphoma

Lymphomas are a group of disorders characterized by malignant neoplasms of the lymph tissue. They occur in adolescents and young adults, as well as persons over 50 years of age. **Clinical Findings:** Malignant lymphomas cause lymph nodes to be large, discrete, nontender, and firm to rubbery. Enlarged nodes usually are unilateral and localized; however, chronic lymphocytic leukemia causes generalized lymphadenopathy. Hodgkin's disease is a malignant lymphoma characterized by a painless, progressive enlargement of lymphoid tissue, usually first evident by the cervical lymph nodes, splenomegaly, and atypical macrophages.

CLINICAL APPLICATION & CLINICAL REASONING

See Appendix E for answers to exercises in this section.

REVIEW QUESTIONS

1 A client describes a recent onset of frequent and severe unilateral headaches that last about 1 hour. The nurse recognizes that these symptoms are consistent with:
   1 Cluster headaches.
   2 Migraine headaches.
   3 Tension headache.
   4 Sinus headache.

2 During a physical examination, the nurse is unable to feel the client's thyroid gland with palpation. The nurse should:
   1 Recognize that this is a normal finding.
   2 Auscultate the thyroid area.
   3 Percuss the anterior neck for thyroid span.
   4 Refer the client for follow-up with an endocrinologist.

3 A 24-year-old female client has a 2-day history of clear nasal drainage. Based on these data, which of the following is the most logical question for the nurse to ask?
   1 "Do you have a foul odor coming from your nose?"
   2 "Have you recently had nosebleeds?"
   3 "Do you snore when sleeping?"
   4 "Do you have allergies?"

4 A 32-year-old woman has a 4-day history of sore throat and difficulty swallowing. The nurse observes tonsils covered with yellow patches, and the tonsils are so large they fill the entire oropharynx and appear to be touching. The nurse documents:
   1 "Tonsils yellow and swollen."
   2 "Enlarged tonsils 4+ with yellow exudate."
   3 "Strep infection to tonsils with 3+ swelling."
   4 "1+ edema of tonsils with pus."

5 When obtaining a health history from a 52-year-old male client with a red lesion at the base of the tongue, the nurse specifically asks the patient about:
   1 Alcohol and tobacco use.
   2 The date of his last dental examination.
   3 The presence of dentures.
   4 A history of pyorrhea.

6 While talking with a client, the nurse suspects that he has hearing loss. Which of the following examination techniques is most accurate for assessing hearing loss?
   1 Whispered voice test.
   2 Rinne test.
   3 Weber's test.
   4 Audiometry test.

7 Which of the following data from the health history of a 42-year-old man should be further evaluated as a possible risk for hearing loss?
   1 "I watch TV in the evenings with my wife and children."
   2 "When I was younger, I wore an earring."
   3 "My primary hobby is carpentry work."
   4 "I have been an accountant for 16 years for an insurance agency."

8 The nurse examines a patient's auditory canal and tympanic membrane with an otoscope. Which of the following is considered an abnormal finding?
   1 The presence of cerumen.
   2 A yellow or amber color to the tympanic membrane.
   3 The presence of a cone of light.
   4 A shiny, translucent tympanic membrane.

9 During the history the client indicates that her eyes have been red and itching. Which additional question will the nurse ask?
   1 "Have you ever had a detached retina?"
   2 "Have you had the pressure in your eyes checked?"
   3 "Do you have seasonal allergies?"
   4 "Do you also have double vision?"

10 How does the nurse assess a client's consensual reaction?
   1 By touching the cornea with a small piece of sterile cotton and observing the change in the pupil size.
   2 By observing the client's pupil size when she or he looks at an object 2 to 3 feet away and then looks at an object 6 to 8 inches away.
   3 By shining a light into the client's right eye and observing the pupillary reaction of the left eye.
   4 By covering one eye with a card and observing the pupillary reaction when the card is removed.

11 What are the characteristics of lymph nodes in clients who have an acute infection?
   1 The lymph nodes are enlarged and tender.
   2 The lymph nodes are round, rubbery, and mobile.
   3 The lymph nodes are hard, fixed, and painless.
   4 The lymph nodes are soft, mobile, and painless.

12 Which of the following is the technique for palpating lymph nodes?
   1 Apply firm pressure over the nodes with the pads of the fingers.
   2 Apply gentle pressure over the nodes with the tips of the fingers.
   3 Apply firm pressure anterior to the nodes with the tips of the fingers.
   4 Apply gentle pressure over the nodes with the pads of the fingers.

SAMPLE DOCUMENTATION

Review the data obtained during an interview and examination by the nurse below.

A 62-year-old man has as the chief complaint vision changes and headaches. He states, "I can't see as well as I used to." Based on the conversation, the nurse notes that he seems to hear well. His last eye examination was 3 years ago. Using the Snellen's chart, the nurse determines that his visual acuity is 20/40 in the right eye, 20/40 in the left eye, and 20/40 with both eyes together. He is 6 feet 4 inches (188 cm) tall and weighs 200 lb (90.9 kg). His facial features are symmetric. He does not have any eye pain, discharge, watering from eyes, excessive blinking, redness or swelling of eyes, or trauma to eyes. His eyebrows, eyelids, and eyelashes are evenly distributed. His visual fields are equal to the nurse's. Both of his pupils are round and they react to light and ac-

62 y/o ♂ CC: "I can't see as well as I used to." PMH of MI, HTN, and arthritis. Medication: aspirin, lisinopril, Indocin.

SUBJECTIVE DATA

C/O blurred vision last 12 mo. Last eye exam 3 yr ago. Ø eye pain, discharge, watering, excessive blinking, redness, or edema. Denies trauma to eye. Reports concern about seeing well enough to drive. Widower, lives alone.

OBJECTIVE DATA

General survey: T 98.6° F (37° C), BP 160/84, HR 78/min, RR 16/min. Ht 6 feet 4 inches (188 cm), wt 200 lb (90.9 kg). Facial structures symmetric.

Eyes: Visual acuity—Right eye 20/40, Left eye 20/40, Both eyes 20/40. Brows, lids, lashes evenly distributed. EOM intact s̄ lid lag or nystagmus. Visual fields—to examiner. Conjunctiva pink s̄ discharge, PERRLA. Ø red reflex d/t opacity of lens.

Ears: Hearing intact, no deformities or lesions noted. Otoscope evaluation deferred.

Nose/Mouth: All mucous membranes in oral cavity and pharynx pink, moist; no lesions noted. Teeth intact, gums tight at base. No nasal discharge noted.

commodation. His conjunctivae appear pink without discharge. His extraocular muscles are intact with no lid lag or nystagmus. The nurse is unable to assess red reflex or perform ophthalmic examination because of opacities of lens. Gums are tight around the teeth; no missing or broken teeth noted. No nasal discharge is noted, the mucous membranes in his oral cavity are pink, moist, and without lesions. His temperature is 98.6° F (37° C), blood pressure is 160/84, heart rate is 78 beats per minute, and respiratory rate is 16 breaths per minute. The client relates that he is worried that his vision will deteriorate to the point where he is unable to drive. He is a widower and lives alone. This client takes lisinopril for hypertension, indomethacin (Indocin) for arthritis, and aspirin for his heart. He had a myocardial infarction 10 years ago.

On the previous page, note how the nurse documented these same data.

CASE STUDY

T. N. is a 25-year-old Native American (Navajo) female who was brought to the clinic by her sister. The following data are collected by the nurse during an interview and assessment.

Interview Data

The client tells the nurse, "My ear is hurting very badly and I also am hot." She adds, "I wanted to go to the clinic yesterday, but my grandmother told me I shouldn't." T. N. tells the nurse, "I have been treated many times for this problem over the last several years by the medicine man. Last night I had drainage from my ears. Grandmother told me this was a sign that the illness was being chased from my body. I did not know what it was, but I felt scared."

Examination Data

- *General survey:* Healthy appearing adult female. Temperature: 101.8° F (38.8° C).
- *External ear examination:* Typical position of ears bilaterally. Left ear pinna red. Dried purulent drainage noted on left external ear and in left external canal. Grimaces when left ear is touched. Right ear unremarkable.
- *Internal canal and tympanic membrane:* Dried drainage noted in left ear canal. TM perforated. Right ear unremarkable.
- *Hearing examination:* Whisper test in right ear 80%; whisper test in left ear 0%.

Clinical Reasoning

1. What data deviate from normal findings, suggesting a need for further investigation?
2. What additional information should the nurse ask or assess for?
3. Based on the data, what risk factors for hearing loss does T. N. have?
4. What nursing diagnoses or collaborative problems should be considered for this situation?

INTERACTIVE ACTIVITIES

Open the interactive student CD-ROM, click on Chapter 11, and choose from the following activities on the menu bar:

- **Multiple Choice Challenge.** Click on the best answer for each question. You will be given immediate feedback, rationale for incorrect answers, and a total score. Good luck!

- **Risk Factors.** Review this patient's history and identify risk factors. Complete your assessment by deciding which risks are modifiable and which are nonmodifiable. You only get one shot, so choose carefully!

- **The Name Game.** Identify each of the anatomic parts of the ear figure shown. Watch out where you place your answer—it won't stick if it's in the wrong place!

- **A Day in the Clinic.** Complete an examination by choosing a technique and an examination area on this client. You'll be able to collect data, document, and compare your answers with those of the experts. Everything you need for a successful assessment is at your fingertips!

- **Printable Lab Guide.** Locate the Lab Guide for Chapter 11, and print and use it (as many times as needed) to help you apply your assessment skills. These guides may also be filled in electronically and then saved and e-mailed to your instructor!

- **Quick Challenge.** Use this critical thinking exercise to assess your skills through case study-style questions, then compare with expert answers!

- **Core Examination Skills Checklists.** Make sure you've got frequently-used exam skills down pat! Use these checklists to help cover all the bases for your examination.

CHAPTER 12

Lungs and Respiratory System

ANATOMY & PHYSIOLOGY

The primary purpose of the respiratory system is to supply oxygen to cells and remove carbon dioxide using the processes of ventilation and diffusion. Ventilation is the process of moving gases in and out of the lungs by inspiration and expiration. Diffusion is the process by which oxygen and carbon dioxide move from areas of high concentration to areas of lower concentration. For example, after inspiration the concentration of oxygen is higher in the alveoli than it is in pulmonary capillaries, causing oxygen to move or diffuse across the alveolar-capillary membrane, where it is carried by erythrocytes to cells. At the cellular level oxygen diffuses into the cells and carbon dioxide diffuses from the cells into the capillaries, where it is carried by erythrocytes to alveoli. Carbon dioxide diffuses from the pulmonary capillaries to the alveoli and is exhaled. The cardiovascular system provides transportation of oxygen and carbon dioxide between alveoli and cells.

STRUCTURES WITHIN THE THORAX

There are three main structures within the thorax or chest: the mediastinum and the right and left pleural cavities. The mediastinum is positioned in the middle of the chest. Within it lie the heart, the arch of aorta, the superior vena cava, the lower esophagus, and the lower part of the trachea. The lungs are contained within the pleural cavities. These cavities are lined with two types of serous membranes: the parietal and visceral pleurae. The chest wall and diaphragm are protected by the parietal pleura, and the lungs are protected by the visceral pleura. A small amount of fluid lubricates the space between the pleurae to reduce friction as the lungs move during inspiration and expiration (Fig. 12-1). The right lung has three lobes and the left has two. Each lobe has a major, oblique fissure dividing the upper and lower portions; however, the right lung has a lesser horizontal fissure dividing the upper lung into upper and middle lobes (Fig. 12-2). Each lung extends anteriorly about 1.5 inches (4 cm) above the first rib into the base of the neck in adults. Posteriorly, the lungs' apices rise to about the level of T1 (first thoracic vertebra), whereas the lower borders, on deep inspiration, expand down to about T12 and, on expiration, rise to about T9 (Fig. 12-3).

EXTERNAL THORAX

A thoracic cage consisting of 12 thoracic vertebrae, 12 pairs of ribs, and the sternum protects most of the respiratory system. All the ribs are connected to the thoracic vertebrae posteriorly. The first seven ribs are also connected to the sternum by the costal cartilages. The costal cartilages of the eighth to tenth ribs are connected immediately superior to the ribs. The eleventh and twelfth ribs are unattached anteriorly; hence their name, the "floating ribs." The tips of the eleventh ribs are located in the lateral thorax, and those of the twelfth ribs are located in the posterior thorax (see Fig. 12-3).

The adult sternum is about 7 inches (17 cm) long and has three components: the manubrium, the body, and the xiphoid

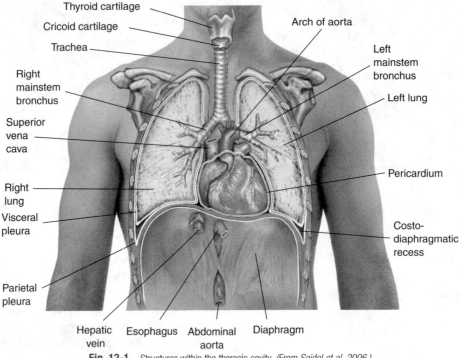

Fig. 12-1   Structures within the thoracic cavity. *(From Seidel et al, 2006.)*

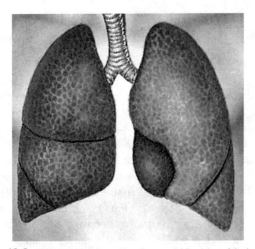

Fig. 12-2   Right and left lung. Note fissures dividing lobes of the lungs.

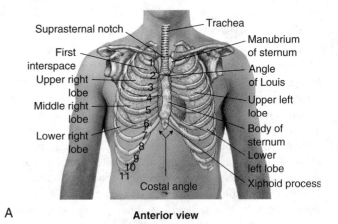

A   **Anterior view**

process. The manubrium and the body of the sternum articulate with the first seven ribs; the manubrium also supports the clavicle. The intercostal space (ICS) is the area between the ribs. The ICS is named according to the rib immediately above it. Thus the first ICS is located between the first and second ribs (see Fig. 12-3, *A*).

MECHANICS OF BREATHING

The diaphragm and the intercostal muscles are the primary muscles of inspiration. During inspiration, the diaphragm contracts and pushes the abdominal contents down while the intercostal muscles help to push the chest wall outward. These combined efforts decrease the intrathoracic pressure, which creates a negative pressure within the lungs compared with the pressure outside the lungs. This pressure difference

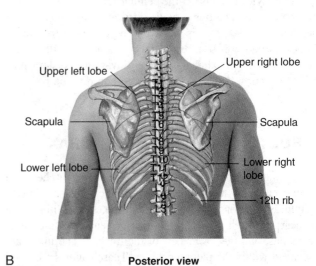

B   **Posterior view**

Fig. 12-3   Thorax and underlying structures. A, Anterior view. **B,** Posterior view.

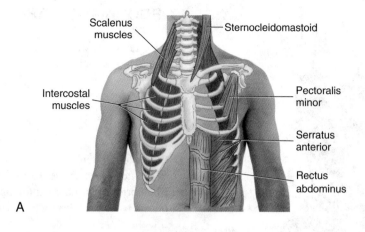

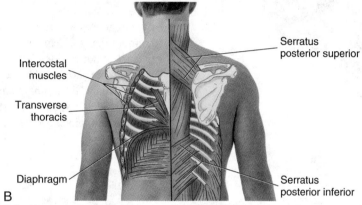

Fig. 12-4 **Muscles involved in ventilation. A,** Anterior view. **B,** Posterior view. *(From Seidel et al, 2006.)*

causes the lungs to fill with air. During expiration the muscles relax, expelling the air as the intrathoracic pressure rises. Accessory muscles that may contribute to respiratory effort include the sternocleidomastoid, scalenus, pectoralis minor, serratus anterior, and rectus abdominis muscles anteriorly and the serratus posterior superior, transverse thoracic, and serratus posterior inferior muscles posteriorly (Fig. 12-4).

During inspiration air is drawn in through the mouth or nose and passes through the pharynx and the larynx to reach the trachea, a flexible tube approximately 4 inches (10 cm) long in the adult. These structures—the nose, pharynx, lar-

ynx, and intrathoracic trachea—make up the upper airway (Fig. 12-5), which has three functions in respiration: to conduct air to the lower airway; to protect the lower airway from foreign matter; and to warm, filter, and humidify inspired air.

The lower airway consists of the trachea, the right and left main stem bronchi, the segmental and subsegmental bronchi, and the terminal bronchioles (Fig. 12-6). The trachea splits into a left and right main stem bronchus at about the level of T4 and T5. The right bronchus is shorter, wider, and more vertical than the left bronchus.

The bronchi are further subdivided into increasingly smaller bronchioles. Each bronchiole opens into an alveolar duct and terminates in multiple alveoli, where gas exchanges occur (Fig. 12-7).

Fig. 12-5 Structures of the upper airway.

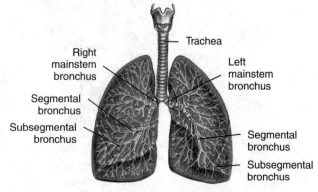

Fig. 12-6 Structures of the lower airway.

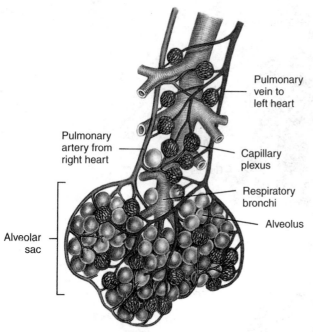

Fig. 12-7 Alveolar sac.

TOPOGRAPHIC MARKERS

Surface landmarks are helpful in locating underlying structures and in describing the exact location of physical findings (Fig. 12-8).

Anterior Chest Wall

- Nipples
- Suprasternal notch: the depression at the ventral aspect of the neck, just above the manubrium
- Manubriosternal junction (angle of Louis): the junction between the manubrium and sternum; useful for rib identification
- Midsternal line: imaginary vertical line through the middle of the sternum
- Costal angle: intersection of the costal margins, usually no more than 90 degrees
- Clavicles: bones extending out both sides of the manubrium to the shoulder; they cover the first ribs
- Midclavicular lines: imaginary vertical lines on the right and left sides of the chest that are "drawn" through the clavicle midpoints, parallel to the midsternal line

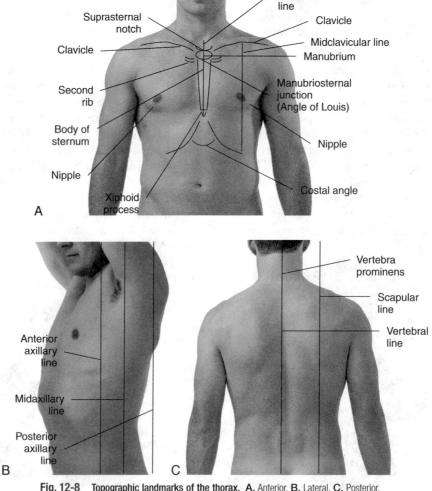

Fig. 12-8 Topographic landmarks of the thorax. **A,** Anterior. **B,** Lateral. **C,** Posterior.

Lateral Chest Wall

- Anterior axillary lines: imaginary vertical lines on the right and left sides of the chest "drawn" from anterior axillary folds through the anterolateral chest, parallel to the midsternal line
- Posterior axillary lines: imaginary vertical lines on the right and left sides of the chest "drawn" from the posterior axillary folds along the posterolateral thoracic wall with abducted lateral arm
- Midaxillary lines: imaginary vertical lines on the right and left sides of the chest "drawn" from axillary apices; midway between and parallel to the anterior and posterior axillary lines

Posterior Chest Wall

- Vertebra prominens: spinous process of C7; visible and palpable with the head bent forward
- Vertebral line: imaginary vertical line "drawn" along the posterior vertebral spinous processes
- Scapular lines: imaginary vertical lines on the right and left sides of the chest "drawn" parallel to the midspinal line; they pass through inferior angles of the scapulae in the upright client with arms at sides

---

LINK TO CONCEPTS *Oxygenation*

The featured concept for this chapter is *Oxygenation.* This concept represents mechanisms that facilitate and impair oxygenation to and from tissues. Several concepts featured in this textbook have an interrelationship with this concept. Because adequate perfusion is necessary to deliver oxygenated blood to tissues and remove metabolic wastes from tissues, this interrelationship is foundational to all others. Intracranial regulation supports respiratory regulation, and adequate oxygenation is needed to support intracranial function. Metabolism, motion, tissue integrity, sleep, and nutrition all require adequate oxygenation for optimal function. These interrelationships are depicted in the model below.

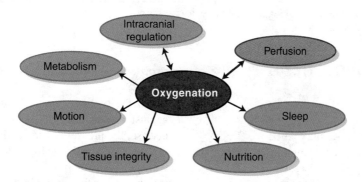

Concept Model: Oxygenation

This model shows the interrelationship of concepts associated with oxygenation. As an example, an individual who has chronic lung disease may have adequate blood perfusion, but poor oxygenation of blood resulting in hypoxia. Low oxygen limits motion (because of activity intolerance), places the individual at risk for nutritional deficits (because of the effects of low oxygen on appetite and food consumption), and potentially impacts the ability to have restful sleep. Having an understanding of the interrelationship of these concepts helps the nurse recognize risk factors and thus increases awareness when conducting a health assessment.

HEALTH HISTORY

RISK FACTORS   *Lung Cancer*

As you conduct a health history related to the respiratory system, it is important to consider common risk factors for lung cancer and follow up with additional questions should risk factors arise.

- *Tobacco smoking:* Smoking is the most important risk factor for lung cancer. (M)
- *Secondhand smoke* (Smoke from other people's cigarette) causes lung cancer in people and animals, (M)
- *Asbestos:* People who work with asbestos are about seven times more likely to die of lung cancer. (M)
- *Environmental exposure in the workplace:* Carcinogens in the workplace include radioactive ores such as radon, arsenic, uranium, coal products, and chemicals such as vinyl chloride, nickel chromates, mustard gas, and chloromethyl ethers. (M)
- *Marijuana:* Marijuana contains more tar than cigarettes and is usually inhaled deeply and the smoke is held in the lungs for a longer time. (M)
- *Personal and family history:* People who have lung cancer are at a higher risk of developing another lung cancer. Brothers, sisters, and children of people who have lung cancer have a slightly higher risk of lung cancer themselves. However, it is difficult so say how much of the excess risk is due to genetic factors versus environmental tobacco smoke.
- *Gender:* Women's lungs may have a genetic predisposition to developing cancer when they are exposed to tobacco smoke.
- *Air pollution:* In some cities air pollution may slightly increase the risk for lung cancer; however, this risk is far less than that caused by smoking. (M)

Data from *www.cdc.gov/cancer/lung,* 2008; *www.cancer.org,* 2008.
M = modifiable risk factor.

GENERAL HEALTH HISTORY

Present Health Status

Do you have any chronic illnesses?
Many chronic illnesses can cause symptoms affecting the respiratory system, including heart disease or renal disease, which may cause pulmonary edema.

Do you have allergies? If so, what are you allergic to? Describe what your symptoms are like. How frequently do you have these symptoms?
The severity of allergies can range from mild seasonal allergies to an anaphylactic allergic reaction. Respiratory symptoms can range from runny nose, nasal congestion, and cough to wheezes and dyspnea. An increased frequency may indicate the onset of new allergies or ineffective therapy for respiratory disease.

Do you have difficulty breathing during your daily activities? If so, describe the difficulty.
Individuals who have no difficulty breathing until they are active may have pulmonary or heart disease that limits the availability of oxygen needed during exertion.

Do you have difficulty breathing when you are sleeping? If so, in what position do you sleep? Do you prop yourself up with pillows to make your breathing easier?
When the body is lying flat, the abdominal contents push against the diaphragm. When individuals have pulmonary disease, the pressure of the abdominal content may increase the work of breathing. Individuals may prop themselves up with pillows to improve their ease of breathing while sleep, which moves the abdominal contents away from the diaphragm.

Are you currently taking any oral medications for a respiratory disorder? If so, what medications are you taking and how effective have they been?
Medications taken to treat respiratory disorders and their effectiveness need to be documented.

Do you use an inhaler? If yes, what medication is in the inhaler, what is the purpose of the medication, and how often do you use it?
Individuals with asthma may use inhalers to prevent symptoms, treat bronchial inflammation, and dilate bronchi. It is important to know how frequently symptoms occur that require use of an inhaler and if the client knows the purpose of each inhaler.

Do you use oxygen at home? If yes, describe what equipment you use, as well as how much oxygen you

use and how often you use it. Does the oxygen relieve your symptoms?

Many individuals with chronic pulmonary disease use oxygen at home. The frequency, amount, and effect help determine the adequacy of this therapy.

Do you smoke, or have you been a smoker in the past? If yes, what do (did) you smoke (cigarettes, cigar, pipe)? How long have you smoked (did you smoke)? How often do you (did you) smoke? Have you ever tried to quit smoking? If yes, describe. What helped you quit? Why do you think your attempt was unsuccessful?

These questions determine the client's smoking history and if there is an interest in quitting. If the client is or has been a smoker, determine the number of pack-years the client has smoked (Box 12-1).

Past Medical History

Have you ever had any problems with your lungs? If yes, describe.

Asking this question may encourage clients to describe symptoms they may be having; these symptoms may or may not have been diagnosed and treated.

Have you been diagnosed with a respiratory disease such as asthma, bronchitis, bronchiectasis, emphysema, cystic fibrosis, lung cancer, tuberculosis, or pneumonia? If yes, please describe.

Background information regarding respiratory problems tells what types of problems the client is likely to experience and what clinical findings to anticipate.

Have you ever had an injury to your chest? Surgery to your chest? If yes, describe.

The incidence of injury or surgery may provide additional information about a possible respiratory or lung problem.

Family History

Is there a family history of lung disease? Cancer? Tuberculosis? Cystic fibrosis? Emphysema? Asthma? If yes, which family member and what is the condition?

Family history may be used to determine risk for the client.

BOX 12-1	**RECORDING TOBACCO USE**

Cigarette use is documented by *pack-years*. A pack-year is the number of years a client has smoked times the number of packs of cigarettes smoked each day. If a client tells you that he or she smoked one-half pack of cigarettes a day for 40 years, it would be recorded as a 20 pack-year smoking history.

Use of pipes, cigars, marijuana, chewing tobacco, or snuff is usually recorded in the amount used daily.

Home Environment

Are there environmental conditions that may affect your breathing at home? If yes, what are they and how do they affect your breathing? Common things to consider include the following:

- Air pollution (near factory, on a busy street, new construction in area)
- Possible allergens in home, such as pets
- Type of heating or air conditioning, including filtering system, humidification, and ventilation
- Hobbies: woodworking, plants, metal work
- Exposure to the smoke of others in your home

A number of respiratory irritants found in or near the home may cause temporary or permanent lung damage. Environmental tobacco smoke (also known as secondhand smoke) has been shown to affect nonsmokers (*www.epa.gov/smokefree/index/html,* 2007).

Occupational Environment

Where do you work? In a factory? Outdoors? In a mine? In a chemical plant? On a farm? In heavy traffic? Are you frequently exposed to dust? Vapors? Chemicals? Paint fumes? Irritants such as asbestos? Known allergens?

The client may be exposed to respiratory irritants in the workplace. These irritants may be risk factors for pulmonary diseases. The client may or may not be aware of the presence of irritants.

If you are exposed to respiratory irritants, do you wear a mask or a respirator mask? Does your work area have a special ventilatory system to clear out pollutants? Do you wear a monitor to evaluate exposure? Do you have periodic health examinations, pulmonary function tests, or x-ray examinations?

Clients may not be able to alter the presence of environmental irritants that are in the work environment. Instead, they must use protective equipment such as masks, respirators, or ventilation hoods to reduce the amount of exposure to respiratory irritants. Regulatory agencies such as the Occupational Safety and Health Administration (OSHA) have guidelines and regulations to reduce the amount of occupational exposure to respiratory irritants (*www.osha.gov,* respiratory protection, 2007).

Travel

Have you recently traveled to foreign countries or areas of the United States where you may have been exposed to uncommon respiratory diseases (e.g., histoplasmosis in the Southeast and Midwest; schistosomiasis or sudden acute respiratory syndrome [SARS] in Southwest Asia, the Caribbean, and Asia)?

Travel to other areas of the country or world may expose clients to infections they have little or no resistance to, increasing their susceptibility to infection.

PROBLEM-BASED HISTORY

Commonly reported problems related to the lungs are cough, shortness of breath, and chest pain with breathing. As with symptoms in all areas of health assessment, a symptom analysis is completed, which includes the location, quality, quantity, chronology, setting, associated manifestations, and alleviating and aggravating factors (see Box 3-3 in Chapter 3).

Cough

When did you first notice the cough? Is the cough constant, or does it come and go? Has the cough changed since you first noticed it?

A cough can be acute (sudden onset and usually lasting less than 3 weeks) or chronic (lasting longer than 3 weeks). Common causes of acute cough are viral infections, allergic rhinitis, acute asthma, acute bacterial sinusitis, or environmental irritants. Chronic cough is commonly caused by postnasal drip, gastroesophageal reflux disease (GERD), asthma, chronic bronchitis, bronchiectasis, cystic fibrosis, chronic interstitial lung disease, smoking (smoker's cough), and sarcoidosis (Spiro, 2003).

Describe your cough. Is it dry? Productive? Hacking? Hoarse?

A description of the cough may provide clues to the cause. For example, viral pneumonia causes a dry cough whereas bacterial pneumonia causes a productive cough.

How often are you coughing up sputum (all of the time or just periodically)? How much sputum do you cough up?

The frequency of sputum production and the time of day most sputum is produced should be explored. Increased sputum in the morning implies an accumulation of sputum during the night and is common with bronchitis. Sputum production with a change in position is suggestive of lung abscess and bronchiectasis. The amount of sputum production can vary from a few teaspoons to a copious amount (a pint or more).

What is the color of the sputum?

The appearance of the sputum is always important to document. Some conditions have characteristic sputum production, such as the following: white or clear sputum may occur with colds, viral infections, or bronchitis; yellow or green sputum may occur with bacterial infections; black sputum may occur with smoke or coal dust inhalation; or rust-colored sputum may occur with tuberculosis or pneumococcal pneumonia. *Hemoptysis* is the expectoration of sputum containing blood. It may vary in severity from slight streaking of blood to frank bleeding.

What is the consistency of the sputum (thick, thin, frothy)?

The consistency of sputum may be described as thin, thick, a gelatin consistency, sticky, or frothy. Pink, frothy sputum

with dyspnea is associated with pulmonary edema. Thick sputum is commonly associated with cystic fibrosis.

Have you noticed if the sputum has an odor?

Foul-smelling (fetid) sputum is typically associated with bacterial pneumonia, lung abscess, or bronchiectasis.

Have you noticed any other symptoms along with the cough, such as shortness of breath, chest pain or tightness with breathing, fever, stuffy nose, noisy respiration, hoarseness, or gagging? Does the cough tire you out? Does it keep you awake at night?

A cough may be a symptom of pulmonary problems, or it may exist in conjunction with other problems. Associated signs and symptoms are important factors to assess when trying to determine the underlying cause of the cough. For example, a cough associated with a fever, shortness of breath, and noisy breath sounds may be indicative of a lung infection, whereas tightness of the chest associated with shortness of breath and a nonproductive cough is more likely to be associated with a problem such as asthma.

Have you done anything to treat the cough yourself such as medications, fluids, or a vaporizer? Have these measures been effective?

Determining what has been used to relieve signs and symptoms may help in understanding the problem and may guide current treatment strategies.

Shortness of Breath

How long have you had shortness of breath? Are you short of breath all the time, or does it come and go?

Shortness of breath, or dyspnea, occurs when breathing becomes difficult. Some conditions, such as pneumonia, may cause sudden onset of shortness of breath; other conditions, such as chronic heart failure, may be associated with a more gradual onset. Some clients may experience shortness of breath at intervals over a period of time. When taking a history from a client who has dyspnea, notice how many words the client can say in between breaths. See Box 12-2 for information about how to document this finding.

How would you describe your shortness of breath? Is it harder to inhale or exhale, or are both equally affected? Do the symptoms interfere with your activities?

Knowing the client's perception of the severity and the extent of disablement, if any, helps understand the extent to which the dyspnea is interfering with the client's daily activities.

BOX 12-2 **CLINICAL NOTES**

An indirect way of assessing the severity of dyspnea is to count the words the client can say between breaths. Normally a person can say 10 to 14 words before taking a breath. A client who has severe dyspnea may take a breath after every third word. This is documented as "three-word dyspnea."

Does anything seem to trigger these episodes or make the shortness of breath worse, such as activity or environmental factors? If this occurs at night, in what position do you sleep? How many pillows do you use to prop behind you? Do you sleep in a recliner? Does changing your position affect the problem?

Causative factors for the dyspnea should be determined. If dyspnea is brought on by activity, find out how much exercise brings on the episode (e.g., number of steps climbed, blocks walked). Positions or other conditions may also initiate dyspnea. *Orthopnea* is difficulty breathing when the individual is lying down. Clients may describe using several pillows to prop themselves up in bed so that they can sleep. The term *three-pillow orthopnea* means the client needs to prop up with three pillows to relieve the dyspnea. *Paroxysmal nocturnal dyspnea* is shortness of breath that awakens the individual in the middle of the night, usually in a panic with the feeling of suffocation. Asthma attacks may be triggered by a specific allergen, which may be external or extrinsic, such as a pet, or internal or intrinsic, such as stress or emotions.

Have you noticed any other problems when you are short of breath? Cough? Chest pain? Break out in a sweat? Swelling of the feet, ankles, or legs?

Shortness of breath may be a problem of the respiratory system, or it may be a symptom associated with the cardiovascular system, such as a severe heart murmur or heart failure that may produce peripheral edema.

When these episodes of shortness of breath occur, what do you do to relieve the symptoms?

Assess the efficacy of treatment and any progression the client has noted. Determining what has been used successfully or unsuccessfully helps in understanding the problem and may guide current treatment strategies.

Chest Pain with Breathing

How long have you had pain in your chest when you breathe? When did this start? Did it start suddenly or gradually? Where do you feel the pain? Does the pain radiate to other areas, such as the neck or arms?

Chest pain caused by respiratory disease is usually associated with chest wall or parietal pleura (e.g., pneumonia). A sharp, abrupt pain associated with deep breathing may be an indication of pleural lining irritation, also called pleuretic chest pain.

What does the pain feel like (viselike, tight, sharp, burning)? On a scale of 0 to 10, how would you rate the intensity of the pain? Is the pain constant, or does it come and go?

Even though the pain is associated with breathing, it is important to evaluate the possibility of the pain being related to a cardiovascular problem.

HEALTH PROMOTION *Tobacco Use*

Cigarette smoking is the single most preventable cause of death and disease in the United States. The majority of all cancers of the lung, trachea, bronchus, larynx, pharynx, oral cavity, and esophagus are caused by tobacco products. Smoking is a leading risk factor for cardiovascular diseases, including myocardial infarction, coronary artery disease, stroke, and peripheral vascular disease. Smoking is also an important risk factor for lung disease, including chronic obstructive pulmonary disease. Environmental smoke (secondhand smoke) affects the health of nonsmokers, particularly children. There is no safe tobacco alternative to cigarettes.

Goals and Objectives—*Healthy People 2010*
Tobacco use is one of the 10 leading health indicators identified by *Healthy People 2010*. The *Healthy People 2010* goal related to tobacco use is to reduce illness, disability, and death related to tobacco use and exposure to secondhand smoke. There are 21 specific objectives, some of which include the following: reduce tobacco use; reduce initiation of tobacco use; increase the average age of first use of tobacco; increase smoking cessation attempts and smoking cessation during pregnancy; reduce the number of children and nonsmokers who are regularly exposed to secondhand smoke; increase smoke-free and tobacco-free environments; reduce the illegal sales rate to minors; eliminate tobacco advertising and promotions that influence adolescents and young adults; reduce the toxicity of tobacco products by establishing a regulatory structure to monitor toxicity; and increase the average federal and state tax on tobacco products.

Recommendations to Reduce Risk (Primary Prevention)
Note: All major health care organizations recommend routine counseling for smoking cessation and recommend against the use of smokeless tobacco.

U.S. Preventive Services Task Force
- Recommend assessment of tobacco use and nicotine dependence for all adolescent and adult clients.
- Counseling for tobacco cessation is recommended on a regular basis for all individuals who use tobacco products. Strategies that can increase effectiveness of counseling include direct face-to-face advice; reinforcement; self-help materials; and community programs for additional help in quitting.
- Counseling regarding the potentially harmful effects of smoking on fetal and child health is recommended for all pregnant women and parents of children.
- The optimal frequency of counseling has not been determined.

Recommendations for Treatment (Tertiary Prevention)
U.S. Preventive Services Task Force
Recommends prescription of nicotine patches or gum as adjunct for selected clients. It is unclear if clonidine is an effective adjunct to tobacco cessation counseling.

Data from US Department of Health and Human Services: Cancer. In *Healthy People 2010: understanding and improving health*, ed 2, Washington, DC, 2000, US Government Printing Office (available at *www.healthypeople.gov*); US Preventive Services Task Force: *Guide to clinical preventive services*, ed 2, 1996 (available at *www.ahrq.gov*).

When it started, was the pain associated with an injury to your ribs or a respiratory infection? Is the pain worse with deep inspiration? Does the pain interfere with your getting enough air?

Injured ribs cause pain when the individual breathes; as a result, the client is likely to have shallow breathing, which may lead to respiratory congestion.

Is there anything that seems to make the pain worse, such as movement or coughing?

Assess for aggravating factors.

Have you done anything to treat the pain, such as applying heat or using pain medication? Have any measures been effective?

Assess self-care behaviors and successful relief of pain.

EXAMINATION

ROUTINE TECHNIQUES

- INSPECT client for general appearance, posture, and breathing effort.
- OBSERVE respirations for rate and quality, ☐ breathing pattern, and chest expansion.
- INSPECT the client's nails, skin, and lips.
- INSPECT the thorax. ☐
- AUSCULTATE the thorax. ☐

SPECIAL CIRCUMSTANCES OR ADVANCED PRACTICE

- PALPATE the trachea.
- PALPATE the chest and thoracic muscles.
- PALPATE the chest wall for expansion

- PALPATE the thoracic wall for vocal (tactile) fremitus. ★
- PERCUSS the thorax for tone. ★
- PERCUSS the thorax for diaphragmatic (respiratory) ★ excursion.
- AUSCULTATE the thorax for vocal sounds (vocal ★ resonance).

EQUIPMENT NEEDED
Stethoscope • Ruler and tape measure • Marking pen to mark diaphragmatic excursion

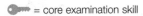 = core examination skill   ★ = advanced practice

PROCEDURES AND TECHNIQUES WITH NORMAL FINDINGS

ABNORMAL FINDINGS

ROUTINE TECHNIQUES

☐ **INSPECT the client for general appearance, posture, and breathing effort.**

The client's general appearance and posture should be relaxed. The posture should be upright. Breathing should be effortless and at a rate that is appropriate for the client's age (Fig. 12-9).

An appearance of apprehension with restlessness, nasal flaring, supraclavicular or intercostal retractions or bulging with expiration, and use of accessory muscles during breathing are all signs of respiratory distress. *Paradoxical chest wall movement* may occur after chest trauma when the chest wall moves in on inspiration and out on expiration. *Tripod position* (leaning forward with the arms braced against the knees, against a chair, or against a bed) also suggests respiratory distress. Tripod position enhances accessory muscle use (Fig. 12-10).

PROCEDURES AND TECHNIQUES WITH NORMAL FINDINGS	**ABNORMAL FINDINGS**

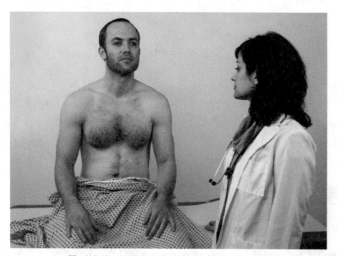

Fig. 12-9   Observing the client for breathing effort.

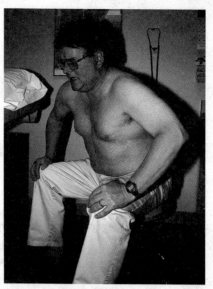

Fig. 12-10   Tripod position.

🔑 **OBSERVE respirations for rate and quality, breathing pattern, and chest expansion.**

Note the respiratory rate. In the adult, passive breathing should occur at a rate of 12 to 20 breaths per minute (this range in respiratory rate is referred to as *eupnea*). The pattern of breathing should be smooth, with an even respiratory depth (Fig. 12-11). The chest wall should symmetrically rise and expand and then relax without effort. A normal variation is abdominal breathing pattern. Men tend to use abdominal breathing (or diaphragmatic breathing) whereas women tend to use more thoracic breathing.

A sigh is another normal variation observed with breathing. It is an occasional interspersed deep breath associated with a normal breathing pattern (Fig. 12-12).

Abnormal breathing patterns are described in Fig. 12-13.

Chest retraction appears when intercostal muscles are drawn inward between the ribs and indicates airway obstruction that may occur during an asthma attack or pneumonia.

Frequent sighing is considered an abnormal finding and may indicate fatigue or anxiety.

Normal   〜〜〜〜〜〜〜

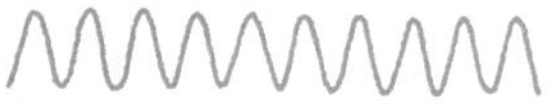

Fig. 12-11   Normal breathing pattern.

Sighing   〜〜〜〜〜〜〜

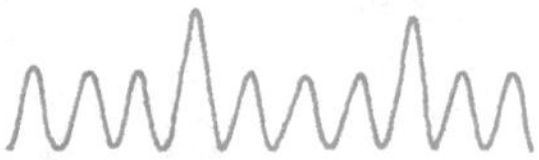

Fig. 12-12   Sigh.

🔑 = core examination skill

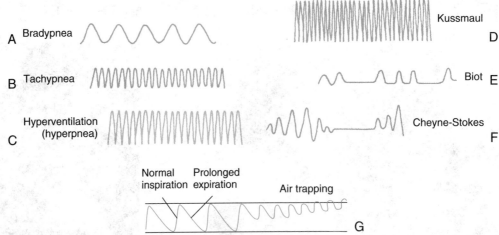

Fig. 12-13   Abnormal breathing patterns. A, *Bradypnea* is a respiratory rate less than 12 breaths per minute. The rate and depth remain smooth and even. **B,** *Tachypnea* is a respiratory rate greater than 20 breaths per minute. The rate and depth remain smooth and even. Tachypnea can be caused by a number of factors, including fever, fear, or activity. **C,** *Hyperventilation* is characterized by increased rate and depth of respiration. **D,** When hyperventilation occurs with ketoacidosis, it is very deep and laborious and is termed *Kussmaul* breathing. **E,** *Biot breathing pattern* is characterized by irregularly interspersed periods of apnea in a disorganized and irregular pattern, rate, or depth. It may be associated with persistent intracranial pressure, respiratory distress, or damage to the medulla. **F,** *Cheyne-Stokes* is characterized by intervals of apnea interspersed with a deep and rapid breathing pattern. This may be seen in clients with severe illness, brain damage, or drug overdose. **G,** *Air trapping* is an abnormal respiratory pattern frequently seen in clients with chronic obstructive pulmonary disease. It is characterized by rapid inspirations with prolonged, forced expirations. Air is not fully exhaled; thus it becomes trapped in the lungs, which eventually leads to a barrel chest. *(Adapted from Seidel et al, 2006.)*

PROCEDURES AND TECHNIQUES WITH NORMAL FINDINGS	ABNORMAL FINDINGS

INSPECT the client's nails, skin, and lips for color.

Skin tones vary among individuals; therefore the general color should be consistent with skin color for that individual. Specifically note the presence of cyanosis or pallor (see Chapters 10 and 13 for details). If there is any question about adequate oxygenation, measure the client's oxygen saturation level using pulse oximetry (see Chapter 4).

Cyanosis or pallor of the nails, skin, or lips may be a sign of inadequate oxygenation of tissues caused by an underlying respiratory or cardiovascular condition. Clubbing of the nails is associated with chronic hypoxia observed in clients with cystic fibrosis or chronic obstructive pulmonary disease (see Fig. 10-10 for finger clubbing).

POSTERIOR THORAX

Move behind the client who is seated on an exam table or on a bed with the back of the gown open (especially for women) or removed.

INSPECT the posterior thorax for shape and symmetry and muscle development.

The thorax should be symmetric. The ribs should slope down at about 45 degrees relative to the spine. Muscle development should be equal. The spinous processes should appear in a straight line. The scapulae should be bilaterally symmetric.

Asymmetry or unequal muscle development is abnormal. Skeletal deformities such as scoliosis or kyphosis may limit the expansion of the chest.

= core examination skill

PROCEDURES AND TECHNIQUES WITH NORMAL FINDINGS	ABNORMAL FINDINGS

AUSCULTATE the posterior and lateral thorax for breath sounds.

Procedure: Instruct the client to sit upright and breathe deeply and slowly through the mouth. Using the diaphragm of the stethoscope, auscultate the client's breath sounds in a systematic manner over the posterior and lateral chest walls (Fig. 12-14, *A* and *B*). Move from the apex to the base, listen during both inspiration and expiration, and compare one side with the other following the landmarks. (Fig. 12-15, *A* and *C*). When auscultating the lateral thorax, ask the client to move his or her arms away from the chest for better access. When thorax auscultation is performed in a hospital setting, the client may be supine rather than sitting up. The lateral and posterior thorax may be auscultated when the client turns to the side or transfers to a chair.

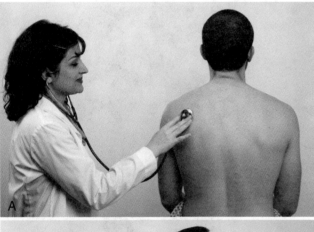

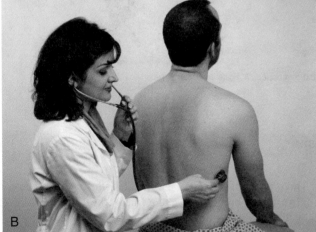

Fig. 12-14 **Auscultating the posterior and lateral chest. A,** Posterior thorax. **B,** Lateral thorax.

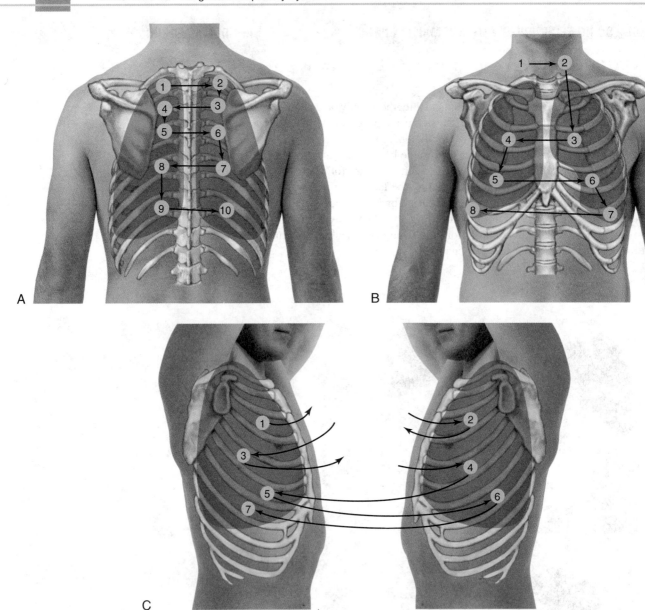

Fig. 12-15   Landmarks for chest auscultation and percussion. **A,** Posterior view. **B,** Anterior view. **C,** Lateral view. *(From Seidel et al, 2006.)*

PROCEDURES AND TECHNIQUES WITH NORMAL FINDINGS

Finding: Breath sounds should be clear to auscultation. Three types of breath sounds are considered normal in various parts of the thorax: vesicular, broncho-vesicular, and bronchial (Fig. 12-16, *B*, and Table 12-1). If an adventitious sound is heard, have the client cough; then repeat the auscultation to see if the sound has changed or disappeared (Box 12-3).

ABNORMAL FINDINGS

Normal breath sounds can be considered abnormal if heard in areas of the lungs where they are not expected. Bronchial breath sounds are abnormal if heard anywhere over the posterior or lateral thorax and may indicate consolidation of the lung, as may be found with pneumonia. (The sound heard will be loud and high pitched. It sounds as if the air source is just under the stethoscope.) Broncho-vesicular breath sounds should be considered abnormal when heard over the peripheral lung areas.

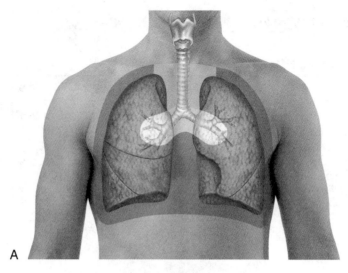

KEY:

■ Bronchovesicular over main bronchi

■ Vesicular over lesser bronchi, bronchioles, and lobes

■ Bronchial over trachea

Fig. 12-16 **Auscultatory sounds.** **A,** Anterior thorax. **B,** Posterior thorax.

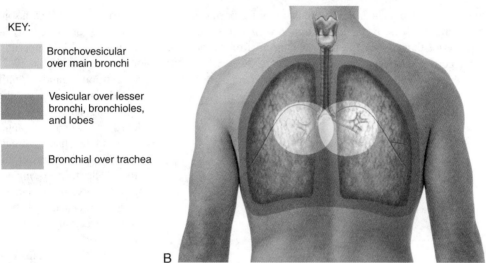

TABLE 12-1 *Characteristics of Breath Sounds*

	BRONCHIAL	BRONCHOVESICULAR	VESICULAR
Pitch	High	Moderate	Low
Intensity	Loud	Medium	Soft
Duration: inspiration and expiration	Insp < Exp 1:2	Insp = Exp 1:1	Insp > Exp 2.5:1
Expected location	Over trachea	First and second intercostal spaces at sternal border anteriorly; posteriorly at T4 medial to scapula	Peripheral lung fields
Abnormal location	Over peripheral lung fields	Over peripheral lung fields	Not applicable

PROCEDURES AND TECHNIQUES WITH NORMAL FINDINGS

ABNORMAL FINDINGS

BOX 12-3 **CLINICAL NOTES**

Before you decide that the client has an adventitious sound, remember that the following may also be causes of sound distortion:

- If you bump the stethoscope tubing against something or if the client touches the tubing, the sound will be distorted.
- If the client is cold and is shivering, the sound will be distorted.
- The stethoscope placed and unintentionally moved on a client's excess chest hair may give a false finding of crackles or pleural friction rub.
- Extraneous environmental noises such as the rustling of a paper gown or drape may sound like crackles or pleural friction rub.

Vesicular breath sounds should be heard over almost all of the posterior lung fields and all of the lateral surfaces. *Bronchovesicular breath sounds* are normally heard in the posterior thorax over the upper center area of the back on either side of the spine between the scapulae.

Adventitious breath sounds (crackles, wheezing, and rhonchi) are extraneous sounds that are superimposed on the breath sounds (Table 12-2). If you hear adventitious sounds, identify the type of sound, the location of the sound (i.e., right lung, left lung, or bilaterally; upper lobes or lower lobes; anterior or posterior) and the phase of breathing in which it is heard (i.e., inspiration or expiration). The term *respiratory stridor* is used to describe a harsh, high-pitched sound associated with breathing that is often caused by laryngeal or tracheal obstruction.

Diminished breath sounds may be heard in clients whose alveoli have been destroyed, which may occur in clients with emphysema. Diminished or absent breath sounds may be heard in clients with collapsed alveoli, which may occur in clients who have atelectasis or are having a severe asthma attack.

TABLE 12-2 *Characteristics of Adventitious Sounds*

ADVENTITIOUS SOUNDS	CHARACTERISTICS	CLINICAL EXAMPLES
Crackles (previously called *rales*) **Fine crackles** 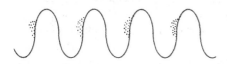	Fine, high-pitched crackling and popping noises (discontinuous sounds) heard during the end of inspiration. Not cleared by cough.	May be heard in pneumonia, heart failure, asthma, and restrictive pulmonary diseases.
Medium crackles 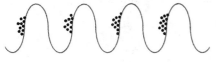	Medium-pitched, moist sound heard about halfway through inspiration. Not cleared by cough.	Same as above, but condition is worse.
Coarse crackles 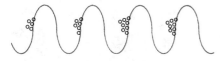	Low-pitched, bubbling or gurgling sounds that start early in inspiration and extend into the first part of expiration.	Same as above, but condition is worse or in terminally ill clients with diminished gag reflex. Also heard in pulmonary edema and pulmonary fibrosis.
Wheeze (also called *sibilant wheeze*) 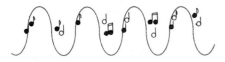	High-pitched, musical sound similar to a squeak. Heard more commonly during expiration, but may also be heard during inspiration. Occurs in small airways.	Heard in narrowed airway diseases such as asthma.
Rhonchi (also called *sonorous wheeze*) 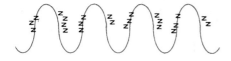	Low-pitched, coarse, loud, low snoring or moaning tone. Actually sounds like snoring. Heard primarily during expiration, but may also be heard during inspiration. Coughing may clear.	Heard in disorders causing obstruction of the trachea or bronchus, such as chronic bronchitis.
Pleural friction rub 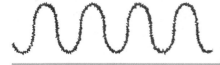	A superficial, low-pitched, coarse rubbing or grating sound. Sounds like two surfaces rubbing together. Heard throughout inspiration and expiration. Loudest over the lower anterolateral surface. Not cleared by cough.	Heard in individuals with pleurisy (inflammation of the pleural surfaces).

PROCEDURES AND TECHNIQUES WITH NORMAL FINDINGS	ABNORMAL FINDINGS

ANTERIOR THORAX

Move in front of the client to assess the anterior thorax.

INSPECT the anterior thorax for shape and symmetry, muscle development, anteroposterior diameter to lateral diameter, and costal angle.

When examining women, limit the time of exposure as much as possible. The thorax should be symmetric. The ribs should slope down at about 45 degrees relative to the spine. Muscle development should be equal. The anteroposterior (AP) diameter of the chest should be approximately half the lateral diameter—

Asymmetry or unequal muscle development is abnormal. In disorders that cause lung hyperinflation such as emphysema, the chest wall may have a barrel-shaped

= core examination skill

PROCEDURES AND TECHNIQUES WITH NORMAL FINDINGS

ABNORMAL FINDINGS

or about a 1:2 ratio of AP to lateral diameter. Thus the distance from the front of the chest to the back of the chest should be half the distance from one side of the chest to the other. Anteriorly the costal angle should be less than 90 degrees (Fig. 12-17).

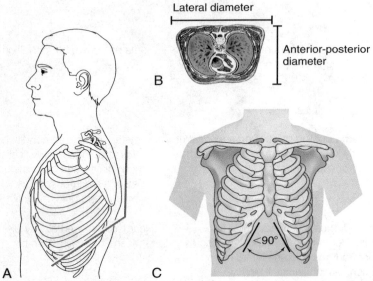

Fig. 12-17   Normal chest findings. A, Angulation of ribs. **B,** AP diameter is about half the lateral diameter. **C,** Costal angle less than 90 degrees. (**A,** *From Barkauskas et al, 1998.*)

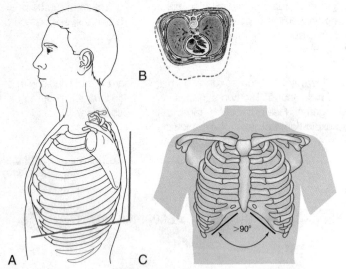

Fig. 12-18   Barrel chest. A, Horizontal ribs. **B,** Increased AP diameter. **C,** Costal angle greater than 90 degrees. (**A,** *From Barkauskas et al, 1998.*)

☞ **AUSCULTATE** the anterior thorax for breath sounds.

Procedure: Follow the same procedure as used to auscultate the posterior thorax. When examining women, you may reach under the gown with the stethoscope to auscultate the thorax while maintaining her modesty. Using the diaphragm of the stethoscope, listen to the client's breath sounds in a systematic manner over the anterior thorax. Auscultate from the apex to the base, during both inspiration and expiration, and compare one side to the other side (Fig. 12-21, *A, B,* and *C*).

☞ = core examination skill

appearance because of an increased AP diameter. In this situation, the ribs are more horizontal, and the chest looks as if it is held in constant inspiration. The costal angle is greater than 90 degrees (Fig. 12-18). Other chest wall skeletal deformities include scoliosis, pectus carinatum (Fig. 12-19), and pectus excavatum (Fig. 12-20).

Adventitious breath sounds (crackles, wheezing, and rhonchi) are extraneous sounds that are superimposed on the breath sounds (see Table 12-2). If you hear adventitious sounds, identify the type of sound, the location of the sound (i.e., right lung, left lung, or bilaterally;

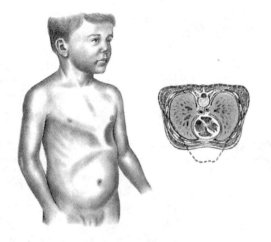

Fig. 12-19   Pectus carinatum, or pigeon chest. Note prominent sternum.

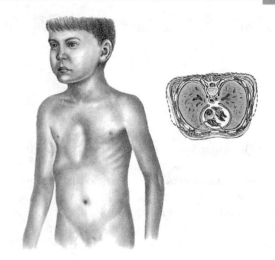

Fig. 12-20   Pectus excavatum, or funnel chest. Note that sternum is indented above xiphoid.

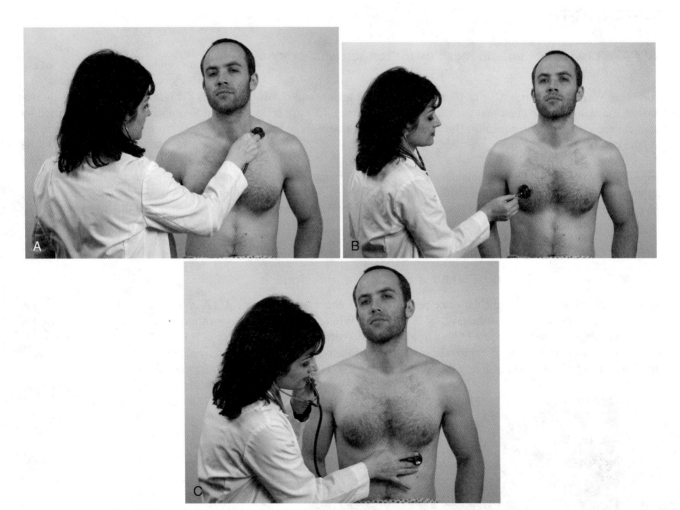

Fig. 12-21   Auscultating the anterior chest. A, Left apex. **B,** Right middle anterior thorax. **C,** Left lower anterior thorax.

PROCEDURES AND TECHNIQUES WITH NORMAL FINDINGS

ABNORMAL FINDINGS

Finding: Vesicular breath sounds should be heard throughout the periphery of the anterior lung fields, including the apex of the lungs above the clavicles. *Bronchovesicular breath sounds* are normally heard over the central area of the anterior thorax around the sternal border. These sounds are heard in an area that approximates where the bronchi split off from the trachea. *Bronchial breath sounds* are normally heard over the trachea and immediately above the manubrium.

SPECIAL CIRCUMSTANCES OR ADVANCED PRACTICE

POSTERIOR THORAX

PALPATE posterior thoracic muscles for tenderness, bulges, and symmetry.

Procedure: With the palmar surface of your fingers, feel the texture and consistency of the skin over the chest and the alignment of vertebrae. Identify areas the client reports as tender or painful. Use both hands simultaneously to compare the two sides of the posterior chest wall.

Finding: The spine should be straight and nontender from C7 through T12. The scapulae should be symmetric and the surrounding musculature well developed. The posterior ribs should be stable and nontender. The posterior rib cage should be symmetric and firm.

PALPATE the posterior chest wall for thoracic expansion.

Procedure: Stand behind the client and place both thumbs on either side of the client's spinal processes at about the level of T9 or T10. While maintaining the thumb position, extend the fingers of both hands laterally (outward) over the posterior chest wall. Instruct the client to take several deep breaths. Observe for lateral movement of both thumbs during the client's inspiration (Fig. 12-22).

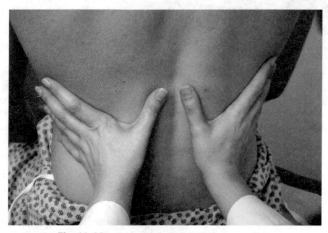

Fig. 12-22 Assessing for posterior thoracic expansion.

upper lobes or lower lobes; anterior or posterior) and the phase of breathing in which it is heard (i.e., inspiration or expiration).

Diminished breath sounds may be heard in clients whose alveoli have been destroyed, which may occur in clients with emphysema. Diminished or absent breath sounds may be heard in clients with collapsed alveoli, which may occur in clients who have atelectasis or are having a severe asthma attack.

Note any crepitus, which feels like a crinkly or crackly sensation under your fingers. This abnormal finding indicates air in the subcutaneous tissue caused by an air leak from somewhere in the respiratory tree. Pleural friction rub may be felt as a coarse, grating sensation during inspiration. It occurs secondary to inflammation of the pleural surface. Muscular development that is asymmetric or an unstable chest wall may indicate a thoracic disorder, such as fractured ribs.

A unilateral or unequal movement of your thumbs suggests asymmetry of expansion, which may be caused by pain, fractured ribs or chest wall injury, pneumonia, and atelectasis or collapsed lung. If unequal chest wall movement is noted, further evaluation is warranted.

PROCEDURES AND TECHNIQUES WITH NORMAL FINDINGS

ABNORMAL FINDINGS

Finding: Both thumbs should move apart symmetrically on the posterior chest wall with each breath.

PALPATE the posterior thoracic wall for vocal (tactile) fremitus.

Procedure: Vocal fremitus is a vibration resulting from verbalizations. You can feel this vibration using the palmar surface of your hand and fingers or the ulnar surfaces of your hands. Place your hands on the posterior thorax over the right and left lung fields following the landmarks shown in Figure 12-23, *A.* Instruct the client to recite "one-two-three" or "ninety-nine" while you systematically palpate the chest wall (from apices to bases [Fig. 12-23, *B*]).

Vibrations feel unequal when comparing sides. Decreased or absent fremitus occurs when the vibrations are blocked, which may occur in clients who have emphysema, pleural effusion, pulmonary edema, or bronchial obstruction. Increased fremitus occurs when the vibrations feel enhanced— sometimes described as a rougher or coarser vibrations. This occurs when lung tissues are congested or consolidated, which may occur in clients who have pneumonia or a tumor.

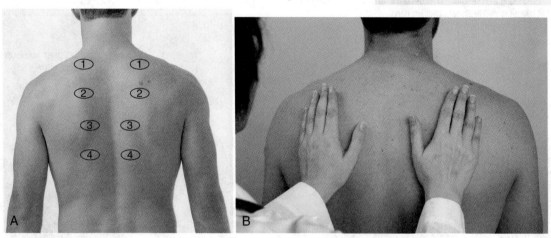

Fig. 12-23 **Assessing for posterior vocal (tactile) fremitus. A,** Hand positions for assessment. **B,** Position hands over both lung fields, making bilateral comparisons.

Finding: The fremitus should feel bilaterally equal, although the quality of the vibrations may vary from person to person because of chest wall density and relative location of the bronchi to the chest wall.

★ PERCUSS the posterior and lateral thorax for tone.

Percussion is the tapping of an object to set the underlying structures in motion and thus produce a sound. If necessary, review the techniques of performing percussion in Chapter 4.

Procedure: Systematically percuss the posterior chest wall following the same pattern that was used for auscultation (see Fig. 12-15, *A* and *C*). To begin, place the client in a sitting position with arms folded in front with head bent forward to move the scapulae laterally, exposing more lung field. Stand behind the client and percuss from above the scapula to the bottom of the ribs. Percuss between the ribs down the thorax from side to side, comparing the two sides as you go (Fig. 12-24). Next compare percussion tones between the left and right lateral thoraces.

Hyperresonance is heard when there is overinflation of the lungs. It has a very loud resonance of low pitch that lasts longer than normal and seems "booming." This may be found in individuals with emphysema. Dull tones may be heard in clients with pneumonia, pleural effusion, or atelectasis.

★ = advanced practice

PROCEDURES AND TECHNIQUES WITH NORMAL FINDINGS

ABNORMAL FINDINGS

Finding: The sound should be resonant, which is loud in intensity, low in pitch, long in duration, and hollow in quality (Table 12-3 and Fig. 12-25, *B*).

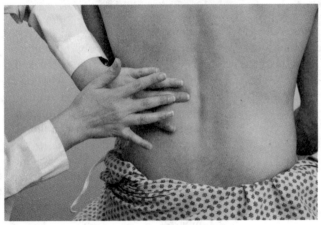

Fig. 12-24 Percussing the posterior thorax using the tip of the middle finger of the right hand to strike the middle finger of the left hand.

TABLE 12-3 *Percussion Tones over the Lungs*

	DESCRIPTION	ADULT PERIPHERAL LUNG
Tone	Description of tone	Resonance
Intensity	Loudness or softness of the tone heard	Loud
Pitch	Number of vibrations per second: Fast vibrations—high pitch Slow vibrations—low pitch	Low
Duration	Length of time a vibration note is sustained	Long
Quality	Subjective assessment of characteristics of tone	Hollow

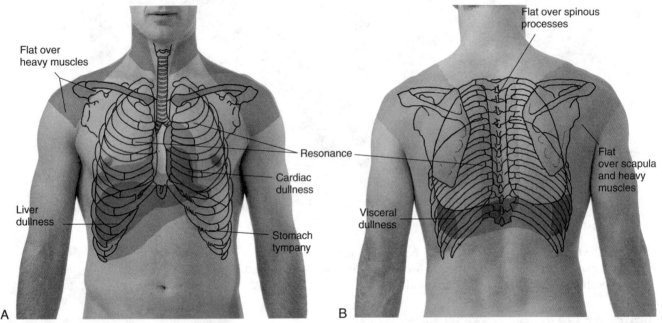

Fig. 12-25 **Percussion tones of the chest. A,** Anterior chest. **B,** Posterior chest.

★ **PERCUSS the thorax for diaphragmatic (respiratory) excursion.**

Diaphragmatic excursion is the movement of the diaphragm with maximum inspiration and expiration. This allows the nurse to estimate the lower lung border during inspiration and expiration.
Procedure: To measure diaphragmatic excursion, follow these steps:
  1. Stand behind the client. Instruct the client to sit upright, inhale deeply, and hold his or her breath. *(Hold your breath at the same time so you can determine the pace of your percussion.)*

★ = advanced practice

PROCEDURES AND TECHNIQUES WITH NORMAL FINDINGS

2. While the client is holding the breath, quickly percuss down the posterior chest wall along the midscapular line to determine the lower border of the lungs. (The percussion tone should change from resonant to dull.)
3. Using a marking pen, make a small line at the level where the percussion tone changed.
4. Tell the client to breathe normally. When ready, instruct the client to *exhale* as much as possible and hold the breath.
5. Repeat the sequence during the client's exhalation. Mark point along the chest wall where the sound changes from resonant to dull at the bottom of the lungs. The difference between the two marks on each side is termed *diaphragmatic excursion* (Fig. 12-26). Repeat the sequence on the other side of the chest.

Finding: The diaphragmatic excursion should be equal bilaterally and measure at least 1 to 2 inches (3 to 5 cm); in well-conditioned individuals it may measure as much as 3 inches (7 to 8 cm).

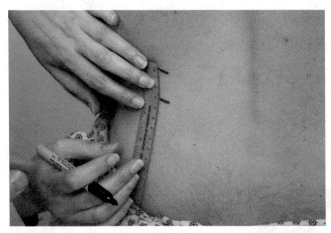

Fig. 12-26 **Measuring amount of diaphragmatic excursion.** Excursion usually measures 3 to 5 cm.

★ **AUSCULTATE the thorax for vocal sounds (vocal resonance).**

When there is an indication of consolidation of the lung, or if there was an abnormal finding when tactile fremitus was performed, evaluate for vocal resonance. This includes three techniques: testing for bronchophony, whispered pectoriloquy, and egophony.

The spoken voice vibrates and transmits sounds through the lung fields. These sounds are normally muffled and cannot be clearly understood. The sound is louder medially and softer at the periphery of the lung.

First, instruct the client to repeat one of the following phrases as you auscultate the posterior thorax to assess vocal resonance: "ninety-nine," "e-e-e," or "one-two-three."

Bronchophony

Procedure: First, instruct the client to repeat one of the following phrases as you auscultate the posterior thorax to assess vocal resonance: "ninety-nine," "e-e-e," or "one-two-three." Using the diaphragm of the stethoscope, systematically auscultate the posterior thorax. As the client repeats either "ninety-nine" or "one-two-three," listen for the response.

Finding: The expected response is a muffled tone such as "nin-nin" or muffled "one-two-three."

ABNORMAL FINDINGS

Any pathologic condition limiting downward lung expansion or diaphragmatic movement results in a decreased diaphragmatic excursion. Examples include pleural effusion, emphysema, atelectasis, abdominal tumor or ascites, and severe pain with injured or fractured ribs.

It is abnormal if the sound is louder and clearer. If there is consolidation or compression of the lung, the sound will actually sound like "ninety-nine" or "one-two-three."

★ = advanced practice

PROCEDURES AND TECHNIQUES WITH NORMAL FINDINGS	ABNORMAL FINDINGS

Whispered Pectoriloquy

Procedure: Perform this procedure when there is a positive finding of bronchophony. It is used to more clearly specify the problem and is referred to as an exaggerated bronchophony. Ask the client to whisper "one-two-three." Systematically auscultate the posterior thorax, listening for the quality of the whispered tones.

Finding: The expected response is a muffled "one-two-three."

An abnormal finding is increased clarity and loudness of the sounds, which may be found in consolidation or compression of the lung.

Egophony

Egophony is the final test for vocal resonance. It evaluates the intensity of the spoken voice.

Procedure: Instruct the client to say "e-e-e" as you auscultate the posterior thorax.

Finding: The expected response is the sound of a muffled "e-e-e."

If there is consolidation of the lung, you may hear changes in intensity and pitch so that the sound appears to be an "a-a-a."

ANTERIOR THORAX

PALPATE the trachea for position.

Procedure: Stand facing the client. Using the thumbs of both hands (or index finger and thumb of one hand), palpate the trachea on the anterior aspect of the neck by placing the thumbs on either side (Fig. 12-27).

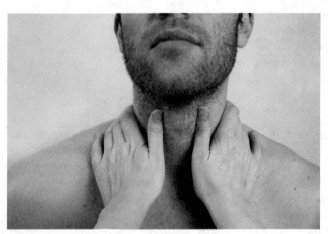

Fig. 12-27   Palpating to evaluate midline position of trachea.

Finding: The trachea should be palpable, midline, and slightly movable.

If the trachea is not midline, it may be an indication of a thorax mass, mediastinal shift, or some degree of lung collapse.

| **PROCEDURES AND TECHNIQUES WITH NORMAL FINDINGS** | **ABNORMAL FINDINGS** |

PALPATE the anterior thoracic muscles for tenderness, bulges, and symmetry.

Procedure: Repeat the same procedure as used for the posterior thorax. With the palmar surface of your fingers, feel the texture and consistency of the skin over the anterior chest. Identify areas the client reports as tender or painful. Use both hands simultaneously to compare the two sides of the posterior chest wall.
Finding: The clavicles should be symmetric and the surrounding musculature well developed. The anterior ribs should be stable and nontender. The rib cage should be symmetric and firm. The sternum and xiphoid should be relatively inflexible.

Note any crepitus, which feels like a crinkly or crackly sensation under your fingers. This abnormal finding indicates air in the subcutaneous tissue caused by an air leak from somewhere in the respiratory tree. Pleural friction rub may be felt as a coarse grating sensation during inspiration. Muscular development that is asymmetric or an unstable chest wall may indicate a thoracic disorder, such as fractured ribs.

PALPATE the anterior chest wall for thoracic expansion.

Procedure: Facing the client, place both thumbs along the coastal margin and the xiphoid process with your palms against the anterolateral chest wall (Fig. 12-28). Instruct the client to take several deep breaths. Observe for lateral movement of both thumbs during the client's inspiration.

A unilateral or unequal movement of your thumbs suggests asymmetry of expansion, which may be caused by pain, fractured ribs or chest wall injury, pneumonia, and atelectasis or collapsed lung.

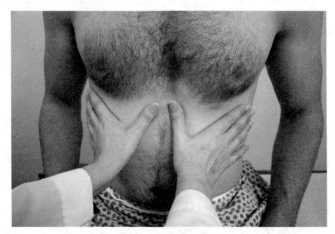

Fig. 12-28 Assessing for anterior thoracic expansion.

Finding: Both thumbs should move apart symmetrically on the anterior chest walls with each breath.

★ PALPATE the anterior thoracic wall for vocal (tactile) fremitus.

Procedure: Repeat the same procedure used for the posterior thorax. Place the palmar side of your hands and fingers or ulnar side of your hands on the anterior thorax over the right and left lung fields. Instruct the client to recite "one-two-three" or "ninety-nine" while you systematically palpate the chest wall (see example in Fig. 12-29).
Finding: The fremitus should feel bilaterally equal, although the quality of the vibrations may vary from person to person because of chest wall density and relative location of the bronchi to the chest wall.

Vibrations feel unequal when comparing sides. Decreased or absent fremitus occurs when the vibrations are blocked, which may occur in clients who have emphysema, pleural effusion, pulmonary edema, or bronchial obstruction. Increased fremitus occurs when the vibrations feel enhanced—sometimes described as a rougher or coarser vibrations. This occurs when lung tissues are congested or consolidated, which may occur in clients who have pneumonia or a tumor.

★ = advanced practice

PROCEDURES AND TECHNIQUES WITH NORMAL FINDINGS

ABNORMAL FINDINGS

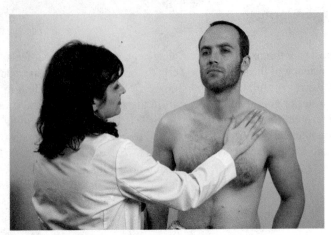

Fig. 12-29   Assessing for anterior vocal (tactile) fremitus.

★ **PERCUSS the anterior thorax for tone.**

Procedure: Repeat the same procedure as used for percussion of the posterior thorax. Systematically percuss the anterior chest wall following the same pattern that was used for auscultation (see Fig. 12-15, *B*). Stand in front of the client. Percuss down the anterior aspects of the thorax, moving from side to side.

Finding: There should be a resonant tone, which is loud in intensity, low in pitch, long in duration, and hollow in quality as shown in Figure 12-25, *A*.

Hyperresonance is heard when there is overinflation of the lungs. It has a very loud resonance of low pitch that lasts longer than normal and seems "booming." This may be found in individuals with emphysema. Dull tones may be heard in clients with pneumonia, pleural effusion, or atelectasis.

★ = advanced practice

AGE-RELATED VARIATIONS

INFANTS, CHILDREN, AND ADOLESCENTS

Assessing the respiratory status of an infant, child, or adolescent usually follows the same sequence as for an adult, although there are a few differences worth noting. The infant must be undressed at least to the diaper to perform an adequate assessment. Keep the infant covered when you are not performing the examination to prevent exposure and cooling. Conduct the examination while the infant is calm, if possible; examination of a crying infant is difficult. By the ages of 2 or 3 years the child is usually cooperative during the respiratory examination. Prior to that age, you need to develop a relationship with the child to improve cooperation

during the exam. Chapter 20 presents further information regarding the respiratory assessment of infants, children, and adolescents.

OLDER ADULTS

Assessing the respiratory status of an older adult follows the same procedures as for an adult, although there are may be structural and functional differences noted. Posterior thoracic stooping or bending or kyphosis may alter the thorax wall configuration and make thoracic expansion more difficult. Chapter 22 presents further information regarding the respiratory assessment of an older adult.

Documenting Expected Findings

Lungs and Respiratory System

Breathing is quiet and effortless at a rate of 16 per minute. Skin, nails, and lips are appropriate color for individual's ethnic background. Thorax is symmetric with ribs sloping downward at about 45 degrees relative to the spine. Muscle development of the thorax is equal bilaterally without tenderness. Thoracic expansion is symmetric bilaterally. Spinous processes are in alignment, scapulae are bilaterally symmetric. The anteroposterior (AP) diameter of the chest is about a 1:2 ratio of AP to lateral diameter. Trachea is midline. Breath sounds are clear with vesicular breath sounds heard over most lung fields, bronchovesicular breath sounds in the posterior chest over the upper center area of the back and around the sternal border, and bronchial breath sounds heard over the trachea.

CLINICAL REASONING *Respiratory System*

At the beginning of a shift, the husband of a 52-year-old woman tells the nurse something seems to be wrong with his wife. She had a nephrectomy for renal cell carcinoma 14 hours ago. She can have nothing by mouth and her last set of vital signs were stable. The man indicates his wife was fine when she came back from surgery, but she has become progressively less responsive over the last few hours.

Noticing: The experienced nurse with extensive postoperative care experience knows that 14 hours following a surgical procedure such as this, the client should not becoming less responsive. The nurse finds that the woman is difficult to arouse and obtains a set of vital signs which include: blood pressure 100/60, pulse 118 (thready), temperature 97.2° F, and respiratory rate 10 with an oxygen saturation of 88% on 2 liters oxygen. Her lungs are clear bilaterally; her respirations are shallow. The nurse notices that her skin is warm, dry, and pale; that her surgical dressing is dry and intact.

Interpreting: Early in the encounter, the nurse considers two possible causes of these findings: medication reaction or hypovolemia, both of which the client is at high risk for. In order to determine if either have any probability of being correct, the nurse gathers additional data.

- How much intravenous fluid has been administered? The woman has an IV of D5 ½ NS (5% dextrose in normal saline) infusing at 125 ml/hour. According the intake and output record, 950 ml IV fluid infused with 620 mL of urine output during the last shift.
- What pain medication is she taking? The woman has a PCA delivering morphine sulfate 1 mg every 10 minutes on demand. The PCA has delivered a total of 15 mg in the last 2½ hours.

The experienced nurse recognizes the adverse effects of morphine (hypotension, respiratory depression and hypoxia as evidenced by low oxygenation saturation and changes in cognition) and interprets this information in the context of a client 14 hours after a nephrectomy.

Responding: The nurse initiates appropriate initial interventions (increase the oxygen delivery and turn off the PCA) and contacts the attending physician to discuss the situation, ensuring the client receives appropriate immediate and follow-up care.

COMMON PROBLEMS & CONDITIONS

INFECTIONS AND INFLAMMATORY CONDITIONS

Acute Bronchitis

An inflammation of the mucous membranes of the bronchial tree caused by viruses or bacteria is called acute bronchitis. **Clinical Findings:** The cough initially is nonproductive, but it may become productive after a few days. Clients may complain of substernal chest pain that is aggravated by coughing. Other clinical manifestations include fever, malaise, and tachypnea. Rhonchi are heard on auscultation, with wheezing heard after coughing (Fig. 12-30).

Pneumonia

This is an infection of the terminal bronchioles and alveoli. It may be caused by bacteria, fungi, viruses, mycoplasma, or

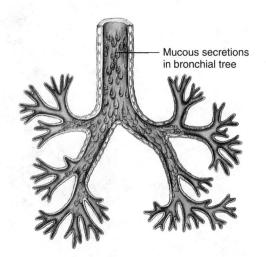

Mucous secretions in bronchial tree

Fig. 12-30 **Bronchitis.** Irritation of the bronchi causes inflammation.

Lobar pneumonia
(right upper lobe)

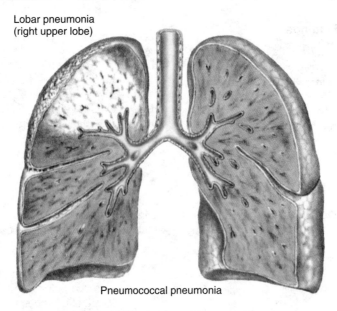

Pneumococcal pneumonia

Fig. 12-31   Right upper lobe pneumonia.

aspiration of gastric secretions. **Clinical Findings:** Viral pneumonia tends to produce a nonproductive cough or clear sputum, whereas bacterial pneumonia causes a productive cough that may produce white, yellow, or green sputum. Other clinical findings include fever, malaise and pleuritic chest pain. Signs of pulmonary consolidation may be noted such as inspiratory crackles, increased tactile fremitus, egophony and whispered pectoriloquy (Fig. 12-31).

Tuberculosis

This contagious, bacterial infection is caused by *Mycobacterium tuberculosis.* This infection is primarily in the lungs, but kidney, bone, lymph node, and meninges can also be in-

volved. **Clinical Findings:** The client is usually asymptomatic during the early stages of the disease. The initial clinical manifestations may consist of fatigue, anorexia, weight loss, night sweats, and fever. A characteristic finding later in the disease is a cough that becomes increasingly frequent, producing a mucopurulent sputum (Fig. 12-32).

Pleural Effusion

An accumulation of serous fluid in the pleural space between the visceral and parietal pleurae is called pleural effusion. **Clinical Findings:** The manifestations depend on the amount of fluid accumulation and the position of the client. If the effusion occurs rapidly and if it is large, there may be dys-

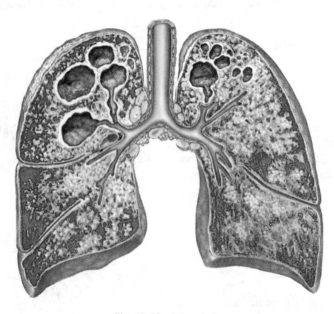

Fig. 12-32   Tuberculosis.

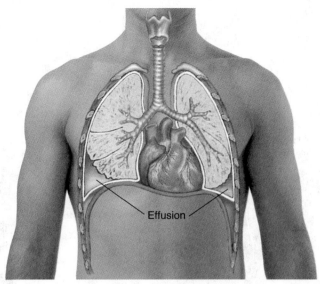

Fig. 12-33 Pleural effusion.

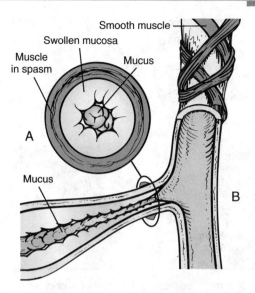

Fig. 12-34 **Factors causing airway obstruction in asthma. A,** Cross section of a bronchiole occluded by muscle spasm, mucosal edema, and mucus. **B,** Longitudinal section of a bronchiole. *(From Lewis, Heitkemper, and Dirksen, 2007. Redrawn from Price and Wilson, 2003.)*

pnea, intercostal bulging, or decreased chest wall movement (Fig. 12-33).

CHRONIC PULMONARY DISEASE

Asthma

This hyperreactive airway disease is a characterized by bronchoconstriction, airway obstruction, and inflammation in response to inhalation of allergens or pollutants, infection, cold air, vigorous exercise, or emotional stress. **Clinical Findings:** Signs include increased respiratory rate with prolonged expiration, audible wheeze, dyspnea, tachycardia, anxious appearance, possible use of accessory muscles, and cough. Expiratory and occasionally inspiratory wheeze and diminished breath sounds are common findings during auscultation (Fig. 12-34).

Emphysema

Destruction of the alveolar walls causes permanent abnormal enlargement of the air spaces in emphysema. **Clinical Findings:** The classic general appearance of a client with advanced emphysema is an underweight individual with a barrel chest who becomes short of breath with minimal exertion. When the client is short of breath, pursed-lip breathing and tripod position are frequently observed. Other clinical findings typically reveal diminished breath and voice sounds, possible wheezing or crackles on auscultation, and decreased diaphragmatic excursion on percussion (Fig. 12-35).

Chronic Bronchitis

This disorder is characterized by hypersecretion of mucus by the goblet cells of the trachea and bronchi resulting in a productive cough for 3 months in each of 2 successive years. It is

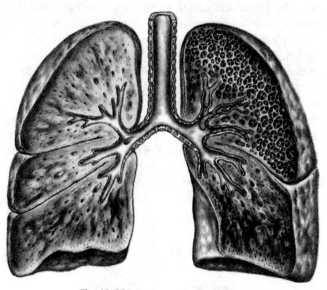

Fig. 12-35 Emphysema in upper left lobe.

caused by irritants such as cigarette smoke and air pollution or by infection. Clinical Findings: Symptoms of chronic bronchitis are productive cough, increased mucus production, and dyspnea. Findings on auscultation are rhonchi, sometimes cleared by coughing. When there is sufficient mucus to occlude alveoli, crackles may be heard (Fig. 12-36).

ACUTE OR TRAUMATIC CONDITIONS

Pneumothorax

Air in the pleural spaces results in a pneumothorax. There are three types of pneumothorax: (1) closed, which may be spontaneous, traumatic, or iatrogenic; (2) open, which occurs fol-

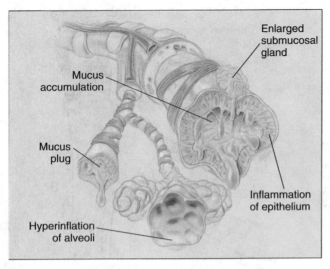

Fig, 12-36   Chronic bronchitis. *(From McCance and Huether, 2002. Modified from Des Jardins and Burton, 1995.)*

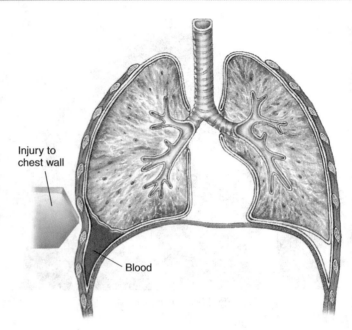

Fig. 12-38   Hemothorax.

lowing penetration of the chest by either injury or surgical procedure; and (3) tension, which develops when air leaks into the pleura and cannot escape. **Clinical Findings:** The signs vary depending on the amount of lung collapse. If there is very minor collapse, the client may be slightly short of breath, anxious, and have chest pain. If a large amount of lung collapses, the client may experience in severe respiratory distress, including dyspnea, tachypnea, and cyanosis. Distant and hyperresonant breath sounds over the affected area are noted on auscultation. Decreased chest wall movement on the affected side may be noted. The client may also have paradoxic chest wall movement, when the chest wall moves in on inspiration and out on expiration. If severe, there may be tracheal displacement toward the unaffected side with a mediastinal shift, termed a tension pneumothorax (Fig. 12-37).

Hemothorax

Blood in the pleural space caused by injury to the chest results in hemothorax, but it also may be a complication of thoracic surgery. **Clinical Findings:** Signs are similar to those described for pneumothorax, although it is common to note distant muffled breath sounds and dullness with percussion over the affected area (Fig. 12-38).

OTHER PULMONARY CONDITIONS

Atelectasis

This disorder refers to collapsed alveoli caused by external pressure from a tumor, fluid, or air in the pleural space (compression atelectasis) or by removal of air from hypoventilation or obstruction by secretions (absorption atelectasis). **Clinical Findings:** The affected lobe has diminished or absent breath sounds. The oxygen saturation may decrease to less than 90% (Fig. 12-39).

Lung Cancer

An uncontrolled growth of anaplastic cells in the lung describes lung cancer. Agents such as tobacco smoke, asbestos, ionizing radiation, and other noxious inhalants can be causative agents. **Clinical Findings:** The most common initial symptom reported is a persistent cough. Weight loss, congestion, wheezing, hemoptysis, labored breathing, or dyspnea are other manifestations that occur with advanced disease. Lung sounds may be normal or diminished over the affected area; if there is a partial obstruction of airways from the tumor, wheezes may be heard. Percussion tones may be normal or may be dull over the tumor, particularly if the cancer is large or the client has associated atelectasis (Fig. 12-40).

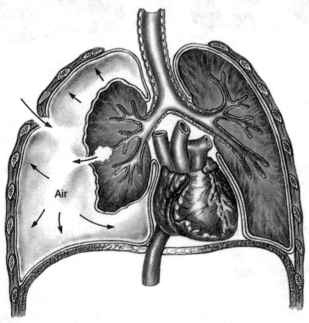

Fig. 12-37   Tension pneumothorax.

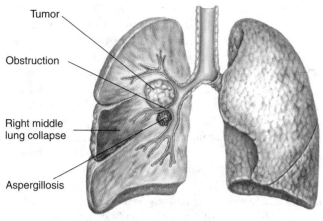

Fig. 12-39 Atelectasis.

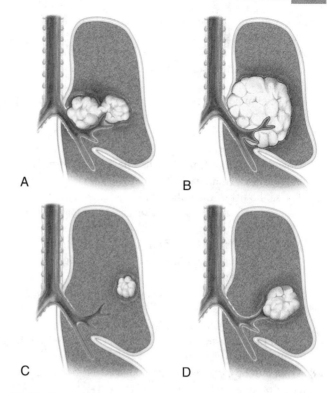

Fig.12-40 **Cancer of the lung. A,** Squamous cell carcinoma. **B,** small cell (oat cell) carcinoma. **C,** Adenocarcinoma. **D,** Large cell carcinoma. *(From Seidel et al, 2006.)*

CLINICAL APPLICATION & CLINICAL REASONING

See Appendix E for answers to exercises in this section.

REVIEW QUESTIONS

1 The nurse suspects a possible viral infection or upper respiratory allergies when the client describes the sputum as:
   1 White.
   2 Clear.
   3 Yellow.
   4 Pink tinged.

2 During inspection of the respiratory system, the nurse documents which finding as abnormal?
   1 Skin color consistent with client's ethnicity.
   2 A 1:2 ratio of anterior-posterior to lateral diameter.
   3 Anterior costal angle is 85 degrees.
   4 Client is leaning forward with the arms braced against the knees,

3 A client has an infection of the terminal bronchioles and alveoli that involves the right lower lobe of the lung. What abnormal findings will be expected?
   1 Dyspnea with diminished breath sounds bilaterally.
   2 Asymmetric chest expansion on the right side.
   3 Fever and tachypnea with crackles over the right lower lobe.
   4 Prolonged expiration with an occasional wheeze in the right lower lobe.

4 On auscultation of a client's lungs, the nurse hears a low-pitched, coarse, loud, and low snoring sound. What term does the nurse use to document this finding?
   1 Rhonchi.
   2 Wheeze.
   3 Crackle.
   4 Pleural friction rub.

5 Which of the following questions will give the nurse further information about the client's complaint of chest pain?
   1 "Have you had your influenza immunization this year?"
   2 "Are there environmental conditions that may affect your breathing at home?"
   3 "How would you describe the chest pain?"
   4 "Has the chest pain been interrupting your sleep?"

6 What finding does the nurse expect when performing tactile fremitus?

1 A vibration of sounds that are equal bilaterally.

2 A change in muscle tone when the client inhales and exhales indicating weakness.

3 The symmetric rise of the thorax as the client speaks indicating equal expansion.

4 Coughing triggered by client speech indicating bronchial irritation.

7 How does the nurse palpate the chest for tenderness, bulges, and symmetry?

1 Use the fist of the dominant hand to gently tap the anterior, lateral, and posterior chest, comparing one side with another.

2 Use the ulnar surface of one hand to palpate the anterior, posterior and lateral chest comparing one side with another.

3 With the tips of the fingers, palpate the skin over the chest and the alignment of vertebrae.

4 With the palmar surface of the fingers of both hands, feel the consistency of the skin over the chest and the alignment of vertebrae.

8 What are the expected breath sounds over the posterior chest of an adult?

1 Vesicular.

2 Bronchovesicular.

3 Bronchial.

4 Bronchoalveolar.

9 Narrowing of the bronchi creates which adventitious sound?

1 Wheeze.

2 Crackles.

3 Rhonchi.

4 Pleural friction rub.

10 During inspection of the thorax, the nurse suspects abnormal thoracic expansion for the client who has:

1 A 4-cm diaphragmatic excursion.

2 A 1:2 ratio AP to lateral diameter.

3 An S-shaped curvature of the spine.

4 A costal angle of 85 degrees.

SAMPLE DOCUMENTATION

Review the data obtained during an interview and examination by the nurse below:

K. B., a 29-year-old male, comes to the emergency department with a 2-hour history of wheezing. He appears anxious. He is sitting leaning forward with his hands braced against his knees, attempting to breathe with mouth open; he is coughing up clear mucus. He is allergic to peanuts, which cause a rash. His sternocleidomastoid muscle retracts when he inhales. Vital signs are as follows: pulse, 132 beats per minute; respiratory rate, 48 breaths per minute; oxygen saturation on room air, 91%; temperature, 100.3° F (37.9° C). His partner indicates that he woke this morning with a "cold" and

has been coughing up sputum. Yesterday he woke up "just fine, no coughing." He has no previous hospitalizations. He has no health problems other than a history of asthma since age 5 years. Earlier today he was jogging until he could not breathe; he "got scared because he could not catch his breath." His chest wall is smooth and in a normal configuration. Retractions are observed on inspiration. Palpation is deferred because of the client's anxious state. His expiration is prolonged. On auscultation, expiratory wheezes are heard bilaterally and diminished breath sounds are heard throughout both lungs. He takes the following medications: Albuterol and Cromolyn sodium by nebulizer; he also uses Proventil inhaler as needed. In the past his breathing has improved after using the Proventil inhaler. He had two puffs just before coming to the clinic, approximately 30 minutes ago, but he is still having difficulty breathing.

Below, note how the nurse documented these same data.

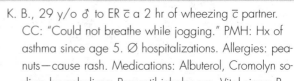

K. B., 29 y/o ♂ to ER c̄ a 2 hr of wheezing c̄ partner. CC: "Could not breathe while jogging." PMH: Hx of asthma since age 5. Ø hospitalizations. Allergies: peanuts—cause rash. Medications: Albuterol, Cromolyn sodium by nebulizer; Proventil inhaler prn. Vital signs: P, 132 beats/min; RR, 48 breaths/min; O₂ on RA, 91%; T, 100.3° F (37.9° C).

SUBJECTIVE DATA

Client reports he woke this A.M. c̄ a "cold" and coughing c̄ mucus production. Jogged today until he could not breathe; got scared. Usually responds well to Proventil inhaler. Had 2 puffs just ā coming to clinic, approx. 30 min ago s̄ relief. No previous hospitalizations for asthma. No other health problems.

OBJECTIVE DATA

29-year-old male appears anxious, sitting in tripod position, using accessory muscles c̄ retractions noted on inspiration. Palpation deferred d/t client's anxious state. Exp. wheezes bil; prolonged exp; ↓ breath sounds throughout.

CASE STUDY

Ms. M. is a 66-year-old woman complaining of shortness of breath. The following initial data are collected.

Interview Data

Ms. M. says that she has had breathing problems "for years" but her breathing is getting worse. She tells the nurse that she gets short of breath with activity, adding that she can do things around the house for only a few minutes before she has to sit down to catch her breath. She says that she can sleep for only a couple of hours at a time. She sleeps best using two pillows to prop her up, but on some nights she just sits in a chair. Ms. M. does not currently use oxygen, but she thinks oxygen would help. She admits to smoking 1.5 packs of cigarettes a day. She has never quit because she says she "just can't do it."

Examination Data

- *General survey:* Alert and slightly anxious female, sitting slightly forward, with moderately labored breathing. Skin is pale with slight cyanosis around the lips and in nail beds. Appears extremely thin.
- *Chest and lungs:* Chest is round shaped and symmetric with increased AP diameter and costal angle greater than 90 degrees. Small muscle mass is noted over chest; ribs protrude. Respiratory rate is 24 and labored. Chest wall expansion with respirations is reduced but symmetric. Sibilant wheezes are auscultated on expiration throughout lung fields. Lung sounds are diminished in lung bases bilaterally. Vocal sounds are muffled bilaterally.

Clinical Reasoning

1. What data deviate from expected findings, suggesting a need for further investigation?
2. What additional information should the nurse ask or assess for?
3. Based on the data, what risk factors does this client have for lung cancer?
4. What nursing diagnoses and collaborative problems should be considered for this situation?

INTERACTIVE ACTIVITIES

Open the interactive student CD-ROM, click on Chapter 12, and choose from the following activities on the menu bar:

- **Multiple Choice Challenge.** Click on the best answer for each of these 15 items. You will be given immediate feedback, rationale for incorrect answers, and a total score. Good luck!

- **Marvelous Matches.** Drag each word or phrase to the appropriate place on the screen. Test your ability to match definitions of abnormal findings or conditions with their names.

- **A Day in the Clinic.** Complete an examination by choosing a technique and examination area for this client. You'll be able to collect data, document, and compare your answers with those of the experts. Everything that you need for a successful assessment is at your fingertips!

- **Symptom Analysis.** Review this client's case study. Choose from the list of questions to ask the client. Practice your clinical skills by taking notes and then ruling out possible causes of her respiratory disorder. See why your analysis is correct or incorrect. Good luck!

- **Printable Lab Guide.** Locate the Lab Guide for Chapter 12, and print and use it (as many times as needed) to help you apply your assessment skills. These guides may also be filled in electronically and then saved and e-mailed to your instructor!

- **Audio Clips: Lung Sounds.** Choose from nine different lung sounds to listen to (as many times as needed) to help you develop your assessment skills.

- **Quick Challenge.** Use this critical thinking exercise to assess your skills through case study-style questions, then compare with expert answers!

- **Core Examination Skills Checklists.** Make sure you've got frequently-used exam skills down pat! Use these checklists to help cover all the bases for your examination.

CHAPTER 13

Heart and Peripheral Vascular System

ANATOMY & PHYSIOLOGY

The cardiovascular system transports oxygen, nutrients, and other substances to the body's tissues and carries metabolic waste products to the kidneys and lungs. This dynamic system is able to adjust to changing demands for blood by constricting or dilating blood vessels and altering the cardiac output.

THE HEART AND GREAT VESSELS

The heart is a pump, about the size of a fist, that beats 60 to 100 times a minute without rest, responding to both external and internal demands such as exercise, temperature changes, and stress. Each side of the heart has two chambers, an atrium and a ventricle. The right side receives blood from the superior and inferior venae cavae and pumps it through the pulmonary arteries to the pulmonary circulation; the left side receives blood from the pulmonary veins and pumps it through the aorta into the systemic circulation.

The upper part of the heart is called the base, and the lower left ventricle is called the apex. The heart lies behind the sternum and above the diaphragm in the mediastinum. It lies at an angle so that the right ventricle makes up most of the anterior surface and the left ventricle lies to the left and posteriorly. The right atrium forms the right border of the heart, and the left atrium lies posteriorly. The pulmonary ar-

teries and aorta are termed the *great vessels*. The aorta curves upward out of the left ventricle and bends posteriorly and downward just above the sternal angle. The pulmonary arteries emerge from the superior aspect of the right ventricle near the third intercostal space (Fig. 13-1).

PERICARDIUM AND CARDIAC MUSCLE

The heart wall has three layers: pericardium, myocardium, and endocardium (Fig. 13-2). The heart is encased in the pericardium, which has a fibrous layer and two serous layers. The fibrous layer, termed the *fibrous pericardium* or *parietal layer,* is a fibrous sac of elastic connective tissue that shields the heart from trauma and infection. One of the serous layers lies next to the fibrous pericardium and the other serous layer lies next to the myocardium. Between the fibrous pericardium and the serous pericardium is the pericardial space, which contains a small amount of pericardial fluid to reduce friction as the myocardium contracts and relaxes. The serous pericardium, also termed the *visceral layer* or *epicardium,* covers the heart surface and extends to the great vessels. The middle layer, or myocardium, is thick muscular tissue that contracts to eject blood from the ventricles. The endocardium lines the inner chambers and valves.

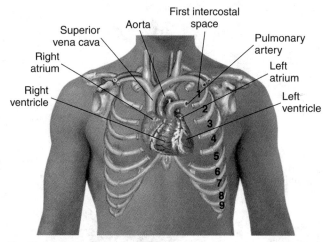

Fig. 13-1 Position of the heart chambers and great vessels. Intercostal spaces 1 to 9 are numbered.

BLOOD FLOW THROUGH THE HEART: THE CARDIAC CYCLE

Four valves govern blood flow through the four chambers of the heart. The tricuspid valve on the right and mitral valve on the left are termed the *atrioventricular* (AV) valves because they separate the atria from the ventricles (Fig. 13-3). The aortic valve opens from the left ventricle into the aorta, while the pulmonic valve opens from the right ventricle into the pulmonary artery. The aortic and pulmonic valves are termed *semilunar* valves because of their half-moon shape.

Diastole

During diastole, the ventricles are relaxed and fill with blood from the atria. The movement of blood from the atria to the

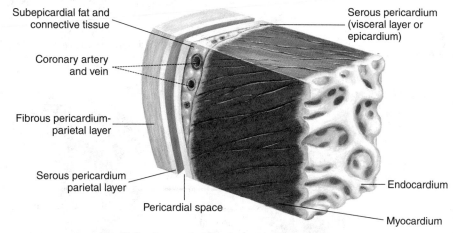

Fig. 13-2 Cross section of cardiac muscle. *(From Canobbio, 1990.)*

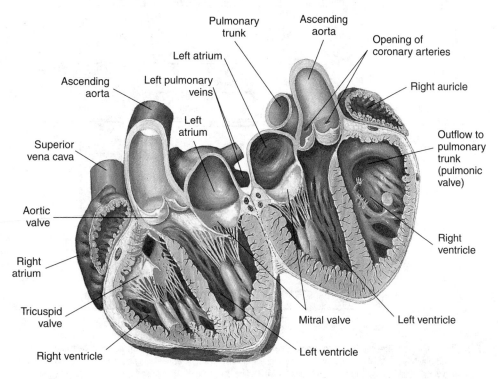

Fig. 13-3 Anterior cross section showing the valves and chambers of the heart. *(From Seidel et al, 2006.)*

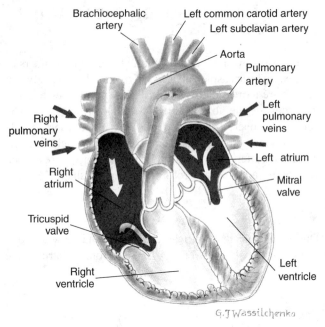

Fig. 13-4 Blood flow during diastole. *(From Canobbio, 1990.)*

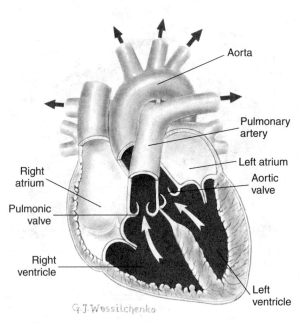

Fig. 13-5 Blood flow during systole. *(From Canobbio, 1990.)*

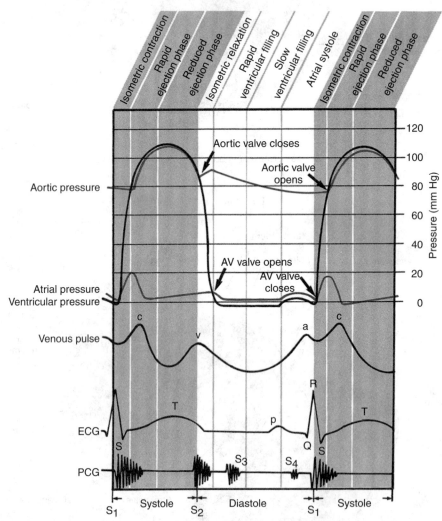

Fig. 13-6 Events of the cardiac cycle showing venous pressure waves, electrocardiograph, and heart sounds in systole and diastole. *a,* Atrial contraction; *AV,* atrioventricular; *c,* carotid artery; *ECG,* electrocardiogram; *PCG,* phonocardiogram; *p,* p wave (atrial contraction); *QRS,* QRS complex (ventricular contraction); S_1, first heart sound; S_2, second heart sound; S_3, third heart sound; S_4, fourth heart sound; *T,* T wave (ventricular repolarization); *v,* venous return coming into the atrium. *(From Seidel et al, 2006.)*

ventricles is accomplished when the pressure of the blood in the atria becomes higher than the pressure in the ventricles. The higher atrial pressures passively open the AV valves, allowing blood to fill the ventricles (Fig. 13-4). About 80% of the blood from the atria flows into relaxed ventricles. A contraction of the atria forces the remaining 20% of the blood into the ventricles. This added atrial thrust is termed the *atrial kick.* At the end of diastole, the ventricles are filled with blood.

Systole

During systole, the ventricles contract, creating a pressure that closes the AV valves, preventing the backflow of blood into the atria. This ventricular pressure also forces the semilunar valves to open, resulting in ejection of blood into the aorta (from the left ventricle) and the pulmonary arteries (from the right ventricle) (Fig. 13-5). As blood is ejected, the ventricular pressure decreases causing the semilunar valves to close. The ventricles relax to begin diastole.

Cardiac Cycle

Figure 13-6 diagrams the events in the cardiac cycle showing the venous pressure waves, electrocardiogram, and heart sounds in systole and diastole. Further discussion about using the electrocardiogram to assess cardiac conduction is found at the end of the examination section (see Fig. 13-32 later in this chapter). The S_3 and S_4 heart sounds are abnormal; however, they are shown in Fig. 13-6 at the point in the cardiac cycle where they would be heard if present.

ELECTRIC CONDUCTION

The heart is stimulated by an electric impulse that originates in the sinoatrial (SA) node in the superior aspect of the right atrium and travels in internodal tracts to the atrioventricular (AV) node. The SA node, termed the *cardiac pacemaker,* normally discharges between 60 and 100 impulses per minute. The electric impulses stimulate contractions of both atria and then flow to the AV node in the inferior aspect of the right atrium. The impulses are then transmitted through a series of branches (bundle of His) and Purkinje fibers in the myocardium, which results in ventricular contraction (Fig. 13-7). The AV node prevents excessive atrial impulses from reaching the ventricles. If the SA node fails to discharge, the AV node can generate ventricular contraction at a slower rate, 40 to 60 impulses per minute. If both SA and AV nodes are ineffective, the bundle branches may stimulate contraction, but at a very slow rate of 20 to 40 impulses per minute.

PERIPHERAL VASCULAR SYSTEM

Arteries, capillaries, and veins provide blood flow to and from tissues. The tough and tensile arteries and their smaller branches, the arterioles, are subjected to remarkable pressure generated

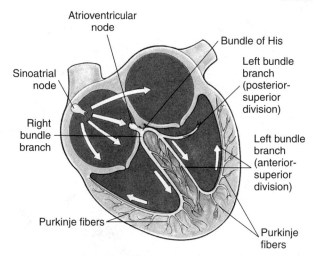

Fig. 13-7 Cardiac conduction. *(From Canobbio, 1990.)*

from the myocardial contraction. They maintain blood pressure by constricting or dilating in response to stimuli. The more passive veins and their smaller branches, the venules, are less sturdy but more expansible, enabling them to act as a reservoir for extra blood, if needed, to decrease the workload on the heart. Pressure within the veins is low, compared with arterial circulation. The valves in each vein keep blood flowing in a forward direction toward the heart. A comparison of the structures of arteries and veins is shown in Fig. 13-8.

LYMPH SYSTEM

The lymph system works in collaboration with the peripheral vascular system in removing fluid from the interstitial spaces. As blood flows from arterioles into venules, oxygen and nutrient-rich fluid is forced out at the arterial end of the capillary into the interstitial space, and then into cells. Waste products from cells flow through the interstitial spaces to the venous end of the capillary.

Excess fluid left in the interstitial spaces is absorbed by the lymph system and carried to lymph nodes throughout the body. Lymphatic fluid is clear, composed mainly of water and a small amount of protein, mostly albumin. Lymph nodes are tiny oval clumps of lymphatic tissue, usually located in groups along blood vessels. In the peripheral vascular system, the lymph node locations of interest are the arm, groin, and leg. The epitrochlear nodes on the medial surface of the arm above the elbow are palpable (Fig. 13-9). These lymph nodes receive fluid via the radial, ulnar, and median lymph vessels. In the upper thigh, the inguinal lymph nodes are superficial; they receive most of the lymph drainage from the great and small saphenous lymphatic vessels in the legs. In men, lymph from the penile and scrotal surfaces drains to the inguinal nodes, but nodes of the testes drain into the abdomen. In the posterior surface of the leg, behind the knee, are the popliteal nodes, which receive lymph from the medial portion of the lower leg (Fig. 13-10). Ducts from the lymph nodes empty into the subclavian veins.

ARTERY   VEIN

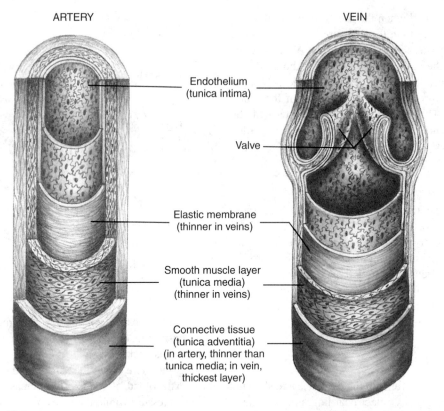

Endothelium
(tunica intima)

Valve

Elastic membrane
(thinner in veins)

Smooth muscle layer
(tunica media)
(thinner in veins)

Connective tissue
(tunica adventitia)
(in artery, thinner than
tunica media; in vein,
thickest layer)

Fig. 13-8   Schematic drawing of artery and vein. Shown are the comparative thickness of three layers (tunica adventitia), muscle layer (tunica media), and lining of endothelium (tunica intima). Note the muscle and outer coats are much thinner in the veins than in the arteries and that veins have valves. *(Modified from Thompson JM et al, 2002.)*

ANTERIOR VIEW   POSTERIOR VIEW

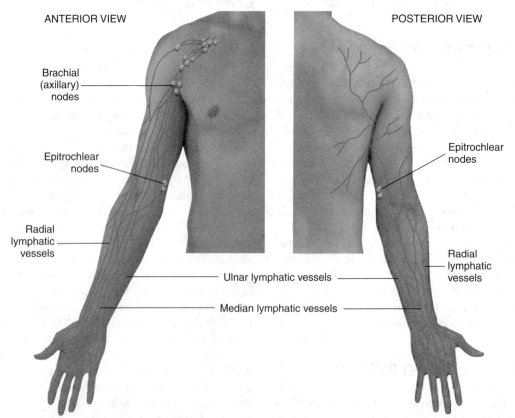

Brachial
(axillary)
nodes

Epitrochlear
nodes

Radial
lymphatic
vessels

Epitrochlear
nodes

Radial
lymphatic
vessels

Ulnar lymphatic vessels

Median lymphatic vessels

Fig. 13-9   System of deep and superficial collecting ducts, carrying lymph from upper extremity to subclavian lymphatic trunk. The only peripheral lymph center is the epitrochlear, which receives some of the collecting ducts from the pathway of the ulnar and radial vessels. *(From Seidel et al, 2006.)*

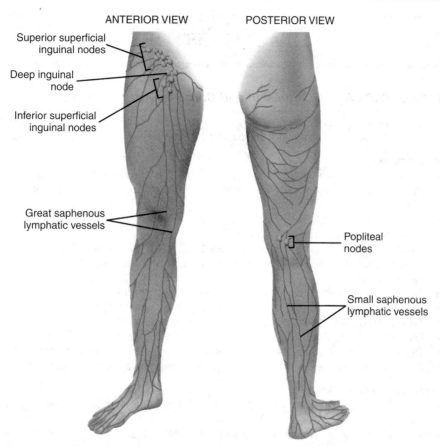

ANTERIOR VIEW   POSTERIOR VIEW

Superior superficial inguinal nodes

Deep inguinal node

Inferior superficial inguinal nodes

Great saphenous lymphatic vessels

Popliteal nodes

Small saphenous lymphatic vessels

Fig. 13-10   Lymphatic drainage of lower extremity. *(From Seidel et al, 2006.)*

LINK TO CONCEPTS   *Perfusion*

The feature concept for this chapter is *Perfusion*. This concept represents mechanisms that facilitate and impair perfusion of oxygenated blood throughout the body. Because all tissues require perfusion of oxygenated blood, all of these physiologic concepts are interrelated—but oxygenation is foundational to all others. Nutrition plays an important interrelated role because of the impact on cardiovascular health. The most important concepts are represented in the model below.

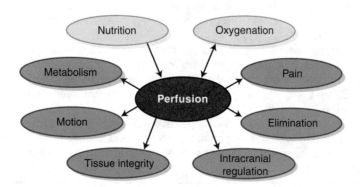

Concept Model: Perfusion

This model shows the interrelationship of concepts associated with perfusion. As an example, an individual who has heart failure has poor perfusion of blood. Pulmonary edema may interfere with oxygenation. Poor perfusion of oxygenated blood results in limits to motion (because of activity intolerance and fatigue), elimination (due to poor perfusion of blood to the kidneys), and potentially results in confusion as a result of poor perfusion of oxygenated blood to the brain. Understanding of the interrelationship of these concepts helps the nurse recognize risk factors and thus increases awareness when conducting a health assessment.

HEALTH HISTORY

RISK FACTORS *Hypertension and Coronary Artery Disease*

As you conduct a health history related to the cardiovascular system, it is important to consider common risk factors associated with hypertension and coronary artery disease.

Hypertension
- *Family history:* When parents have hypertension, their children have a greater risk.
- *Race:* African Americans are twice as likely to develop high blood pressure as Caucasians.
- *Gender:* Men have a greater risk than women.
- *Age:* Risk increases with age.
- *Obesity:* Overweight people are more likely to develop hypertension. (M)
- *Cigarette smoking:* Nicotine constricts blood vessels, increasing the workload of the heart. (M)
- *Elevated serum lipids:* Plaques accumulate within the arteries. (M)
- *Alcohol:* Excessive intake is strongly associated with hypertension. (M)
- *Excessive sodium intake:* Sodium retains water, increasing blood volume. (M)
- *Physical inactivity:* Contributes to obesity and elevated serum lipids. (M)
- *Diabetes mellitus:* Causes atherosclerosis and other factors that narrow vessels. (M)
- *Persistent stress:* Causes increased sympathetic nervous system stimulation. (M)

Coronary Artery Disease
- *Heredity:* When parents have coronary artery disease, their children have a greater risk.
- *Race:* African Americans have more severe high blood pressure than Caucasians and have higher risk of heart disease
- *Gender:* Men have a greater risk than women. Even after menopause, when women's death rate from heart disease increases, it is not as great as men.
- *Age:* Risk increases with age. Over 83% of people who die of coronary artery disease are 65 or older.
- *Smoking:* Smokers' risk of developing coronary heart disease is 2 to 4 times that of nonsmokers. Exposures of other people's smoke increases the risk of heart disease for nonsmokers.(M)
- *Hypertension:* High blood pressure increases the heart's workload, causing the myocardium to thicken and become stiffer. It also increases the risk for myocardium infarction and heart failure. When hypertension exists with obesity, smoking, high blood cholesterol, or diabetes, the risk of heart attack increase several times. (M)
- *Elevated serum cholesterol:* Risk of coronary artery disease increases as blood cholesterol rises. (M)
- *Obesity:* People who have excess body fat, especially at the waist, are more likely to develop heart disease, even if they have no other risk factors. (M)
- *Physical inactivity:* An inactive lifestyle is a risk factor for coronary heart disease. Regular moderate-to-vigorous physical exercise helps prevent heart and blood vessel disease. (M)
- *Diabetes mellitus:* Even when glucose levels are under control, diabetes increases the risk of heart disease, but the risks are greater if blood glucose is not well controlled. About 75% of people with diabetes die from some form of heart or blood vessel disease.

Data from *www.americanheart.org,* 2008.
M = modifiable risk factor.

GENERAL HEALTH HISTORY

Present Health Status

Do you have any chronic illnesses, such as diabetes mellitus, renal failure, chronic hypoxia, or hypertension? If yes, describe.
Chronic illnesses can cause symptoms affecting the cardiovascular system when they increase the workload of the heart by narrowing peripheral vessels (diabetes, hypertension), increase the fluid volume to be pumped (diabetes, renal failure), or increase the heart rate and cause pulmonary capillary vasoconstriction (chronic hypoxia).

Are you taking any medications? If yes, what are you taking, and when did you start taking the medications? Have you had any side effects from these medications? Do you take them as prescribed?
Medications may be taken to treat cardiovascular problems or may cause side effects affecting the cardiovascular system. For example, tricyclic antidepressants, phenothiazines, or lithium can cause dysrhythmias; hormonal contraceptives can cause thrombophlebitis; corticosteroids can cause sodium and fluid retention; and theophylline can cause tachycardia and dysrhythmias.

What over-the-counter drugs do you take? Do you take an aspirin on a regular basis to help thin your blood? Do you take herbs? How often do you use herbs or drugs?
These nonprescription drugs may affect the cardiovascular system. For example, aspirin prevents platelet aggregation to reduce clot formation. Decongestants containing pseudoephedrine may aggravate hypertension. Ayurvedic herbs can act as a cardiac stimulant, while others act as a cardiac depressant.

Do you use cocaine? Other street drugs? How often do you use these drugs?
Cocaine use has been associated with myocardial infarction and stroke.

Do you exercise? If yes, what kind of exercise? How often do you exercise? How much time do you spend exercising? If no, have you ever exercised? What motivated you to start in the past? What influenced you to stop your exercising?
Physical activity for at least 30 minutes five times weekly increases energy and improves self-esteem, as well as preventing coronary artery disease, hypertension, and obesity.

Clients who no longer exercise should be encouraged to resume an exercise program. Exploring reasons for stopping can begin the problem-solving process to determine what can motivate them to start again.

How would you describe your personality type? How do you deal with stress?
Stress and persistent intensity are risk factors for heart disease. (Observe the client as he or she responds, and throughout the examination, to detect stress or intensity.) Clients who are frequently in psychological stressful environments should be encouraged to use several strategies to relieve stress and to change their perceptions of the situations so that they are perceived as less stressful.

How often do you take time to relax? What do you do to relax? Hobbies? Sports? Meditation? Yoga? Music?
Physical relaxation can relieve stress and reduce blood pressure.

Describe your usual eating habits. How often do you eat red meat? How much red meat do you eat at a meal? Do you monitor your fat and salt intake? Do you eat whole grains each day?
Selecting foods consistent with the food pyramid provides balanced nutrition. Calories from fat should be limited to 20% of daily calories with 10% limited to saturated fat. Frequent consumption of large servings of red meat is associated with high cholesterol. A serving of red meat is 4 oz and should be limited to three times weekly. Whole grains (e.g., cereals) have been found to reduce heart disease.

Do you drink alcoholic beverages? What type of alcohol do you drink? How much? How often?
Excessive alcohol intake has been associated with hypertension, as well as the development of cardiomyopathy. Moderate alcohol intake is defined as two drinks per day for men and one drink per day for women and those over 65 years of age. One drink is defined as 12 oz of beer, 5 oz of wine, or 1.5 oz of 80-proof distilled spirits.

Do you consume caffeine? In coffee? Chocolate? Soft drinks? How much caffeine do you consume? How often?
Excessive caffeine intake can cause tachycardia, which can increase the workload of the heart.

Do you smoke or have you been a smoker in the past? If yes, what forms of tobacco do (did) you use (cigarettes, cigars, pipe, marijuana, smokeless or chewing tobacco)? How often do you use tobacco? Have you ever quit smoking? If yes, how did you accomplish it and for what length of time? Are you interested in quitting smoking?
Nicotine in tobacco causes vasoconstriction, which may decrease blood flow to extremities and increase blood pressure, both of which increase the workload on the heart. Clients who previously have successfully stopped their tobacco use may be more easily convinced to repeat their success. Clients must be interested in stopping tobacco use; otherwise, there is little motivation to change behavior. Perhaps educating them about the negative effects of nicotine on the cardiovascular system will provide some motivation.

Past Medical History

As a child did you have congenital heart disease or heart defect?

Data from past medical history gives information about clinical findings to anticipate.

During childhood did you have "growing pains," unexplained joint pains? Recurrent tonsillitis? Rheumatic fever? Heart murmur?

These questions relate to diagnosis of rheumatic fever that may have contributed to rheumatoid arthritis or rheumatic heart disease, which gives information about clinical findings to anticipate.

Have you been told that you have high levels of cholesterol or elevated triglycerides?

High levels of serum lipids line the arteries, which may impede blood flow to tissues and increases workload on the heart.

Have you ever had surgery on your heart? On your blood vessels? If so, what procedure was done? When was it done? How successful was the surgery?

Knowledge of past surgical procedures may provide additional information about possible cardiovascular problems. These data also explain the presence of scars you will observe on examination.

Have you ever had any tests on your heart? Electrocardiogram (EKG or ECG), stress EKG, or other heart tests? When were the tests performed? What did the tests reveal? What, if any, treatment did you receive?

These tests provide objective measures that provide baseline data on the health of the client's heart.

Family History

Is there anyone in your family who has a history of diabetes, heart disease, hyperlipidemia, or hypertension, especially among young and middle-aged relatives? Is so, who?

These conditions are risk factors for heart disease and have familial tendencies, especially among first-degree relatives.

PROBLEM-BASED HISTORY

The focus of the history includes descriptions of chest pain, shortness of breath, cough, urinating during the night (nocturia), fatigue, fainting (syncope), swelling of the extremities, and leg pain. As with symptoms in all areas of health assessment, a symptom analysis is completed that includes the location, quality, quantity, chronology, setting, associated manifestations, and alleviating and aggravating factors (see Box 3-3 in Chapter 3).

Chest Pain

Where are you feeling the chest pain? What does the pain feel like? Does the pain radiate to any location? How severe is the pain on a scale of 0 to 10?

The origin of chest pain may be pulmonary, musculoskeletal, or gastrointestinal rather than cardiac. Table 13-1 describes different types of chest pain. If clients indicate that they are having active chest pain, the nurse assesses quickly to determine the need for immediate treatment.

Angina is an important symptom of coronary artery disease, which indicates myocardial ischemia due to a lack of oxygen to meet the myocardium's demand. Women may experience pain or discomfort in the center of the chest or in the arms, back, neck, jaw or stomach (*www.nhlbi.nih.gov,* 2008).

When did the pain start? Is the pain intermittent or constant? If intermittent, how long does it last?

These questions help distinguish different types of chest pain. See Table 13-1, Differentiation of Chest Pain.

What symptoms have you noticed along with the pain? Sweating? Turning pale or gray? Heart skipping beats or racing? Shortness of breath? Nausea or vomiting? Dizziness? Anxiety?

These associated symptoms frequently accompany a myocardial infarction in men. The symptoms reported by women may include sweating, nausea, light headedness, or shortness of breath as warning signs of a myocardial infarction (*www. nhlbi.nih.gov,* 2008).

What factors preceded the pain? Exercise? Rest? Highly emotional situations? Eating? Sexual intercourse?

Chest pain that begins during exertion such as exercise and then diminishes after exertion may indicate an inability of the coronary arteries to provide adequate blood to the myocardium during exertion.

What makes the pain worse? Moving the arms or neck? Deep breathing? Lying flat? Exercise?

The chest pain from pericarditis is aggravated by deep breathing, coughing, or lying supine. Chest pain from muscle strain may be aggravated by movement of arms.

What relieves the pain? Rest? Nitroglycerin? How many nitroglycerin tablets does it take to relieve chest pain?

These questions assess for alleviating factors. Chest pain that is relieved by nitroglycerin may be caused by myocardial ischemia, whereas chest pain that is not relieved by four or more nitroglycerin tablets taken 5 minutes apart may be caused by myocardial infarction.

TABLE 13-1 *Differentiation of Chest Pain*

CAUSE	LOCATION	QUALITY OF PAIN	QUANTITY OF PAIN	CHRONOLOGY	ASSOCIATED MANIFESTATIONS	AGGRAVATING FACTORS	ALLEVIATING FACTORS
Stable angina	Precordial or retrosternal, radiates to L > R arm, jaw, interscapular or epigastrium not above C3 or below T10	Pressure, burning, dull, or sharp	Variable, usually worse with activity	>1 min or <1 hr	Dyspnea, diaphoresis, palpitations, nausea, weakness	Physical exertion, emotional stress, cold	Rest, nitroglycerin, beta-blocker, calcium channel blocker
Unstable angina/ myocardial infarction	Precordial or retrosternal, radiates to L > R arm, jaw, interscapular or epigastrium not above C3 or below T10	Pressure, squeezing, crushing; burning, dull, or sharp	10 of 10 on pain scale	Sudden onset or progressing <30-40 min for unstable angina, >1 hr to 2-3 days for MI	Dyspnea, diaphoresis, palpitations, nausea, weakness	Chest pain during exercise or at rest	Beta-blocker, aspirin, heparin, oxygen
Cocaine-induced chest pain	Similar to myocardial infarction	Sharp, pressure-like, squeezing	Severe 8 to 10 of 10 on pain scale	Gradual onset over minutes lasting minutes to hours	Tachycardia, tachypnea, hypertension	During and shortly after cocaine use	Nitroglycerin or calcium channel blockers
Mitral valve prolapse	Anywhere in chest, localized or diffuse; does not radiate	Variable, often sharp or "kick"	Variable within same client	Sudden, recurrent onset. Lasts seconds or persists for days	Often asymptomatic; palpitations when lying on left side, dyspnea, dizziness	Usually nonexertional, occasionally positional	Position change, nitroglycerin, analgesics
Acute pericarditis	Precordial, posterior neck, trapezius muscle	Boring, oppressive, pleuritic, or positional	Moderate, 4 to 6 of 10 on pain scale	Onset hours to days, lasts hours to weeks	Fever, dyspnea, orthopnea, friction rub	Reclining	Leaning forward
Panic disorder	Localized retrosternally, abdomen	Tightness, vague, diffuse; unrelated to exertion	May be described as disabling	Lasts 30 min or more	Hyperventilation, fatigue, anorexia, emotional strain	Emotional strain	Variable by client
Peptic ulcer disease	Epigastric radiating to lower bilateral chest (T6 to T10)	Burning, gnawing	Moderate, 4 to 6 of 10 on pain scale	Gradual, recurrent onset, lasts hours	Nausea, abdominal tenderness	Empty stomach	Food, antacids, histamine₂ (H₂) blocker
Esophageal reflux	Midepigastric to xiphoid area, C7 to T12, radiates to neck, ear, or jaw	Burning, pressure-like, squeezing	Moderate to severe	Spontaneous onset, lasts minutes to days	Dysphagia	Spicy or acidic meal, alcohol, lying supine	Oral fluids, belching, antacids, nitroglycerin, H₂ blocker
Costochronditis (inflammation of rib or cartilage)	Second to fourth costochondral junction, xiphoid, radiates to precordium, arms, shoulders	Variable	Variable	Gradual onset, constant pain lasts for days	None	Coughing, deep breathing, laughing, sneezing	Localized heat, analgesics, antiinflammatories

Adapted with permission from Hill B, and Geraci SA: A diagnostic approach to chest pain based on history and ancillary evaluation, *Nurse Pract* 23(4):20-45, 1998 © Springhouse Corporation. www.springnet.com.

Shortness of Breath

How long have you had shortness of breath? Do you feel short of breath now?

Dyspnea may be caused by respiratory or cardiac problems. A gradual onset may be caused by heart failure that develops slowly from backup of fluid from the heart into the alveoli.

When does the shortness of breath happen? How often does it occur? How long does it last?

These questions determine the frequency and duration of dyspnea as well as the extent to which dyspnea interferes with daily activities and the extent to which daily activities cause dyspnea.

Does the shortness of breath interfere with your daily activities? How many level blocks can you walk before you become short of breath? How many blocks could you walk 6 months ago?

Dyspnea that interferes with activities of daily living may require the client to use supplemental oxygen. If the distance the client can to walk is decreased, it is a sign that the dyspnea is getting worse. Notice if the client has to take a breath in middle of sentences (see Box 12-2 in Chapter 12).

Do you have any other symptoms with the shortness of breath (e.g., do your feet swell during the day when you are up)?

Dependent edema seen in the ankles or feet may develop because of right-sided heart failure.

What makes the shortness of breath worse? Walking upstairs? Lying down? How many pillows do you require when you lie down to sleep? Do you sleep in a recliner?

Walking up stairs increases the workload of the heart. When dyspnea becomes worse on lying down, the term *orthopnea* is used. Orthopnea occurs when a person must sit up or stand to breathe easily. The number of pillows necessary to relieve the orthopnea is documented (e.g., *two-pillow orthopnea* means the client must elevate his or her chest with two pillows to breathe easily). Some clients sleep in a recliner for elevation rather than using pillows.

When these episodes of shortness of breath occur, what do you do to breathe more easily?

Determine the effectiveness of the action(s) to relieve dyspnea. This information may be helpful in planning future treatment strategies.

Cough

When did your cough start? How often do you cough? Do you cough up anything? What does it look like?

Coughing up blood (hemoptysis) is a symptom of mitral stenosis, as well as of pulmonary disorders. White, frothy sputum may be a sign of pulmonary edema that occurs with left-sided heart failure.

Is your cough associated with position (more coughing when lying down), with anxiety, or with talking or activity? What makes it worse? What actions do you take to relieve the cough?

Coughing more when lying down may indicate heart failure. Knowing how the client relieves the cough may help identify treatment strategies.

Urinating During the Night

For how long have you been getting up during the night to urinate? How many times a night do you get up to urinate?

Nocturia occurs with heart failure in persons who are ambulatory during the day. Lying down at night creates a fluid shift by gravity that promotes the reabsorption of fluid and increases the need to urinate. Taking a diuretic prior to bedtime may also contribute to nocturia. This can be resolved by changing the time the diuretic is taken.

What have you done to prevent this from happening? How successful have your efforts been?

Stopping fluid intake within a few hours of bed or changing time of taking diuretic may help prevent nocturia. This information may guide future teaching and treatment strategies.

Fatigue

When do you notice fatigue? Was the onset sudden or gradual? Is the fatigue worse in the morning or evening? Are you too tired to take part in normal activities?

When cardiac output is decreased, fatigue results. It is generally worse in the evening. In a study of 515 women who had myocardial infarctions, 71% reported unusual fatigue, 48% reported sleep disturbance, and 42% reported dyspnea. Many women in the study reported indigestion and weakness in the arms, but there was variability in the frequency and severity of symptoms (*www.nih.gov,* 2003). Fatigue from other causes—for example, psychogenic (depression or anxiety)—occurs all day or is worse in the morning and varies by location. Fatigue from anemia lasts all day. Fatigue from anemia and heart disease occurs gradually, whereas fatigue from acute blood loss occurs more rapidly.

Do you take iron pills? Do you eat foods with iron, such as green leafy vegetables and liver? For women: Do you have a heavy menstrual flow?

These questions relate to iron deficiency anemia, which can cause fatigue. Women may have iron deficiency from monthly blood loss.

Have you had any other symptoms associated with the fatigue, such as rapid heart rate, headache, pale skin, sore tongue or lips, or changes in your nails?

Fatigue and exertional dyspnea are manifestations of mild anemia and heart failure. Additional signs of tachycardia—headache; pallor; brittle, spoon-shaped nails; glossitis (inflammation of the tongue); and cheilitis (inflammation of the lips)—occur with moderate to severe anemia.

Have you noticed any unusual feelings in your feet and hands, muscle weakness, or trouble thinking?
Neurologic symptoms in addition to those described previously may indicate anemia from vitamin B$_{12}$ deficiency.

Fainting

What were you doing just before you fainted? Did you feel dizzy? Did you lose consciousness?
A brief lapse of consciousness is termed *syncope*. When syncope occurs with activity or position changes and causes dizziness, it may be due to hypotension or inadequate blood flow to the brain.

Has this happened to you before? How often has this occurred?
These questions determine frequency of syncope.

Was fainting preceded by any other symptoms? Nausea? Chest pain? Headache? Sweating? Rapid heart rate? Confusion? Numbness? Hunger? Ringing in your ears?
These questions attempt to determine whether the cause of fainting is a cardiovascular, a neurologic, or an inner ear problem. It may be due to small emboli in the cerebral circulation. Emboli may be the result of atrial fibrillation, valvular disease, or cardiac dysrhythmias. Cerebral emboli may cause a stroke, resulting in reports of headache, confusion, and numbness. Ask about tinnitus to rule out Ménière's disease.

HEALTH PROMOTION *Cardiovascular Disease*

Cardiovascular disease is the leading cause of death and a major cause of disability in the United States, contributing to increases in health care costs. Cardiovascular diseases include coronary artery disease and myocardial infarction, stroke, hypertension, hyperlipidemia, and peripheral vascular diseases.

Goals and Objectives—*Healthy People 2010*
The overall *Healthy People 2010* goal related to cardiovascular disease is to improve cardiovascular health and quality of life through the prevention, detection, and treatment of risk factors; early identification and treatment of heart attacks and strokes; and prevention of recurrent cardiovascular events.

Recommendations to Reduce Risk (Primary Prevention)
American Heart Association
Smoking cessation (see Health Promotion: Tobacco Use in Chapter 12).
Diet: (a) Limit intake of high-cholesterol, saturated fats; (b) promote diet high in fruits, vegetables, and grains; (c) limit alcohol intake to two or fewer drinks per day for men and no drinks or one drink per day for women; and (d) limit salt intake to less than 6 g/day.
Weight: Achieve and maintain a desirable body weight (body mass index [BMI] between 18.5 and 24.9).
Low-dose aspirin: 75 to 160 mg/day for those with higher risk for cardiovascular disease.
Physical activity: At least 30 minutes of moderate intensity physical activity on most days of the week.
Blood pressure control.
Blood lipid management.
Diabetes management: See Health Promotion/Health Protection: Diabetes Mellitus in Chapter 9.

Screening Recommendations (Secondary Prevention)
U.S. Preventive Services Task Force
Blood pressure screening:
    Recommends screening for hypertension for all children and adults. Optimal interval for screening has not been

determined and is left to clinical discretion. It is suggested that blood pressure measurement be performed during office visits for children and adolescents. For normotensive adults, blood pressure measurement is suggested at least every 2 years; for adults with known hypertension, more frequent intervals are recommended.
Lipid-level screening:
    Strongly recommends routine screening for men age 35 and older and women age 45 and older for lipid disorders.
    Recommends screening for younger adults (men 20 to 35 years and women 20 to 45 years) for lipid disorders if they have other risk factors for CHD (family history of cardiovascular disease before age 50 in male relatives or age 60 in female relatives; family history of hyperlipidemia; diabetes; and multiple other risk factors, including tobacco use, hypertension).
    Optimal interval for screening is uncertain; reasonable options include every 5 years (more frequently for individuals who have lipid levels warranting therapy and less frequently for individuals at low risk who have repeatedly low or normal lipid levels).

Tertiary Prevention
American Heart Association
Antihypertensive agents are recommended as appropriate for those with hypertension.
Lipid-lowering drug therapy is recommended as appropriate for those with elevated low-density lipoprotein cholesterol.
Hypoglycemic therapy is recommended as appropriate for those with diabetes mellitus.

Data from Pearson et al: AHA guidelines for primary prevention of cardiovascular disease and stroke: 2002 update, *Circulation* 106:388-391, 2002; US Department of Health and Human Services: *Healthy People 2010: understanding and improving health,* ed 2, Washington, DC, 2000, US Government Printing Office (available at *www.healthypeople.gov*); US Preventive Services Task Force: *Guide to clinical preventive services,* ed 3, 2003 (available at *www.ahrq.gov*).

Swelling of Extremities

Where is the swelling located? Arms or Legs? Unilateral or bilateral?

Edema of both legs may be caused by fluid overload from systemic disease (e.g., heart failure, renal failure, or liver disease). Unilateral edema of an extremity may be lymphedema caused by occlusion of lymph channels (e.g., elephantiasis or trauma) or surgical removal of lymph channels (e.g., after mastectomy). Localized edema of one leg may be caused by venous insufficiency from varicosities or thrombophlebitis

What makes the swelling go away? Does elevating your arms or feet reduce the swelling? Does the swelling disappear after a night's sleep?

Edema that increases during the day and decreases at night or with elevation may be related to venous stasis that may occur with right-sided heart failure. Compression garments for the arms or legs may reduce lymphedema or venous insufficiency.

Are there any symptoms associated with the swelling? Shortness of breath? Weight gain? Warmth? Discoloration?

Dyspnea may be due to heart failure. Weight gain occurs anytime there is fluid retention regardless of cause. Warmth and redness may indicate an inflammatory process, whereas discoloration and ulceration may indicate ischemia.

For women: Is the swelling associated with your menstrual period?

Hormonal contraceptives may be associated with thrombophlebitis, which may cause unilateral leg edema. Changes in estrogen and progesterone blood levels can contribute to fluid retention, resulting in dependent edema.

Leg Cramps or Pain

Describe the pain and its location. Feet? Calf? Thighs? Buttocks? How severe is the pain on a scale of 0 to 10? What makes the pain worse? What relieves the pain?

Pain from arterial insufficiency is commonly felt in the calf but may occur in other locations mentioned. Arterial insufficiency produces pain that worsens with activity, especially prolonged walking. Leg pain that occurs while walking and that is relieved by rest is termed *intermittent claudication*. This occurs when the artery is about 50% occluded. As the insufficiency becomes worse, the client reports pain when walking that is not relieved after rest. This is termed *rest pain*. Leg pain caused by arterial insufficiency is worse when legs are elevated and improves when legs are in a dependent position. By contrast, pain due to venous insufficiency intensifies with prolonged standing or sitting in one position. Pain is worse when legs are in a dependent position and is relieved when legs are elevated. Discomfort increases throughout the day, being worse at the end of the day.

Have you noticed any changes in the skin of your legs, such as coldness, pallor, hair loss, sores, redness or warmth over the veins, or visible veins?

These signs may indicate arterial insufficiency of the legs.

EXAMINATION

ROUTINE TECHNIQUES

ASSESS General Appearance
- INSPECT for general appearance, skin color, and ⚷ breathing effort.

ASSESS the Peripheral Vascular System
- PALPATE temporal and carotid pulses.
- INSPECT jugular vein.
- MEASURE blood pressure. ⚷
- INSPECT and PALPATE the upper extremities. ⚷
- PALPATE upper extremity pulses. ⚷
- INSPECT and PALPATE the lower extremities. ⚷
- PALPATE lower extremity pulses. ⚷

ASSESS the Heart
- INSPECT the anterior chest wall.
- PALPATE apical pulse. ⚷
- AUSCULTATE heart sounds. ⚷
- INTERPRET the Electrocardiogram of the conduction of the heart.

SPECIAL CIRCUMSTANCES OR ADVANCED PRACTICE

ASSESS the Peripheral Vascular System
- AUSCULTATE the carotid arteries.
- ESTIMATE jugular venous pressure. ★
- PALPATE the epitrochlear lymph nodes.
- PALPATE the lower extremities.
- PALPATE the inguinal lymph nodes.
- CALCULATE the ankle-brachial index.
- ASSESS for varicose veins. ★

ASSESS the Heart
- PALPATE the precordium. ★
- PERCUSS the heart borders. ★

EQUIPMENT NEEDED
Stethoscope • Sphygmomanometer • Tape measure • Penlight • Tongue blade and ruler • Marking pen or pencil and centimeter ruler (optional) • Doppler and conductivity gel

⚷ = core examination skill   ★ = advanced practice

PROCEDURES AND TECHNIQUES WITH NORMAL FINDINGS	ABNORMAL FINDINGS

ROUTINE TECHNIQUES

ASSESS General Appearance

INSPECT the client for general appearance, skin color, and breathing effort.

Observe the client. He or she should appear at ease and relaxed with skin color appropriate for race and regular, unlabored respirations.

Dyspnea, cyanosis, pallor, and use of accessory muscle to breathe are abnormal findings.

ASSESS the Peripheral Vascular System

PALPATE temporal and carotid pulses for amplitude.

Procedure: For the temporal pulse, palpate over the temporal bone on each side of the head lateral to each eyebrow to assess perfusion and pain (Figs. 13-11 and 13-12).

For the carotid pulse, palpate along the medial edge of the sternocleidomastoid muscle in the lower third of the neck to assess perfusion. Palpate one carotid pulse at a time to avoid reducing blood flow to the brain (Figs. 13-13 and 13-14, and also see Fig. 13-12).

Findings: See Box 13-1, left column.

Tenderness and edema may be found in temporal arteritis. (See Box 13-1, right column.)

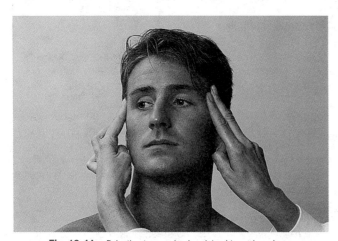

Fig. 13-11 Palpating temporal pulses lateral to each eyebrow.

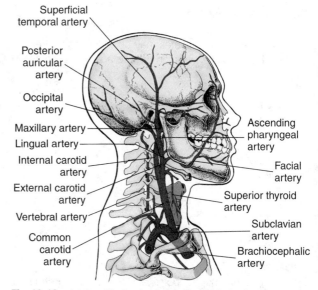

Superficial temporal artery

Posterior auricular artery

Occipital artery

Maxillary artery

Lingual artery

Internal carotid artery

External carotid artery

Vertebral artery

Common carotid artery

Ascending pharyngeal artery

Facial artery

Superior thyroid artery

Subclavian artery

Brachiocephalic artery

Fig. 13-12 Arteries of the head and neck. *(From Thibodeau and Patton, 1999.)*

= core examination skill

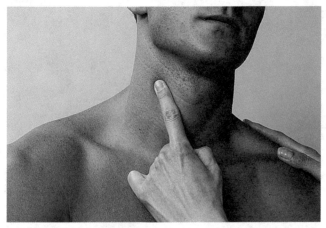

Fig. 13-13   Palpating carotid pulse in the lower third of the neck.

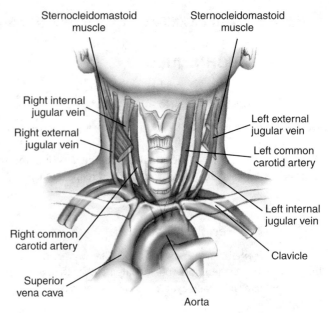

Fig. 13-14   Right and left common carotid arteries that are palpated. *(From Barkauskas, 2002.)*

BOX 13-1 | PALPATING PULSES

Palpate arteries using the finger pads of the first two fingers and applying light pressure. If you press too hard, you will obscure the pulse. Note the rate, rhythm, amplitude, and contour of each pulse. Comparing pulses on each side of the body is customary. When you are unable to palpate a pulse, use a Doppler to amplify the sounds of the pulse (see Fig. 4-21).

Procedures and Techniques

Rate
60 to 100 beats/min (athletes may be as low as 50 beats/min). Pulse rates in women tend to be 5 to 10 beats/min faster than men.

Rhythm
Regular, that is, equal spacing between beats.

Amplitude
Easily palpable, smooth upstroke. Compare the strength of upper extremity pulses with lower extremity and the left with the right.
Pulse amplitude ratings:
0+   Absent
1+   Diminished, barely palpable
2+   Normal
3+   Full volume
4+   Full volume, bounding hyperkinetic

Contour (Outline of the Pulse that is Felt)
Smooth and rounded, a series of unvaried, symmetric pulse strokes.
Note: There may be a slight transient increase in rate during inspiration, especially in clients younger than 40.

Abnormal Findings

Rates above 100 beats/min (tachycardia) or below 60 beats/min (bradycardia) are typically abnormal, although recent exertion, smoking, or anxiety will elevate the rate.

Irregular rhythms without any pattern should be noted. Coupled beats (two beats that occur close together) are abnormal also.
When you palpate an irregular pulse rhythm, note whether there is a pattern to the irregularity. For example, pulses of clients who have premature ventricular contractions (PVC) may have a pattern to the irregularity such as an extra beat every third heart beat. This is documented as a *regular irregularity.* By contrast, pulses of clients who have atrial fibrillation may not have any pattern to the irregularity. This is documented as an *irregular irregularity.*

Note any exaggerated or bounding upstroke or, conversely, pulses that are weak, small, or thready, or where the peak is prolonged. Upstrokes should not vary (seen in pulsus alternans). The force of the beat should not be reduced during inspiration (paradoxic pulse).

PROCEDURES AND TECHNIQUES WITH NORMAL FINDINGS

ABNORMAL FINDINGS

INSPECT the jugular vein for pulsations.

The external jugular vein provides information about the right atrial pressure. *Procedure:* Elevate the head of the bed until venous pulsation in the external jugular vein is seen above the clavicle, close to the insertion of the sternocleido-mastoid muscles. The angle may be 30 to 45 degrees or as high as 90 degrees if venous pressure is elevated. Elevate the client's chin slightly and tilt the head away from the side being examined. Use a penlight to create tangential light across the jugular veins and observe for pulsations (Fig. 13-15).

Finding: The vein itself is not visible, only the pulsations.

Note any fluttering or oscillating of the pulsations. Note irregular rhythms or unusually prominent waves (Fig. 13-16). These may indicate right-sided heart failure.

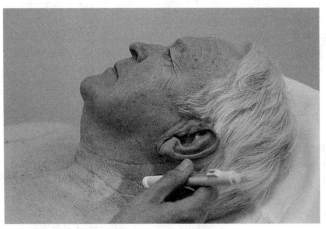

Fig. 13-15   Tangential light to view jugular veins and pulsations.

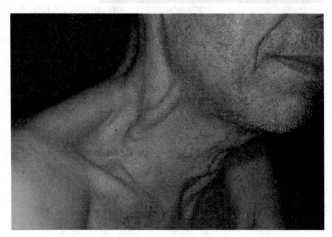

Fig. 13-16   Neck vein distention. *(From Swartz, 2006.)*

MEASURE blood pressure.

(See Chapter 4 for procedure.) The blood pressure frequently is taken in both arms during an initial visit for comparison. Blood pressure varies with gender, body weight, and time of day, but the upper limits for adults are less than 120 mm Hg systolic, less than 80 mm Hg diastolic, and 30 to 40 mm Hg pulse pressure. The pressure should not vary more than 5 to 10 mm Hg systolic between the two arms (Fig. 13-17).

Note elevated systolic or diastolic pressures (hypertension) and lowered systolic or diastolic pressures (hypotension). Also note significant discrepancies in measurements between the two arms.

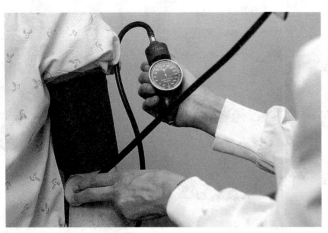

Fig. 13-17   Assessing blood pressure.

= core examination skill

PROCEDURES AND TECHNIQUES WITH NORMAL FINDINGS

ETHNIC & CULTURAL VARIATIONS

African Americans have generally higher blood pressure readings than whites. These higher readings are thought to be related to differences in renin activity and the regulation of angiotensin II, which acts as a vasoconstrictor. African Americans also retain sodium and chloride better in heat-related situations than do whites.

If the client offers a history of dizziness or is taking antihypertensive medications, measure the client's blood pressure and heart rate while he or she is supine, sitting, and standing. The blood pressure is usually lower in the supine position than sitting. The blood pressure taken when standing may be lower than it is when sitting by 10 to 15 mm Hg systolic and 5 mm Hg diastolic.

INSPECT and PALPATE the upper extremities for skin turgor.
Pinch an area of the skin between your finger and thumb and then release the skin. It should immediately fall back into place. Skin turgor should be elastic without tenting or edema (see Fig. 10-5).

ABNORMAL FINDINGS

A decrease in systolic blood pressure greater than 20 mm Hg and symptoms such as dizziness indicate orthostatic (postural) hypotension. Diastolic pressure may decrease also. This may be due to a fluid volume deficit, drugs (e.g., antihypertensives), or prolonged bed rest.

When the skin does not immediately fall back into place, it is termed *tenting* and is an indication of reduced fluid in the interstitial space from fluid volume deficit. When the indentation of the thumb or finger remains in the skin, it is termed *pitting edema* and is an indication of excess fluid in the interstitial space (Fig. 13-18). Refer to Table 13-2 for interpretation of edema.

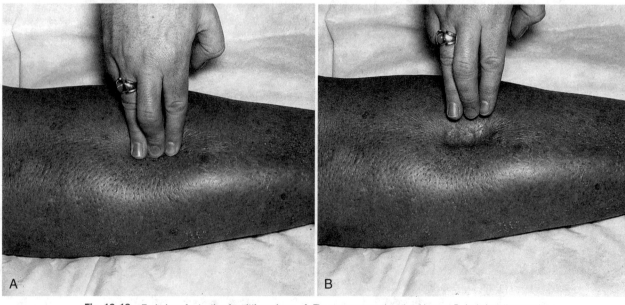

Fig. 13-18   Technique for testing for pitting edema. A, The nurse presses into the shin area. **B,** An indentation remains after the fingers are lifted when pitting edema is present. *(From Swartz, 2006.)*

= core examination skill

TABLE 13-2 *Pitting Edema Scale*

SCALE	DESCRIPTION	"MEASUREMENT"*
1+	A barely perceptible pit	2 mm (3/32 in)
2+	A deeper pit, rebounds in a few seconds	4 mm (5/32 in)
3+	A deep pit, rebounds in 10-20 seconds	6 mm (1/4 in)
4+	A deeper pit, rebounds in >30 seconds	8 mm (5/16 in)

+1　　2 mm　　+2　　4 mm　　+3　　6 mm　　+4　　8 mm

G.J. Wassilchenko

Descriptions column data from Kirton C: Assessing edema, *Nursing 96* 26(7):54, 1996.
Illustrations from Canobbio MM: *Cardiovascular disorders,* St. Louis, 1990, Mosby.
*"Measurement" is in quotation marks because depth of edema is rarely actually measured but
is included as a frame of reference.

PROCEDURES AND TECHNIQUES WITH NORMAL FINDINGS

INSPECT and PALPATE the upper extremities for symmetry, skin integrity, color, and temperature, capillary refill, and color and angle of the nail beds.

Procedure: Compare the sizes of the upper and lower arms for symmetry and examine the skin color. Use the back of your hand to assess skin temperature. Assess capillary refill by gently squeezing pads of fingers or nails until they blanche. Release pressure and observe capillary refill, that is, how many seconds it takes for the original color to appear.

Findings: Arms should appear symmetric without edema. Skin should be intact without pallor or redness. Nail beds should be pink, with an angle of 160 degrees at the nail bed. Capillary refill should be 2 seconds or less.

ABNORMAL FINDINGS

When one arm is larger in circumference than the other, it could be due to lymphedema. Thickening skin, skin tears, and ulceration are abnormal findings. Arterial insufficiency may cause cold extremities in a warm environment and is abnormal. Note marked pallor or mottling when the extremity is elevated or any ulcerated finger tips. A capillary refill time greater than 2 seconds indicates poor perfusion. Clubbing of fingers (angle of nail disappears, becoming greater than 160 degrees) indicates chronic hypoxia (Fig. 13-19).

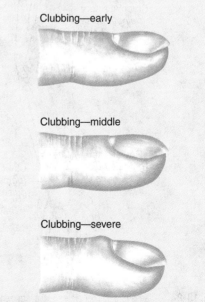

Clubbing—early

Clubbing—middle

Clubbing—severe

Fig. 13-19 Clubbing of fingers. *(From Canobbio, 1990.)*

= core examination skill

PROCEDURES AND TECHNIQUES WITH NORMAL FINDINGS

PALPATE brachial and radial pulses for rate, rhythm, amplitude, and contour.

Procedure: For the brachial pulse, palpate in the groove between the biceps and triceps muscle just medial to the biceps tendon at the antecubital fossa (in the bend of the elbow) (Figs. 13-20 and 13-22).

For the radial pulse, palpate at the radial or thumb side of the forearm at the wrist (Fig. 13-21; see Fig. 13-22).

Findings: The left column of Box 13-1 has expected findings for pulses.

ABNORMAL FINDINGS

See the right column of Box 13-1 for abnormal findings. Clients who take certain medications, such as beta-adrenergic antagonists and digoxin, may have slow pulse rates because of the medication.

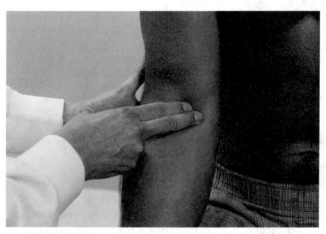

Fig. 13-20 Palpating brachial pulse at the antecubital fossa.

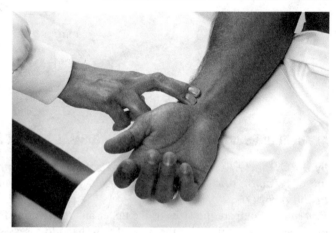

Fig. 13-21 Palpating radial pulse on the thumb side of the forearm at the wrist.

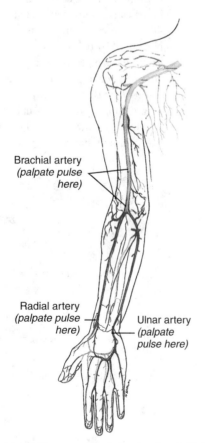

Brachial artery
(palpate pulse here)

Radial artery
(palpate pulse here)

Ulnar artery
(palpate pulse here)

Fig. 13-22 Arteries of the upper extremity that are palpated. *(Modified from Francis and Martin, 1975.)*

FREQUENTLY ASKED QUESTIONS

Why aren't all pulses assessed for rate, rhythm, contour, and amplitude?

The rate and rhythm of all pulses will be the same because the pulse is generated from the contraction of the myocardium. Radial pulses are the ones most frequently assessed for rate, rhythm, contour, and amplitude. Dorsalis pedis pulses are routinely palpated for assessment of lower extremity perfusion. Palpation of other pulses is performed to ensure that the tissues distal to those pulses are perfused with blood.

PROCEDURES AND TECHNIQUES WITH NORMAL FINDINGS

ABNORMAL FINDINGS

INSPECT and PALPATE the lower extremities for skin turgor.

Pinch an area of the skin between your finger and thumb and then release the skin as was performed on the upper extremities. It should immediately fall back into place, indicating elasticity. Skin turgor should be elastic without tenting or edema (see Fig. 10-5).

When the skin does not immediately fall back into place, it is termed *tenting* and is an indication of reduced fluid in the interstitial space from fluid volume deficit. When the indentation of the thumb or finger remains in the skin, it is termed *edema* and is an indication of excess fluid in the interstitial space (see Fig. 13-18). Refer to Table 13-2 for interpretation of edema.

INSPECT and PALPATE the lower extremities for symmetry, skin integrity, color, and temperature, hair distribution, capillary refill, color and angle of nail beds, tenderness, and superficial veins.

Procedure: Follow the same procedures performed on the upper extremities for assessment of symmetry, integrity, color, and temperature and capillary refill. Observe the hair distribution. Some women shave leg hair, but others do not. With the client's legs dependent, observe for superficial veins that appear dilated. Palpate the legs lightly for tenderness.

Findings: Legs should appear symmetric without edema or superficial veins. The skin should be intact without pallor or redness. The skin should feel warm without tenderness. Capillary refill should be 2 seconds or less. Nails should be pink, with an angle of 160 degrees at the nail bed.

Abnormalities are similar to those described for the upper extremities. Note marked pallor or mottling when the extremity is elevated or any ulcerated digit tips. Arterial insufficiency may cause a decrease in or lack of hair peripherally or skin that appears thin, shiny, and taut. Note if there is tenderness on palpation or the sensation of "stocking anesthesia," wherein the legs feel numb in a pattern resembling stockings. Note if there are distended veins in the anteromedial aspect of the thigh and lower leg or on the posterolateral aspect of the calf from the knee to the ankle. Varicose veins appear as dilated, often tortuous veins when legs are in a dependent position.

If edema is anticipated, measure the circumference of both thighs and calves with a tape measure as a baseline. Measure the same distance from the top of the patella to mark the location on the thigh for measuring the circumference. Measure the other leg in the same location. Use the same procedure for measuring the circumference of the calf. Compare the measurements of each leg: they should be similar. There should be distention of veins in the dependent position, and the venous valves may appear as nodular bulges. The veins collapse with elevation of the limbs. A positive Homan's sign (pain in the calf on forced dorsiflexion) was previously considered an indicator of thrombophlebitis, but it is positive in only 10% of clients with deep vein thrombosis and false positives are frequent (Church, 2000).

Impaired venous blood flow may cause edema (see Fig. 13-18). Note any edema of one or both legs (especially if one calf appears larger than the other), tenderness on palpation, warmth, or redness (see Table 13-2). Clients who are immobile with reduced sensation, such as clients with spinal cord injury, may manifest an increase in thigh circumference as the first sign of deep vein thrombosis. When one leg is larger in circumference than the other, it could be due to lymphedema. Chronic venous stasis may be bilateral (Fig. 13-23).

If arterial insufficiency is suspected, have the client lie down. Elevate his or her legs 12 inches (30 cm) above the level of the heart. Then ask the client to flex and dorsiflex the feet for 60 seconds. The feet should exhibit mild pallor. Next have the client sit up and dangle the legs. Original color should return in about 10 seconds, with the foot veins filling up in about 15 seconds. (*Note:* This

Note any marked pallor in one or both feet, any delayed return of color or mottled appearance, delay in filling of the veins, or marked redness in the dependent foot (or hand). Use the 5 P's to

PROCEDURES AND TECHNIQUES WITH NORMAL FINDINGS

can also be done with the arms and hands.). Calculate the ankle-brachial index when additional data are needed as described later in this chapter

🗝 *PALPATE femoral, popliteal, posterior tibial, and dorsalis pedis pulses for amplitude.*

Procedure: For the femoral pulse, palpate below the inguinal ligament, midway between the symphysis pubis and anterior superior iliac to assess for perfusion. To find the femoral pulse, move inward toward the genitalia. You can locate the anatomy using the mnemonic NAVEL: *N*, nerve; *A*, artery; *V*, vein; *E*, empty space; *L*, lymph. Firm compression may be needed for obese clients (Figs. 13-24 and 13-28).

remember abnormal findings: pulseless, pale, paresthesia, pain, and poikilothermia (cold).

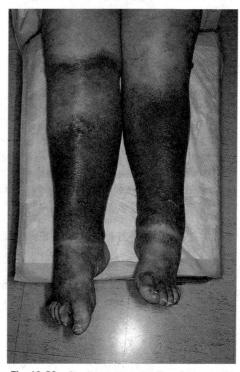

Fig. 13-23   Chronic venous stasis. *(From Swartz, 2006.)*

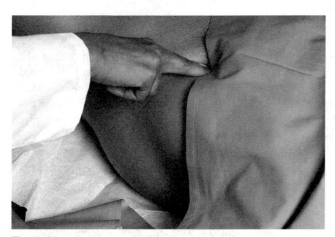

Fig. 13-24   Palpating femoral pulse below the inguinal ligament between the symphysis pubis and anterior superior iliac crest. *(From Canobbio, 1990.)*

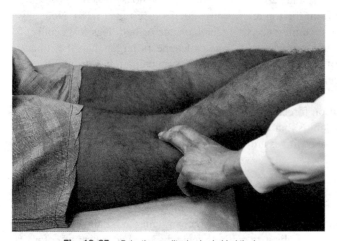

Fig. 13-25   Palpating popliteal pulse behind the knee.

🗝 = core examination skill

PROCEDURES AND TECHNIQUES WITH NORMAL FINDINGS

For the popliteal pulse, palpate the popliteal artery behind the knee in the popliteal fossa to assess perfusion (Figs. 13-25 and 13-28). This pulse may be difficult to find. Having the client in the prone position and flexing the leg slightly may help in finding this pulse.

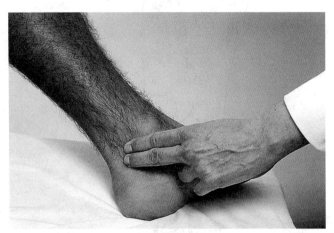

Fig. 13-26   Palpating posterior tibial pulse on the inner aspect of the ankle.

For the posterior tibial artery, palpate on the inner aspect of the ankle below and slightly behind the medial malleolus (ankle bone) to assess for perfusion (Figs. 13-26 and 13-28).

For the dorsalis pedis artery, palpate lightly over the dorsum of the foot between the extension tendons of the first and second toes to assess for perfusion (Figs. 13-27 and 13-28).

Findings: See Box 13-1, left column.

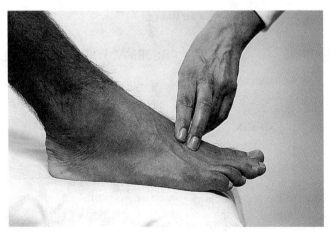

Fig. 13-27   Palpating dorsalis pedis pulse on top of the foot between the first and second toes.

ABNORMAL FINDINGS

See Box 13-1, right column.

Impaired peripheral pulses may indicate arterial insufficiency.

FREQUENTLY ASKED QUESTIONS

How can the nurse assess perfusion if there is a cast or dressing over the pulse site?
Capillary refill time of less than 2 seconds and warm skin validate that there is blood flow to the area. An area that is pale, blue, or black or that is painful or numb to the client is not receiving adequate blood supply.

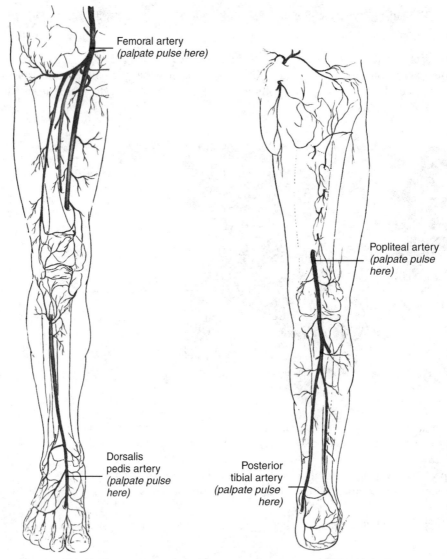

Fig. 13-28 Arteries of the leg that are palpated. *(From Francis and Martin, 1975.)*

PROCEDURES AND TECHNIQUES WITH NORMAL FINDINGS

ASSESS THE HEART

INSPECT the anterior chest wall for contour, pulsations, lifts, heaves, and retractions.

Provide modesty and privacy while inspecting the female client's unclothed chest. Use tangential light to inspect the client's chest at eye level. The chest should be rounded and symmetric. Slight retraction medial to the left midclavicular line at the fourth or fifth intercostal space is expected; this is the apical pulse. This location may be documented as LSB 5ICS. See Box 13-2 for abbreviations of topographic landmarks.

The apical pulse may be visible only when the client sits up and leans forward, bringing the heart closer to the anterior chest. It may be obscured by obesity, large breasts, or muscularity.

ABNORMAL FINDINGS

Note any sternal depression or asymmetry. A retraction is noted when some of the tissue is pulled into the chest on the precordium. Marked retraction of apical space may indicate pericardial disease or right ventricular hypertrophy. Box 13-3 has definitions of lifts, heaves, thrills, and retraction.

Apical pulsation may be observed after exertion, in hyperthyroidism, or in left ventricular hypertrophy. Pulsations may be displaced left, right, or downward because of cardiac anomalies or change in heart size.

BOX 13-2	ABBREVIATIONS FOR TOPOGRAPHIC LANDMARKS
ICS	intercostal space
RICS	right intercostal space
LICS	left intercostal space
SB	sternal border
RSB	right sternal border
LSB	left sternal border
MCL	midclavicular line
RMCL	right midclavicular line
LMCL	left midclavicular line

BOX 13-3   DEFINITIONS OF LIFT, HEAVE, THRILL, AND RETRACTION

A *lift* feels like a more sustained thrust than an expected apical pulse and is felt during systole. A *heave* is a more prominent thrust of the heart against the chest wall during systole. Lifts and heaves may occur from left ventricular hypertrophy due to increased workload. A *thrill* is a palpable vibration over the precordium or artery: it feels like fine, palpable, rushing vibration. A thrill is associated with aortic valve stenosis. *Retraction* of the chest is a visible sinking in of tissues between and around the ribs. Retraction begins in the intercostal spaces. It occurs with increased respiratory effort. If additional effort is needed to fill the lungs, supraclavicular and infraclavicular retraction may be seen.

PROCEDURES AND TECHNIQUES WITH NORMAL FINDINGS

ABNORMAL FINDINGS

PALPATE apical pulse for location.

With the client in a sitting position, palpate over the apex of the heart at the fifth intercostal space, left midclavicular line, using the fingertips (Fig. 13-29). This is the point of maximal impulse (PMI) that corresponds to the left ventricular apex. If the PMI cannot be palpated in this position, repeat the procedure with the client lying supine and also on the left side.

If the client has ventricular hypertrophy, the myocardium is enlarged, which may move the PMI laterally. Clients who have chronic obstructive lung disease have overinflated lungs, which may displace the PMI downward and to the right (Swartz, 2006).

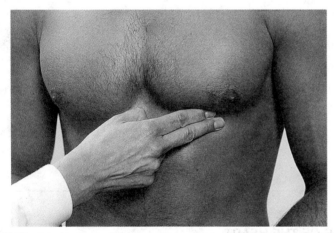

Fig. 13-29   Palpating the apical pulse at the fourth or fifth intercostal space, left midclavicular line.

AUSCULTATE S$_1$ and S$_2$ heart sounds for rate, rhythm, pitch, and splitting.

Procedure: Box 13-4 describes a technique for locating intercostal spaces for auscultation of the heart. All five areas should be auscultated, first with the diaphragm using firm pressure and then with the bell using light pressure. The sounds are generated by valve closure and are best heard where blood flows away from the valve instead of directly over the valve area (Fig. 13-30). Heart sounds may be low pitched, making them difficult to hear (Box 13-5). When first learning heart sounds, you may want to close your eyes to concentrate on each specific sound (i.e., selective listening). Begin with the client sitting upright. A systematic approach is used to listen in the five auscultatory areas, with the client breathing normally and then holding the breath in expiration. This allows you to hear the heart sounds better. Using the diaphragm, begin with the aortic valve area (second ICS, right sternal border [RSB]) (Fig. 13-31, *A*), then the pulmonic valve area (second ICS, LSB) (Fig. 13-31, *B*), then Erb's point (third ICS, LSB) (Fig. 13-31, *C*), then the tricuspid valve area (fourth ICS, LSB)

= core examination skill

PROCEDURES AND TECHNIQUES WITH NORMAL FINDINGS	ABNORMAL FINDINGS

(Fig. 13-31, *D*), and finally the mitral valve area/apical pulse (fifth ICS, left midclavicular line [MCL]) (Fig. 13-31, *E*). Repeat the auscultation of the five areas using the bell of the stethoscope. Box 13-6 has a tip to help you remember which valves you are listening to.

BOX 13-4 **TECHNIQUE FOR LOCATING INTERCOSTAL SPACES FOR AUSCULTATION OF THE HEART**

A systematic approach is needed for this assessment. Some nurses begin at the apex and proceed upward toward the base of the heart, whereas others begin at the base and proceed downward toward the apex. The sequence is irrelevant as long as the assessment is systematic. Listen first with the diaphragm to hear high-pitched sounds, then with the bell to hear low-pitched sounds.

- When auscultating from base to apex, begin at the second intercostal space (ICS). Locate this ICS by palpating the right sternoclavicular joint (where the right clavicle joins the sternum).
- Palpate the first rib and then move down to palpate the space between the first and second ribs: this is the first ICS.
- Continue palpating downward to the space between the second and third ribs. This is the second ICS at the right sternal border (RSB), the auscultatory site for the aortic valve area. This is not the anatomic site of the aortic valve, but the site on the chest wall where sounds produced by the valve are heard best.
- Moving to the left side of the sternum at the second ICS, the area for auscultating the pulmonic valve area is found.
- Remaining at the LSB, move the stethoscope down to the third ICS, which is called *Erb's point,* an area to which pulmonic or aortic sounds frequently radiate. The fourth ICS, LSB is over the tricuspid valve area.
- At the fifth ICS, move the stethoscope laterally to the left midclavicular line, where the mitral valve area is located.

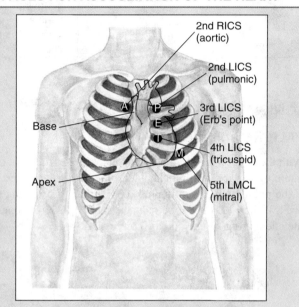

2nd RICS (aortic)
2nd LICS (pulmonic)
3rd LICS (Erb's point)
4th LICS (tricuspid)
5th LMCL (mitral)
Base
Apex

BOX 13-5 **LOW- AND HIGH-PITCHED SOUNDS OF THE HEART**

In Chapter 4 you read that the heart had low-pitched (low-frequency) sounds best heard with the bell of the stethoscope and that breath sounds were high pitched (high frequency), best heard with the diaphragm of the stethoscope. In this chapter you read that S_1 is lower in pitch than S_2 or that S_2 is higher in pitch than S_1 and that bruits are low pitched. How can both statements be true? The pitch of the sounds is relative, depending on which sounds you are comparing. When comparing breath sounds with heart sounds, heart sounds are low pitched. However, when comparing the sounds of S_1 with S_2, the pitch of S_1 is lower than S_2. Now, if you compared the pitch of breath sounds to the pitch of S_2, you would find S_2 is low pitched. These sounds could be put on a continuum from high to low pitch. Breath sounds would be high pitched, S_2 would be a lower pitch than breath sounds but higher than S_1, and S_1 would be the lowest pitch of all three sounds.

FREQUENTLY ASKED QUESTIONS

Why do nurses listen at the right sternal border for the aortic valve when it is located in the left chest?

The sounds made by valves closing are projected away from the valve location. The sounds of the valves closing is heard more accurately over the area on the chest where blood flows after passing through the valve. The arrows in Fig. 13-19 show the direction of the blood flow from the valves.

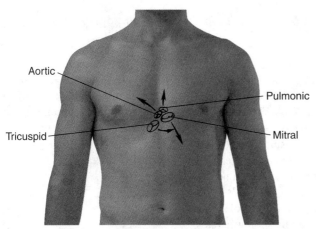

Fig. 13-30 Transmission of closure sounds from the heart valves.

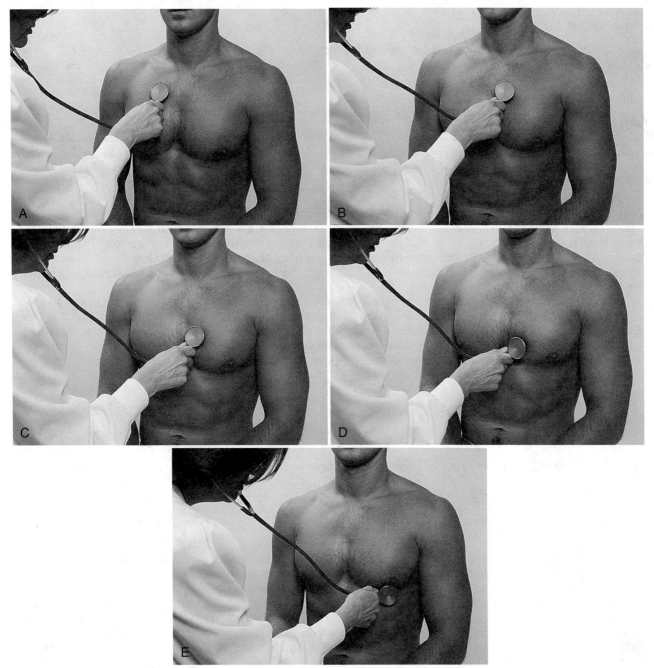

Fig. 13-31 **Position for cardiac auscultation. A,** Aortic area. **B,** Pulmonic area. **C,** Erb's point. **D,** Tricuspid area. **E,** Mitral area.

| PROCEDURES AND TECHNIQUES WITH NORMAL FINDINGS | ABNORMAL FINDINGS |

ASSESS Heart Rate

Count the number of heart beats (S_1 and S_2) heard for one minute for the apical rate. First heart sound (S_1) is made by the closing of the mitral (M1) and tricuspid (T1) valves. (When the heart sounds are described as *lubb-dubb*, the *lubb* represents S_1.) S_1 indicates the beginning of systole. This heart sound should be heard at all sites. S_1 is louder than S_2 at the apex over the tricuspid valve (fourth left ICS) and the mitral valve (fifth left MCL). S_1 is usually lower in pitch than S_2; it is almost synchronous with the carotid pulse. The second heart sound (S_2) is made by the closing of the aortic (A2) and pulmonic (P2) valves. It is described as the *dubb* of *lubb-dubb* and indicates the beginning of diastole. Normal range is 60 to 100 beats/min; conditioned athletes may have slower rates. Normally the heart rate is regular, that is, an equal space between beats.

Rates greater than 100 or less than 60 beats/min are abnormal. Note any irregular rhythm, sporadic or extra beats, or pauses between beats.

See Box 13-1, right column, for abnormal findings.

ASSESS Rhythm

When listening to each heart beat, notice the spacing between beats. There should be equal spacing between each beat.

See Box 13-1, right column, for abnormal findings. Table 13-3 describes abnormal heart sounds.

TABLE 13-3   *Abnormal Heart Sounds*

Abnormal heart sounds and murmurs are described by where they occur in the cardiac cycle. The normal sequence of events in the cardiac cycle can be diagrammed as follows:

$$S_1 \rightarrow \text{systole} \rightarrow S_2 \rightarrow \text{diastole} \rightarrow S_1 \rightarrow \text{etc.}$$

To determine if an abnormal sound occurs in systole or diastole, determine if the sound occurs after S_1 or after S_2.
- During diastole, when 80% of the blood in the atria rapidly fills the ventricles, a third heart sound may be heard (S_3). It is often heard at the apex. An S_3 occurs just after the S_2 and lasts about the same time as it takes to say "me too." The "me" is the S_2 and the "too" is the S_3. An S_3 is normal in children and young adults. However, when an S_3 is heard in adults over 30 years of age, it signifies fluid volume overload to the ventricle that may be due to heart failure or mitral or tricuspid regurgitation (Swartz, 2006).
- At the end of diastole, when atrial contraction completes the filling of the ventricle, a fourth heart sound may be heard (S_4). An S_4 occurs just before the S_1 and lasts about the same time as it takes to say "middle." The "mi" is the S_4 and the "ddle" the S_1. An S_4 is normal in children and young adults. However, when an S_4 is heard in adults over 30 years of age, it signifies a noncompliant or "stiff" ventricle. Hypertrophy of the ventricle precedes a noncompliant ventricle. Also, coronary artery disease is a major cause of a stiff ventricle. Useful mnemonics for remembering the cadence and pathophysiology of the third and fourth heart sounds (Swartz, 2006) are as follows.

SLOSH'ing-in	SLOSH'ing-in	SLOSH'ing-in
S_1 S_2 S_3	S_1 S_2 S_3	S_1 S_2 S_3
a-STIFF'-wall	a-STIFF'-wall	a-STIFF'-wall
S_4 S_1 S_2	S_4 S_1 S_2	S_4 S_1 S_2

Another way to remember the cadence of the S_3 and S_4 heart sounds is using the words "Kentucky" and "Tennessee."

Ken-tuck-y	Ken-tuck-y	Ken-tuck-y
S_1 S_2 S_3	S_1 S_2 S_3	S_1 S_2 S_3
Ten-ness-ee	Ten-ness-ee	Ten-ness-ee
S_4 S_1 S_2	S_4 S_1 S_2	S_4 S_1 S_2

Thus the third and fourth heart sounds can be abnormal when they occur in adults over 30. Both sounds occur in diastole.
- The opening *snap* caused by the opening of the mitral or tricuspid valves is another abnormal sound heard in diastole when either valve is thickened, stenotic, or deformed. The sounds are high-pitched and occur early in diastole.
- In systole, *ejection clicks* may be heard if either the aortic or pulmonic valve is stenotic or deformed. The aortic valve ejection click is heard at either apex or base of the heart and does not change with respiration. The less common pulmonic valve ejection click is heard over the second or third left ICS. It increases with expiration and decreases with inspiration.
- *Pericardial friction rubs* are caused by inflammation of the layers of the pericardial sac. A rubbing sound is usually present in both diastole and systole and is best heard over the apical area.

PROCEDURES AND TECHNIQUES WITH NORMAL FINDINGS

ASSESS Pitch

Note the pitch of the heart sounds. Pitch is the quality of the sound dependent on the relative speed of the vibrations by which it is produced. The first and second heart sounds have low and high pitches, respectively (see Box 13-5).

ASSESS Splitting

Notice whether there is one sound or two for each S_1 and S_2 sound. While the closing of two valves create each heart sound, you should hear only one sound indicating that the valves are closing at the same time.

TABLE 13-4 *Listening to Murmurs*

When you identify a heart murmur, consider the following variables for documentation

Timing and duration	At what part of the cycle is the murmur heard? Is it associated with S_1 or with S_2, or is it continuous?
Pitch	Is it a low or high pitch? Low pitches are best heard with the bell of the stethoscope.
Quality	Refers to the type of sound, including a harsh sound, a raspy machine-like sound, or a vibratory, musical, or blowing sound.
Intensity	Murmur intensity refers to how loud the murmur is: • Grade I is barely audible in a quiet room. • Grade II is quiet but clearly audible. • Grade III is moderately loud. • Grade IV is loud and associated with a thrill. • Grade V is very loud, and a thrill is easily palpable. • Grade VI is very loud, and a thrill is palpable and visible.
Location	Where is the sound heard loudest? Most often, it will be over one of the five anatomic landmarks used to auscultate heart sounds.
Example of documentation	S_1, grade II, low-pitch murmur auscultated at fifth ICS, MCL. No thrill palpable.

ICS, Intercostal space; *MCL,* midclavicular line.

ABNORMAL FINDINGS

An abnormality may be present when the first heart sound seems accented, diminished, or muffled, or when intensity varies with different beats.

When the mitral and tricuspid valves do not close at the same time, S_1 sounds as if it were split into two sounds instead of one. Splitting is heard occasionally in the tricuspid area with deep inspiration and varies from beat to beat, occasionally heard as a narrow split. Note that the fourth heart sound is sometimes mistaken for the splitting of the first heart sound.

Table 13-4 describes variables when a murmur is heard. Table 13-5 describes murmurs caused by valvular defects.

Systolic Murmur. A murmur occurring during the ventricular ejection phase of the cardiac cycle is termed a *systolic murmur.* Most systolic murmurs are caused by obstruction of the outflow of the semilunar valves or by incompetent AV valves. The vibration is heard during all or part of systole. Other causes of systolic murmurs are structural deformities of the aorta or pulmonary arteries, anemia, and thyrotoxicosis (hyperthyroidism). A ventricular septal defect results in a murmur classified as pansystolic or holosystolic because it occupies all of systole.

Diastolic Murmur. A murmur occurring in the filling phase of the cardiac cycle is termed a *diastolic murmur.* Incompetent semilunar valves or stenotic AV valves create diastolic murmurs. These murmurs almost always indicate heart disease. Early diastolic murmurs usually result from insufficiency of a semilunar valve or dilation of the valvular ring. Mid- and late-diastolic murmurs are generally caused by stenosed mitral and tricuspid valves that obstruct blood flow.

TABLE 13-5   *Murmurs Caused by Valvular Defects*

TYPE	DETECTION	QUALITY/PITCH
Systolic Ejection Murmur	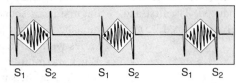	
Aortic stenosis	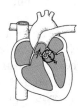 Bell, heard over aortic valve area; ejection sound at second right intercostal border. Radiates to neck, down left sternal border.	Medium pitch, coarse, with crescendo-decrescendo pattern. Pitch low.
Pulmonic stenosis	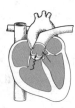 Bell, heard over pulmonic valve; radiates left to neck; thrill at second and third left intercostal spaces.	Same as for aortic stenosis. Pitch medium.
Diastolic Regurgitant Murmur	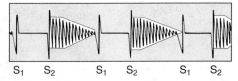	
Aortic regurgitation	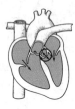 Diaphragm, client sitting and leaning forward. Second right intercostal space radiates to left sternal border.	Blowing in early diastole. Pitch high.
Pulmonic regurgitation	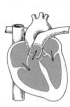 Diaphragm, client sitting or leaning forward. Third and fourth left intercostal spaces.	Blowing. Pitch high or low.

TABLE 13-5   *Murmurs Caused by Valvular Defects—cont'd*

TYPE	DETECTION	QUALITY/PITCH
Diastolic Murmur	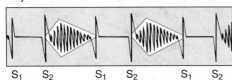	
Mitral stenosis 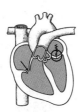	Bell at apex with client in left lateral decubitus position.	Low rumble more intense in early and late diastole. Pitch low.
Tricuspid stenosis 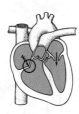	Bell over tricuspid area.	Similar to mitral stenosis but louder on inspiration. Pitch low.
Holosystolic Murmur	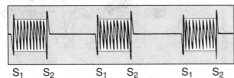	
Mitral regurgitation 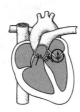	Diaphragm at apex, radiates to left axilla or base.	Harsh blowing quality. Pitch high.
Tricuspid regurgitation 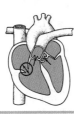	Diaphragm at fifth intercostal space, left lower sternal border.	Blowing. Pitch high.

Systole Diastole

S_1 S_2 S_1 S_2 S_1 S_2

PROCEDURES AND TECHNIQUES WITH NORMAL FINDINGS

INTERPRET the electrocardiogram of the conduction of the heart.

The electrical conduction of the heart can be seen on an electrocardiogram (EKG) to assess rate and rhythm. This assessment tool is called an EKG rather than an ECG to avoid errors because the sound of ECG is similar to that of EEG (electroencephalogram). Figure 13-32, *A*, shows the EKG reflections of one cardiac cycle. The P wave represents the atrial contraction or depolarization. The QRS complex represents the ventricular contraction or depolarization. The atrial repolarization occurs at the same time, but is overshadowed by the ventricular contraction. The T wave represents the repolarization of the ventricle. Figure 13-32, *B*, shows the time intervals of each part of the cardiac cycle. Figure 13-32, *C*, shows which part of the heart is represented by the wave or complex.

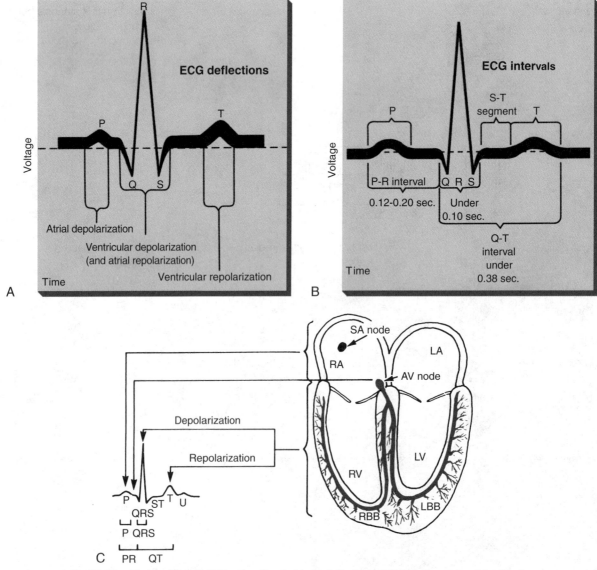

Fig. 13-32　**Electrocardiogram (EKG) and cardiac electrical activity. A,** Ideal EKG deflections represent depolarization and repolarization of cardiac muscle tissue. **B,** Principal EKG interval among P, QRS, and T waves. Note that the RP interval is measured from the start of the P wave to the end of the Q wave. **C,** Schematic representation of EKG and its relationship to the cardiac electrical activity. *AV,* Atrioventricular; *LA,* left atrium; *LBB,* left bundle branch; *LV,* left ventricle; *RA,* right atrium; *RBB,* right bundle branch; *RV,* right ventricular, *SA,* sinoatrial. (*A, B, From Thibodeau GA, Patton KI:* Anatomy and physiology, *ed 4, St Louis, 1999, Mosby.* **C,** *From Thibodeau GA:* Anatomy and physiology, *St Louis, 1987, Mosby.*)

| PROCEDURES AND TECHNIQUES WITH NORMAL FINDINGS | ABNORMAL FINDINGS |

SPECIAL CIRCUMSTANCES OR ADVANCED PRACTICE

ASSESS the Peripheral Vascular System

AUSCULTATE the carotid artery for bruits.

Using the bell of the stethoscope, auscultate the carotid artery. Ask the client to hold his or her breath while you listen. You should hear no sound over these arteries (Fig. 13-33).

Bruits are low-pitched blowing sounds usually heard during systole that indicate occlusion of the vessel.

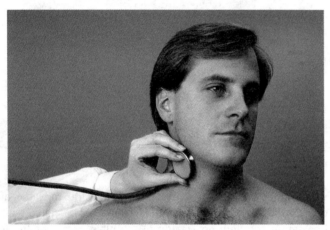

Fig. 13-33   Auscultating the carotid artery. *(From Canobbio, 1990.)*

★ *ESTIMATE jugular venous pressure for pulsations.*

Procedure: With the client's head elevated, identify the highest level at which jugular vein pulsations are visible, and then identify the manubriosternal joint (angle of Louis). Use a tongue blade or ruler to create an imaginary line from the highest venous pulsation to the manubriosternal angle. Measure the vertical distance between the tongue blade and the manubriosternal angle to estimate jugular venous pressure in centimeters (Fig. 13-34). This pressure should not rise more than 1 inch (2.5 cm) above the sternal angle. (*Note:* If you cannot find the jugular vein, have the client lie down flat for a few minutes so that it will distend.)

Findings: Pulsations should be regular, soft, and of a wavelike quality. The level of pulsation decreases with inspiration, and the pulsation increases in recumbent position.

Note if the jugular venous pressure exceeds 1 inch (2.5 cm) above the level of the manubrium. *Note:* If venous pressure is elevated (meaning that the vein is distended up to the neck), raise the client's head until the highest jugular pulsation can be detected. The distance in inches above the sternal angle and the angle at which the client is reclining should be recorded. Also note if other veins in the neck, shoulder, or upper chest are distended. Note any fluttering or oscillating of the pulsation. Note irregular rhythms or unusually prominent waves.

★ = advanced practice

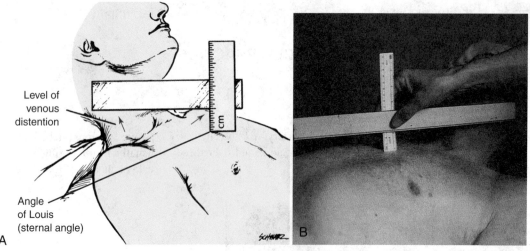

Level of venous distention

Angle of Louis (sternal angle)

A

B

Fig. 13-34   Measuring jugular venous pressure. *(From Barkauskas et al, 2002.)*

PROCEDURES AND TECHNIQUES WITH NORMAL FINDINGS

ABNORMAL FINDINGS

PALPATE epitrochlear lymph nodes for size, consistency, mobility, borders, tenderness, and warmth.

Flex the client's arm to a 90-degree angle and palpate below the elbow posterior to the medial condyle of the humerus (Fig. 13-35). Compare the sizes of the upper and lower arms for symmetry. The arms should be symmetric with no palpable lymph nodes.

Enlarged, firm, warm, movable, and tender nodes may be associated with infection of the ulnar aspect of the forearm and the fourth and fifth fingers.

When one arm is larger in circumference than the other, it could be due to lymphedema.

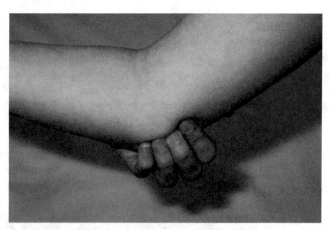

Fig. 13-35   Palpation for epitrochlear lymph nodes is performed in the depression above and posterior to the medial condyle of the humerus. *(From Seidel et al, 2003.)*

PALPATE inguinal lymph nodes for size, consistency, mobility, borders, tenderness, and warmth.

With the client in the supine position, lightly palpate with finger pads in the area just below the inguinal ligament and on the inner aspect of the thigh at the groin (Fig. 13-36). It may not be possible to palpate them at all, but they should be smooth and soft if they can be felt. Moving inward toward the genitalia, you can locate the anatomy using the mnemonic NAVEL: *N,* nerve; *A,* artery; *V,* vein; *E,* empty space; *L,* lymph nodes. Compare the sizes of the upper and lower legs for symmetry.

The inguinal nodes are small, mobile nodes, some of which may be nontender. The upper and lower legs should be symmetric.

Enlarged, tender, firm, warm, and freely movable nodes indicate an inflammatory process distal to these nodes, such as in the leg, vulva, penis, or scrotum.

When one leg is larger in circumference than the other, it could be due to lymphedema.

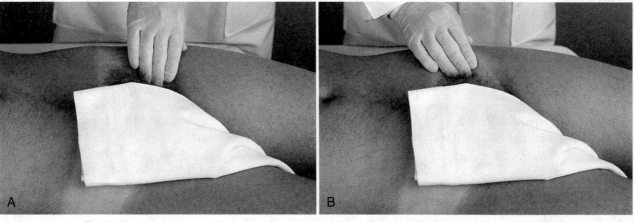

Fig. 13-36 **A,** Palpation of inferior superficial inguinal (femoral) lymph nodes. **B,** Palpation of superior superficial inguinal lymph nodes. *(From Seidel et al, 1999.)*

PROCEDURES AND TECHNIQUES WITH NORMAL FINDINGS

ABNORMAL FINDINGS

CALCULATE the ankle brachial index (ABI) to estimate arterial occlusion.

Procedure: With the client in a supine position, take the brachial blood pressure in both arms using Doppler sound. Apply the blood pressure cuff above the brachial artery. Apply conductive gel over the radial pulse. Pump up the blood pressure cuff until you can no longer hear the radial pulse by Doppler. Then increase the pressure 20 mm Hg more. Slowly release the pressure in the cuff until you hear the pulse again. The value from the manometer is the systolic pressure. Repeat the procedure on both legs. Apply the blood pressure cuff to the ankle and use the dorsalis pedis pulse for the Doppler sounds. Divide the posterior tibial (ankle) systolic pressure by the brachial systolic blood pressure for each side.

Findings: The expected value of ABI is greater than 0.9.

The client who has peripheral vascular disease has impaired peripheral perfusion that is reflected in an ABI less than normal. An ABI less than 0.9 indicates peripheral vascular disease; an ABI less than 0.6 is associated with intermittent claudication; an ABI less than 0.25 is associated with rest pain; and an ABI less than 0.2 reflects severe ischemia leading to gangrene (data from *www. fpnotebook.com,* 2003).

★ *PERFORM Trendelenburg's test to evaluate competence of venous valves in clients who have varicose veins.*

With the client in a supine position, lift one leg above the level of the heart to allow veins to empty, then assist the client to stand. If veins are competent, veins fill slowly. Repeat the test on the other leg.

If the veins fill rapidly, the valves may be incompetent, and varicose veins may be present.

ASSESS the Heart

★ *PALPATE the precordium for pulsations, thrills, lifts, and heaves.*

Supine is the preferred position for cardiac palpation; however, the sitting position may be necessary to feel impulses. Using the palmar surface of your hand and finger pads, gently palpate the anterior chest, allowing the movements of the chest to lift the hands. Palpate systematically from the base to the apex or from the apex to the base.

Observe whether the entire chest seems to lift or heave with the heartbeat. A lift or heave may indicate left ventricular enlargement.

★ = advanced practice

PROCEDURES AND TECHNIQUES WITH NORMAL FINDINGS

Palpate the base of the heart (Fig. 13-37, *A*).

Palpate the left sternal border (LSB) (Fig. 13-37, *B*) with the heel of the hand over the third, fourth, and fifth left intercostal spaces (ICS) (see Box 13-3).

Palpate the apex of the heart at the fifth ICS midclavicular line (Fig. 13-37, *C*). The apical impulse has small amplitude, is of brief duration, and is no larger than 2 to 3 cm in diameter.

Palpate the epigastric area for pulsations. There may be an aortic pulsation.

ABNORMAL FINDINGS

Pulsations may indicate an aortic aneurysm. A thrill may be associated with a murmur from a disorder of the aortic or pulmonic valve.

Sustained lifts or palpations may indicate right ventricular hypertrophy; pulsations may indicate pulmonary hypertension. A thrill is associated with pulmonic valve stenosis.

Forceful pulsation, displaced laterally or downward, is associated with increased cardiac output or left ventricular hypertrophy. Presence of a thrill may indicate a murmur.

Bounding pulsations may indicate abdominal aortic aneurysm or aortic valve regurgitation.

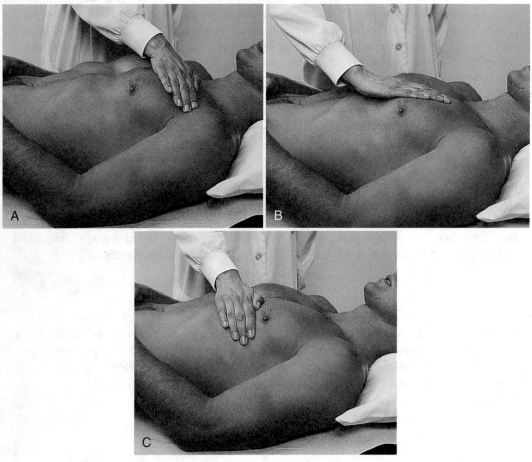

Fig. 13-37   **Palpation of precordium. A,** Palpating base. **B,** Palpating left sternal border. **C,** Palpating apex.

PROCEDURES AND TECHNIQUES WITH NORMAL FINDINGS

★ *PERCUSS the heart borders for the heart size.*
(NOTE: This is an optional assessment technique because echocardiogram provides more precise information.) Percussion is performed at the third, fourth, and fifth ICS from the left anterior axillary line to the right anterior axillary line. The expected finding is a change from resonance to dullness about 6 cm lateral to the left of the sternum. The areas of dullness are marked with a pencil and the distance from the sternum measured with a ruler. Percussion of the heart may be difficult with obese or large-breasted clients.

ABNORMAL FINDINGS

Deviation of the left border further to the left is associated with dilated left ventricle, right pneumothorax, or pericardial effusion. Deviation of the left border to the right is associated with dextrocardia or left pneumothorax.

★ = advanced practice

AGE-RELATED VARIATIONS

INFANTS, CHILDREN, AND ADOLESCENTS

There are several differences in the assessment of the cardiovascular system for infants and young children. For example, the equipment used to measure blood pressure is smaller, the sequence of the exam may be different, and findings may differ based on anatomical differences. Assessment of the older child and adolescent follows the same procedures and reveals similar expected findings. One exception in the examination is the electrocardiogram, which is not typically performed.

Chapter 20 presents further information regarding the cardiovascular assessment of infants, children, and adolescents.

OLDER ADULTS

Assessing the cardiovascular status of an older adult usually follows the same procedures as for an adult. Expected variations may be found in heart rate and blood pressure. Chapter 22 presents further information regarding the cardiovascular assessment of an older adult.

Documenting Expected Findings

Heart and Peripheral Vascular System

The client is sitting in a relaxed position, with regular respirations; BP 120/68, jugular pulsations visible without distention; extremities are symmetric in size; skin is intact, and has elastic turgor, is warm with color appropriate for client without pallor or redness; pulses 70 beats per minute, regular rhythm, smooth contour with pulse amplitude 21; capillary refill <2 seconds in all extremities; nail beds pink with angle 160 degrees. Chest is rounded and symmetric without lifts, heaves, or pulsations; PMI at 5th ICS, MCL, S_1 louder at the apex and S_2 louder at the base, regular rate and rhythm without murmurs or extra sounds. Electrocardiogram shows sinus rhythm in Lead II.

CLINICAL REASONING   *Cardiovascular System*

A 67-year-old man with a long-standing history of emphysema and hypertension presents to the emergency department with a history of shortness of breath and productive cough that has progressed over the last 2 days. He also complains of being very tired, and having no appetite. The nurse obtains a set of vital signs which include: blood pressure 128/92, pulse 122, temperature 99.1° F, and respiratory rate 26 and labored.

Noticing: Although an experienced nurse would expect a client with COPD to be dyspneic and have a cough, this client reports increasing shortness of breath and a productive cough, both an apparent change from his baseline. The experienced nurse understands that clients with COPD are at increased risk for pneumonia and for congestive heart failure; either of these might result in decreased PO_2, and indeed the nurse measures his oxygen saturation at 84% on room air. The nurse notices that the client's skin is warm and slightly diaphoretic.

Interpreting: Early in the encounter, the nurse considers two possible causes of the shortness of breath and cough: pneumonia, heart failure, or both. In order to determine if either have any probability of being correct, the nurse gathers additional data:

- What is the color and character of the sputum? The man tells the nurse it is "whitish and bubbly."
- Is there evidence of excessive fluid? The man has 2+ pitting edema in his legs and feet; the man is wearing house slippers. When asked about this, he tells the nurse he can't put on his shoes.
- The nurse proceeds to auscultate his heart and lung sounds. His lungs have crackles bilaterally; an S3 heart sound is auscultated.

The experienced nurse not only recognizes heart failure by the clinical signs (increased respiratory rate and effort, bilateral crackles, S_3 heart sound, peripheral edema) and symptoms (fatigue, shortness of breath), but interprets this information in the context of an older adult with hypertension and emphysema.

Responding: The nurse initiates appropriate initial interventions (oxygen delivery and obtaining intravenous access), and notifies the emergency department health care provider of the situation, ensuring the client receives appropriate immediate and follow-up care.

COMMON PROBLEMS & CONDITIONS

CARDIAC DISORDERS

Valvular Heart Disease

An acquired or congenital disorder of a heart valve is called valvular heart disease (VHD). It can be characterized by a heart valve that either does not open completely (stenotic valve) or one that does not close completely (incompetent valve). Rheumatic fever and endocarditis account for most cases of acquired VHD. **Clinical Findings:** See Table 13-5.

Angina Pectoris

Chest pain that is due to ischemia of the myocardium is called angina pectoris. It is usually caused by atherosclerosis within the coronary arteries. Angina can occur during activity, stress, or exposure to intense cold because of an increased demand on the heart. Angina can also occur during rest as a result of spasms of the coronary arteries. **Clinical Findings:** Clients describe the pain as squeezing, suffocating, or constricting. There may be significant hypertension, although hypotension may also occur. The duration of the angina is important to determine. If the angina is precipitated by exertion and the client rests promptly, it may last for less than 3 minutes. If the angina follows a heavy meal or is caused by anger, it may last 15 to 20 min-

utes. Angina lasting more than 30 minutes is unusual and may indicate unstable angina or developing myocardial infarction (Massie and Amidon, 2003).

Myocardial Infarction

This condition occurs when myocardial ischemia is sustained resulting in death of myocardial cells (necrosis). The left ventricle is more commonly affected, but the right ventricle may also be affected. **Clinical Findings:** Clients describe the pain as the worst chest pain ever experienced, a pain that lasts longer than 5 minutes; it may radiate to the left shoulder, jaw, arm, or other areas of the chest; and it is not relieved by rest or nitroglycerin. Dysrhythmias are common. Heart sounds may be distant with a thready pulse. Women report different symptoms prior to a myocardial infarction. They report pain or discomfort in the center of the chest, as well as shortness of breath, cold sweat, nausea, vomiting, or lightheadedness (*www.nhlbi.nih.gov,* last accessed Sept 14, 2007).

Heart Failure

When either ventricle fails to pump blood efficiently into the aorta or pulmonary arteries, the condition is termed *heart failure*. Heart failure may occur in the left ventricle or right ventricle, or both.

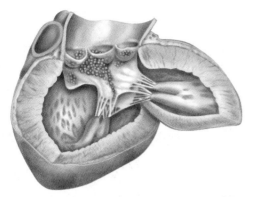

Fig. 13-38 Bacterial endocarditis. *(From Seidel et al, 2003. Modified from Canobbio, 1990.)*

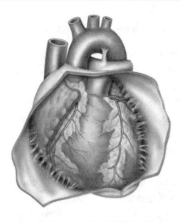

Fig. 13-39 Pericarditis. *(From Seidel et al, 2006. Modified from Canobbio, 1990.)*

Left ventricular failure

This cardiac condition is caused by (1) increased resistance that occurs with aortic stenosis or hypertension when the ventricle can no longer compensate effectively for the increased workload or (2) weakening of the left ventricular contraction that occurs after a myocardial infarction when the death of myocardial cells causes an ineffective contraction. Because the left ventricle cannot pump sufficient blood forward, some of the blood backs up into the left atrium and eventually into the pulmonary capillaries, causing pulmonary edema. **Clinical Findings:** The client complains of fatigue and shortness of breath, including orthopnea, dyspnea on exertion (DOE), and paroxysmal nocturnal dyspnea (PND). Findings may reveal precordial movement, displaced apical pulse and palpable thrill, S_3, and systolic murmur at apex. In the acute phase the client usually has crackles bilaterally from pulmonary edema.

Right ventricular failure

This cardiac condition is caused by hypertrophy from pulmonary hypertension or from necrosis from a myocardial infarction. The failure of the right ventricle to pump blood into the pulmonary arteries causes a backflow of blood into the inferior and superior venae cavae. Right ventricular failure caused by pulmonary disease, termed *cor pulmonale*, is discussed in Chapter 12. **Clinical Findings:** Findings may include precordial movement at the xiphoid or left sternal border, elevated jugular venous pressure, dependent peripheral edema, S_3 at lower left sternal border, systolic murmur, and weight gain.

Infective Endocarditis

An infection of the endothelial layer of the heart, including the cardiac valves, is called infective endocarditis. This infection develops when the endocardial surface is damaged by turbulent blood flow as a result of valvular heart disease, congenital lesions, or direct injury from intravenous lines or injections, cardiac catheterization, or artificial valves (Fig. 13-38). **Clinical Findings:** Heart sounds are normal during the early infection. In late infection, a murmur is heard if valve damage occurs.

Pericarditis

Inflammation of the parietal and visceral layers of the pericardium and outer myocardium is termed *pericarditis*. It may be idiopathic or the result of myocardial infarction, uremia, cancer, trauma, infections, cardiac surgery, or an autoimmune reaction (Fig. 13-39). **Clinical Findings:** Two classic findings are pericardial friction rub and chest pain. A pericardial friction rub develops as the inflamed layers of pericardium move against each other. The friction rub is best heard with the client leaning forward so that the heart is closer to the chest wall. Listen in the second, third, or fourth intercostal spaces at the left sternal border or at the apex; it is louder during inspiration. The chest pain is described as a sharp pleuritic pain that is aggravated by deep breathing, lying supine, or coughing.

PERIPHERAL VASCULAR DISEASE

Hypertension

A diagnosis of hypertension is based on the mean of two or more properly measured seated blood pressure readings on each of two or more occasions that are above 120/80 mm Hg in an adult over 18 years of age. Pressure in the arteries can become elevated due to constriction of the blood vessels or fluid volume overload or both. **Clinical Findings:** Normal blood pressure values are less than 120 mm Hg systolic and less than 80 mm Hg diastolic. Criteria for hypertension are shown in Box 13-7 (*www.nhlbi.nih.gov/guidelines*, 2003). Since there no specific symptoms of hypertension, periodic screening is important.

BOX 13-7	**CLASSIFICATION OF BLOOD PRESSURE FOR ADULTS AGE 18 AND OLDER**		
Category*	**Systolic (mm Hg)**		**Diastolic (mm Hg)**
Normal	<120	and	<80
Prehypertension	120-139	or	80-89
Stage 1 hypertension	140-159	or	90-99
Stage 2 hypertension	>160	or	>100

Modified from National Heart, Lung, and Blood Institute: The seventh report of the Joint Commission on Prevention, Detection, Evaluation and Treatment of High Blood Pressure (JNC VII), available at *www.nhlbi.nih.gov/guidelines*, May 2003.

Venous Thrombosis and Thrombophlebitis

When a thrombus (clot) develops within a vein it is called a *venous thrombosis*. In contrast, thrombophlebitis is inflammation of a vein that may or may not be accompanied by a clot. The triad of venous stasis, damage to the inner layer of veins, and hypercoagulability usually is responsible for both venous thrombosis and thrombophlebitis. Either may occur in the lower extremity, usually in deep veins. **Clinical Findings:** Thromboses are sometimes recognized by dilated superficial veins, edema and redness of the involved extremity, and increased circumference of the involved leg. In the upper extremity, venous thrombosis and thrombophlebitis may occur in superficial veins and are recognized by redness, warmth, and tenderness over the affected area. Veins may be visible and palpable (Fig 13-40).

Aneurysm

A localized dilation of an artery caused by weakness in the arterial wall is referred to as an aneurysm. They occur anywhere along the aorta as well as iliac and cerebral vessels (Fig 13-41). **Clinical Findings:** Clinical findings depend on the location of the aneurysm. Thoracic aneurysms are usually asymptomatic with deep, diffuse chest pain reported by some clients. Aneurysms of the aorta and aortic arch can produce hoarseness from pressure on the laryngeal nerve or dysphagia from pressure on the esophagus. Abdominal aortic aneurysms are most common. They may be asymptomatic and discovered on routine examination or with an ultrasound or computed tomography performed for another reason. A pulsatile mass may be palpated in the

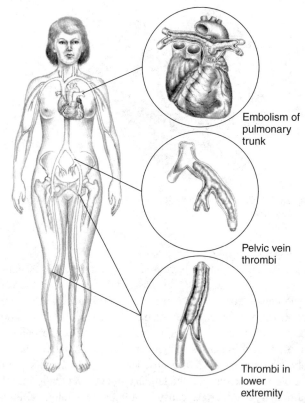

Embolism of pulmonary trunk

Pelvic vein thrombi

Thrombi in lower extremity

Fig. 13-40   Sites of venous thrombosis. *(From Canobbio, 1990.)*

periumbilical area. A thrill or bruit may be noted over the aneurysm (Wipke-Tevis and Rich, 2004). Cerebral aneurysms can cause intracranial hemorrhages and the manifestations directly related to the size and location of the bleed.

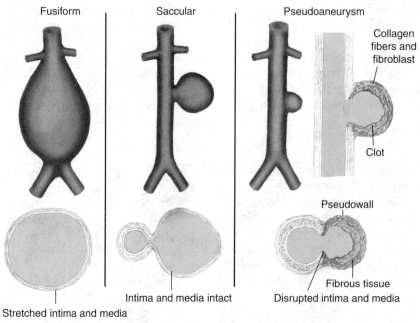

Fusiform   Saccular   Pseudoaneurysm

Collagen fibers and fibroblast

Clot

Pseudowall

Fibrous tissue
Disrupted intima and media

Intima and media intact

Stretched intima and media

Fig. 13-41   Arterial aneurysm. *(From Canobbio, 1990.)*

CLINICAL APPLICATION & CLINICAL REASONING

See Appendix E for answers to exercises in this section.

REVIEW QUESTIONS

1 The nurse is listening to the client's heart at the LSB second ICS. Which area is being auscultated?
   1 Erb's point.
   2 Mitral area.
   3 Aortic area.
   4 Pulmonic area.

2 A client complains of pain in the calf when walking. What is a question the nurse should ask in relation to the calf pain for further data?
   1 "Does your calf also swell when this pain occurs?"
   2 "Does the pain go away when you stop walking?"
   3 "Do you become short of breath when you are walking?"
   4 "Do you feel dizzy when the pain occurs?"

3 Which client has the greatest risk for hypertension? The client who is:
   1 An Asian man who is 5 feet 5 inches (165 cm) tall, weighs 125 lb (56.7 kg), and complains of a headache over his forehead and eyes.
   2 A Cheyenne Indian woman who complains of a gnawing, burning epigastric pain radiating to her neck and jaw.
   3 An African American man who has type 2 diabetes mellitus, exercises once a month, and drinks two to three alcoholic drinks a night with dinner.
   4 A Caucasian woman who has a family history of heart disease and complains of pain in her chest when she takes a deep breath.

4 When a client complains of chest pain, what question is pertinent to ask to gain additional data?
   1 "What were you doing when the pain first occurred?"
   2 "What does the pain feel like?"
   3 "Do you have episodes of shortness of breath?"
   4 "Has anyone in your family ever had a similar pain?"

5 How does a nurse determine jugular vein pulsations?
   1 Elevate the head of the bed about 90 degrees and look for the jugular vein pulsation parallel to the sternocleidomastoid muscle as the head of the bed is slowly lowered.
   2 Look for jugular vein pulsations at the jaw line as the client turns from supine to a side-lying position.
   3 Elevate the head of the bed until the external jugular vein pulsation is seen above the clavicle.
   4 Position the client supine and ask him or her to cough. Look for the jugular vein pulsations during the cough.

6 The nurse assesses the posterior tibial pulse by lightly palpating:
   1 Behind the knee in the popliteal fossa.
   2 The inner aspect of the ankle below and slightly behind the medial malleolus.
   3 Over the dorsum of the foot between the extension tendons of the first and second toes.
   4 The outer side of the ankle below and slightly behind the lateral malleolus.

7 On auscultation the nurse recognizes which finding as normal?
   1 A low-pitched blowing sound is heard over the abdominal aorta.
   2 A high-pitched vibration is heard over the base of the heart.
   3 The S_1 heart sound is louder at the apex of the heart.
   4 The S_3 heart sound sounds like "Ken-tuck-y."

8 What is the most accurate technique for detecting a deep vein thrombosis?
   1 Dorsiflex the calf and note if the client complains of pain.
   2 Elevate one leg above the level of the heart to determine if the veins empty.
   3 Palpate the pulses distal to the areas of the suspected thrombosis.
   4 Measure the thigh circumference to detect an increase from the baseline.

9 Each of the following clients has had consistent blood pressure readings during the last three clinic visits. Which client has a blood pressure consistent with normal findings?
   1 Mr. P., whose blood pressure has been 110/78.
   2 Ms. J., whose blood pressure has been 140/90.
   3 Mr. Q., whose blood pressure has been 130/76.
   4 Ms. Y., whose blood pressure has been 120/80.

10 While inspecting the legs of a male client, the nurse notes the skin is shiny and taut with little hair growth. What additional data would the nurse find to indicate that this client has peripheral arterial disease?
   1 Pitting edema of one or both feet or legs.
   2 Increased circumference in the thighs bilaterally.
   3. Pale, cool legs with diminished to absent dorsalis pulses.
   4 Pain when legs are dependent that is relieved when legs are elevated.

SAMPLE DOCUMENTATION

Review the data below obtained by the nurse during an interview and examination:

R. D. is a 45-year-old man who came to the office today for an annual physical examination as required by his employer. He has no complaints. He is married with two teenage sons. He says that he does not have time to exercise. He does not take any medications, does not drink alcohol, and does not use street drugs. He is allergic to codeine.

R. D. is an alert, cooperative, healthy-appearing man. Height is measured as 6 feet 1 inch (185 cm); weight is measured as 190 lb (86 kg). Vital signs are as follows: temperature, 98.5° F (36.9° C); pulse, 76 beats per minute; respiratory rate, 16 breaths per minute; blood pressure, 150/95 mm Hg, right arm—sitting; 148/97 mm Hg, left arm—sitting.

His father had a myocardial infarction (MI) at age 47 and died from a second MI at age 54. His paternal grandfather died of a heart attack at age 65; his paternal grandmother died of breast cancer at age 50. He says, "Heart attacks just run in my family."

There are no lifts, heaves, or pulsations on inspection or palpation. The point of maximal impulse is palpable at the fifth intercostal space at the midclavicular line, S_1 heart sound is loudest at apex, and S_2 heart sound is loudest at base; regular rate and rhythm without murmur or S_3 or S_4. He is employed full time as an engineer. He has worked for this company for 1 year. He likes his job, but becomes stressed with deadlines every 2 to 3 months.

Brachial, radial, and dorsalis pedis pulses are 2+, symmetric. No carotid bruits are heard. Currently he smokes one-half pack of cigarettes per day. He has a 10 pack-year history. He states that he is interested in stopping smoking because there are "so few places I can smoke anymore." Capillary refill is less than 2 seconds. His extremities appear dry and feel warm. He has the usual male hair distribution, and skin turgor is elastic. He had an appendectomy at age 15 and a vasectomy at age 44. He does not remember his last medical examination; his last dental examination was 2 years ago.

On the right, note how the nurse documented these same data.

CASE STUDY

Howard is a 56-year-old man complaining of difficulty breathing. The following initial data are collected.

Interview Data

Howard does not know exactly when his breathing difficulty started, but it has gotten noticeably worse the last couple of days. His father died of a heart attack at age 60. Howard plays golf twice a week; however, he tells the nurse that this

R. D. is a 45-y/o ♂ for annual PE.

SUBJECTIVE DATA

No complaints. Appendectomy at 15, vasectomy at 44. Does not remember last PE; last dental examination, 2 years ago. Father had MI at 47, died from MI at 54. PGF died of MI at 65; PGM died of breast cancer at 50. "Heart attacks just run in my family." Married c̄ two teenage sons. Employed FT as engineer, worked for this company 1 yr. Likes his job, but stressful c̄ deadlines q2-3mo. Does not have time to exercise. Smokes ½ pack of cigarettes/day; has a 10 pack-year hx. Interested in stopping smoking. Allergic to codeine. Does not take medications, drink alcohol, or use street drugs.

OBJECTIVE DATA

General survey: Alert, cooperative, healthy-appearing. ♂
Vital signs: T 98.5° F (36.9° C); P 76/min; RR 16/min; BP 150/95 mm Hg, right arm—sitting; 148/97 mm Hg, left arm—sitting. Ht (measured), 6 feet 1 inch (185 cm); wt (measured), 190 lb (86 kg).
Heart: No lifts, heaves, or pulsations on inspection or palpation. PMI palpable at fifth ICS, MCL, S_1 loudest at apex, and S_2 loudest at base; RRR s̄ murmur or S_3 or S_4.
Pulses: Brachial, radial, and dorsalis pedis 2+, symmetric. No carotid bruits.
Lower extremities: Warm, dry, elastic turgor, cap refill <2 seconds; usual male hair distribution.

last week he has "just felt too tired to do anything." Howard says that he has not been able to sleep very well at night because of his breathing difficulty. He adds, "I keep coughing out this bubbly looking phlegm." Howard denies taking any medications. He says that he does not smoke or drink alcoholic beverages.

Examination Data

- *General survey:* Alert, anxious, cooperative, well-groomed male. Appears stated age. Breathing is labored.
- *Vital signs:* Temperature, 98.8° F (37.1° C); pulse, 120 beats/min; respiration, 26 breaths/min; blood pressure, 142/112 mm Hg, right arm; 144/110 mm Hg, left arm.
- *Pulses:* All pulses palpable 2+. No carotid bruits bilaterally.
- *Neck:* Jugular distension and pulsation noted with client in supine position.
- *Lower extremities:* Skin warm and dry, without cyanosis. Even hair distribution. 2+ pitting edema noted bilaterally; no lesions present.

Clinical Reasoning

1. What data deviate from normal findings, suggesting a need for further investigation?
2. What additional information should the nurse ask or assess for?
3. Based on these data, what risk factors for coronary artery disease does this client have?
4. What nursing diagnoses and collaborative problems should be considered for this situation?

INTERACTIVE ACTIVITIES

Open the interactive student CD-ROM, click on Chapter 13, and choose from the following activities on the menu bar:

- **Multiple Choice Challenge.** Click on the best answer of each of these 15 items. You will be given immediate feedback, rationale for incorrect answers, and a total score. Good luck!

- **Risk Factors.** Click on the risk factors that place this client at risk for cardiovascular disease. Can you identify them?

- **A Day in the Clinic.** Complete an examination by choosing a technique and an examination area for this client. You'll be able to collect data, document, and compare your answers with those of the experts. All that you need for a successful assessment is at your fingertips!

- **Printable Lab Guide.** Locate the Lab Guide for Chapter 18, and print and use it (as many times as needed) to help you apply your assessment skills. These guides may also be filled in electronically and then saved and e-mailed to your instructor!

- **Audio Clips: Heart Sounds.** Choose from 18 different heart sounds to listen to (as many times as needed) to help you develop your assessment skills.

- **Quick Challenge.** Use this critical thinking exercise to assess your skills through case study-style questions, then compare with expert answers!

- **Core Examination Skills Checklists.** Make sure you've got frequently-used exam skills down pat! Use these checklists to help cover all the bases for your examination.

CHAPTER **14**

Abdomen and Gastrointestinal System

ANATOMY & PHYSIOLOGY

The abdominal cavity, the largest cavity in the human body, contains the stomach, small and large intestines, liver, gallbladder, pancreas, spleen, kidneys, ureters, bladder, and adrenal glands, as well as major vessels (Figs. 14-1 and 14-2). In women the uterus, fallopian tubes, and ovaries are located within the abdominal cavity. Lying outside the abdominal cavity, but a vital part of the gastrointestinal (GI) system, is the esophagus.

PERITONEUM, MUSCULATURE, AND CONNECTIVE TISSUE

The abdominal lining, the peritoneum, is a serous membrane forming a protective cover. It is divided into two layers: the parietal peritoneum and the visceral peritoneum. The parietal peritoneum lines the abdominal wall, and the visceral peritoneum covers organs. The space between the parietal peritoneum and visceral peritoneum is the peritoneal cavity. It usually contains a small amount of serous fluid to reduce friction between abdominal organs and their membranes.

The rectus abdominis muscles form the anterior border of the abdomen, and the vertebral column and lumbar muscles form the posterior border. Lateral support is provided by the internal and external oblique muscles. The external oblique

aponeurosis is a strong membrane that covers the entire ventral surface of the abdomen and lies superficial to the rectus abdominis. Fibers from both sides of the aponeurosis interlace in the midline to form the linea alba. The linea alba is a tendinous band that protects the midline of the abdomen between the rectus abdominis muscles. This band extends from the xiphoid process to the symphysis pubis. The abdomen is bordered superiorly by the diaphragm and inferiorly by the superior aperture of the lesser pelvis (Fig. 14-3).

ALIMENTARY TRACT

From the mouth to the anus, the adult alimentary tract extends 27 feet (8.2 m) and includes the esophagus, stomach, small intestine, large intestine, rectum, and anal canal (see Fig. 14-1). Its main functions are to ingest and digest food; to absorb nutrients, electrolytes, and water; and to excrete waste products. Products of digestion are moved along the digestive tract by peristalsis, under the control of the autonomic nervous system. The alimentary tract begins with the esophagus, a tube about 10 inches (25.4 cm) long connecting the pharynx to the stomach, extending just posterior to the trachea, through the mediastinal cavity and diaphragm. The usual pH of the esophagus is between 6 and 8.

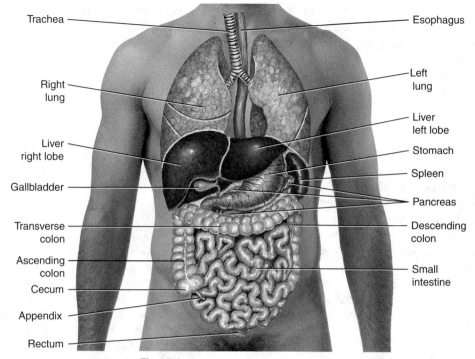

Fig. 14-1 Anatomy of the gastrointestinal system.

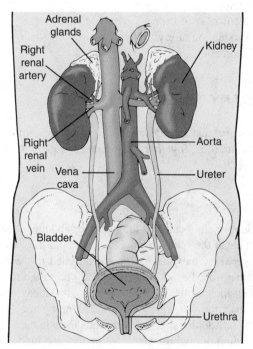

Fig. 14-2 Anatomy of the urinary system and major vessels of the abdominal cavity. *(From Lewis, Heitkempner, and Dirksen, 2000.)*

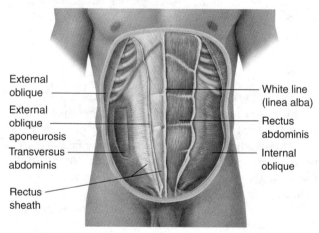

Fig. 14-3 Muscles of the abdomen. *(From Seidel et al, 2006.)*

breaks down proteins, converting them to peptones and amino acids, and gastric lipase acts on emulsified fats to convert triglycerides to fatty acids and glycerol. The stomach also liquefies food into chyme and propels it into the duodenum of the small intestine. The usual pH of the stomach ranges from 2 to 4. The pyloric sphincter regulates the outflow of chyme into the duodenum.

Stomach

The stomach is a hollow, flask-shaped, muscular organ located directly below the diaphragm in the left upper quadrant. Contents from the esophagus enter the stomach through the lower esophageal sphincter and mix with digestive enzymes and hydrochloric acid. Gastric acid continues the breakdown of carbohydrates that began in the mouth. Pepsin

Small Intestine

The longest section of the alimentary tract, the small intestine, is about 21 feet (6.4 m) long, beginning at the pyloric orifice and joining the large intestine at the ileocecal valve. In the small intestine, ingested food is mixed, digested, and absorbed. The small intestine is divided into three segments: the duodenum, jejunum, and ileum. The duodenum occupies the first 1 foot (30 cm) of the small intestine and forms a C-shaped curve around the head of the pancreas. Absorption occurs through the intestinal villi of the duodenum, jejunum (8 feet [2.4 m] long), and ileum (12 feet [3.6 m] long). The ileocecal valve between the ileum and the large intestine prevents backward flow of fecal material (see Fig. 14-1).

Large Intestine (Colon) and Rectum

The large intestine is about 5 feet (1.5 m) long, consisting of cecum, appendix, colon, rectum, and anal canal. The ileal contents empty into the cecum through the ileocecal valve; the appendix extends from the base of the cecum. The colon is divided into three parts: ascending, transverse, and descending. The end of the descending colon turns medially and inferiorly to form the S-shaped sigmoid colon. The rectum extends from the sigmoid colon to the pelvic floor, where it continues as the anal canal, terminating at the anus. The large intestine absorbs water and electrolytes. Feces are formed in the large intestine and held until defecation (see Fig. 14-1).

ACCESSORY ORGANS

Accessory organs of the gastrointestinal tract are the salivary glands, liver, gallbladder, and pancreas. Salivary glands are described in Chapter 11.

Liver

The liver is the largest organ in the body, weighing about 3.5 lb (1.6 kg). It lies under the right diaphragm, spanning the upper quadrant of the abdomen from the fifth intercostal space to slightly below the costal margin (see Fig. 14-1). The rib cage covers a substantial portion of the liver; only the lower margin is exposed beneath it. The liver is divided into right and left lobes.

This complex organ has a variety of functions, including the following:
- Bile production and secretion
- Transfer of bilirubin from the blood (conjugated or direct) to the gallbladder (unconjugated or indirect)
- Protein, carbohydrate, and fat metabolism
- Glucose storage in the form of glycogen
- Production of clotting factors and fibrinogen
- Synthesis of most plasma proteins (albumin and globulin)
- Detoxification of a variety of substances, including drugs and alcohol
- Storage of certain minerals (iron and copper) and vitamins (A, B_{12}, and other B-complex vitamins)

Gallbladder

The gallbladder is a pear-shaped sac, 3 inches (7.6 cm) long, attached to the inferior surface of the liver (see Fig. 14-1). It concentrates and stores bile produced in the liver. The cystic duct combines with the hepatic duct to form the common bile duct, which drains bile into the duodenum. Bile in feces creates the characteristic brown color.

Pancreas

The pancreas lies in the upper left abdominal cavity, immediately under the left lobe of the liver, behind the stomach (see Fig. 14-1). It has both endocrine and exocrine functions. Endocrine secretions include insulin, glucagon, and gastrin for carbohydrate metabolism. Exocrine secretions contain bicarbonate and pancreatic enzymes that flow into the duodenum to break down proteins, fats, and carbohydrates for absorption.

Spleen

The spleen is a highly vascular, concave, encapsulated organ about the size of a fist, situated in the upper left quadrant of the abdomen between the stomach and diaphragm. It is composed of two systems: the white pulp (consisting of lymphatic nodules and diffuse lymphatic tissue) and the red pulp (consisting of venous sinusoids) (see Fig. 14-1). Its main functions include the following:
- Storage of 1% to 2% of erythrocytes and platelets
- Removal of old or agglutinated erythrocytes and platelets
- Activation of B and T lymphocytes
- Production of erythrocytes during bone marrow depression

URINARY TRACT

The urinary tract includes the kidneys, ureters, urinary bladder, and urethra. Together, they remove water-soluble waste materials.

Kidneys

The kidneys are located in the posterior abdominal cavity on either side at the spinal levels of T12 through L3, where they are covered by the peritoneum and attached to the posterior abdominal wall. Each kidney is partially protected by the ribs and a cushion of fat and fascia. The right kidney is slightly lower than the left, due to displacement by the liver (see Fig. 14-2). Additional kidney functions include the following: (1) secretion of erythropoietin to stimulate red blood cell production; (2) secretion of renin to activate the renin-angiotensin-aldosterone system; and (3) production of a biologically active form of vitamin D. The nephron regulates fluid and electrolyte balance through an elaborate microscopic filter and pressure system that eventually produces urine.

Ureters

The urine formed in the nephrons flows from the distal tubes and collecting ducts into the ureters and on into the bladder through peristaltic waves. Each ureter is composed of long, intertwining muscle bundles that extend for approximately

12 inches (30 cm) to insertion points at the base of the bladder (see Fig. 14-2).

Bladder

The bladder, a sac of smooth muscle fibers, is located behind the symphysis pubis in the anterior half of the pelvis (see Fig. 14-2). The bladder contains an internal sphincter, which relaxes in response to a full bladder. Generally, when the bladder's urine volume reaches about 300 ml, moderate distention is felt; a level of 450 ml causes discomfort. For voiding to occur, the external sphincter relaxes voluntarily and urine exits through the urethra, which extends out of the base of the bladder to the external meatus.

VASCULATURE OF THE ABDOMEN

In the abdomen, the descending aorta travels through the diaphragm just to the left of midline until it branches into the two common iliac arteries at about the level of the umbilicus. Perfusion of the kidneys is provided by the right and left renal arteries, which branch off of the descending aorta. Blood is returned to the right side of the heart from the abdomen in the inferior vena cava, which parallels the abdominal aorta (see Fig. 14-2). Several veins empty into the inferior vena cava. These include the hepatic portal system, which is composed of veins that drain the intestines, pancreas, stomach, and gallbladder, as well as the renal veins, which drain the kidneys and ureters.

HEALTH HISTORY

RISK FACTORS *Abdominal Cancers*

As you conduct a health history related to the abdomen, it is important to consider common risk factors associated with cancer and follow up with additional questions should they exist.

Esophageal Cancer
- *Age:* Risk increases with age, with the peak between 70 and 80 years.
- *Gender:* Men have a rate three times that of women.
- *Race:* African Americans are 2.5 times more likely to develop esophageal cancer than whites.
- *Tobacco:* The longer a person smokes, the greater the risk. (M)
- *Alcohol:* Long-term alcohol intake increases risk. Alcohol and smoking together raises a person's risk more than using either alone. (M)
- *Barrett's esophagus:* This condition is associated with long-term gastroesophageal reflux. (M)
- *Diet:* Deficits in fruits and vegetables, particularly vitamin A, vitamin C, and riboflavin. (M)

Stomach Cancer
- *Age:* The rate of people over 65 years is 15 times that of people under 65 years.
- *Gender:* Twice as common in men.
- *Race:* Highest rates are seen in Asians/Pacific Islanders. Rates are higher in Hispanics and African Americans than in non-Hispanic whites.
- *Blood type:* For unknown reasons, people with blood type A have a greater risk.
- *Family history:* Risk is higher in those with a family history of stomach cancer.
- *Previous stomach surgery:* Risk is higher in those who have had surgery to treat peptic ulcer disease.
- *Infection:* Infection with *Helicobacter pylori* is a cause of peptic ulcer disease.
- *Diet:* Eating large amounts of smoked foods, salted fish and meat, and pickled vegetables increases risk. (M)
- *Tobacco:* The longer a person smokes, the greater the risk of proximal stomach cancer. (M)
- *Alcohol:* Long-term alcohol intake increases risk. Alcohol and smoking together raises a person's risk more than using either alone. (M)

Colon Cancer
- *Age:* 90% of people with colon cancer are over 50 years old.
- *Family history:* Having a first-degree relative with colorectal cancer increases one's risk.
- *Ethnicity:* Jews of Eastern European descent have the highest rate.
- *Preexisting condition:* Personal history of chronic inflammatory bowel disease.

M = modifiable risk factor.
Data from *www.cancer.org,* 2007.

Continued

RISK FACTORS *Abdominal Cancers—cont'd*

Colon Cancer—cont'd
- *Diabetes mellitus:* This increases risk 30% to 40%. (M)
- *Tobacco:* Smokers are 30% to 40% more likely than nonsmokers to die from colorectal cancer. (M)
- *Alcohol:* Heavy intake of alcohol increases risk. (M)
- *Obesity:* Increases risk. (M)
- *Diet:* Diet high in animal fat increases risk. (M)

Liver Cancer
- *Gender:* Men develop liver cancer several times more often than women.
- *Hepatitis:* Hepatitis B and C infections increase risk.
- *Cirrhosis:* Cirrhosis is common related to alcoholism.
- *Tobacco:* A strong link exists between smoking and liver cancer.

Pancreatic Cancer
- *Age:* Most clients are between 60 and 80 years old when diagnosed.
- *Gender:* Men are more likely to develop this cancer.
- *Tobacco:* About 30% of pancreatic cancer cases are thought to be directly related to cigarette smoking. (M)
- *Diet:* Diet high in meats and fats increases risk. (M)
- *Diabetes mellitus:* Pancreatic cancer is more common in people with diabetes mellitus. (M)
- *Family history:* In about 5% to 10% of cases there is an inherited tendency for this cancer.

Bladder Cancer
- *Tobacco:* The greatest risk factor for bladder cancer is smoking. (M)
- *Age:* The average age at diagnosis is 68 years.
- *Gender:* Men get bladder cancer at a rate two to three times greater than women.
- *Race:* Whites are two times more likely to develop bladder cancer than are African Americans and Hispanic Americans.
- *Chronic bladder inflammation:* Urinary tract infections, kidney stones, and bladder stones are linked to bladder cancer.

M = modifiable risk factor.
Data from *www.cancer.org,* 2007.

Questions regarding nutrition and eating habits are asked in the general evaluation of the client in Chapter 9.

GENERAL HEALTH HISTORY

Present Health Status

Do you have any chronic diseases that affect your gastrointestinal or urinary systems? If yes, describe.
Some chronic diseases may affect the gastrointestinal (GI) or urinary systems, such as diabetes mellitus. Diseases such as chronic hepatitis or cirrhosis may impair the liver's ability to metabolize nutrients and drugs.

Do you take any medications? If yes, what do you take and how often? Are you taking the medications as they were prescribed?
Both prescription and over-the-counter medications should be documented. Medications may cause GI side effects. Since drugs are metabolized in the liver, clients with liver diseases may not metabolize drugs well, which causes increased blood levels of these drugs.

Do you drink alcohol? If so, how much? How often? When was your last drink (of alcohol)?
Alcohol is a risk factor for peptic ulcer disease; esophageal, stomach, and colon cancer; pancreatitis, and cirrhosis. Alcoholism may damage the liver, the organ that metabolizes alcohol.

Do you smoke? If so, how much and for how long? Have you considered stopping or cutting down?
Cigarette smoking is a risk factor for peptic ulcer disease, as well as most cancers of the GI system.

How often do you have a bowel movement? When was your last bowel movement? What are the color and consistency of the stool?
Frequency of bowel movement is individual for each person. The frequency, color and consistency of stool are documented as baseline data. This question also gives the client an opportunity to describe disorders of the colon such as diarrhea, constipation, dark or light stools, or blood in stool.

Do you ever experience the leaking of urine? When does this occur? Do you ever use pads, tissue, or cloth in your underwear to catch urine?

Many clients, particularly women, do not report incontinence unless asked about it, often because of embarrassment. Nurses should ask at least one screening question to identify clients who have urinary incontinence (Dougherty et al, 2000). *Stress incontinence* is the most common type and is characterized by involuntary loss of small amounts of urine caused by physical exertion such as coughing, sneezing, jogging, and lifting. *Urge incontinence* is associated with a sudden strong urge to void. People can have both types of incontinence.

Past Medical History

Have you had problems with your abdomen or digestive system in the past? Esophagus? Stomach? Intestines? Liver? Gallbladder? Pancreas? Spleen? If yes, describe.

History of GI disorders may provide insight into findings to anticipate at this visit. These data give clues to client's education needs about reducing risk for other disease involving these body systems, such as cancers.

Have you had surgery of your abdomen or urinary tract? If yes, describe. Has the surgery required that you change any of your former routines, such as changes in the food you can eat or changes in bowel or urinary elimination? How have you been able to cope with having an ostomy?

Clients who have had gastrectomies may have changed the amount and frequency of meals, as well as the foods they eat. Clients may have a colostomy or an ileostomy after surgery for such disorders as colon cancer or ulcerative colitis. Clients who have had bladder cancer may have an ileal conduit as an alternative route for urine excretion. Any of these surgeries require that the client change an appliance over the stoma. This question conveys concern about their adjustment to this change in their body.

Have you had problems with your urinary tract in the past? If yes, describe.

History of urinary disorders may provide insight into findings to anticipate at this visit. These data also give clues to client's education needs about reducing risk for other diseases involving these body systems, such as urinary tract infection and cancers.

Family History

In your family, is there a history of diseases of the GI system such as gastroesophageal reflux disease (GERD)? Peptic ulcer disease? Stomach cancer? Colon cancer?

Family history may be used to determine clients' risk factors for GI disorders.

In your family, is there a history of diseases of the urinary tract such as kidney stones? Kidney cancer? Bladder cancer?

Family history may be used to determine clients' risk factors for urinary disorders.

PROBLEM-BASED HISTORY

Specific areas of assessment of the abdomen and GI system include abdominal pain, nausea and vomiting, indigestion, abdominal distention, change in bowel habits, jaundice, and problems with urination. As with symptoms in all areas of health assessment, a symptom analysis is completed, which includes the location, quality, quantity, chronology, setting, associated manifestations, and aggravating and alleviating factors (see Box 3-3 in Chapter 3).

Abdominal Pain

How long have you had abdominal pain? Where is it located? When did you first feel the pain? What activity were you doing when the pain occurred?

Time, location, and activity when pain occurs are important to diagnosis. Sudden, severe pain that awakens the client may be associated with acute perforation, inflammation, or torsion of an abdominal organ.

Describe the pain. Is it constant, or does it come and go? Have you had episodes of this pain before? Did the pain start suddenly?

Table 14-1 differentiates various types of abdominal pain. Pain description is helpful in determining the cause of the abdominal pain. Intense pain may be caused by a stone in the biliary tract or ureter, rupture of a fallopian tube from an ectopic pregnancy, or inflammation such as peritonitis following perforation of a gastric ulcer. Visceral pain arises from the GI tract and pancreas and may be described as an ache and well defined due to tumor growth, or it may be cramping, diffuse, and poorly localized due to obstruction.

Has the pain changed its location since it started? Do you feel the pain in any other parts of your body?

Pain radiation patterns are shown in Table 14-1. Pain from acute appendicitis starts around the umbilicus and radiates to the right lower quadrant. Back pain is associated with abdominal aneurysms or duodenal ulcers. Pain from gallbladder disease may be felt in the right shoulder.

Is the pain worse when your stomach is empty? Is it affected by eating? Is the pain worse at night or during the day?

Patterns of GI pain may help identify the cause. For example, the pain of duodenal ulcer may awaken the client from sleep. Pain in gastroenteritis and irritable bowel disease is worse in the presence of food because peristalsis is stimulated, which causes pain.

What relieves the pain? Is there any particular position that relieves the pain?

TABLE 14-1 *Differentiation of Abdominal Pain*

CAUSE	CLIENT CHARACTERISTICS	QUALITY	LOCATION	ASSOCIATED SYMPTOMS	AGGRAVATED BY	ALLEVIATED BY	FINDINGS
Gastroesophageal reflux	Any age	Gnawing, burning	Midepigastric; may radiate to jaw	Weight loss	Recumbency, bending, stooping	Antacids, sitting up	Hyperactive bowel sounds
Gastroenteritis	Any age	Crampy	Diffuse	Nausea and vomiting, fever, diarrhea	Food	Some relief with vomiting, diarrhea	
Gastritis	Alcoholism	Constant, burning	Epigastric	Hemorrhage, nausea and vomiting, diarrhea, fever	Alcohol, food, salicylates	Antacids	Epigastric tenderness on palpation or percussion
Peptic ulcer	30-50 years; more males than females	Gnawing, burning	Epigastric, back, and upper abdomen Gastric 1-2 hr after meals Duodenal 2-4 hr after meals, midmorning, midafternoon, and middle of the night	Nausea, vomiting, weight loss	Stress, alcohol; gastric ulcer aggravated by food; duodenal ulcers by empty stomach	Food, antacids—duodenal ulcers only	
Pancreatitis	Alcoholism, cholelithiasis	Steady, severe to mild, knifelike, sudden onset	LUQ and epigastric; radiates to back	Nausea and vomiting, diaphoresis	Lying supine	Leaning forward	Abdominal distention, bowel sounds, diffuse rebound
Appendicitis	Any age; peak 10-20 yr	Colicky, progressing to constant	Umbilicus, moving to RLQ	Vomiting, constipation, fever	Moving, coughing	Lying still	Rebound tenderness RLQ, positive obturator, positive iliopsoas
Cholecystitis or cholelithiasis	Adults; more females than males	Colicky, progressing to constant	RUQ radiates to right scapula	Nausea and vomiting, dark urine, light stools, jaundice	Fatty foods, drugs		Tender to palpation or percussion of RUQ
Ectopic pregnancy	History of menstrual irregularity	Sudden onset, persistent pain	Lower quadrant	Tender adnexal mass, vaginal bleeding			Palpable mass on affected side
Diverticular disease	Older adults	Intermittent cramping	LLQ	Constipation, diarrhea	Eating	Bowel movement, passing flatus	Palpable mass in LLQ
Irritable bowel disease	Young women	Crampy, recurrent, sharp, burning	LLQ	Mucus in stools		May be relieved by defecation	Colon tender on palpation
Intestinal obstruction	Older adults; those with prior abdominal surgery	Colicky, sudden onset	May be localized or generalized	Vomiting, constipation			Hyperactive bowel sounds in small obstruction

LLQ, Left lower quadrant; *LUQ,* left upper quadrant; *RLQ,* right lower quadrant; *RUQ,* right upper quadrant.

A particular position may relieve abdominal pain, for example pain from pancreatitis may be relieved in the knee-chest position. Colicky pain from a gallbladder or kidney stone may be relieved with restless movement. The pain of appendicitis is relieved by lying very still.

Is the pain associated with other symptoms, such as stress, fatigue, nausea and vomiting, gas, eating certain foods, fever, chills, constipation, diarrhea, rectal bleeding, frequent urination, or vaginal or penile discharge?

Identifying symptoms associated with pain may assist in determining the cause.

For females: Is the pain associated with your menstrual period? When was your last menstrual period? Could you be pregnant?

Dysmenorrhea (pain associated with menstruation) may cause lower abdominal pain and vomiting because of the increase in prostaglandin. An ectopic pregnancy may cause abdominal pain.

Nausea and Vomiting

How long have you been experiencing nausea or vomiting? How often does this occur?

Vomiting has many causes, and gaining additional details helps determine the cause.

How much do you vomit? What does the vomitus look like? Does it contain blood? Does it have an odor?

The characteristics of the vomitus may help determine its cause. Acute gastritis leads to vomiting of stomach contents, whereas obstruction of the bile duct results in greenish-yellow vomitus, and an intestinal obstruction may have a fecal odor to the vomitus. Stomach or duodenal ulcers or esophageal varices may cause blood in vomitus (hematemesis).

For females: Could you be pregnant?

Pregnancy should be ruled out as a cause of nausea and vomiting. Pregnant women have high serum levels of chorionic gonadotropin, which stimulates vomiting.

Do you have nausea without vomiting?

Nausea without vomiting is a common symptom of pregnant clients or those with metastatic disease.

What foods have you eaten in the last 24 hours? Where did you eat? How long after you ate did you vomit? Has anyone else who ate with you had these symptoms over the same time period?

These questions are asked to detect food poisoning or stomach influenza.

Do you have other symptoms with the nausea or vomiting? Pain? Constipation? Diarrhea? Change in color of stools? Change in color of urine? Fever or chills?

Knowing associated symptoms may help determine the cause of nausea and vomiting. For example, liver disease may change stool color from brown to clay colored. Infection such as hepatitis may cause fever and chills.

Indigestion

How long after eating do you have indigestion or heartburn? Where do you feel the discomfort? In your stomach? Chest? How long has this been happening? How often does this occur?

Heartburn felt in the chest, over the esophagus, or in the stomach that occurs after eating may indicate gastroesophageal reflux disease (GERD).

What makes the symptoms worse? Does a change in position, such as lying down, affect your indigestion?

Heartburn caused by GERD or hiatal hernia is often worse when the client lies down because the gastric acids move by gravity toward the esophagus.

What relieves these symptoms? Do you take antacids or acid blockers?

When antacids relieve pain, excessive acid can be part of the cause of the indigestion.

Are there any other symptoms associated with the heartburn? Radiating pain? Sweating? Light-headedness?

Knowing associated symptoms may help determine the cause of indigestion. Angina or myocardial infarction may be the cause of the "indigestion-like" symptoms. Questions about radiating pain to the arms or jaw, along with other questions, are asked with these cardiovascular disorders in mind.

Abdominal Distention

How long has your abdomen been distended? Does it come and go? Is it related to eating? What relieves the distention?

Distention associated with eating is intermittent and relieved by passing gas. Constipation contributes to distention and develops slowly, but is not relieved without bowel movement. Distention caused by ascites is a progressive process and increases abdominal girth.

Are there other symptoms associated with the abdominal distention? Vomiting? Loss of appetite? Weight loss? Change in bowel habits? Shortness of breath? Pain?

Vomiting may indicate intestinal obstruction as a cause of distention. Loss of appetite is associated with cirrhosis and malignancy. Shortness of breath is associated with heart failure, and ascites is associated with chronic liver disease.

Change in Bowel Habits

Describe the change in your bowel movements. Change in frequency? Change in consistency of feces? When did you first notice the change? How long has this been happening? What does the stool look like: bloody, mucoid, fatty, watery?

Changes in bowel habits can be related to a number of factors, including changes in diet, activity, stress, and medications. A change in bowel habits is one of the seven warning signs of cancer.

Are there other associated symptoms to the change in bowel habits, such as increased gas, pain, fever, nausea, vomiting, abdominal cramping, diarrhea? Is there a time of day when the change occurs, such as after eating or at night?

Knowing associated symptoms may help determine the cause of the change in bowel function. Some foods cause increased gas, fever suggests inflammation or infection, and abdominal cramping with diarrhea may indicate gastroenteritis.

Yellow Discoloration of Eyes or Skin (Jaundice)

When did you first notice the yellow discoloration of your skin or eyes? Has it become more noticeable?

Jaundice indicates elevated serum bilirubin that can be caused by liver disease or obstruction of bile flow from gallstones.

Is the yellow discoloration of your skin or eyes associated with abdominal pain? Loss of appetite? Nausea? Vomiting? Fever?

Fever, nausea, vomiting, and loss of appetite are also symptoms of hepatitis.

In the last year, have you had a blood transfusion or tattoos? Are you using any intravenous drugs? Do you eat raw shellfish, for example, oysters? Have you traveled abroad in the last year? Where? Did you drink unclean water?

These are possible sources of transmission of the hepatitis virus.

Has the color of your urine or stools changed?

Urine changing from amber to brown and stools changing from brown to clay colored suggest high serum bilirubin that occurs with liver disease or obstruction of the common bile duct.

Problems with Urination

Describe the change in your urination. What is your usual pattern of urination? Have you felt any pain or burning when urinating? Are you urinating frequently in small amounts (frequency) or feeling you cannot wait to urinate (urgency)? If yes, when did this begin?

Pain, burning, or frequency may indicate a bladder infection. Loss of muscle tone may cause incontinence, particularly in

---

HEALTH PROMOTION   *Colorectal Cancer*

Colorectal cancer is the third most common cause of cancer and the second leading cause of cancer-related death in men and women. An estimated 147,000 new cases and 56,700 deaths were projected for 2004. Individuals with greatest risk for colorectal cancer include those with a history suggestive of familial polyposis or hereditary nonpolyposis colorectal cancer, those with a personal history of ulcerative colitis, and those with a previous history of colorectal cancer. Other important risk factors include diet high in fat and low in fiber, obesity, and sedentary lifestyle. Smoking and excessive alcohol intake are also thought to be connected.

Goals and Objectives—*Healthy People 2010*
The overall *Healthy People 2010* goal related to cancer is to reduce the number of new cancer cases, as well as illness, disability, and death caused by cancer. Three specific objectives are related to colorectal cancer: reduce the death rate from colorectal cancer, increase the proportion of adults who are screened for colorectal cancer, and increase the number of primary care providers who counsel clients about blood stool tests for colorectal screening.

Recommendations to Reduce Risk (Primary Prevention)
American Cancer Society
Prevention is possible because most colon cancers develop from adenomatous polyps. Polyps are precancerous growths in the colon and rectum. Removing polyps can lower a person's risk of developing cancer (see screening recommendations).

An individual can lower risk of developing colorectal cancer by managing controllable risk factors, such as diet and physical activity. Information to share with clients includes the following:

- Consume diet high in fruits, vegetables, and whole-grain foods; limit intake of high-fat foods.
- Participate in moderate to vigorous activity for 30 minutes on 5 days or more a week.
- Attain and maintain a healthy weight.

For individuals with average risk: Beginning at age 50, both men and women should have one of the following screening tests done:

- Fecal occult blood test (FOBT) annually
- Flexible sigmoidoscopy every 5 years
- FOBT yearly plus sigmoidoscopy every 5 years
- Double-contrast barium enema every 5 years
- Colonoscopy every 10 years

Digital rectal examination is recommended to be done in conjunction with a sigmoidoscopy, colonoscopy, or double-contrast barium enema.

For individuals with higher risk, screening should begin earlier.

From *www.cancer.org*, 2007; US Department of Health and Human Services: *Healthy People 2010: understanding and improving health*, ed 2, Washington, DC, 2000, US Government Printing Office (available at *www.healthypeople.gov*).

women. Men who have an enlarged prostate may have some of these same symptoms (see Chapter 18).

Have you had associated symptoms such as fever, chills, and back pain?

These symptoms may indicate a kidney disorder such as pyelonephritis or kidney stones.

Describe the color of the urine. Is there blood in the urine?

Dark amber urine is associated with kidney or liver disease. Blood in the urine is associated with menstrual periods in women or with kidney disease.

Have you had an unexpected weight gain? Have you noticed swelling in your ankles at the end of the day or shortness of breath? Are you urinating less?

These clinical manifestations may indicate renal failure, when kidney dysfunction causes fluid retention.

EXAMINATION

ROUTINE TECHNIQUES

- OBSERVE the client's general behavior and position. 🔑
- INSPECT the abdomen. 🔑
- AUSCULTATE the abdomen. 🔑
- PALPATE the abdomen lightly. 🔑
- PALPATE the abdomen deeply.

SPECIAL CIRCUMSTANCES OR ADVANCED PRACTICE

- PERCUSS the abdomen. ★
- PERCUSS the liver. ★
- PERCUSS the spleen. ★
- PALPATE around the umbilicus.
- PALPATE the liver.
- PALPATE the gallbladder. ★
- PALPATE the spleen. ★
- PALPATE the kidneys. ★
- PERCUSS the kidneys.
- ASSESS the abdomen for fluid. ★
- ELICIT abdominal reflexes. ★
- ASSESS for abdominal pain due to inflammation.
- ASSESS the abdomen for floating mass. ★

EQUIPMENT NEEDED
Stethoscope • Penlight • Tape measure • Small ruler • Marking pen

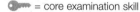 = core examination skill   ★ = advanced practice

PROCEDURES AND TECHNIQUES WITH NORMAL FINDINGS

ROUTINE TECHNIQUES

OBSERVE client's general behavior and position.

The client should appear relaxed, sitting or lying quietly with slow, even respirations.

ABNORMAL FINDINGS

Note abnormal findings such as emaciation, obesity, marked restlessness, or a rigid posture, the knees drawn up, facial grimacing, and rapid, uneven, or grunting respirations. Clients with pancreatitis may prefer the knee-chest position; those with peritonitis or appendicitis may lie very still; those with colicky gallstones or ureteral stones may rock back and forth.

PROCEDURES AND TECHNIQUES WITH NORMAL FINDINGS	ABNORMAL FINDINGS

⚷ INSPECT the abdomen for skin color, surface characteristics, contour, and surface movements.

Direct a light source at a right angle to the client's long axis. Skin color may be paler than other parts of the skin, because of lack of exposure.

Surface characteristics should be smooth. There may be silver-white striae, scars, and a very faint, fine vascular network present. The umbilicus should be centrally located (Fig. 14-4).

Jaundice indicates elevated serum bilirubin; erythema may indicate inflammation; bruises may indicate trauma or low platelet count; and striae may indicate abdominal distention.

Note prominent venous patterns or engorgement of the veins around the umbilicus. Glistening or taut appearance is associated with ascites. The umbilicus should not be displaced upward, downward, or laterally, nor should a hernia be visible around or slightly above the umbilicus. Note if the umbilicus is inflamed or has drainage.

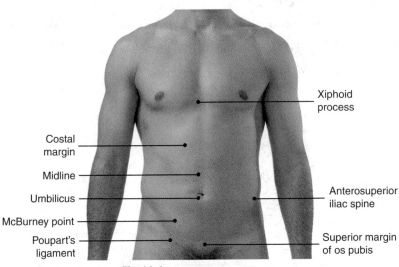

Costal margin
Midline
Umbilicus
McBurney point
Poupart's ligament
Xiphoid process
Anterosuperior iliac spine
Superior margin of os pubis

Fig. 14-4   Landmarks of the abdomen.

Contour is usually sunken, although it may protrude slightly, especially in overweight and obese clients. Adjusting the light source to form shadows may highlight small changes in the contour. Evaluate symmetry by viewing the abdomen from two additional angles: standing behind the client's head and squatting at the side to view the abdomen at eye level. Ask the client to take a deep breath and hold it. The contour of the abdomen should remain smooth and symmetric.

With the client lying supine, ask him or her to cough to increase intraabdominal pressure while you inspect for a sudden bulge.

When abdominal distention is noted, place a measuring tape around the abdomen at the level of the superior iliac crests to measure the abdominal girth (circumference). This provides an objective measure to assess the increase or decrease in abdominal distention.

Check for marked concavity, which is associated with general wasting signs or anteroposterior rib expansion.

Bulges during coughing indicate an abdominal hernia: ventral, umbilical, inguinal, or femoral (Swartz, 2006).

Abdominal distention may result from the "seven F's"—fat (obesity), fetus (pregnancy), fluid (ascites), flatulence (gas), feces (constipation), fibroid tumor, or fatal tumor. Note any bulges or masses, particularly of the liver or spleen. Abdominal or incisional hernias can also create bulges of the abdomen.

Inspect the surface for movements. Peristalsis is usually not visible, but there may be an upper midline pulsation visible in thin individuals. The abdomen should move smoothly and evenly with respirations. Generally females exhibit thoracic movements during inhalation, whereas males exhibit abdominal movements. Ask the client to raise his or her head without using the arms for support. The rectus abdominis muscles become prominent, and a midline bulge may appear. Areas of bulges considered normal variations are pregnancy and marked obesity.

Note visible peristalsis or marked pulsations. The area of pulsation is not palpated because it may indicate an abdominal aneurysm, a weakening in the wall of the abdominal aorta. Grunting or labored movements or restricted abdominal movements with respirations should be recorded.

⚷ = core examination skill

PROCEDURES AND TECHNIQUES WITH NORMAL FINDINGS

ABNORMAL FINDINGS

When examining a client with an ileostomy or colostomy, remove the bag if needed for inspection. The stoma should appear red and moist. The area where the ostomy attaches to the skin should appear well healed and without lesions, irritation, or areas of excoriation. The stool characteristics depend on the location of the ostomy. Clients with an ileostomy (small-bowel area) have stool that is of a thick liquid consistency. If the client has had a transverse (upper colon) level colostomy, the stool is mushy. If the client's colostomy is in the area of the descending or sigmoid (lower) colon, the stool is more solid.

The stoma appears pale from ischemia or brown or black from necrotic tissue. The skin around the stoma is excoriated and tender, with or without exudate.

AUSCULTATE the abdomen for bowel sounds.

Be sure to auscultate *before* palpating and percussing the abdomen so that the presence or absence of bowel sounds or pain is not altered. A quiet environment may be necessary. Box 14-1 lists the anatomic correlates of the quarters of the abdomen (Fig. 14-5). Box 14-2 shows an alternative way to section the abdo-

Report any absence of sound after listening for several minutes in each quadrant. Decreased or absent bowel sounds occur with mechanical obstruction or paralytic ileus as well as with peritonitis and bowel obstruction. Audible sounds produced by hyperactive peristalsis is termed *borborygmi*, and create rumbling, gurgling, and high-pitched tinkling sounds. Although increased peristalsis is associated with diarrhea, laxative use, and gastroenteritis, true borborygmi are more intense and episodic sounds associated with intestinal obstruction.

BOX 14-1 ANATOMIC CORRELATES OF THE QUADRANTS OF THE ABDOMEN

Right Upper Quadrant	**Left Upper Quadrant**
Liver and gallbladder	Left lobe of liver
Pylorus	Spleen
Duodenum	Stomach
Head of pancreas	Body of pancreas
Right adrenal gland	Left adrenal gland
Portion of right kidney	Portion of left kidney
Portions of ascending and transverse colon	Portions of transverse and descending colon

Right Lower Quadrant	**Left Lower Quadrant**
Lower pole of right kidney	Lower pole of left kidney
Cecum and appendix	Sigmoid colon
Portion of ascending colon	Portion of descending colon
Bladder (if distended)	Bladder (if distended)
Right ureter	Left ureter
Right ovary and salpinx	Left ovary and salpinx
Uterus (if enlarged)	Uterus (if enlarged)
Right spermatic cord	Left spermatic cord

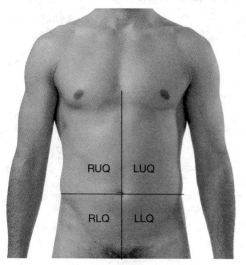

Fig. 14-5 Quadrants of the abdomen.

= core examination skill

PROCEDURES AND TECHNIQUES WITH NORMAL FINDINGS

ABNORMAL FINDINGS

men for examination using nine regions (Fig. 14-6). Use the diaphragm of the stethoscope and press lightly. Listen in a systematic progression, such as from right upper quadrant (RUQ) to left upper quadrant (LUQ) to left lower quadrant (LLQ) and finally to right lower quadrant (RLQ). Bowel sounds should be noted every 5 to 15 seconds. The duration of a single bowel sound may range from 1 second to several seconds. The sounds are high-pitched gurgles or clicks, although this varies greatly.

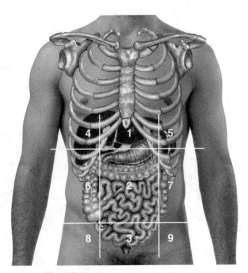

Fig. 14-6   Nine regions of the abdomen.

BOX 14-2	**ANATOMIC CORRELATES OF THE NINE REGIONS OF THE ABDOMEN**	
Right Hypochondriac Right lobe of liver Portion of gallbladder Portion of duodenum Portion of right kidney Right adrenal gland	**Epigastric** Pyloric end of stomach Duodenum Pancreas Portion of liver Portion of gallbladder	**Left Hypochondriac** Stomach Spleen Tail of pancreas Upper pole of left kidney Left adrenal gland
Right Lumbar Ascending colon Lower half of right kidney Portion of duodenum and jejunum	**Umbilical** Lower duodenum Jejunum and ileum Transverse colon	**Left Lumbar** Descending colon Lower half of left kidney Portions of jejunum and ileum
Right Inguinal Cecum Appendix Ileum (lower end) Right ureter Right spermatic cord Right ovary	**Hypogastric** Ileum Bladder Uterus (in pregnancy)	**Left Inguinal** Sigmoid colon Left ureter Left spermatic cord Left ovary

| **PROCEDURES AND TECHNIQUES WITH NORMAL FINDINGS** | **ABNORMAL FINDINGS** |

AUSCULTATE the abdomen for arterial and venous vascular sounds.

Listen with the bell of the stethoscope. Listen over aorta and renal, iliac, and femoral arteries for bruits. They make "swishing" sounds, occur during systole, and are continuous regardless of the client's position (Fig. 14-7). Also listen with the bell over the epigastric region and around the umbilicus for a venous hum, a soft, low-pitched, and continuous sound. Normally vascular sounds are not heard.

A bruit indicates a turbulent blood flow caused by narrowing of a blood vessel. Bruits over the aorta suggest an aneurysm. Two sound patterns may indicate renal arterial stenosis: soft, medium- to low-pitched murmurs heard over the upper midline or toward the flank or epigastric bruits that radiate laterally. Venous hums are rare and are associated with portal hypertension and cirrhosis.

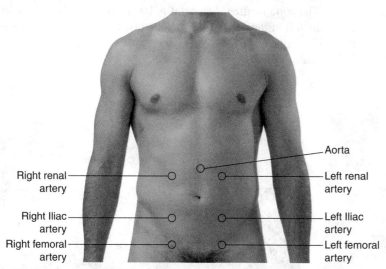

Fig.14-7   Sites to auscultate for bruits: renal arteries, iliac arteries, aorta, and femoral arteries.

PALPATE the abdomen lightly for tenderness, muscle tone, and surface characteristics.

Palpate all quadrants of the abdomen. Use the pads of the fingertips to depress the abdomen 1 to 2 cm (Fig. 14-8). Some nurses reduce ticklishness by sliding their hands into each palpation position to maintaining contact with the client's skin.

No tenderness should be present, and the abdominal muscles should be relaxed, although anxious clients may have some muscle resistance on palpation. Note consistent tension as you move across the smooth surface. When the client has abdominal pain, palpate over the area of pain last.

Note any cutaneous tenderness or hypersensitivity. Note superficial masses or localized areas of rigidity or increased tension. Rigidity is associated with peritoneal irritation and may be diffuse or localized.

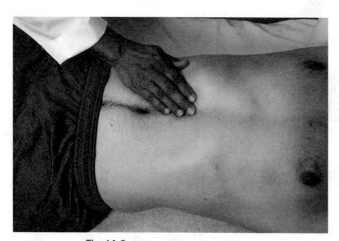

Fig. 14-8   Light palpation of the abdomen.

= core examination skill

PROCEDURES AND TECHNIQUES WITH NORMAL FINDINGS	**ABNORMAL FINDINGS**

PALPATE the abdomen deeply for tenderness, masses, and aortic pulsation.

Palpate all quadrants. Use either the distal flat portions of the finger pads (Fig. 14-9) and press gradually and deeply 4 to 6 cm into the palpation area, or use a bimanual technique, with the lower hand resting lightly on the surface and the upper hand exerting pressure for deep palpation (Fig. 14-10). Observe for facial grimaces during palpation that may indicate areas of tenderness. Ask the client to breathe slowly through the mouth to facilitate muscle relaxation. When the client has abdominal pain, palpate over the area of pain last. The aorta is often palpable at the epigastrium, as well as above and slightly to the left of the umbilicus (Fig. 14-11). The borders of the rectus abdominis muscles can be felt, as can the sacral promontory and feces in the ascending or descending colon.

Note any pain that is present in local or generalized areas. The client may respond to pain by using muscle guarding, facial grimaces, or pulling away from the nurse. Abnormal findings include masses that descend during inspiration, lateral pulsatile masses (abdominal aortic aneurysm), laterally mobile masses, and fixed masses.

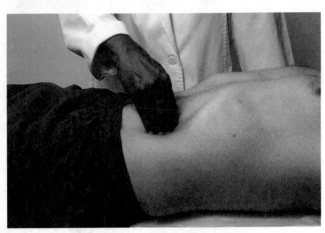

Fig. 14-9   Deep palpation of the abdomen.

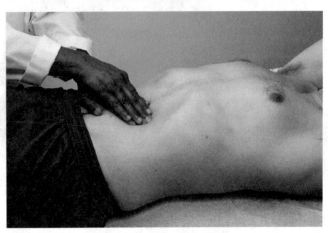

Fig. 14-10   Deep bimanual palpation.

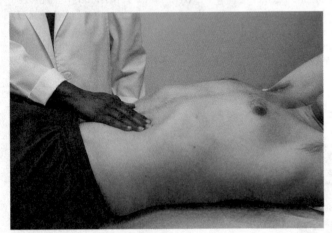

Fig. 14-11   Palpating the aorta.

| PROCEDURES AND TECHNIQUES WITH NORMAL FINDINGS | ABNORMAL FINDINGS |

SPECIAL CIRCUMSTANCES OR ADVANCED PRACTICE

★ PERCUSS the abdomen for tones.

Percuss all quadrants for tones, using indirect percussion to assess density of abdominal contents. (Develop a routine for the percussion process to ensure that all areas are covered [Fig. 14-12].) Percuss in each quadrant for tympany and dullness. Tympany is the most common percussion tone heard and is due to the presence of gas. The suprapubic area may be dull when the urinary bladder is distended. See Chapter 4 for the procedures for percussion.

Note any marked dullness in a localized area that may indicate an abdominal mass.

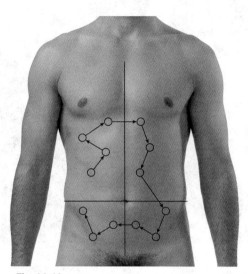

Fig. 14-12   Systematic route for abdominal percussion.

★ PERCUSS the liver to determine span and descent.

Procedure:
1. Beginning below the level of the umbilicus at the right midclavicular line (RMCL), percuss upward until the tone changes from a tympany to a dull percussion tone indicating the liver border. Mark the border with a pen. The lower border is usually at the costal margin or slightly below it (Fig. 14-13, *A*) (see also Fig. 14-4).
2. Beginning over the lung in the RMCL, percuss the intercostal spaces downward until the tone changes from resonant to dull, indicating the upper liver border. Mark the location with a pen. The upper border usually begins in the fifth to seventh intercostal space (Fig. 14-13, *B*).
3. Measure the span between the two lines using a ruler or tape measure to estimate the midclavicular liver span.
4. To assess the liver descent, ask the client to take a deep breath and hold it; then percuss upward from the stomach to the RMCL.

Findings: Normally the midclavicular liver span is 2.5 to 4.5 inches (6 to 12 cm) (Fig. 14-13, *C*). Liver span correlates with body size and gender; large people and men tend to have larger spans. The lower border of the liver should descend downward 0.75 to 1.25 inches (2 to 3 cm).

Note when the lower border of the liver exceeds 0.75 to 1.25 inches (2 to 3 cm) below the costal margin. This indicates an enlarged liver (hepatomegaly), which is associated with cirrhosis and hepatitis. Note when dullness extends above the fifth intercostal space, indicating hepatomegaly. Also, clients with chronic obstructive pulmonary disease may have a flat diaphragm, which makes percussion of the upper border of the liver difficult. Obesity can make percussion difficult. Note if the liver fails to move with inspiration or if movement is less than 0.75 inch (2 cm).

★ = advanced practice

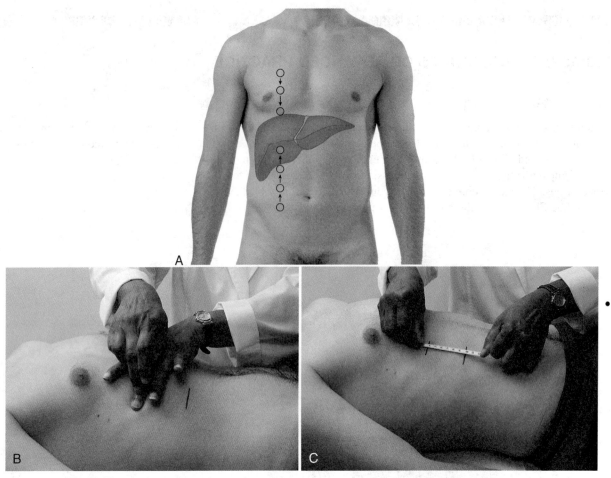

Fig. 14-13   **A,** Liver percussion route. **B,** Percussion method of estimating size of liver in the midclavicular line. **C,** Distance between the two marks measured in estimating the liver span in midclavicular line is usually 2.5 to 4.5 inches (6 to 12 cm).

PROCEDURES AND TECHNIQUES WITH NORMAL FINDINGS	ABNORMAL FINDINGS

★ **PERCUSS the spleen for size.**

With the client lying supine, percuss in the lowest intercostal space just posterior to the left midaxillary line (LMAL) (Fig. 14-14). Try to outline the spleen by percussing in several directions from dullness to resonance or tympany. Normally the spleen cannot be percussed, or you may hear a small area of splenic dullness at the sixth to the tenth intercostal spaces. A full stomach and feces in the transverse or descending colon may mimic dullness of splenic enlargement. Percuss the lowest intercostal space in the left anterior axillary line before and after the client takes a deep breath. The area is usually tympanic.

Splenic enlargement may indicate infection or trauma. Note whether the tympany changes to dullness on inspiration. An enlarged spleen is brought forward on inspiration to produce a dull percussion note.

PALPATE around the umbilicus for bulges, nodules, and the umbilical ring.

The umbilical ring should feel round with no irregularities or bulges. The umbilicus itself may be inverted or slightly everted.

Note if the umbilical ring is incomplete or soft in the center. Note any bulges from an umbilical hernia.

★ = advanced practice

PROCEDURES AND TECHNIQUES WITH NORMAL FINDINGS

ABNORMAL FINDINGS

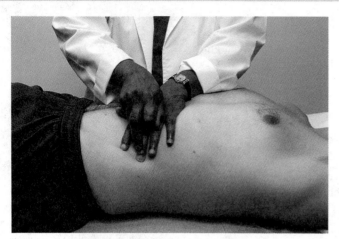

Fig. 14-14 Percussion of the spleen.

PALPATE the liver for lower border and tenderness.

Two techniques may be used to palpate the liver.

One technique begins by placing the left hand under the eleventh and twelfth ribs to lift the liver closer to the abdominal wall. Place your right hand parallel to the right costal margin and press down and under the costal margin (Fig. 14-15, *A* and *B*) (see also Fig. 14-4). Ask the client to take some deep breaths. The border and contour of the liver are often not palpable. The liver may "bump" against the right fingers during inspiration, especially in thin clients.

A very enlarged liver may lie under the nurse's hand as it extends downward into the abdominal cavity. Note any irregular surfaces or edges, as well as any tenderness. The client may complain of pain when taking a deep breath during this assessment.

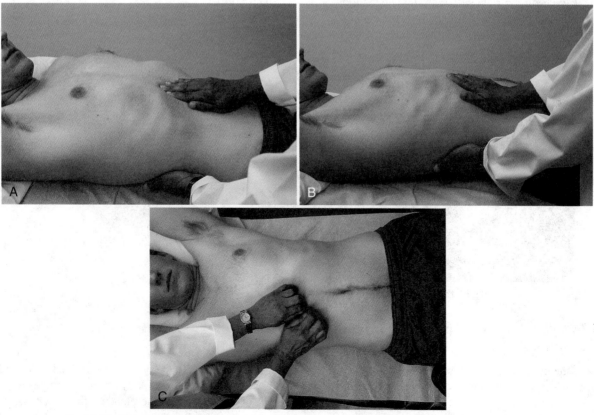

Fig. 14-15 **Methods of palpating the liver. A,** Fingers are extended, with tips on right midclavicular line below the level of liver tenderness and pointing toward the head. **B,** Fingers parallel to the costal margin. **C,** Fingers hooked over the costal margin.

PROCEDURES AND TECHNIQUES WITH NORMAL FINDINGS

ABNORMAL FINDINGS

Another technique is called the "hooking" technique. Stand on the client's right side facing the feet. Place your hands side by side at the right costal margin and curve your fingers to "hook" them under the costal margin (Fig. 14-15, *C*). Ask the client to take a deep breath, and you may feel the liver "bump" against your fingers during inspiration The border of the liver should feel smooth. No tenderness should be present.

★ PALPATE the gallbladder for tenderness.

Palpate below the liver margin at the right lateral border of the rectus abdominis muscle for the gallbladder. A healthy gallbladder is not palpable.

A palpable, tender gallbladder may indicate cholecystitis. Test for cholecystitis by asking the client to take in a deep breath during deep palpation. Cholecystitis is suspected if the client experiences pain and abruptly stops inhaling during palpation (Murphy's sign). A nontender, enlarged gallbladder suggests common bile duct obstruction.

★ PALPATE the spleen for border and tenderness.

Standing at the client's right side, reach across the client to place the palm surface of your left hand under the client's left flank at the costovertebral angle and exert pressure upward to elevated the left rib cage and move the spleen anteriorly. Press the palm surface of your right hand gently under the left anterior costal margin (Fig. 14-16). Press your fingertips inward toward the spleen as the client takes a deep breath and try to feel the tip of the spleen as it descends during inspiration. The spleen it is normally not palpable.

An alternative strategy for spleen palpation is to perform the procedure with the client lying on the right side with the legs and knees flexed. Stand on the client's right and place your left hand over the client's left costovertebral angle while pressing your right hand under the left anterior costal margin.

A palpable spleen will feel like a firm mass that bumps against the nurse's fingers. Spleen tenderness may indicate infection or trauma.

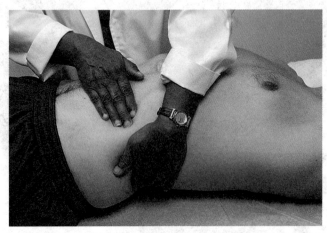

Fig. 14-16 Palpation of the spleen.

★ PALPATE the kidneys for presence, contour, and tenderness.

Normally the kidney is not palpable and is excluded from the routine health assessment unless data from the history indicate a need.

Tenderness is associated with kidney trauma or infection (e.g., pyelonephritis or glomerulonephritis).

★ = advanced practice

PROCEDURES AND TECHNIQUES WITH NORMAL FINDINGS	**ABNORMAL FINDINGS**

Left kidney: Stand to the client's right side with the client in a supine position. Place the left hand at the left posterior costal angle (left flank) and the right hand at the client's left anterior costal margin (see Fig. 14-4). Ask the client to take a deep breath, and elevate the client's left flank with your left hand and palpate deeply with your right hand (Fig. 14-17). Occasionally the lower pole of the kidney can be felt during inhalation in thin clients, but rarely in the average client. The contour should be smooth with no tenderness.

Right kidney: Repeat the same maneuver on the right side, which is easier to palpate because it lies lower than the left kidney. The lower pole of the right kidney may be palpated during inspiration as smooth, firm, and nontender.

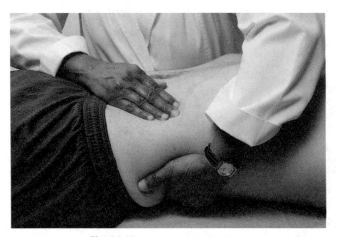

Fig. 14-17 Palpation of the left kidney.

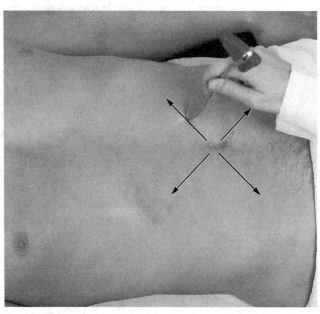

Fig. 14-18 Eliciting superficial abdominal reflexes. Stroke the upper abdominal area upward, away from the umbilicus, and the lower umbilicus area downward, away from the umbilicus. *(From Seidel et al, 2003.)*

★ **ELICIT abdominal reflexes for presence.**

Elicit the abdominal reflexes by stroking each quadrant with the end of a reflex hammer or tongue blade (Fig. 14-18). For upper abdominal reflexes, stroke upward and away from the umbilicus; for lower abdominal reflexes, stroke downward and away from the umbilicus. The expected response to each stroke is contraction of the rectus abdominis muscle and movement of the umbilicus toward the side stroked.

Diminished reflexes may be found in clients who are obese or have been pregnant. An absence of reflexes is associated with disease of the motor tracts of the spinal cord.

★ = advanced practice

PROCEDURES AND TECHNIQUES WITH NORMAL FINDINGS

ABNORMAL FINDINGS

PERCUSS the kidneys for costovertebral angle (CVA) tenderness.

Approach the client from behind as he or she is seated. One method for percussion is the direct approach. Use direct percussion to tap each CVA with the ulnar surface of the dominant fist (Fig. 14-19, *A*). An alternative method is to use indirect percussion. Place the palmar surface of the nondominant hand over the CVA, and tap the dorsum of that hand with the dominant fist (Fig. 14-19, *B*). The client should perceive a thud but no pain. Figure 14-20 shows the underlying anatomy of the kidney in relation to the CVA or the flank.

Costovertebral angle tenderness or severe pain may indicate pyelonephritis, glomerulonephritis, or nephrolithiasis (kidney stones).

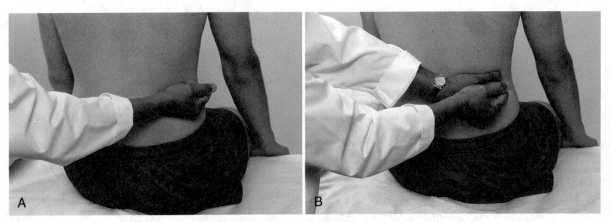

Fig. 14-19   Fist percussion of costovertebral angle for kidney tenderness. **A,** Direct percussion. **B,** Indirect percussion.

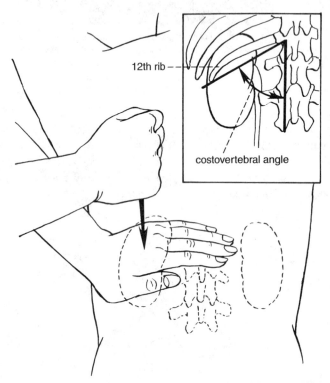

12th rib

costovertebral angle

Fig. 14-20   Anatomic drawing showing landmarks for indirect percussion of the costovertebral angle. *(From Polaski and Tatro, 1996.)*

PROCEDURES AND TECHNIQUES WITH NORMAL FINDINGS

ABNORMAL FINDINGS

★ **ASSESS the abdomen for fluid.**

If fluid is suspected within the abdomen, perform the following tests:

Shifting dullness: Ask the client to lie supine so that any fluid pools in the lateral (flank) area. Percuss the abdomen. Draw lines on the abdomen to indicate the midline tympany (the expected tone) in contrast to lateral dullness (tone created by fluid). Then have the client turn to the right side and repeat percussion. Listen as the tympanic tone shifts to the upper (left) side and the area of dullness rises toward the midline (Fig. 14-21). Finally, have the client turn to the left lateral position and percuss. Listen as the dullness rises toward the midline.

Fluid wave: The client lies supine. You will need the hand of another nurse or the client to be placed sideways in the middle of the client's abdomen to stop the transmission of a tap across the skin (Fig. 14-22). Place your hands on either side of the abdomen. Use your fingertips to sharply strike one side of the abdomen. Feel for the fluid wave with the other hand on the opposite side of the abdomen.

Movement of dullness as the client shifts position reflects the shift of fluid in the peritoneal cavity (ascites).

If ascites is present, the tap causes a fluid wave through the abdomen (Fig. 14-23).

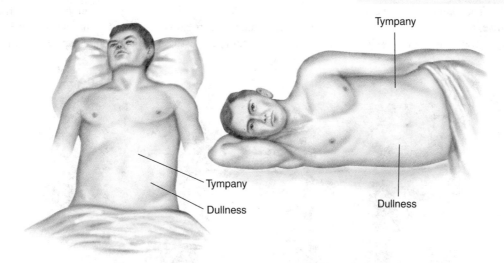

Fig. 14-21 **Testing for shifting dullness.** Dullness shifts to the dependent side. *(From Seidel et al, 2006.)*

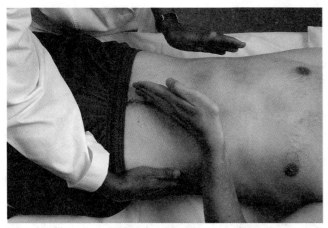

Fig. 14-22 **Testing for fluid wave.** Strike one side of the abdomen sharply with the fingertips. Feel for the impulse of a fluid wave with the other hand.

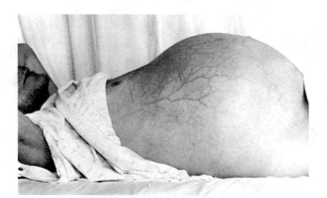

Fig. 14-23 **Massive ascites in an individual with cirrhosis.** Distended abdomen, dilated upper abdominal veins, and inverted umbilicus are classic manifestations. *(From Prior, Silberstein, and Stang, 1981.)*

★ = advanced practice

PROCEDURES AND TECHNIQUES WITH NORMAL FINDINGS

ASSESS the abdominal pain due to inflammation.

If the client has abdominal pain that you suspect is due to inflammation, test for *rebound tenderness* as follows: Press down firmly at a 90-degree angle to the abdomen in an area away from the point of pain. Press inward deeply (Fig. 14-24), then release your fingers quickly. A response that indicates no pain is for the client to report less pain the when the pressure is released than when the pressure is exerted.

Testing for *McBurney sign* is a test for appendicitis. Palpate McBurney point, which is located halfway between the umbilicus and the right anterior iliac crest (see Fig 14-4). Press firmly into the abdomen, and release pressure quickly. Absence of pain is a negative McBurney sign.

When acute appendicitis is suspected, perform the *iliopsoas muscle test.* With the client supine, place your hand over the lower right thigh. Ask the client to raise the right leg, flexing at the hip. Push down to resist the raising of the leg (Fig. 14-25). When the client reports no pain from the pressure on the iliopsoas muscle, the test is negative.

When a ruptured appendix or pelvic abscess is suspected, perform the *obturator muscle test.* The client lies supine and flexes the right hip and knee to 90 degrees. The nurse, holding the leg just above the knee and at the ankle, rotates the leg medially and laterally (Fig. 14-26). If the client has no pain, the test is negative.

ABNORMAL FINDINGS

Rebound tenderness is present if the client experiences more pain when pressure is released than when pressure is exerted and indicates peritoneal inflammation (see Table 14-1).

Positive rebound tenderness over McBurney point indicates appendicitis.

An inflamed appendix may irritate the lateral iliopsoas muscle. When the client reports RLQ pain to pressure against the raised leg, the iliopsoas muscle test is positive.

Pain in the hypogastric region is a positive sign indicating irritation of the obturator muscle, which may be caused by a ruptured appendix or pelvic abscess.

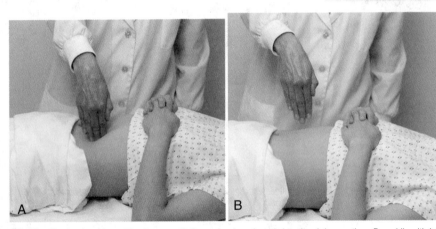

Fig. 14-24 **Testing for rebound tenderness. A,** Press deeply and gently into the abdomen; then, **B,** rapidly withdraw the hand and fingers.

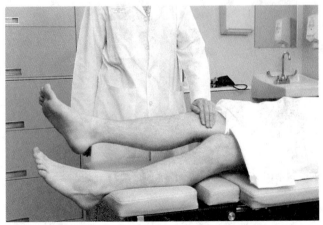

Fig. 14-25 Iliopsoas muscle test. *(From Doughty and Jackson, 1993.)*

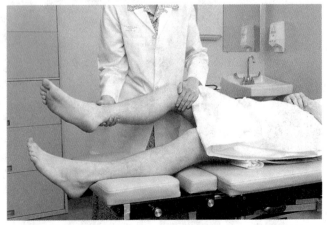

Fig. 14-26 Obturator muscle test. *(From Doughty and Jackson, 1993.)*

PROCEDURES AND TECHNIQUES WITH NORMAL FINDINGS

★ **ASSESS the abdomen for floating mass.**

Ballottement is a palpation technique used to determine a floating mass. Ballottement can be performed with one or two hands.

Place one hand perpendicular to the abdomen and push in toward the mass with fingertips at a 90-degree angle (Fig. 14-27, *A*). A freely movable mass will float upward and touch the fingertips as fluids and other structures are displaced.

When using the bimanual method, place one hand on the anterior abdomen to push down. The other hand is placed against the flank to push up and palpate the mass to determine presence and size (Fig. 14-27, *B*).

ABNORMAL FINDINGS

A floating mass may be an abnormal growth or a fetal head.

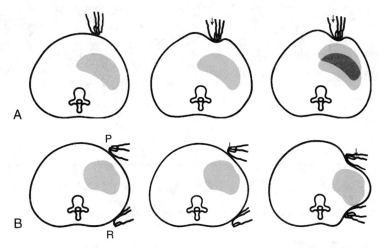

Fig. 14-27   Ballottement technique. A, Single-handed ballottement. Push inward at a 90-degree angle; if the object is freely movable, it will float upward to touch the fingertips. **B,** Bimanual ballottement. P, Pushing hand; R, Receiving hand. *(From GI series, 1981, Whitehall-Robins Healthcare.)*

Documenting Expected Findings

Abdomen and Gastrointestinal System

The abdomen is smooth, flat, and lighter color than extremities, with smooth, symmetric contour and no visible peristalsis. The umbilicus is midline and rectus abdominis muscles become prominent when head raised. Bowel sounds present in all quadrants with no vascular sounds. No tenderness, masses, or aortic pulsations to light or deep abdominal palpation. Umbilical ring feels round with no irregularities or bulges. Tympany heard over abdomen and spleen, and dullness over suprapubic area. Liver spans 3.0 inches at the midclavicular line, the lower border descends downward 1 inch. Liver border feels smooth without tenderness. Gallbladder, spleen, and kidneys not palpable. Abdominal reflexes present in each quadrant. No CVA tenderness.

★ = advanced practice

CLINICAL REASONING *Gastrointestinal System*

A 46-year-old female with a long-standing history of alcoholism presents to the emergency department with severe abdominal pain that has been constant for the last 12 hours. She is screaming in pain and demanding morphine. Her other symptoms include nausea and vomiting.

Noticing: The experienced nurse immediately recognizes that clients with long history of alcoholism are at risk for gastrointestinal (GI) inflammation and bleeding, as well as liver disorders such as cirrhosis. The nurse also knows that two inflammatory disorders affecting the gut can cause extreme pain—pancreatitis and gastritis. The pain is described as knifelike and it radiates to her back. The client's bowel sounds are hypoactive; the abdomen is distended, firm, and tender with palpation. The nurse obtains a set of vital signs that include: blood pressure 102/58, pulse 120, temperature 37.7° C (100° F), respiratory rate 24, oxygen saturation 96%. Her skin is warm and slightly diaphoretic.

Interpreting: Early in the encounter, the nurse considers two possible causes for this client's abdominal pain and presenting findings: gastritis with GI bleeding or pancreatitis. In order to determine if either has any probability of being correct, the nurse gathers additional data.

- What is the color and character of the emesis and stool? The woman tells the nurse her vomit is yellowish green; sometimes she just has "dry heaves." The woman describes the stool from her last bowel movement as "light brown."
- Are there aggravating and alleviating factors? The woman indicates that nothing relives the pain, but any movement makes it worse.

The experienced nurse not only recognizes pancreatitis by the clinical signs (severe, unrelieved, knifelike pain that radiates to the back) and symptoms (nausea, vomiting), but interprets this information in the context of an adult with a history of alcohol abuse.

Responding: The nurse initiates appropriate initial interventions (oxygen, IV access, pain control) and notifies the emergency department provider of the situation, ensuring the client receives appropriate immediate and follow-up care.

AGE-RELATED VARIATIONS

INFANTS, CHILDREN, AND ADOLESCENTS

Assessment techniques are the same for infants, children, and adolescents. There are several differences in the assessment findings in infants based on anatomical differences. Children and adolescents may resist abdominal palpation because they are ticklish. Chapter 20 presents further information for assessing the gastrointestinal and renal systems of infants, children, and adolescents.

OLDER ADULTS

Procedures and techniques for assessing the gastrointestinal and renal systems of an older adult are the same as for the younger adult. Chapter 22 presents further information regarding the assessments of these systems for this age group.

COMMON PROBLEMS & CONDITIONS

ALIMENTARY TRACT

Gastroesophageal Reflux Disease

Flow of gastric secretions into the esophagus is termed *gastroesophageal reflux disease* (GERD). It is caused by weakening of the lower esophageal sphincter or increased intraabdominal pressure. **Clinical Findings:** Clients complain of heartburn, regurgitation, and dysphagia (difficulty swallowing) that are aggravated by lying down and relieved by sitting up, antacids, and eating.

Hiatal Hernia

A protrusion of the stomach through the esophageal hiatus of the diaphragm into the mediastinal cavity is termed *hiatal hernia* (Fig. 14-28). Muscle weakness is a primary factor in developing this type of hernia. **Clinical Findings:** Clinical

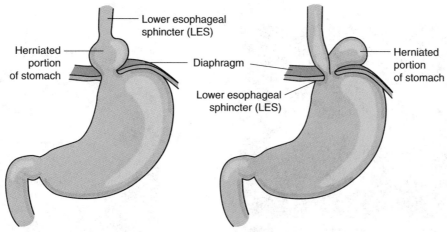

Fig. 14-28 **Hiatal hernia.** **A,** Sliding hernia. **B,** Paraesophageal. *(From Phipps, Sands, and Marek, 1999.)*

manifestations are the same as those of GERD: heartburn, regurgitation, and dysphagia.

Peptic Ulcer Disease

An ulcer occurring in the lower end of the esophagus, in the stomach, or in the duodenum is termed *peptic ulcer.* Duodenal ulcer is the most common form, caused by a break in the duodenal mucosa that scars with healing (Fig. 14-29). Gastric and duodenal ulcers may result from infection with *Helicobacter pylori.* Gastric ulcers also are caused by stress and medications such as corticosteroids, aspirin, and NSAIDs. **Clinical Findings:** Clients with gastric ulcers complain of burning pain in the left epigastrium and back 1 to 2 hours after eating. Clients with duodenal ulcers complain of burning pain 2 to 4 hours after eating and at midmorning, at midafternoon, and in the middle of the night, with pain relief after taking antacids or eating.

Crohn's Disease

This chronic inflammatory bowel disease (IBD) is also called regional enteritis or regional ileitis (Fig. 14-30). Inflammation may occur from mouth to anus, but it commonly affects the terminal ileum and colon. Affected mucosa is ulcerated, with presence of fistulas, fissures, and abscesses that may form adjacent to healthy bowel segments. **Clinical Findings:** Clients complain of severe abdominal pain, cramping, diarrhea, nausea, fever, chills, weakness, anorexia, and weight loss.

Ulcerative Colitis

This chronic inflammatory bowel disease (IBD) starts in the rectum and progresses through the large intestine (Fig. 14-31). The submucosa becomes engorged, and mucosa becomes ulcerated and denuded with granulation tissue; it may progress to colon cancer. **Clinical Findings:** Clients complain of severe abdominal pain, fever, chills, anemia, and weight loss. The client experiences profuse watery diarrhea of blood, mucus, and pus.

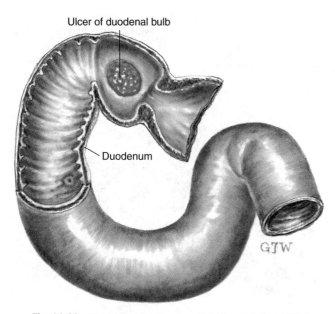

Fig. 14-29 Duodenal peptic ulcer. *(From Doughty and Jackson, 1993.)*

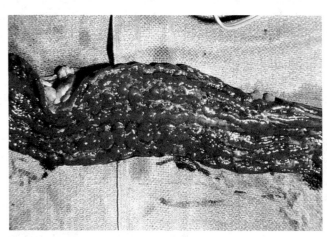

Fig. 14-30 Crohn's disease showing deep ulcers and fissures, creating "cobblestone" effect. *(From Doughty and Jackson, 1993.)*

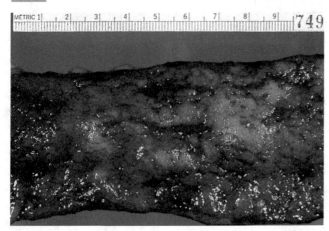

Fig. 14-31 Ulcerative colitis showing severe mucosal edema and inflammation with ulcerations and bleeding. *(From Doughty and Jackson, 1993.)*

Diverticulitis

Inflammation of diverticula is termed *diverticulitis.* Diverticula are herniations through the muscular wall in the colon (Fig. 14-32). Presence of fecal material through the thin-walled diverticula causes inflammation and abscesses. **Clinical Findings:** Clients complain of cramping pain in the LLQ, nausea, vomiting, and altered bowel habits, usually constipation. The abdomen may be distended and tympanic, with decreased bowel sounds and localized tenderness.

HEPATOBILIARY SYSTEM

Viral Hepatitis

This inflammation of the liver results from different viruses. **Clinical Findings:** Common symptoms are anorexia, vague abdominal pain, nausea, vomiting, malaise, and fever. An enlarged liver and spleen are classic findings. Jaundice, tan-colored stools and dark urine may also be reported.

Cirrhosis

This condition is a chronic degenerative disease of the liver in which diffuse destruction and regeneration of hepatic parenchymal cells occur. Figure 14-33 illustrates the cobblestone appearance of the cirrhotic liver that results in impaired liver function and impaired blood flow. Causes of cirrhosis include viral hepatitis, biliary obstruction, and alcohol abuse. **Clinical Findings:** The liver becomes palpable and hard. Associated signs include ascites, jaundice, cutaneous spider angiomas, dark urine, tan-colored stools, and spleen enlargement. End-stage cirrhosis is characterized by hepatic encephalopathy and coma.

Cholecystitis with Cholelithiasis

Inflammation of the gallbladder is termed *cholecystitis,* and when gallstones are present, the condition is termed *cholelithiasis* (Fig. 14-34). The bile duct becomes obstructed either

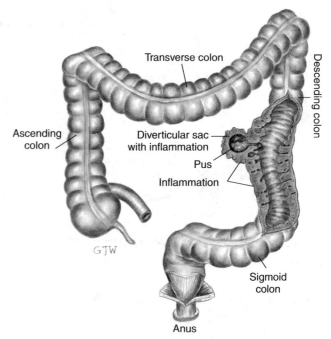

Fig. 14-32 Diverticulosis (diverticulitis). *(From Doughty and Jackson, 1993.)*

by edema from inflammation or by gallstones. **Clinical Findings:** The primary symptom is RUQ colicky pain that may radiate to midtorso or right scapula. Other indications include indigestion and mild transient jaundice.

PANCREAS

Pancreatitis

Acute or chronic inflammation of the pancreas resulting from autodigestion of the organ is called pancreatitis. It can be caused by alcoholism or by obstruction of the sphincter of Oddi by gallstones. See Fig. 14-34, which shows how the location of gallstones could move to obstruct the flow of digestive enzymes from the pancreas. **Clinical Findings:** Clients complain of pain, described as steady, boring, dull, or sharp, that radiates from the epigastrium to the back. Clients

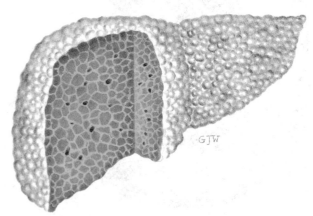

Fig. 14-33 Cirrhosis of the liver. *(From Doughty and Jackson, 1993.)*

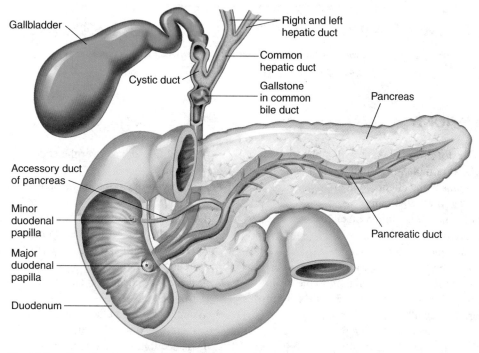

Fig. 14-34 The gallstone in the common bile duct causes biliary colic and may cause jaundice when the bile cannot flow from the liver and gallbladder to the duodenum. *(Courtesy Kissane, 1990. From Thibodeau and Patton, 2002.)*

prefer the fetal position with knees to the chest. Other manifestations include nausea and vomiting, weight loss, steatorrhea, and glucose intolerance.

URINARY SYSTEM

Urinary Tract Infections

These infections may involve the urinary bladder (cystitis), the urethra (urethritis), or the renal pelvis (pyelonephritis). Most urinary tract infections result from gram-negative organisms such as *Escherichia coli, Klebsiella, Proteus,* or *Pseudomonas* that originate from the client's own intestinal tract and ascend through the urethra to the bladder. **Clinical Findings:** Symptoms of urethritis include frequency, urgency, and dysuria. Symptoms of cystitis are the same as those of urethritis plus signs of bacturia and perhaps fever. Clients with pyelonephritis complain of flank pain, dysuria, nocturia, and frequency. Manifestations in older adults include confusion or delirium with or without fever.

Nephrolithiasis

The formation of stones in the kidney pelvis is termed *nephrolithiasis* (Fig. 14-35). Factors contributing to stone formation may be metabolic, dietary, genetic, or climatic. Urinary stasis and urinary infection are important variables in the development of stones. **Clinical Findings:** Signs include fever and hematuria. A symptom is flank pain that may radiate to the groin and genitals.

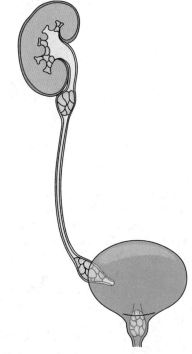

Fig. 14-35 Most common locations of renal calculi formation. *(From Phipps, Sands, and Marek, 1999.)*

CLINICAL APPLICATION & CLINICAL REASONING

See Appendix E for answers to exercises in this section.

REVIEW QUESTIONS

1 When taking a history from a client with a history of pancreatitis who is complaining of abdominal pain, the nurse specifically asks the client about?
   1 Which foods aggravate the pain.
   2 Recent travel outside the United States.
   3 Recent change in bowel habits.
   4 Severity of pain and speed of onset.

2 The nurse is interviewing a client with a history of flank pain, fever chills, and pain radiating to the groin. Which of the following examination techniques is most appropriate for this client?
   1 Percussion of the costovertebral angle.
   2 Deep palpation of the abdomen.
   3 Testing for rebound tenderness.
   4 Auscultation of all four quadrants of the abdomen.

3 A client reports a gnawing, burning in the midepigastric area that is aggravated by bending over or lying down. The nurse asks further questions of the client to detect possible:
   1 Peptic ulcer disease.
   2 Pancreatitis.
   3 Gastroesophageal reflux disease.
   4 Cholecystitis.

4 The nurse palpates the abdomen with the knowledge that which organs are located in the RUQ?
   1 Liver and gallbladder.
   2 Stomach and spleen.
   3 Uterus, if enlarged, and right ovary.
   4 Right ureter and ascending colon.

5 A nurse performing an abdominal examination on a 37-year-old woman would document which finding as abnormal?
   1 Nonpalpable spleen or kidneys.
   2 Bowel sounds every 15 seconds in the lower quadrants
   3 Bulges when coughing.
   4 Silver-white striae and a faint vascular network.

6 A 50-year-old client asks how he can reduce his risk of colon cancer. The nurse teaches the client that:
   1 A diet high in animal protein reduces the risk.
   2 Regular exercise to reduce body fat helps prevent colon cancer.
   3 Taking antacids for heartburn can help prevent colon cancer.
   4 Daily vitamin C intake helps reduce the risk.

7 Which is an expected finding of an abdominal examination of an adult?
   1 Tympanic percussion tones over the bladder.
   2 Venous hum over the epigastrium on auscultation.

3 High-pitched gurgles every 5 to 15 seconds on auscultation.
4 Swishing sounds over the abdominal aorta on auscultation.

8 What technique does the nurse use to palpate a client's abdomen?
   1 Asks the client to breathe slowly though the mouth.
   2 Uses the heel of the hand to perform deep palpation.
   3 Uses the left hand to lift the rib cage away from the abdominal organs.
   4 Depresses the abdomen 1 to 2 inches for light palpation.

9 When assessing a client's abdomen, the nurse uses assessment techniques in which order?
   1 Inspection, palpation, percussion, and auscultation.
   2 Inspection, auscultation, palpation, and percussion.
   3 Auscultation, inspection, percussion, and palpation.
   4 Palpation, auscultation, inspection, and percussion.

10 While taking a client's history, the nurse suspects that the client has appendicitis. Which assessment techniques can the nurse use to confirm his suspicion?
   1 Gently perform fist percussion over the right costovertebral angle.
   2 Ask the client to place her hand on the abdomen while the nurse taps one side of the abdomen and palpates the other side.
   3 Palpate the left lower quadrant at a 90-degree angle, then quickly release your hand.
   4 Lying supine, the client flexes her right knee and hip and the nurse taps on the sole of the client's right foot.

SAMPLE DOCUMENTATION

Review the data obtained during an interview and examination by the nurse below:

An alert, cooperative 55-year-old man is complaining of epigastric pain; he is holding his hand on his stomach. He reports having a gnawing pain in his stomach for 2 weeks that does not radiate. He has smoked one pack of cigarettes per day for 40 years. His pain is worse before meals and is relieved somewhat after meals. He has a bowel movement every day and his stools are soft, but "much darker than usual—almost black." Bowel sounds are heard in all quadrants. He has been taking antacids with some relief of the epigastric pain. The spleen is not tender to palpation, and his kidneys are not palpable. His superficial reflexes are intact. He complains about fatigue and shortness of breath with activity since pain onset. He drinks a fifth of whiskey per week.

He is employed full time at an insurance company. He is married with two children. Vital signs are as follows: blood pressure, 140/80 mm Hg; pulse, 88 beats/min; respirations, 18; temperature, 98.8° F (37.1° C). Height (stated), 6 feet 3 inches (190 cm); weight (measured), 180 lb (82 kg). He has a history of hypertension managed by diet and exercise. He is allergic to iodine. His abdomen is scaphoid, soft, with no scars. The aorta is midline and there are no bruits. His epigastrium is tender on deep palpation. His liver span is 9 cm in the right midclavicular line, and 2 cm of the liver is palpable. He denies having any nausea and vomiting. He has no costovertebral tenderness. His stool specimen is guaiac positive. He takes one aspirin daily and nonsteroidal inflammatory drugs twice a day for arthritis. He says that he experiences occasional stress at work and minimal stress at home.

Below, note how the nurse documented these same data.

55 y/o ♂ with epigastric pain.

Subjective Data

Alert, cooperative man reports a 2 wk hx of nonradiating, gnawing epigastric pain. Pain worse a̅c̅ relieved somewhat p̅c̅ by antacids. Denies N&V. Has BM every other day, stools soft, but "much darker than usual—almost black." Reports fatigue and SOB since pain onset. Hx of osteoarthritis; HTN managed c̅ diet and exercise. Allergies: iodine. Current medications: daily ASA, NSAIDs bid for arthritis. 40 pack-year smoking hx; drinks a fifth of whiskey/wk. Employed full time at an insurance company; married with two children. Reports occasional stress at work, minimal stress at home.

Objective Data

General survey: VS: BP, 140/80 mm Hg; HR, 88 beats/min; RR, 18/min; T, 98.8° F (37.1° C). Ht (stated), 6 feet 3 inches (190 cm); wt (measured), 180 lb (82 kg).

Abdomen: Scaphoid, soft, no scars; aorta midline with no bruits; BS×4, epigastrium tender to deep palpation; liver span 9 cm RMCL; liver palpable 2 cm, nontender; spleen and kidneys nonpalpable; superficial reflexes intact; no CVA tenderness. Stool is guaiac positive.

CASE STUDY

Katie is a 22-year-old woman complaining of abdominal pain. The following data are collected by the nurse during an interview and examination.

Interview Data

Katie tells the nurse that the pain started yesterday evening and has gotten progressively worse. She describes the pain as "really bad." The pain is constant and located in her right lower abdomen, toward her umbilicus. She says that her pain feels a little better if she stays curled up and does not move. She tells the nurse that she is in good health and that she has never had a problem with her stomach. Katie indicates that normally she has a good appetite and can eat anything—except for now. She says she ate breakfast and lunch yesterday, but by dinnertime she was nauseated and had no appetite. She has not eaten anything since. She has had no recent weight changes, but she would like to weigh about 5 lb less than she currently does. Katie smokes a half pack of cigarettes daily. She does not drink alcoholic beverages, and she takes no medication. She denies discomfort or problems with urination, describing her urine as "usual looking."

Examination Data

- *General survey:* Alert and anxious female in moderate distress lying in a fetal position on the examination table, with her eyes closed. Appears well nourished. Her skin is hot.
- *Inspection:* Abdomen is flat and symmetric. No lesions or scars are noted. No surface movements are seen except for breathing.
- *Auscultation:* Bowel sounds are absent.
- *Palpation:* Tympany is noted over most of abdominal surface; dullness over liver. Midclavicular liver span is 4 inches.
- *Light palpation:* Demonstrates pain and guarding in right lower quadrant. Unable to palpate deep structures because of excessive abdominal discomfort. Demonstrates positive rebound tenderness in right lower quadrant.

Clinical Reasoning

1. What data deviate from normal findings, suggesting a need for further investigation?
2. What additional information should the nurse ask or assess for?
3. Based on the data, what risk factors for cancers in the abdomen does this client have?
4. What nursing diagnoses and collaborative problems should be considered for this situation?

💿 INTERACTIVE ACTIVITIES

Open the interactive student CD-ROM, click on Chapter 14, and choose from the following activities on the menu bar:

- **Multiple Choice Challenge.** Click on the best answer for each of these items. You will be given immediate feedback, rationale for incorrect answers and a total score. Good luck!

- **Tummy Toss-up.** Test your knowledge of anatomy by dragging anatomic parts and dropping them in their correct location.

- **A Day in the Clinic.** Complete an examination by choosing a technique and an examination area for this client. You'll be able to collect data, document, and compare your answers with those of the experts. Everything you need for a successful assessment is at your fingertips.

- **Symptom Analysis.** Review this client's case study. Choose from the list of questions to ask the client. Practice your clinical skills by taking notes and then ruling out possible causes. See why your analysis is correct or incorrect. Good luck!

- **Printable Lab Guide.** Locate the Lab Guide for Chapter 14, and print and use it (as many times as needed) to

help you apply your assessment skills. These guides may also be filled in electronically and then saved and e-mailed to your instructor!

- **Quick Challenge.** Use this critical thinking exercise to assess your skills through case study-style questions, then compare with expert answers!

- **Core Examination Skills Checklist.** Make sure you've got frequently-used exam skills down pat! Use these checklists to help cover all the bases for your examination.

Musculoskeletal System

ANATOMY & PHYSIOLOGY

The musculoskeletal system provides both support and mobility for the body and protection for internal organs. This system also produces blood cells and stores minerals such as calcium and phosphorus.

SKELETON

Functions of bones include support for soft tissues and organs, protection of organs such as the brain and spinal cord, body movement, and hematopoiesis. Bones are continually remodeling and changing the collagen and mineral composition to accommodate stress placed on them. The function of each bone dictates its shape and surface features. For example, long bones act as levers and have a flat surface for the attachment of muscles with grooves at the end for passage of tendons or nerves. Examples of long bones are the humerus, femur, fibula, and phalanges. Short bones, such as carpal and tarsal bones, are cube shaped. Flat bones make up the cranium, ribs, and scapula. The vertebrae are irregular bones.

The human skeleton has two major divisions: the axial and appendicular skeletons. The axial skeleton includes the facial bones, auditory ossicles, vertebrae, ribs, sternum, and hyoid bone; the appendicular skeleton includes the scapula and clavicle, as well as the bones of the pelvis and legs. The subsequent discussion of bone is organized by these divisions.

SKELETAL MUSCLES

Skeletal muscles are composed of muscle fibers that attach to bones to facilitate movement. Although some skeletal muscles move by reflex, all are under voluntary control. Skeletal muscle fibers are arranged parallel to the long axis of bones to which they attach, or they are obliquely attached. Muscles attach to a bone, ligament, tendon, or fascia.

JOINTS

Joints are articulations where two or more bones come together. They help hold the bones firmly while allowing movement between them.

Joints are classified in two ways: by the type of material between them (fibrous, cartilaginous, or synovial) and by their degree of movement. Immovable joints are synarthrodial (e.g., the suture of the skull); slightly movable joints are amphiarthrodial (e.g., the symphysis pubis); and freely movable joints are diarthrodial (e.g., the knee and the distal interphalangeal [DIP] joint of the distal fingers.

Diarthrodial joints are further classified by their type of movement. Only the diarthrodial joints have one or more ranges of motion. See Table 15-1 in the examination section of this chapter for types of movement of each diarthrodial joint. Hinge joints permit extension and flexion; examples are the knee, elbow, and fingers. Some hinge joints

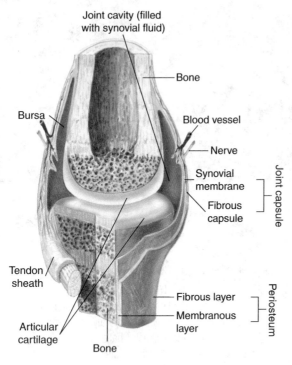

Fig. 15-1 Structures of a synovial joint (the knee). *(From Mourad, 1991.)*

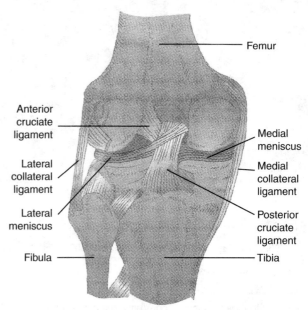

Fig. 15-2 **A posterior view of the left knee.** The medial collateral ligament prevents the knee from going into too much valgus during stress (inward). The lateral collateral ligament prevents the knee from going into too much varus during stress (outward). *(From Black and Matassairin-Jacobs, 1997.)*

allow hyperextension; however, there is variability among individuals—not all hinge joints are able to hyperextend. Pivot joints permit movement of one bone articulating with a ring or notch of another bone, such as the head of the radius, which articulates with the radial notch of the ulna. The ends of saddle-shaped bones articulate with each other: the base of the thumb is the only example. Condyloid or ellipsoidal joints consist of the condyle of one bone that fits into the elliptically shaped portion of its articulating bone. For instance, the distal end of the radius articulates with three wrist bones. Ball-and-socket joints are made of a ball-shaped bone that fits into a concave area of its articulating bone (e.g., the head of the femur fits into the acetabulum within the pelvis). Gliding joints permit movement along various axes through relatively flat articulating surfaces, such as joints between two vertebrae.

Diarthrodial joints are synovial joints because they are lined with synovial fluid (Fig. 15-1). Synovial fluid lubricates the joint to facilitate its movement in various directions. Some synovial joints such as the knee also have a disk called the meniscus, which is a pad of cartilage that cushions the joint. These joints have a covering surrounding them, called the joint capsule, which is an extension of the periosteum of the articulating bone. Ligaments also encase the capsule to add strength.

LIGAMENTS AND TENDONS

The difference between ligaments and tendons is more functional than structural. Ligaments are strong, dense, flexible bands of connective tissue that hold bones to bones (Fig. 15-2).

They can provide support in several ways: by encircling the joint, by gripping it obliquely, or by lying parallel to the bone ends, across the joint. They can simultaneously allow some movements while restricting others.

Conversely, tendons are strong, nonelastic cords of collagen located at the ends of muscles to attach them to bones (see Fig. 15-1). Tendons support bone movement in response to skeletal muscle contractions, transmitting remarkable force at times from the contracting muscles to the bone without sustaining injury themselves.

CARTILAGE AND BURSAE

Cartilage is a semismooth, gel-like supporting tissue that is strong and able to support weight. The upper seven pairs of ribs are connected directly to the sternum by costal cartilage. The flexibility of the cartilage allows the thorax to move when the lungs expand and contract. Cartilage also reinforces respiratory passages such as the nose, larynx, trachea, and bronchi. Cartilage forms a cap over the ends of long bones, providing a smooth surface for articulation (see Fig. 15-1). Because it contains no blood vessels, cartilage receives nutrition from the synovial fluid forced into it during movement and weight-bearing activities. For this reason, weight-bearing activity and joint movement are essential to maintaining cartilage health.

Bursae are small sacs in the connective tissues adjacent to selected joints such as the shoulders (the glenohumeral joint) and knees. Each bursa is lined with synovial membrane containing synovial fluid that acts as a lubricant to reduce friction when a muscle or tendon rubs against another muscle, tendon, or bone (see Fig. 15-1).

AXIAL SKELETON AND SUPPORTING STRUCTURES

Skull and Neck

The six bones of the cranium (one frontal, two parietal, two temporal, and one occipital) are fused together. The face consists of 14 bones, which include two nasal, a frontal, two lacrimal, a sphenoid, two zygomatic, two maxillary, and a mandible, which is movable. The neck is supported by the cervical vertebrae, ligaments, and the sternocleidomastoid and trapezius muscles, with its greatest mobility at the level of C4-5 or C5-6. The type of movement permitted includes flexion, extension, and hyperflexion, as well as lateral, flexion, and rotation. The sternocleidomastoid muscle stretches from the upper sternum and anterior clavicle to the mastoid process; the trapezius links the scapula, the lateral third of the clavicle, and the vertebrae, extending to the occipital prominence.

Trunk and Pelvis

The trunk is formed by the vertebrae, ribs, and sternum of the axial skeleton, as well as the scapula and clavicle of the appendicular skeleton. The pelvis is part of the appendicular skeleton. Fig. 15-3 shows the bones of the trunk and pelvis, and Fig. 15-4 shows the muscles. The spine is composed of 7 cervical, 12 thoracic, 5 lumbar, and 5 sacral vertebrae (see Fig. 16-8, spinal column). The cervical, thoracic, and lumbar vertebrae are separated from each other by fibrocartilaginous disks, whereas the sacral vertebrae are fused. The vertebral joints, separated by disks, glide slightly over one another's surfaces, permitting flexion, hyperextension, lateral bending, and rotation. The cervical joints are most active.

APPENDICULAR SKELETON AND SUPPORTING STRUCTURES

Upper Extremities

The bones of the upper extremities are shown in Fig. 15-5 and the muscles are shown in Fig. 15-6.

Shoulder and Upper Arm

The shoulder joint, also called the glenohumeral joint, consists of the point where the humerus and the glenoid fossa of the scapula articulate (Fig. 15-7). The acromial and coracoid processes (see Fig. 15-3) and surrounding ligaments protect this ball-and-socket joint and permit flexion, extension, and hyperextension, abduction and adduction, and internal and external rotation. Besides the glenohumeral joint, two other joints contribute to shoulder movement: the acromioclavicular joint (between the acromial process and the clavicle) and the sternoclavicular joint (between the sternal manubrium and the clavicle).

Elbow, Forearm, and Wrist

The elbow joint consists of the humerus, radius, and ulna enclosed in a single synovial cavity protected by ligaments

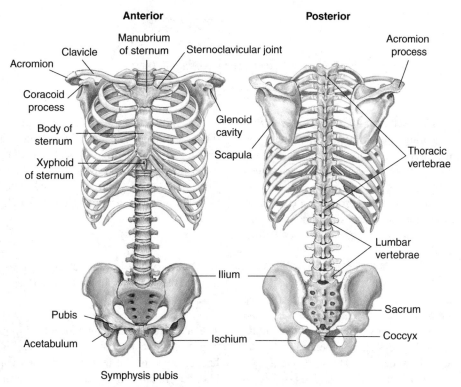

Fig. 15-3 Bones of the trunk and pelvis. *(From Mourad, 1991.)*

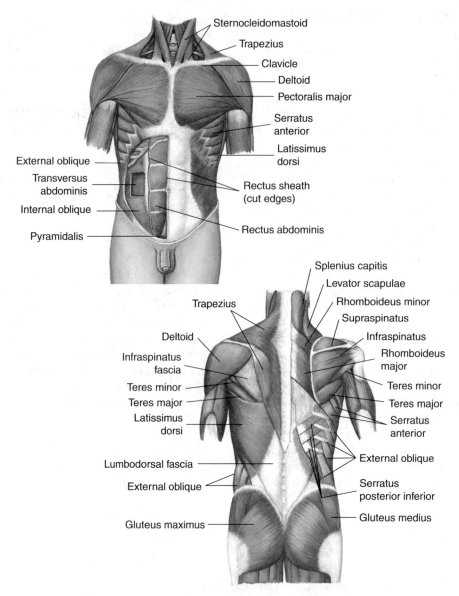

Fig. 15-4   Muscles of the trunk and pelvis. *(From Mourad, 1991.)*

and a bursa between the olecranon and the skin (see Fig. 15-5). The elbow is a hinge joint; it permits extension, flexion, and sometimes hyperextension. Pronation and supination of the forearm are provided also. The wrist joins the radius and the carpal bones with articular disks of the wrist, ligaments, and a fibrous capsule to form a condyloid joint. This joint permits flexion, extension, and hyperextension, as well as radial and ulnar flexion, also called radial and ulnar deviation.

Hand

There are small, subtle movements or articulations within the hand between the carpals and metacarpals, between the metacarpals and proximal phalanges, and between the middle and distal phalanges (see Fig. 15-5). Ligaments protect the diarthrotic joints, which allow flexion, extension, and hyperextension. The fingers are able to flex and extend, as well as

abduct and adduct. The names of joints in the hands describe their location. For example, the distal joint of the fingers is called the distal interphalangeal (DIP) joint; the middle joint of each finger is called the proximal interphalangeal (PIP) joint; and the joint that attaches the metacarpal to the carpal is called the metacarpophalangeal (MCP) joint.

Lower Extremities

The bones of the lower extremities are shown in Fig. 15-8, and the muscles are shown in Fig. 15-9.

Hip and Thigh

The acetabulum and femur form the hip joint, protected by a fibrous capsule and three bursae. Three ligaments help stabilize the head of the femur in the joint capsule (Fig. 15-10). Like the shoulder, this is a ball-and-socket joint that provides

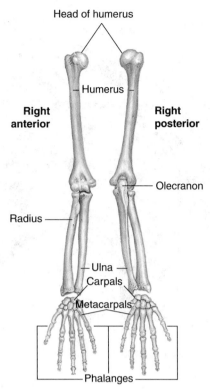

Fig. 15-5 Bones of the upper extremities. *(From Mourad, 1991.)*

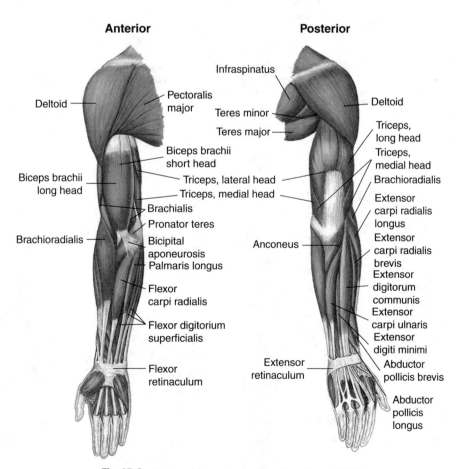

Fig. 15-6 Muscles of the upper extremities. *(From Mourad, 1991.)*

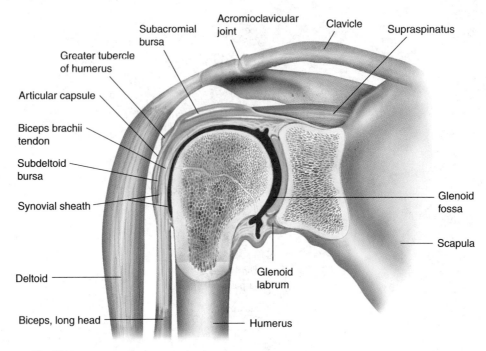

Fig. 15-7   Structures of the glenohumeral and acromioclavicular joint of the shoulder. *(From Seidel et al, 2006.)*

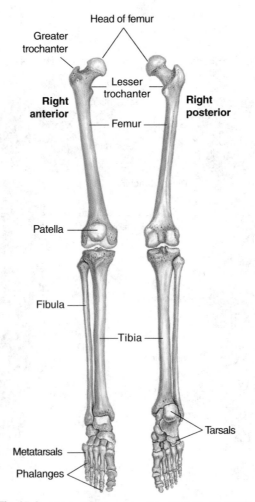

Fig. 15-8   Bones of the lower extremities. *(From Mourad, 1991.)*

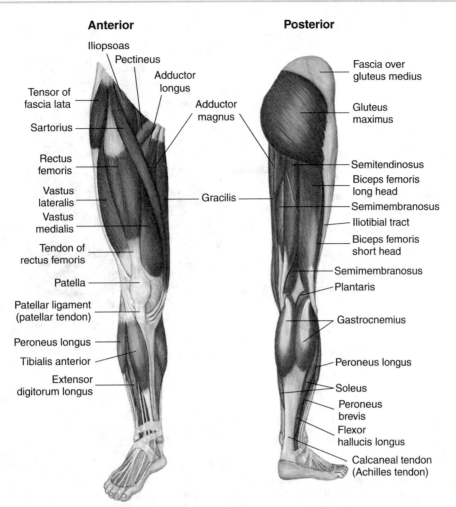

Anterior

- Iliopsoas
- Pectineus
- Adductor longus
- Tensor of fascia lata
- Adductor magnus
- Sartorius
- Rectus femoris
- Vastus lateralis
- Gracilis
- Vastus medialis
- Tendon of rectus femoris
- Patella
- Patellar ligament (patellar tendon)
- Peroneus longus
- Tibialis anterior
- Extensor digitorum longus

Posterior

- Fascia over gluteus medius
- Gluteus maximus
- Semitendinosus
- Biceps femoris long head
- Semimembranosus
- Iliotibial tract
- Biceps femoris short head
- Semimembranosus
- Plantaris
- Gastrocnemius
- Peroneus longus
- Soleus
- Peroneus brevis
- Flexor hallucis longus
- Calcaneal tendon (Achilles tendon)

Fig. 15-9   Muscles of the lower extremities. *(From Mourad, 1991.)*

flexion, extension and hyperextension, abduction and adduction, internal and external rotation, and circumduction.

Knee and Lower Leg

The knee is a hinge joint that serves as the point of articulation between the femur, the tibia, and the patella (see Fig. 15-1). The knee has medial and lateral menisci (disk-shaped fibrous cartilage) that cushion the tibia and the femur and connect to the articulated capsule. Ligaments provide stability; the bursae reduce friction on movement between the femur and the tibia. Movements of this joint include flexion, extension, and sometimes hyperextension.

Ankle and Foot

The ankle joint, or tibiotalar joint, forms a hinge joint, permitting flexion, called dorsiflexion, and extension in one plane, called plantar flexion. Protective medial and lateral ligaments join the tibia, fibula, and talus to form the tibiotalar joint. Smaller joints within the ankle permit a pivot or rotation movement, producing inversion and eversion, as well as adduction and abduction. These joints are the subtalar (talocalcaneal) joint and the talonavicular (transverse tarsal) joint (Fig. 15-11).

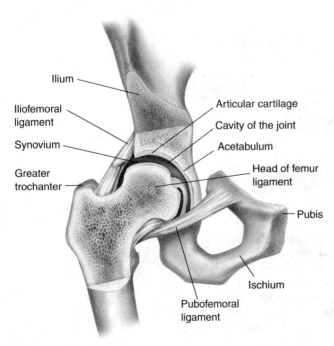

- Ilium
- Iliofemoral ligament
- Synovium
- Greater trochanter
- Articular cartilage
- Cavity of the joint
- Acetabulum
- Head of femur ligament
- Pubis
- Ischium
- Pubofemoral ligament

Fig. 15-10   Structures of the hip. *(Modified from Thompson et al, 2002.)*

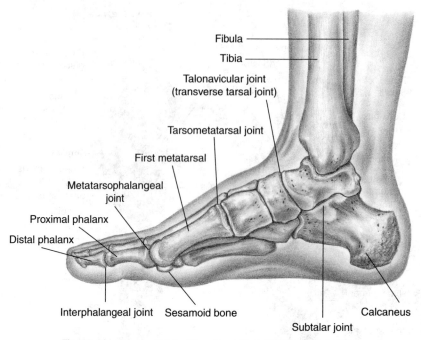

Fig. 15-11   Bones and joints of the ankle and foot. *(From Seidel et al, 2003.)*

LINK TO CONCEPTS   *Motion*

The feature concept for this chapter is *Motion.* This concept represents mechanisms that facilitate and impair mobility. Several concepts featured in this textbook have an interrelationship with this concept. Motion depends on the delivery of oxygenated blood to tissues and coordination of movement regulated by the brain, spinal cord, and peripheral nerves. Motion can cause pain and thus limit movement. Adequate nutrition is needed for motion, and motion is needed for the procurement and preparation of food. Elimination is impacted by motion as is the maintenance of tissue integrity. These interrelationships are depicted in the model below.

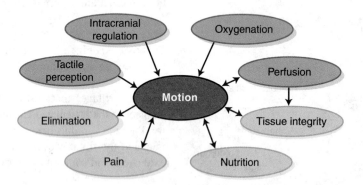

Concept Model: Motion

This model shows the interrelationship of concepts associated with motion. As an example, over time excessive body weight damages the joints causing pain with movement. This pain may limit the walking the person does, which may limit such activities as shopping for food as well as limit exercise performed. Others who have limited mobility may develop constipation and possible skin breakdown because of extended pressure on tissue. An understanding of the relationship of these concepts helps the nurse recognize risk factors and thus increases awareness when conducting a health assessment.

Five metatarsal bones form the sole of the foot. Like the names of joints in the hands, the names of joints in the feet describe their location. For example, the joint between the distal phalanx and the proximal phalanx is called the interphalangeal joint; the joint between the proximal phalanx and the first metatarsal is called the metatarsophalangeal joint; and the joint that attaches the first metatarsal to the tarsals is called the tarsometatarsal joint (see Fig. 15-11).

The foot has a gliding joint that allows inversion and eversion. The toes are condyloid joints that allow flexion and extension, as well as abduction and adduction.

ETHNIC & CULTURAL VARIATIONS

A number of racial variations have been noted in the anatomy of the skeleton and of the skeletal muscles. Long bones are generally longer, narrower, and denser in African Americans, particularly African American males. They are thus less subject to osteoporosis and other diseases involving the loss of bone density.

HEALTH HISTORY

RISK FACTORS *Musculoskeletal System*

As you conduct a health history related to the musculoskeletal system, it is important to consider common risk factors associated with this system and follow up with additional questions should risk factors exist.

Temporomandibular Joint (TMJ) Dysfunction[a]
- *Gender:* Females between puberty and menopause account for 90% of cases.
- *Mechanical factors:* Malocclusion, or "bad bite," puts stress on muscles of mastication. Bruxism (grinding of the teeth), abnormal bite, and faulty dentures can lead to TMJ dysfunction. (M)

Gout[b]
- *Gender:* Men have a higher risk.
- *Family history:* About 20% of clients with gout have a positive family history.
- *Alcohol:* Alcohol use is highly associated with gout, particularly binge drinking, which has been shown to increase uric acid levels. (M)
- *Obesity:* There is a link between high uric acid levels and body weight. Gaining more than 30 lbs or more than ideal body weight during adulthood increases risk. (M)
- *Hypertension:* Between 25% and 50% of clients who have gout also have hypertension; however, the association is unclear. Use of diuretics also is highly associated with gout. (M)
- *Chronic diseases* such as diabetes mellitus, hyperlipidemia and arteriosclerosis increase risk of gout.
- *Medications* such as thiazide diuretics used to treat hypertension and low dose aspirin can increase uric acid levels.

Osteoarthritis (OA)[c]
- *Gender:* OA occurs in women over age 45 years more than in men, but it occurs in men under 45 years more than in women.
- *Weight:* Being overweight puts stress on joints. (M)
- *Repeated cartilage damage:* Overuse of joints increases risk. (M)
- *Joint injury:* Injury to the knee or hip increases risk. (M)
- *Physical inactivity:* Lack of exercise weakens muscles that support joints. (M)

Osteoporosis[d]
- *Age:* Bone density decreases beginning at age 35 years.
- *Gender:* Women have less bone tissue and lose it more readily than men.
- *Race:* Whites and Asians have increased risk.
- *Bone structures and body weight:* Small-boned and thin women (under 127 lb) are at greater risk.

[a] Data from *www.tmj.org*, 2002.
[b] Data from *www.mayoclinic.com/health/gout*, 2005
[c] Data from *www.biomedicalabs.com/osteoarthritis*, 2007.
[d] Data from *www.nof.org/prevention/risk*, 2007 (National Osteoporosis Foundation).
M = modifiable risk factor.

Continued

RISK FACTORS   *Musculoskeletal System—cont'd*

- *Family history:* A family history of osteoporosis increases risk.
- *Lifestyle:* Cigarette smoking, excessive alcohol intake, consuming inadequate calcium, and performing inadequate weight-bearing exercises increase the risk. (M)
- *Medications to treat chronic diseases:* Some medications have side effects that lead to osteoporosis, including glucocorticoids, methotrexate, thyroid hormone, antacids containing aluminum, cyclosporin A, and heparin. (M)
- *Estrogen:* Estrogen deficiency from menopause, surgical removal of ovaries (oophorectomy), and being underweight increases risk. (M)

M = modifiable risk factor.

GENERAL HEALTH HISTORY

Present Health Status

Do you have any chronic diseases? Loss of bone density or osteoporosis?
Chronic diseases may affect mobility and activities of daily living.

Do you take any medications? If yes, what do you take and how often? Are you taking medications as they were prescribed? Are you taking any medications to prevent loss of bone density?
Both prescription and over-the-counter medications should be documented. Clients may not report musculoskeletal problems if they are being successfully treated with medications. Many medications for musculoskeletal problems (aspirin, nonsteroidal antiinflammatory drugs, narcotics, tranquilizers, or sleep aids) can cause adverse side effects and may increase risk of injury.

Have you noticed any changes in your ability to move around or participate in your usual activities? Have you noticed any changes in your muscle strength? What do you do to adapt to these changes?
If there are changes, they can be diagnosed and treated at an early stage, or they can generate a discussion about how to prevent further changes. The health care provider needs to determine how the client is adapting to these changes to determine the impact of these changes on the client's quality of life.

What do you do for exercise? How often do you exercise and for what period of time? Do you smoke cigarettes? If yes, how many and how often? Do you drink alcohol? If yes, how much and how often?
These questions identify the client's learning needs for health promotion and assess for risk factors for osteoporosis.

Do you play sports? If yes, which ones and how often? How do you protect yourself from injury while exercising or playing sports?

These questions assess for risk for injury. Adults should protect themselves from injury (e.g., stretching before running, wearing a bike helmet, and wearing elbow pads and wrist guards for in-line skating).

Do you lift, push, or pull items or bend or stoop frequently as a part of your daily routine either at home or at work? How do you protect yourself from muscle strain or injury?
Many musculoskeletal injuries are due to heavy lifting and repetitive and forceful motions that may be prevented with proper body mechanics, appropriate help when lifting, and use of protective equipment.

Past Medical History

Have you ever had any accidents or trauma that affected the bones or joints, including fractures, strains of the joints, sprains, and dislocations? If yes, when? Have you noticed any continuing problems or difficulties that seem related to this previous incident?
Previous injury can leave residual problems such as muscle weakness, decreased range of motion, or impaired mobility.

Have you ever had surgery on any bones, joints, or muscles? If yes, describe the procedure(s), when it (they) occurred, and what the outcome was.
The incidence of surgery may provide additional information about possible musculoskeletal problems and the findings to anticipate during assessment.

Family History

In your family, is there a history of curvature of the spine or back problems? If yes, describe.
Family history may be used to determine client's risk for vertebral disorders.

In your family, is there a history of arthritis—rheumatoid arthritis, osteoarthritis, or gout?
Family history may be used to determine the client's risk for a form of arthritis.

PROBLEM-BASED HISTORY

Commonly reported problems related to the musculoskeletal system are pain, problems with movement, and problems with daily activities. As with symptoms in all areas of health assessment, a symptom analysis is completed, which includes the location, quality, quantity, chronology, setting, associated manifestations, and alleviating and aggravating factors (see Box 3-3 in Chapter 3).

Pain

Where do you feel the pain? When did you first notice the pain? Is the pain related to movement? Describe how the pain feels. How severe is the pain on a scale of 0 to 10, with 10 being the worst pain possible?

Joint pain is the most common musculoskeletal symptom for which clients seek help. Pain is felt in and around the joint and may be accompanied by edema and erythema, indicating inflammation. Bone pain typically is described as "deep," "dull," "boring," or "intense." Bone pain frequently is not related to movement unless the bone is fractured, in which case the pain is described as sharp. Muscle pain is described as "crampy." Muscle pain associated with weakness suggests a primary muscular disorder.

Did the pain occur suddenly? When during the day do you feel the pain?

Sudden onset of pain and erythema in the great toe, ankle, and lower leg suggests gout (also called gouty arthritis). Pain from rheumatoid arthritis and tendonitis may awaken the client, especially when the client is lying on the affected limb. Clients with rheumatoid arthritis often have morning stiffness lasting 1 to 2 hours. By contrast, clients with osteoarthritis experience pain when weight bearing that is relieved by rest.

Does the pain move from one joint to another? Has there been any injury, overuse, or strain of muscles or joints? Were you ill before the onset of pain?

Some disorders cause migratory arthritis, in which pain moves among joints (e.g., acute rheumatic fever, leukemia, or juvenile arthritis). Viral illnesses can cause muscle aches and pain (myalgia).

What makes the pain worse? Does the pain change according to the weather?

Learning what makes the pain worse may help in diagnosing the disorder. Arthritis pain may become worse with changes in the barometric pressure. Movement usually makes joint pain worse except in rheumatoid arthritis, in which movement may reduce pain.

What have you done to relieve the pain? How effective has it been?

Knowing what relieves pain may help selection of pain-relief strategies.

Problems with Movement

How long have you had problems with movement? Are your joints swollen, red, or hot to the touch? Is the movement in your joints limited?

Acute inflammation such as arthritis or gout produces erythema, warmth, and edema. Decreased range of motion occurs in injury to the cartilage or capsule or with muscle contracture or edema.

Have you had a recent sore throat?

Joint pain that occurs 10 to 14 days after a sore throat may be associated with rheumatic fever.

Do you feel any weakness in your muscles? If yes, which muscles? How long have you had this weakness? Does the weakness become worse as the day progresses?

Muscle weakness may be due to altered nerve innervation or muscle contraction disorder. Atrophied muscles may be due to prolonged lack of use (e.g., atrophy occurs from disuse when an extremity is casted). Proximal muscle weakness is usually a myopathy, whereas distal weakness is usually a neuropathy.

Have you noticed your knees or ankles giving way when you put pressure on them? If yes, when does this occur? How often does it occur?

This may indicate joint instability that may occur from chronic inflammation or joint trauma. Safety must be a concern of the client when a joint gives way.

Have your joints felt as if they are locked and will not move? If yes, when does this occur? How often does it occur? What relieves the locking? What makes it worse?

This may indicate joint instability that may occur from chronic inflammation or joint trauma. Safety must be a concern of the client when a joint gives way.

Problems with Daily Activities

What activities are limited? To what extent are your daily activities limited? How do you compensate for this limitation?

- **Bathing (getting in and out of the tub, turning faucets on or off)?**
- **Toileting (urinating, defecating, ability to raise or lower yourself onto or off of the toilet)?**
- **Dressing (buttoning, zipping, fastening openings behind your neck, hooking your brassiere, pulling a dress or shirt over your head, pulling up your pants, tying shoes, having shoes fit your feet)?**
- **Grooming (shaving, brushing teeth, brushing or combing hair, washing and drying hair, applying makeup)?**
- **Eating (preparing meals, pouring, holding utensils, cutting up food, bringing food to your mouth, drinking)?**

- **Moving around (walking, going up or down stairs, getting in or out of bed, getting out of the house)?**
- **Sleeping?**
- **Communicating (writing, talking, using the telephone)?**

Any impaired mobility or function may cause a self-care deficit. It is important to identify which activities are impaired, to what extent, and how the client compensates. For example, a client who reports hip pain when putting on shoes may have degenerative disease, which is aggravated by externally rotating the hip (Swartz, 2006).

For clients who have chronic disability or a crippling disease: How has your illness affected your interactions with your family? How has it affected your relationships with friends?

Assess for disturbance of self-esteem, body image, or role performance; loss of independence; or social isolation. Maintaining social relationships is an important aspect of therapy.

HEALTH PROMOTION   *Osteoporosis*

Osteoporosis is defined as a bone mineral density (BMD) more than 2.5 standard deviations below the mean for young healthy adult women. It is estimated that half of all postmenopausal women will have an osteoporosis-related fracture during their lives. The risk for fracture increases as bone density decreases. Bone density decreases in women following menopause because of hormonal changes. BMD has been identified as one of the primary predictive factors for osteoporosis-related fractures.

Goals and Objectives—*Healthy People 2010*
The *Healthy People 2010* goal is to prevent illness and disability related to osteoporosis, along with arthritis and back conditions. Two specific objectives are related to osteoporosis: reduce the proportion of adults with osteoporosis and reduce the proportion of adults who are hospitalized for vertebral fractures associated with osteoporosis.

Recommendations to Reduce Risk (Primary Prevention)
National Osteoporosis Foundation
- Suggests counseling clients to eat a balanced diet rich in calcium and vitamin D. Calcium intake should be between 1000 and 1300 mg per day; vitamin D intake should be between 400 and 800 IU per day.
- Encourage clients to engage in weight-bearing exercise.
- Encourage clients to avoid smoking and excessive alcohol use.

Screening Recommendations (Secondary Prevention)
U.S. Preventive Services Task Force
- Recommends routine screening for osteoporosis for women age 65 and older.
- For women at increased risk of osteoporotic fracture, routine screening should begin at age 60. Increased risk factors include low body weight (less than 70 kg) and no current use of estrogen therapy.
- Optimal intervals for repeated screening are not established. A minimum of 2 years may be needed to reliably measure a change in BMD.
- Measurement of BMD is considered accurate as a screening method for osteoporosis and the risk for fractures.

In *Healthy People 2010: understanding and improving health,* ed 2, Washington, DC, 2000, US Government Printing Office (available at *www.healthypeople.gov*); US Preventive Services Task Force: *Guide to clinical preventive services,* ed 3 (available at *www.ahrq.gov*).

HEALTH PROMOTION   *Low Back Pain*

Back pain is one of the leading causes for individuals to seek health care. It is estimated that 60% to 80% of adults in the United States suffer from low back pain at some point in their lives; up to 50% experience back pain within a given year. Although back pain appears to be equally common in men and women, impairment from back and spine conditions is more common in women. Back pain accounts for one of every five workplace injuries or illnesses. Occupation-related back injury most commonly results from repetitive lifting.

Goals and Objectives—*Healthy People 2010*
The overall *Healthy People 2010* goal related to low back pain is to prevent illness and disability related to chronic back conditions. One specific objective is related to low back pain: reduce activity limitation resulting from back conditions.

Recommendations to Reduce Risk (Primary Prevention)
American Academy of Orthopaedic Surgeons
Recommends informing clients about risk factors for back injury and ways to prevent back pain. Specific suggestions for prevention of back pain include the following:
- Use the correct lifting and moving techniques.
- Engage in regular exercise to keep back muscles strong and flexible.
- Maintain proper posture; poor posture puts a strain on the lower back.
- Maintain proper body weight to avoid straining back muscles.
- Maintain a positive attitude about job/home life; persons who are unhappy at work or home have more back problems and take longer to recover than persons who have a positive attitude.

Data from American Academy of Orthopaedic Surgeons website (available at *www.aaos.org*); US Department of Health and Human Services. In *Healthy People 2010: understanding and improving health,* ed 2, Washington, DC, 2000, US Government Printing Office (available at *www.healthypeople.gov*).

EXAMINATION

ROUTINE TECHNIQUES	SPECIAL CIRCUMSTANCES OR ADVANCED PRACTICE
• INSPECT axial skeleton and extremities.	• PERFORM Phalen's test and TEST for Tinel's sign. ★
• INSPECT muscles. ⚷	• PERFORM the drop arm test. ★
• PALPATE bones.	• ASSESS for knee effusion. ★
• OBSERVE each major joint and adjacent muscles. ⚷	• ASSESS for knee stability ★
• TEST muscle strength and compare sides. ⚷	• ASSESS for hip flexion contracture. ★
	• ASSESS for nerve root compression.

Equipment Needed
Tape measure • Goniometer

⚷ = core examination skill   ★ = advanced practice

PROCEDURES AND TECHNIQUES WITH NORMAL FINDINGS	ABNORMAL FINDINGS

In each specific musculoskeletal region the nurse performs the same skills: inspect the skeleton and muscles; palpate bones, joints, and muscles; observe range of motion; and test muscle strength.

ROUTINE TECHNIQUES

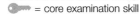 **INSPECT axial skeleton and extremities for alignment, contour, symmetry, size, and gross deformities.**

Observe the client standing upright and straight from the front, back, and sides (Fig. 15-12). He or she should stand erect. The body appears relatively symmetric when one side is compared with the other. The spine should be straight with normal curvatures (cervical concave, thoracic convex, lumbar concave) (see Fig. 15-12, *C*). The knees should be in a straight line between the hips and ankles, and the feet should be flat on the floor and pointing directly forward.

Irregular posture or any asymmetry or misalignment warrants further assessment.

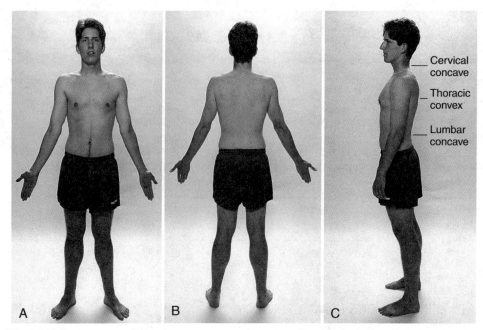

Cervical concave

Thoracic convex

Lumbar concave

A   B   C

Fig. 15-12   Inspection of overall body posture. Note the even contour of the shoulders, level scapulae and iliac crests, alignment of the head over the gluteal folds, and symmetry and alignment of extremities. **A,** Anterior view. **B,** Posterior view. **C,** Lateral view showing normal cervical concave, thoracic convex, and lumbar concave curves of the spine.

PROCEDURES AND TECHNIQUES WITH NORMAL FINDINGS

INSPECT muscles for size and symmetry.

Muscle size should appear relatively symmetric bilaterally. (No person has exact side-to-side symmetry.) Muscle circumference can be measured with a cloth or paper tape measure to provide a baseline for future comparisons and to make side-to-side comparisons. The dominant side usually is slightly larger than the nondominant side. To ensure consistency of measurement, record the number of centimeters or inches above or below the joint where the muscle was measured or include a diagram such as the one shown in Fig. 15-13, *B*. Measurement differences less than 1 cm usually are not significant.

ABNORMAL FINDINGS

Atrophy of muscle mass bilaterally may indicate lack of nerve stimulation, such as a spinal cord injury or malnutrition. Unilateral muscle atrophy may be from disuse, from pain on movement, or after removal of a cast. Fasciculations (muscle twitching of a single muscle group) may be caused by side effects of drugs. Fasciculations are localized, whereas spasms (involuntary muscle contractions) tend to be more generalized.

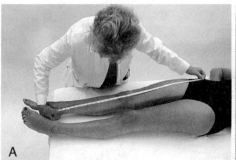

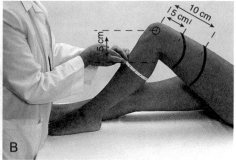

Fig. 15-13   Sites at which a limb is measured. A, Measure limb length from the anterior superior iliac spine to the medial malleolus. **B,** Measurement of the lower leg at 5 cm below the patella and of the upper leg at 5 and 10 cm above the patella. Exact location of measurement should be noted for future comparison.

= core examination skill

PROCEDURES AND TECHNIQUES WITH NORMAL FINDINGS

PALPATE bones for tenderness; joints for tenderness, heat, and edema; and muscles for tenderness, heat, edema, and tone.

Using the pads of the thumbs and fingers of both hands, palpate both of the client's shoulders simultaneously. Compare one side with the other. Systematically move distally palpating the muscles and bones of the arms, elbows, and hands. Use the dorsum of your hands to detect temperature. Use the same technique for palpating the legs from the hips to the toes. Bones should be nontender on palpation. No tenderness or edema should be detected on palpation of joints or muscles. Muscles should feel firm, not hard or soft. The joints and muscle should be the same temperature as the surrounding tissue

OBSERVE range of motion for major joints and adjacent muscles for tenderness on movement, joint stability, and deformity.

Ask the client to perform range of motion actively. Table 15-1 shows range of motion for diarthrodial joints. You may need to demonstrate active range of motion for the client. When you move the client's joints passively through the full range of motion, do not force movement of a joint when it is painful or spastic. There should be full range of motion actively and passively with joint stability but without tenderness, heat, edema, crepitus, deformity, or contracture.

ABNORMAL FINDINGS

Tenderness, heat, or edema over bones, joints, or muscles may indicate tumor, inflammation, or trauma. Muscle atrophy may be evident by a decrease in muscle tone.

Differences found between active and passive range of motion may indicate an actual muscle weakness or a joint disorder (e.g., arthritis or joint effusion). Limited range of motion may indicate inflammation such as arthritis; fluid in the joint; or contracture of muscle, ligament, or capsule. By contrast, increased mobility of a joint may indicate connective tissue disruption, tear of a ligament, or a fracture. *Crepitus* is a crackling sound produced by bone fragments or articular surfaces rubbing together (e.g., osteoarthritis). Crepitus is also heard in chondromalacia patellae that occurs after knee injury. Joint instability or deformity may indicate a number of disorders, including muscle weakness, fracture, inflammation, strained ligaments, or meniscus tear.

= core examination skill

TABLE 15-1 *Range of Motion for Diarthrodial Joints*

BODY PART	TYPE OF JOINT	TYPE OF MOVEMENT	BODY PART	TYPE OF JOINT	TYPE OF MOVEMENT
Neck and cervical spine	Pivotal	Flexion: bring chin to rest on chest Extension: return head to erect position Hyperextension: bend head back as far as possible			Internal rotation: with elbow flexed, rotate shoulder by moving arm until thumb is turned inward and toward back External rotation: with elbow flexed, move arm until thumb is upward and lateral to head
		Lateral flexion: tilt head as far as possible toward each shoulder			
		Rotation: turn head as far as possible to right and left			Circumduction: move arm in full circle. Circumduction is combination of all movements of ball-and-socket joint
Shoulder	Ball and socket	Flexion: raise arm from side position forward to position above head	Elbow	Hinge	Flexion: bend elbow so that lower arm moves toward its shoulder joint and hand is level with shoulder Extension: straighten elbow by lowering hand Hyperextension: bend lower arm back as far as possible. Not all elbows hyperextend
		Extension: return arm to position at side of the body Hyperextension: move arm behind body, keeping elbow straight	Forearm	Pivotal	Supination: turn lower arm and hand so that palm is up Pronation: turn lower arm so that palm is down
		Abduction: raise arm to side to position above head with palm away from head Adduction: lower arm sideways and across body as far as possible	Wrist	Condyloid	Flexion: move palm toward inner aspect of the forearm Extension: move fingers so that fingers, hands, and forearm are in same plane Hyperextension: bring dorsal surface to hand back as far as possible

From Potter PA, Perry AG: *Basic nursing: essentials for practice*, ed 5, St Louis, 2003, Mosby.

TABLE 15-1   *Range of Motion for Diarthrodial Joints—cont'd*

BODY PART	TYPE OF JOINT	TYPE OF MOVEMENT	BODY PART	TYPE OF JOINT	TYPE OF MOVEMENT
					Hyperextension: move leg behind body

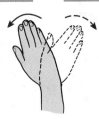

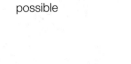

Fingers — Condyloid hinge

Hyperextension: bring dorsal surface to hand back as far as possible
Radial flexion: bend wrist medially toward thumb
Ulnar flexion: bend wrist laterally toward fifth finger
Referred to as radial/ulnar deviation
Flexion: make fist
Extension: straighten fingers
Hyperextension: bend fingers back as far as possible

Abduction: spread fingers apart
Adduction: bring fingers together

Abduction: move leg laterally away from body
Adduction: move leg back toward medial position and beyond if possible

Internal rotation: turn knee toward the inside
External rotation: turn knee toward the outside

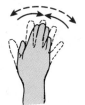
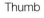
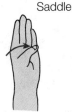

Thumb — Saddle

Flexion: move thumb across palmar surface of hand
Extension: move thumb straight away from hand
Abduction: extend thumb laterally (usually done when placing fingers in abduction and adduction)
Adduction: move thumb back toward hand
Opposition: touch thumb to each finger of same hand

Circumduction: move leg in circle

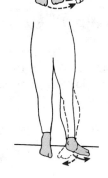

Knee — Hinge

Flexion: bring heel back toward back of thigh
Extension: return heel to floor

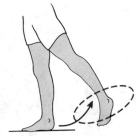

Hip — Ball and socket

Flexion: move leg forward and up
Extension: move leg back beside other leg

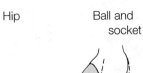
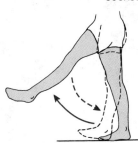
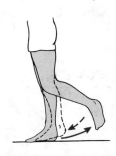

Continued

TABLE 15-1 *Range of Motion for Diarthrodial Joints—cont'd*

BODY PART	TYPE OF JOINT	TYPE OF MOVEMENT	BODY PART	TYPE OF JOINT	TYPE OF MOVEMENT
Ankle	Hinge	Dorsiflexion: move foot so that toes are pointed upward Plantar flexion: move foot so that toes are pointed downward	Toes	Condyloid	Flexion: curl toes downward Extension: straighten toes Abduction: spread toes apart Adduction: bring toes together
Foot	Gliding	Inversion: turn sole of foot medially Eversion: turn sole of foot laterally			

PROCEDURES AND TECHNIQUES WITH NORMAL FINDINGS

When a joint seems to have increased or decreased range of motion, use a goniometer to measure the angle (Fig. 15-14; Box 15-1). With the joint in neutral position or fully extended, flex the joint as far as possible and measure the angles of greatest flexion and extension.

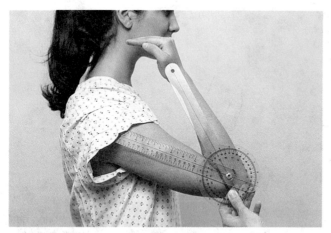

Fig. 15-14 Use of goniometer to measure joint range of motion.

ABNORMAL FINDINGS

BOX 15-1 **HOW TO USE A GONIOMETER**

A goniometer looks like a protractor with two long arms (see Fig. 15-14). Place the 0 setting of the goniometer over the middle of a joint that is in neutral position. The middle of one arm of the goniometer is aligned with the extremity proximal to that joint, and the other arm is aligned with the middle of the distal joint. Keeping the 0 at the middle of the joint, move the distal joint through its range of motion and notice the degrees of flexion, extension, or hyperextension on the goniometer.

PROCEDURES AND TECHNIQUES WITH NORMAL FINDINGS

ABNORMAL FINDINGS

➤ TEST muscle strength and compare sides.

Testing muscle strength may be performed as part of the musculoskeletal or neurologic system examination. Ask the client to flex the muscle being evaluated and then to resist when you apply opposing force against the muscles. Screening tests for strength are listed in Table 15-2. There are three scales used to determine the functional level (or "measure") of muscles, and each requires a subjective assessment of muscle strength. These scales are the Lovett scale, grading, and percent of normal. Grading is commonly used. Criteria for grading and recording muscle strength using these scales are described in Table 15-3. Expect muscle strength to be 5, bilaterally symmetric, with full resistance to opposition. The client's muscle strength is documented as 5/5 with the client's value in the numerator and the expected value in the demoninator.

Muscle weakness may indicate a muscular or joint disease or atrophy from disuse. A muscle strength of 1/5 means that the client has slight muscle contraction, with 1 representing the client's value and 5 representing the expected value.

TABLE 15-2 *Screening Tests for Muscle Strength*

MUSCLES TESTED	CLIENT ACTIVITY	NURSE'S ACTIVITY
Ocular musculature		
Lids	Close eyes tightly	Attempt to resist closure
Eye muscles	Track object in six cardinal positions	
Facial musculature	Blow out cheeks	
	Place tongue in cheek	Assess pressure in cheeks with fingertips
	Stick out tongue, move it to right and left	Assess pressure in cheek with fingertips
		Observe strength and coordination of thrust and extension
Neck muscles	Extend head backward	Push head forward
	Flex head forward	Push head backward
	Rotate head in full circle	Observe mobility, coordination
	Touch shoulders with head	Observe range of motion
Deltoid	Hold arms upward	Push down on arms
Biceps	Flex arm	Pull to extend arm
Triceps	Extend arm	Push to flex arm
Wrist musculature	Extend elbow	Push to flex
	Flex elbow	Push to extend
Finger muscles	Extend fingers	Push dorsal surface of fingers
	Flex fingers	Push ventral surface of fingers
	Spread fingers	Hold fingers together
Hip musculature	In supine position raise extended leg	Push down on leg above knee
Hamstring, gluteal, abductor, and adductor muscles of leg	Sit and perform alternate leg crossing	Push in opposite direction of crossing limb
Quadriceps	Extend leg	Push to flex leg
Hamstring	Bend knees to flex leg	Push to extend leg
Ankle and foot muscles	Bend foot up (dorsiflexion)	Push to plantar flexion
	Bend foot down (plantar flexion)	Push to dorsiflexion
Antigravity muscles	Walk on toes	
	Walk on heels	

Adapted from Barkauskas VH et al: *Health and physical assessment,* ed 3, St Louis, 2002, Mosby.

➤ = core examination skill

TABLE 15-3   *Criteria for Grading and Recording Muscle Strength*

FUNCTIONAL LEVEL	LOVETT SCALE	GRADE	PERCENT OF NORMAL
No evidence of contractility	Zero (0)	0	0
Evidence of slight contractility	Trace (T)	1	10
Complete range of motion with gravity eliminated	Poor (P)	2	25
Complete range of motion with gravity	Fair (F)	3	50
Complete range of motion against gravity with some resistance	Good (G)	4	75
Complete range of motion against gravity with full resistance	Normal (N)	5	100

From Barkauskas VH et al: *Health and physical assessment,* ed 3, St Louis, 2002, Mosby.

PROCEDURES AND TECHNIQUES WITH NORMAL FINDINGS

ABNORMAL FINDINGS

EXAMINATION OF SPECIFIC MUSCULOSKELETAL REGIONS

OBSERVE gait for conformity, symmetry, and rhythm.

Ask the client to walk across the room and back. Expected findings are conformity (ability to follow gait sequencing of both stance and swing), regular smooth rhythm, symmetry in length of leg swing, smooth swaying, and smooth, symmetric arm swing.

An unstable or exaggerated gait, limp, irregular stride length, arm swing that is unrelated to gait, or any other inability to maintain straight posture or asymmetry of body parts requires further assessment. When unequal leg length is suspected, measure the leg from the anterior superior iliac spine to the medial malleolus (see Fig. 15-13, *A*).

INSPECT musculature of the face and neck for symmetry.

Client is in a sitting position. Inspection of the client's facial symmetry began during the interview. Ask client to open and close his or her mouth.

Asymmetric facial or neck musculature may indicate previous or current facial fractures or previous facial surgery.

PALPATE each temporomandibular joint for movement, sounds, and tenderness.

Use the pads of the first two fingers in front of the tragus of each ear to palpate the temporomandibular joint (TMJ) with the mouth closed and open. The mandible should move smoothly and painlessly. An audible or palpable snapping or clicking in the absence of other symptoms is not unusual (Fig. 15-15, *A*).

Pain or crepitus of the TMJ with locking or popping may indicate a TMJ disorder.

OBSERVE jaw for range of motion.

Ask the client to open and close the mouth. It should open between 1.25 and 2.5 inches (between 3 and 6 cm) between upper and lower teeth. Ask the client to move the jaw side to side; the mandible should move 1 to 2 cm in each direction (Fig. 15-15, *B*). Motion should be smooth and without pain. Finally, the client should be able to protrude and retract the chin without difficulty or pain.

Difficulty opening the mouth or limited range of motion may result from injury or arthritic changes. Pain in the TMJ may indicate malocclusion of teeth or arthritic changes.

= core examination skill

PROCEDURES AND TECHNIQUES WITH NORMAL FINDINGS

ABNORMAL FINDINGS

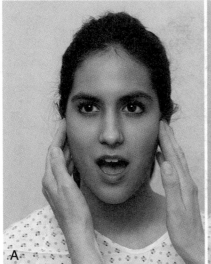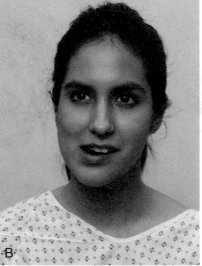

Fig. 15-15 A, Palpation of temporomandibular joint. **B,** Lateral range of motion in the temporomandibular joint.

PALPATE the neck for pain.

Use the pads of thumbs and fingers to palpate the neck muscles and lymph nodes. The neck is soft and firm, without masses, pain, or spasms.

Pain on palpation may indicate inflammation of the muscle (myositis). Masses may be enlarged lymph nodes, indicating inflammation or neoplasm. Neck spasm may indicate nerve compression or psychologic stress.

OBSERVE the neck for range of motion.

Ask the client to flex the chin to the chest. It should move to a point 45 degrees from midline. Ask the client to hyperextend the head, if possible; it should reach 55 degrees from midline (Fig. 15-16, *A*). Have the client laterally bend his or her head to the right and the left. Range should be 40 degrees from midline in each direction (Fig. 15-16, *B*). Have the client rotate the chin to the shoulders, first to the right and then to the left. It should reach 70 degrees from midline (Fig. 15-16, *C*).

Range of motion may be impaired by pain or muscle spasms. Hyperextension and flexion may be limited because of cervical vertebral disk herniation or osteoarthritic changes. Pain, numbness, or tingling reported during range of motion may indicate compression of cervical spinal root nerves.

TEST the neck muscles for strength.

To assess muscle strength of the neck, ask the client to repeat the rotation of the head against resistance of your hand to test strength of the sternocleidomastoid muscle (Fig. 15-17, *A*). Ask the client to flex the chin to the chest and maintain the position while you palpate the sternocleidomastoid muscle and try to manually force the head upright. If muscle strength is present, you should be unable to force the head upright (Fig. 15-17, *B*).

Have the client extend the head and maintain position while you try to manually force the head upright to assess the trapezius muscle strength (Fig. 15-17, *C*). If muscle strength is 5/5, you should be unable to force the head upright.

If you can break the muscular flexion before the anticipated point, the client has muscle weakness.

= core examination skill

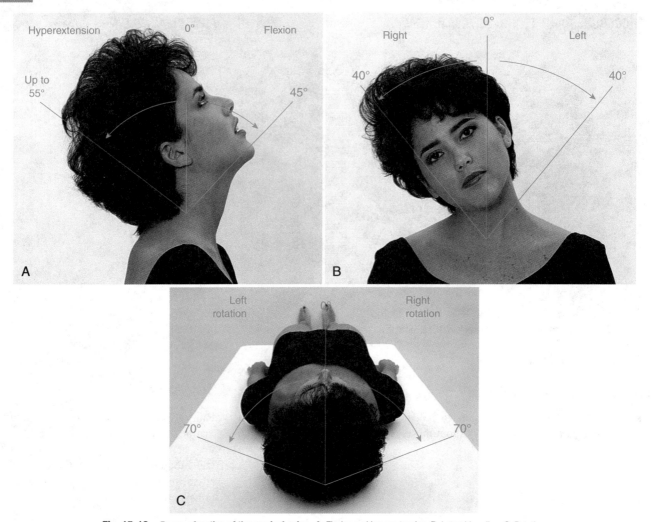

Fig. 15-16   Range of motion of the cervical spine. A, Flexion and hyperextension. **B,** Lateral bending. **C,** Rotation.

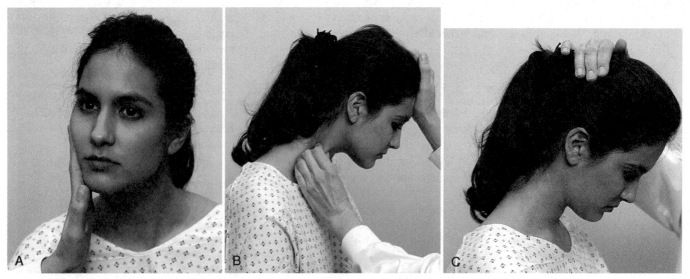

Fig. 15-17   Examining the strength of the sternocleidomastoid and trapezius muscles. A, Rotation against resistance. **B,** Flexion with palpation of the sternocleidomastoid muscle. **C,** Extension against resistance.

PROCEDURES AND TECHNIQUES WITH NORMAL FINDINGS

🗝 **INSPECT** the shoulders and cervical, thoracic, and lumbar spine for alignment and symmetry.

Ask the client to stand; while you stand to the side of the client, observe the cervical concave, the thoracic convex, and the lumbar concave (see Fig. 15-12, *C*). Note the landmarks on the back: spinous processes protruding slightly at C7 and T1, paravertebral muscles, and the alignment across the iliac crests at L4 and the posterior superior iliac spine at S2 (Fig. 15-18). Ask the client to touch the toes. Move behind the client to inspect the spine. Vertebrae should be aligned, indicating a straight spine. Shoulders should be level or at equal heights. (While the client is bending forward, you will perform the next assessment.)

ABNORMAL FINDINGS

Deviation of the spine or asymmetry of shoulder or iliac height is an abnormal finding. *Kyphosis* is a posterior curvature (convexity) of the thoracic spine (Fig. 15-19, *B*), *lordosis* is an anterior curvature (concavity) of the spine (Fig. 15-19, *C*), and *scoliosis* is a lateral curvature of the spine (Fig. 15-19, *E* and *F*). Curvature of the spine may create asymmetry of the shoulders.

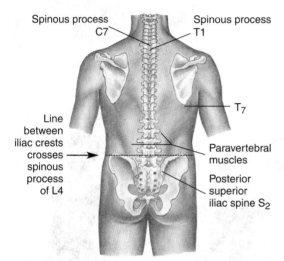

Fig.15-18 Landmarks of the back. *(From Seidel et al, 2003.)*

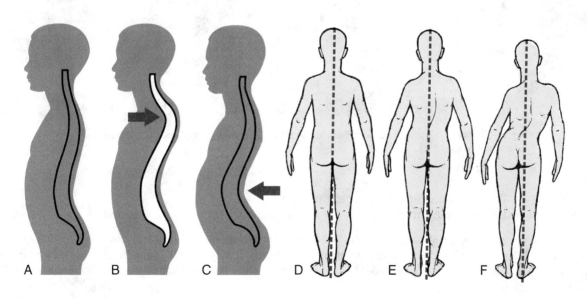

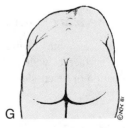

Fig. 15-19 **Defects of the spinal column. A,** Normal spine. **B,** Kyphosis. **C,** Lordosis. **D,** Normal spine in balance. **E,** Mild scoliosis. **F,** Severe scoliosis, not in balance. **G,** Rib hump and flank asymmetry seen in flexion. *(Modified from Hilt and Schmitt, 1975. In Hockenberry et al, 2003.)*

🗝 = core examination skill

| **PROCEDURES AND TECHNIQUES WITH NORMAL FINDINGS** | **ABNORMAL FINDINGS** |

 OBSERVE range of motion of the thoracic and lumbar spine.

The client should be able to reach 75 degrees of flexion while touching his or her toes (Fig. 15-20, *A*). Document how close the client gets to the floor by measuring from fingertips to the floor (e.g., 6 inches from the floor). Some clients are unable to touch the floor because of tight hamstrings and leg muscles or obesity. These are considered normal variations.

Observe for range of motion as the client hyperextends the spine; it should reach 30 degrees back from the neutral position (extension) (Fig. 15-20, *B*).

Ask the client to bend laterally right and left. (NOTE: It may be necessary to stabilize the client's hips.) He or she should be able to reach 35 degrees of flexion both ways from midline (Fig. 15-20, *C*).

Have the client rotate the upper trunk (you may need to stabilize pelvis) to the right and left; he or she should achieve 30 degrees of rotation in both directions from a directly forward position (Fig. 15-20, *D*).

ABNORMAL FINDINGS

Flexion less than 75 degrees with pain or muscle spasm is abnormal.

Impaired range of motion during hyperextension or lateral flexion may be due to pain from muscle strain or spasms or a herniated vertebral disk.

Impaired range of motion during rotation may be due to pain from muscle strain or spasms.

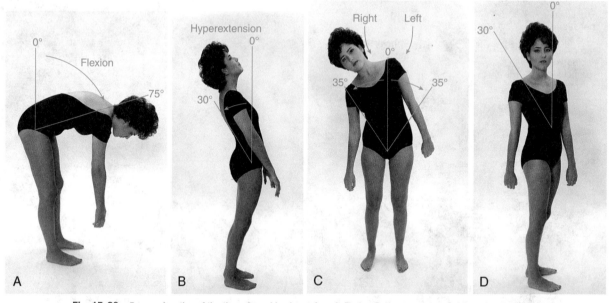

Fig. 15-20 **Range of motion of the thoracic and lumbar spine. A,** Flexion. **B,** Hyperextension. **C,** Lateral bending. **D,** Rotation of the upper trunk.

PALPATE the posterior neck, spinal processes, and paravertebral muscles for alignment and tenderness.

Stand behind the client. Use the pads of the thumbs and fingers for palpation. The posterior neck and spine should be straight and nontender. (NOTE: It may be helpful to have the client hunch his or her shoulders forward and slightly flex the neck [Fig. 15-21]).

Misalignment may be due to muscle weakness. Tenderness may be due to inflammation such as myositis or herniated vertebral disk.

PERCUSS the spinal processes for tenderness.

First tap each process with one finger, and then lightly tap each side of the spine with the ulnar surface of your fist. No muscle spasm or tenderness should be noted on palpation or percussion.

Tenderness may be due to inflammation such as myositis or herniated vertebral disk. Muscle spasm may be due to muscle strain.

 = core examination skill

PROCEDURES AND TECHNIQUES WITH NORMAL FINDINGS	ABNORMAL FINDINGS

INSPECT the shoulders and shoulder girdle for equality of height and contour.

Facing the client, who is in a seated position, inspect scapulae and clavicles, as well as the acromioclavicular junction, for equality of height and symmetry.

Observe the trapezius muscle for shape and size. All structures should be smooth, regular, and bilaterally symmetric. Right and left shoulders should be level, rounded, and firm, with smooth contour and no bony prominences. Each shoulder should be equidistant from the vertebral column. Note any erythema, edema, or nodules.

Shoulder joints may have some deformity from trauma, arthritic changes, or scoliosis.

PALPATE the shoulders for firmness, fullness, tenderness, and masses.

Use the pads of the thumbs and fingers to palpate the acromioclavicular joint and humerus, as well as the trapezius, biceps, triceps, and deltoid muscles. Compare one side to the other side. These areas should be nontender, smooth, firm and full without masses, and bilaterally symmetric. The muscles of the dominant arm may be slightly larger.

Tenderness may be due to inflammation of the muscles, overwork of unconditioned muscles, or sports injuries.

TEST the trapezius muscles for strength.

Ask the client to shrug the shoulders while you attempt to push them down (Fig. 15-22). This also tests function of cranial nerve XI (CN XI; spinal accessory).

Weakness of the trapezius muscles may indicate compressed spinal nerve root or compression of the spinal accessory cranial nerve (CN XI).

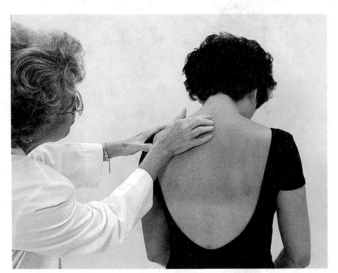

Fig. 15-21   Palpation of the spinal processes of the vertebrae.

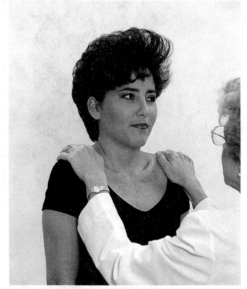

Fig. 15-22   Test strength of the trapezius muscle with the shrugged shoulder movement.

= core examination skill

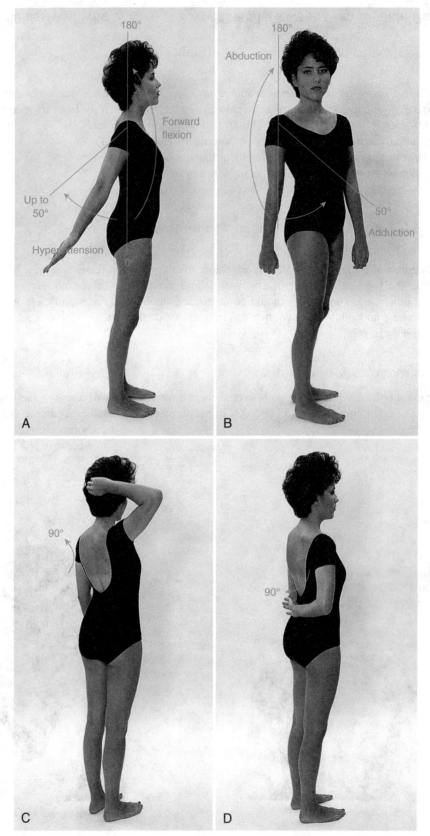

Fig. 15-23   Range of motion of the shoulders. A, Forward flexion and hyperextension. **B,** Abduction and adduction.
C, External rotation and abduction. **D,** Internal rotation and adduction.

PROCEDURES AND TECHNIQUES WITH NORMAL FINDINGS	ABNORMAL FINDINGS

OBSERVE the shoulders for range of motion.

Ask the client to extend the arms straight up beside the ears. The arms should reach 180 degrees from resting neutral position, be bilaterally equal, and cause no discomfort (Fig. 15-23, *A*).

Ask the client to hyperextend the arms backward. They should reach 50 degrees, be bilaterally equal, and cause no discomfort.

Ask the client to lift both arms laterally over his or her head. Expected shoulder abduction is 180 degrees. Then ask the client to swing each arm across the front of the body. Expected adduction is 50 degrees (Fig. 15-23, *B*).

To test external rotation, have the client place the hands behind the head with elbows out. A range of 90 degrees is normal; movement should be bilaterally equal and without discomfort (Fig.15-23, *C*).

To test internal rotation, ask the client to place the hands at the small of the back. Range should be 90 degrees, with movements bilaterally equal and without discomfort (Fig. 15-23, *D*).

Limited range of motion, pain with movement, crepitations, and asymmetry are abnormal findings. Degenerative joint changes or sports injuries may impair range of motion.

TEST the arms for muscle strength.

Have the client hold the arms up while you try to push them down. Remember to compare one side with the other. They should be strong bilaterally so that you cannot move them out of position. Use criteria in Table 15-3 for grading.

To test triceps muscle strength, ask the client to extend the arm while you resist by pushing the arm to a flexed position (Fig. 15-24, *A*). Expected muscle strength is recorded as 5/5 (see Table 15-4).

To test biceps strength, have the client try to flex the arm while you try to extend his or her forearm. You should be unable to move the arm out of position, and strength should be equal bilaterally, documented as 5/5 (Fig. 15-24, *B*).

Abnormal findings include unequal response, weak response, muscular spasm, and pain. These findings may be due to joint or muscle inflammation, trauma, or sports injuries.

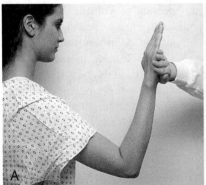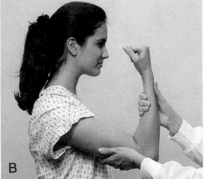

Fig. 15-24   Testing muscle strength of arms. A, Testing triceps muscle strength. **B,** Testing biceps muscle strength.

= core examination skill

PROCEDURES AND TECHNIQUES WITH NORMAL FINDINGS

PALPATE the elbows for tenderness, edema, and nodules.

Hold the client's lower arm in your nondominant hand while using the pads of the thumb and fingers of the dominant hand to palpate the olecranon process and lateral epicondyle (Fig. 15-25). Repeat the procedure on the other side. The elbows should be smooth without nodules, edema, or discomfort over the groove on either side.

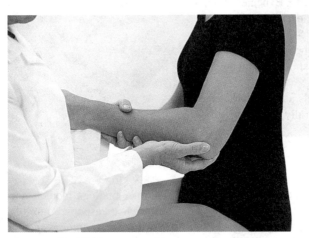

Fig. 15-25   Palpation of the olecranon process grooves.

OBSERVE the elbows for range of motion.

Ask the client to flex and extend the elbow; 160 degrees of full movement should be present bilaterally without discomfort (Fig. 15-26, *A*).

Assess pronation and supination of the elbow by having the client rotate the hands palms up and palms down (pronate and supinate); 90 degrees should be achieved in each direction, and the movements should be bilaterally equal and without discomfort (Fig. 15-26, *B*).

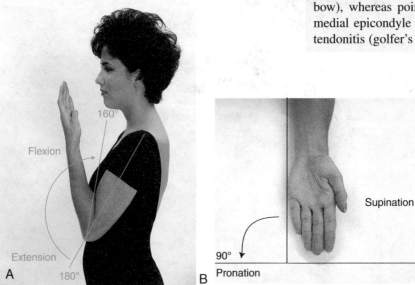

Fig. 15-26   Range of motion of the elbow. A, Flexion and extension. **B,** Palm up, supination; palm down, pronation.

ABNORMAL FINDINGS

Abnormal findings include edema, subcutaneous nodules, point tenderness, and palpable nodes. Subcutaneous nodules at pressure points of the ulnar surface may indicate rheumatoid arthritis.

Note any limitation of motion, asymmetry of movement, or pain at the elbow. Subcutaneous nodules just inferior to the olecranon process (elbow joint) may indicate rheumatoid arthritis. Tenderness or pain with pronation and supination of the elbow and point tenderness on the lateral epicondyle may indicate lateral tendonitis or epicondylitis (tennis elbow), whereas point tenderness on the medial epicondyle may indicate medial tendonitis (golfer's elbow).

= core examination skill

PROCEDURES AND TECHNIQUES WITH NORMAL FINDINGS

INSPECT the joints of the wrists and hands for position, contour, and number of digits.

Compare the right wrist and hand with the left. They should be smooth, firm, and symmetric, with no edema or deformities. The hand with five digits is aligned with the wrist, and fingers are aligned with wrist and forearm (Fig. 15-27).

ABNORMAL FINDINGS

Missing fingers are recorded. Swan-neck and boutonniére deformities of interphalangeal joints may be related to rheumatoid arthritis (Fig. 15-28). Osteoarthritis may cause Bouchard's nodes in the PIP joints, whereas Heberden's nodes form in the DIP joints (Fig. 15-29).

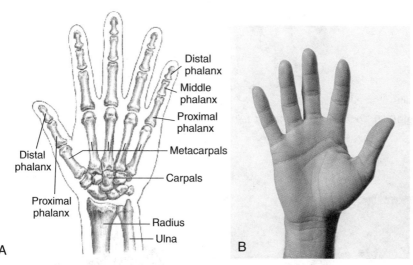

A

- Distal phalanx
- Middle phalanx
- Proximal phalanx
- Metacarpals
- Carpals
- Distal phalanx
- Proximal phalanx
- Radius
- Ulna

B

Fig. 15-27 **A,** Bony structures of the right hand and wrist. Note alignment of fingers with the radius. **B,** Palmar aspect of right hand. (**A,** From Seidel et al, 2003.)

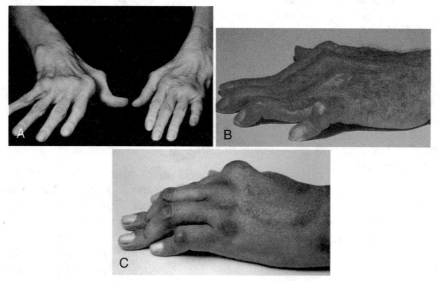

Fig. 15-28 **A,** Ulnar deviation and subluxation of metacarpophalangeal joints. **B,** Swan-neck deformity. **C,** Boutonnière deformity. (**A and B,** Reprinted from the Clinical slide collection of the rheumatic diseases, copyright 1991, 1995, 1997. Used with permission of the American College of Rheumatology. **C,** From Seidel et al, 2006.)

= core examination skill

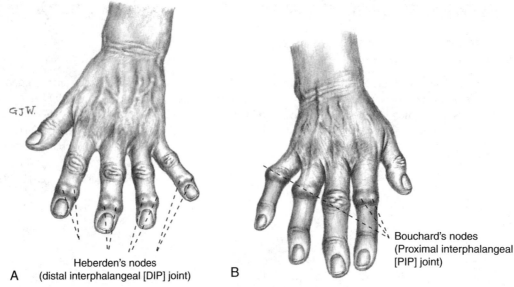

A Heberden's nodes
(distal interphalangeal [DIP] joint)

B

Bouchard's nodes
(Proximal interphalangeal
[PIP] joint)

Fig. 15-29 Osteoarthritis. *(From Mourad, 1991.)*

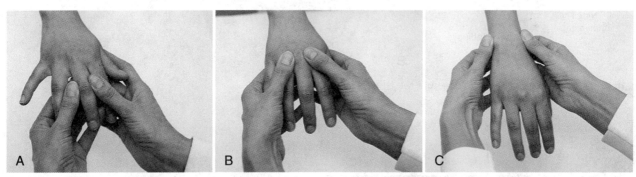

Fig. 15-30 Palpation of joints of the hand and wrist. **A,** Interphalangeal joints. **B,** Metacarpophalangeal joints. **C,** Radiocarpal groove.

PROCEDURES AND TECHNIQUES WITH NORMAL FINDINGS

PALPATE each joint of the hand and wrist for surface characteristics and tenderness.

Palpate the interphalangeal joints with your thumb and index finger. Palpate the metacarpophalangeal joints with both thumbs. Palpate the wrist and radiocarpal groove with your thumbs on the dorsal surface and your fingers on the palmar surface. Joint surfaces should be smooth, without nodules, edema, or tenderness (Fig. 15-30).

ABNORMAL FINDINGS

Painful, edematous DIP or PIP joints are found in osteoarthritis. A firm mass over the dorsum of the wrist may be a ganglion. Rheumatoid arthritis may cause wrists and PIP joints to appear hot, tender, painful, deformed, and edematous.

PROCEDURES AND TECHNIQUES WITH NORMAL FINDINGS

ABNORMAL FINDINGS

TEST for muscle strength and OBSERVE for range of motion of wrists and fingers.

First, ask the client to extend and spread the fingers (both hands) while you attempt to push the fingers together (Fig. 15-31, *A*). The response should be symmetric, to full flexion and extension, without discomfort, and with sufficient muscle strength to overcome the resistance you apply.

Next, have the client grip your first two fingers on each hand. The response should be bilaterally equal and the grip tight and full flexion (Fig. 15-31, *B*).

Weak muscle strength and impaired range of motion may accompany rheumatoid arthritis and osteoarthritis. Fractures of metatarsals or phalanges may weaken the muscle strength.

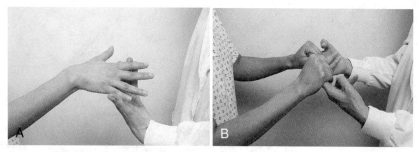

Fig. 15-31   **A,** Assessment of finger strength. **B,** Assessment of grip strength.

= core examination skill

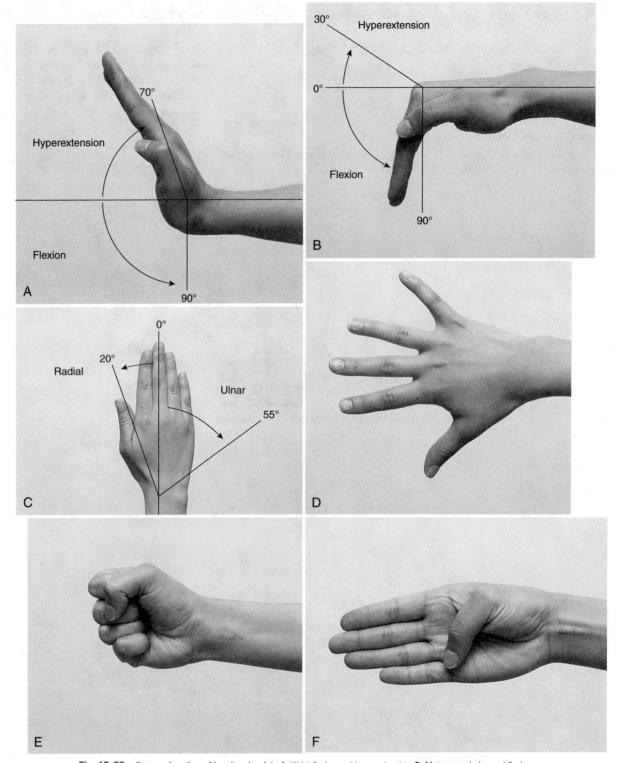

Fig. 15-32   Range of motion of hand and wrist. A, Wrist flexion and hyperextension. **B,** Metacarpophalangeal flexion and hyperextension. **C,** Wrist radial and ulnar deviation. **D,** Finger abduction. **E,** Finger flexion: fist formation. **F,** Finger extension: thumb to each fingertip and to base of little finger.

PROCEDURES AND TECHNIQUES WITH NORMAL FINDINGS	**ABNORMAL FINDINGS**

Observe the range of motion of wrists as the client bends the hand up at the wrist (hyperextension to 70 degrees), flexes the hand down at the wrist (palmar flexion of 90 degrees) (Fig. 15-32, *A*), and flexes the fingers up and down at the metacarpophalangeal joints (flexion of 90 degrees, hyperextension of 30 degrees) (Fig. 15-32, *B*). Then, with the client's palms flat on the table, ask the client to turn them outward and inward (ulnar deviation of 50 to 60 degrees, radial deviation of 20 degrees) (Fig. 15-32, *C*), spread the fingers apart (Fig. 15-32, *D*), and then make a fist (abduction of 20 degrees, fist tight) (Fig. 15-32, *E*), and touch the thumb to each finger (opposition) and to the base of the fifth finger (able to perform all motions) (Fig. 15-32, *F*). These findings should be bilaterally equal.

Abnormal findings include unequal response, weak response, muscular spasm, and pain. The findings may be due to joint or muscle inflammation.

INSPECT the hips for symmetry.

Ask the client to stand. Look at the symmetry of the hips anteriorly and posteriorly. The hips should be the same height and symmetric. You may need to move the client's clothing aside to visualize the hips.

Asymmetric hips may occur from curvature of the spine.

PALPATE the hips for stability and tenderness.

Assist the client to a supine position. Use the iliac crests and greater trochanter of the femur as landmarks (see Fig. 15-18). Palpate iliac crests to determine if they are symmetric. Findings should be bilaterally symmetric hips that are stable and painless.

Osteoarthritis or hip dislocation may cause pain and hip instability.

OBSERVE the hips for range of motion.

Assist the client to a supine position. To evaluate hip range of motion, ask the client to alternately pull each knee up to the chest. The client should achieve 120-degree flexion from the straight, extended position (Fig. 15-33, *A*).

Next, have the client raise the leg to flex the hip as far as possible without bending the knee. Results should be 90 degrees from the straight extended position (Fig. 15-33, *B*).

To test external hip rotation (Patrick test), ask the client to place the heel of one foot on the opposite patella. Apply gentle pressure to the medial aspect of the flexed knee as the client externally rotates the hip until the knee or lateral thigh touches the examination table. Repeat the procedure with the other hip. Rotation should reach 45 degrees from the straight midline position (Fig. 15-33, *C*).

To test the hip for internal rotation, ask the client to flex the knee and turn medially (inward) as you pull the heel laterally (outward) to test internal hip rotation. Rotation should reach 40 degrees from the straight midline position (Fig. 15-33, *D*).

Ask the client to move one leg laterally with the knee straight to test abduction and medially to test adduction. The expected range for abduction is up to 45 degrees; the expected range for adduction is up to 30 degrees (Fig. 15-33, *E*).

Assist the client to a prone position. Test hyperextension of the hip by raising the leg upward with the knee straight. The expected range of movement is up to 30 degrees (Fig. 15-33, *F*). This assessment can also be performed with the client in the standing position.

Osteoarthritis and hip dislocation also impair hip range of motion. Vertebral compression of spinal nerves may cause back or leg pain during hip flexion with leg extension.

= core examination skill

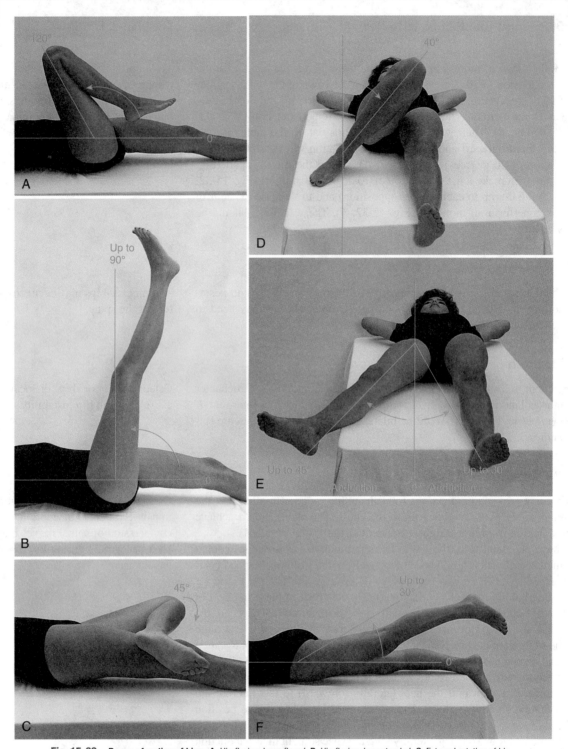

Fig. 15-33 **Range of motion of hips.** **A,** Hip flexion, knee flexed. **B,** Hip flexion, leg extended. **C,** External rotation of hip. **D,** Internal rotation of hip. **E,** Abduction and adduction of hip. **F,** Hyperextension of hip, leg extended.

PROCEDURES AND TECHNIQUES WITH NORMAL FINDINGS	ABNORMAL FINDINGS

TEST the hips for muscle strength.

Assist the client to a supine position. Ask him or her to attempt to raise the legs while you try to hold them down. Evaluate one leg at a time, noting if the response is bilaterally strong and if you are unable to interfere with the movement.

Abnormal findings include unequal response, weak response, muscular spasm, and pain. These findings may be due to joint or muscle inflammation, trauma, or sports injuries.

TEST the leg muscles for strength.

To test the quadriceps with the client sitting, have the client extend the legs at the knee while you attempt to flex the knee. Strength should be bilaterally equal, and you should be unable to flex the knee. Compare one side with the other. Use criteria from Table 15-3 for grading muscle strength.

   To evaluate the hamstrings with the client sitting, have the client attempt to bend his or her knee while you attempt to straighten it. Strength should be bilaterally equal, and you should be unable to flex the knee (Fig. 15-34).

Abnormal findings include unequal response, weak response, muscular spasm, and pain. These findings may be due to joint or muscle inflammation, trauma, or sports injuries.

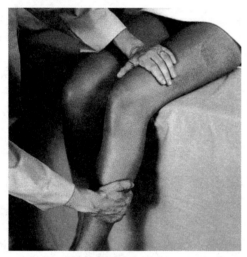

Fig. 15-34   Assessment of hamstring muscle strength. Client flexes knee while examiner tries to straighten it. *(From Barkauskas et al, 2002.)*

INSPECT the knees for symmetry and alignment.

The knees should be lined up with the tibia and ankle without medial or lateral deviation.

Knees that appear edematous and warm, bowlegged (genu varum), knock-kneed (genu valgum), thick, boggy (spongy), or inflamed are abnormal findings.

PALPATE the knees for contour, tenderness, and edema.

First, palpate the suprapatellar pouch on each side of the quadriceps with the thumb and fingers of one or both hands. Compare one side with the other. The knees should feel smooth, nonedematous, and nontender.

   Next, with the knee flexed to 90 degrees, palpate over the medial and lateral aspects of the tibiofemoral joint space. These areas should be nonedematous and nontender. Palpate the popliteal space for contour, tenderness, and edema. It should be smooth and nontender.

Abnormal findings include bogginess, thickening, tenderness, or pain that may occur from rheumatoid arthritis, osteoarthritis, or bursitis. Edema of the suprapatellar pouch may indicate synovitis.

= core examination skill

PROCEDURES AND TECHNIQUES WITH NORMAL FINDINGS	ABNORMAL FINDINGS

OBSERVE the knees for range of motion.

Evaluate the range of motion by having the client flex the knees (Fig. 15-35). Flexion should reach 130 degrees from the straight extended position without discomfort or difficulty. If the knee is able to hyperextend, it should reach 15 degrees from the extended position (midline).

A decrease in the range of motion may occur as a result of a form of arthritis, trauma, or ligament, tendon, or meniscus injury.

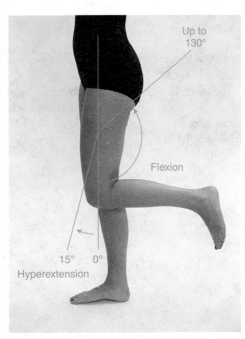

Up to 130°

Flexion

15°   0°
Hyperextension

Fig. 15-35   Flexion and hyperextension of knee.

INSPECT the ankles and feet for contour, alignment, and number of toes.

The ankles should be smooth, with no deformity. The feet are in straight position aligned with the long axis of the lower leg with five toes that are extended and straight on each foot.

Abnormal findings include misalignment of the feet with the ankle or leg or amputation or deformity of toes. Medial deviation of the toes, hallux valgus (Fig. 15-36), claw toes, hammer toes, and calluses are abnormal findings as well.

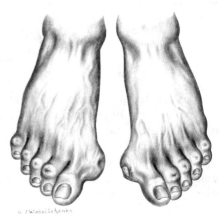

Fig. 15-36   Hallux valgus with bunions and hammer toes. *(From Mourad, 1991.)*

= core examination skill

PROCEDURES AND TECHNIQUES WITH NORMAL FINDINGS

ABNORMAL FINDINGS

PALPATE the ankles and feet for contour, edema, and tenderness.

Use the pads of the thumbs and fingers to palpate the ankle, heel, and joints using both hands to palpate one foot at a time. These structures should be smooth, nonedematous, and nontender.

Abnormal findings include tenderness (diffuse versus pinpoint), inflammation, ulcerations, and nodules. Localized pain in one heel may indicate a bone spur. Pain in both feet that is worse on arising may indicate plantar fasciitis.

OBSERVE the ankles and feet for range of motion.

To evaluate the range of motion of both feet and ankles, have the client dorsiflex and plantar flex the foot. Dorsiflexion should reach 20 degrees from midline, and plantar flexion should reach 45 degrees from midline (Fig.15-37, *A*). Then have the client invert and evert the foot. (NOTE: You may need to stabilize the heel during these maneuvers.) Eversion (turning the foot outward at the ankle) is 20 degrees and inversion (turning the foot inward at the ankle) is 30 degrees from midline position (Fig. 15-37, *B*). Next, ask the client to rotate the ankle, turning the foot away from and then toward the other foot while you stabilize the leg. Expect abduction of 10 degrees and adduction of 20 degrees (Fig. 15-37, *C*). Finally, have the client flex and extend the toes. These should be active movements. All movements should be bilaterally equal and performed without discomfort.

Limitations in range of motion, pain, crepitations, and asymmetry are abnormal findings. Tightening or trauma to the Achilles tendon may cause plantar flexion.

TEST the ankle and feet muscles for strength.

Ask the client to walk on his or her toes, then heels, followed by walking on the inside of the feet (eversion) and finally walking on the outside of the feet (inversion).

Abnormal findings include unequal response, weak response, muscular spasm, and pain. These findings may be due to joint or muscle inflammation, trauma, or sports injuries.

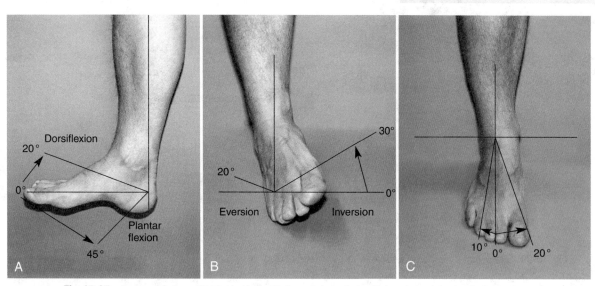

Fig. 15-37   **Range of motion of the ankle. A,** Dorsiflexion and plantar flexion. **B,** Inversion and eversion. **C,** Abduction and adduction. *(From Seidel et al, 2003.)*

= core examination skill

| PROCEDURES AND TECHNIQUES WITH NORMAL FINDINGS | ABNORMAL FINDINGS |

SPECIAL CIRCUMSTANCES OR ADVANCED PRACTICE

★ **ASSESS for carpal tunnel syndrome.**

The test for *Phalen's sign* is performed by asking the client to flex both wrists and press the dorsum of the hands against each other for 1 minute (Fig. 15-38). No report of numbness, tingling, or pain is a negative test.

A positive Phalen's sign occurs if the client complains of numbness, pain, or paresthesia over the palmar surface of the hand and the first three fingers and part of the fourth. This positive finding may indicate carpal tunnel syndrome.

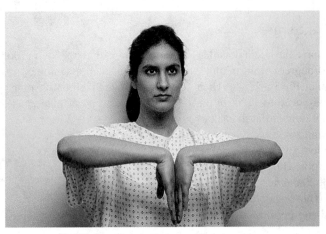

Fig. 15-38   Phalen's test for carpal tunnel syndrome.

The test for *Tinel's sign* is performed by tapping on the median nerve where it passes through the carpal tunnel under the flexor retinaculum (carpal ligament) and volar carpal ligament. No report of tingling sensation is a negative Tinel's sign (Fig. 15-39).

A positive Tinel's sign occurs when the client reports a tingling sensation or pain radiating from the wrist to the hand along the median nerve. This positive finding may indicate carpal tunnel syndrome.

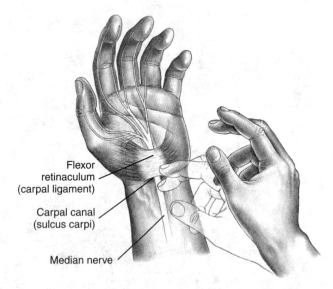

Flexor
retinaculum
(carpal ligament)

Carpal canal
(sulcus carpi)

Median nerve

Fig. 15-39   Tinel's sign for carpal tunnel syndrome. *(From Seidel et al, 2006.)*

★ = advanced practice

| **PROCEDURES AND TECHNIQUES WITH NORMAL FINDINGS** | **ABNORMAL FINDINGS** |

★ ASSESS for rotator cuff damage.

Rotator cuff damage can be determined with the drop arm test. Abduct the client's affected arm and ask the client to lower the arm slowly. The expected response is a slow, controlled adduction of the arm.

Inability to lower the arm slowly and smoothly or severe shoulder pain while adducting the arm may indicate rotator cuff damage.

★ ASSESS for knee effusion.

Two tests evaluate the presence of fluid in the knee joint. The *bulge sign* tests for small effusions of the knee. Assist the client to a supine position. Elicit the bulge sign by extending the knee and milking the medial aspect upward two or three times. Then tap on the lateral side of the patella. No fluid waves or bulging should be seen on the opposite side of the joint (Fig. 15-40).

The second test, *ballottement,* is used for larger effusions. With the knee extended, apply downward pressure on the suprapatellar pouch with the thumb and fingers of one hand, and with the other hand push the patella firmly against the femur. Release the pressure from the patella, but leave your fingers in contact with the knee to detect any fluid wave (Fig. 15-41).

If fluid is present, fluid waves are palpable on the opposite side of the joint. Fluid in a joint (effusion) is an accumulation of serous exudate as part of an inflammatory process such as osteoarthritis.

Palpation of a fluid wave after release of pressure against the patella is ballottement, indicating excess fluid in the knee joint.

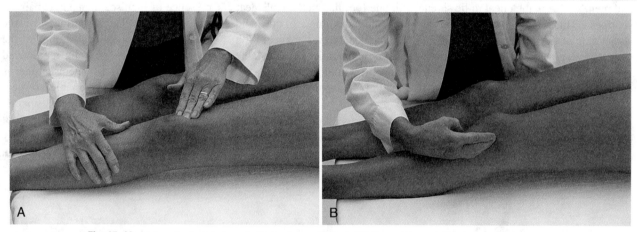

Fig. 15-40 **Bulge sign to detect small effusion in knee joint. A,** Milk the medial aspect of the knee two or three times. **B,** Then tap the lateral side of the patella.

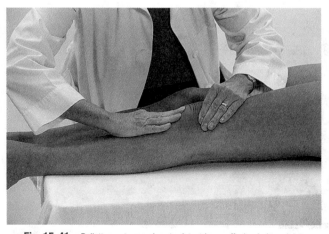

Fig. 15-41 Ballottement procedure to detect large effusion in knee joint.

★ = advanced practice

PROCEDURES AND TECHNIQUES WITH NORMAL FINDINGS	**ABNORMAL FINDINGS**

★ **ASSESS for knee stability.**

With the client in supine position, assess knee stability provided by *collateral and cruciate ligaments* (see Fig. 15-2). Assess the lateral collateral ligament by placing one hand against the medial aspect of the knee joint to keep it from moving and using your other hand to grasp the ankle. Adduct the lower leg (Fig. 15-42, *A*). Normally there is little lateral motion at the knee. To test the medial collateral ligament, place your hand on the lateral aspect of the knee, grasp the ankle, and abduct the lower leg. Repeat the procedure on the other knee if indicated.

Assess the *anterior and posterior cruciate ligaments* using the drawer test. The client remains in supine position with the hip flexed 45 degrees and the knee flexed with the foot flat on the examination table. Sit on the client's foot to stabilize it. Instruct the client to relax the muscles in the flexed leg. It is important to be sure that the hamstrings are relaxed by palpating them at the back of the knee. Using both hands, jerk the head of the tibia forward (open drawer) to assess the anterior cruciate ligament and push backward (closed drawer) to assess the posterior cruciate ligament (Fig. 15-42, *B*). Repeat the procedure on the other knee if indicated. You should not be able to displace the knee from its position.

Perform *McMurray's test* to evaluate the presence of a damaged medial or lateral meniscus. Ask the client to lie supine with one foot flat on the table near the buttocks. This flexes the knee. Place the thumb and index finger of one hand on either side of the joint space to maintain flexion and stabilize the knee. With the other hand, grasp the client's heel, raise the lower leg parallel with the table (knee will be flexed 90 degrees), and rotate the knee. External rotation tests the lateral meniscus, and internal rotation tests the medial meniscus (Fig. 15-43).

Movement of the knee medially or laterally suggests collateral ligament damage, which often results from trauma to the knee.

When the tibia can be pulled anteriorly more than 2 cm from the femur, injury to the anterior cruciate ligament may be indicated. When the tibia can be pushed posteriorly from the femur, an injury to the posterior cruciate ligament may be indicated.

A positive McMurray's test in the presence of meniscal damage is pain on the medial or lateral surfaces of the knee, audible click or locking of the knee on movement, or pain reproduced along the joint lines. If meniscal tear is present, the client is unable to bear weight or flex the knee. Medial meniscus tear is more common than lateral meniscus tear. A meniscal tear frequently occurs with twisting of the knee playing sports.

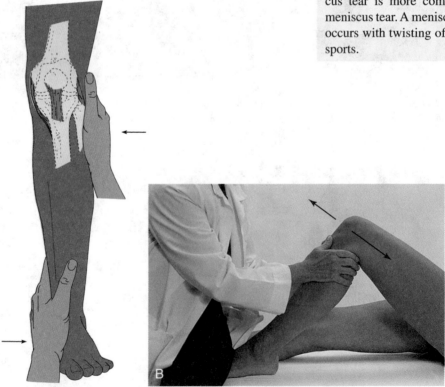

Fig. 15-42   **Assessing knee stability. A,** Assessing collateral ligaments. **B,** Drawer test for assessing anterior and posterior cruciate ligaments. (*A, From Greenberger and Hinthorn, 1993.*)

★ = advanced practice

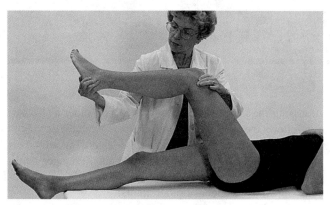

Fig. 15-43 **Examination of the knee with McMurray's test.** Knee is flexed, stabilized with thumb and index finger; with the other hand rotate and extend the lower leg.

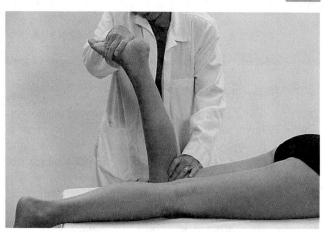

Fig. 15-44 Examination of the knee with the Apley test.

PROCEDURES AND TECHNIQUES WITH NORMAL FINDINGS

When the client complains of knee locking, perform the *Apley test* to detect meniscal tear. With the client in prone position, flex the knee 90 degrees. Press down on the client's foot so that the tibia is firmly against the femur; then rotate the knee externally. No pain or locking is a negative test (Fig. 15-44).

★ **ASSESS for hip flexion contractures.**

Perform the *Thomas test* to evaluate flexion contractures of the hip. Have the client lie supine and ask him or her to fully extend one leg on the table and flex the other knee up to the chest as far as possible. Observe if the extended leg remains flat on the table when the other leg is flexed, which indicates a negative Thomas test (Fig. 15-45).

ASSESS for nerve root compression.

To evaluate for nerve root irritation or lumbar disk herniation, perform *straight leg raises*. With the client supine, raise one leg, keeping the knee straight. Tightness of the hamstring may be reported, but no pain should be felt (Fig. 15-46).

ABNORMAL FINDINGS

Pain, locking of the knee, or clicking during rotation of the knee is a positive Apley test, indicating meniscal tear.

Lifting of the extended leg off the table in response to the other leg being flexed indicates a hip flexion contracture. Record the degree of flexion.

Pain in the back of the leg with 30 to 60 degrees of elevation indicates pressure on a peripheral nerve by an intervertebral disk.

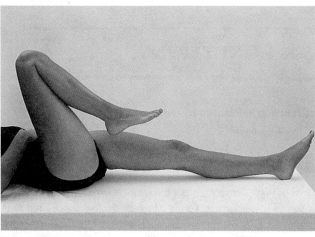

Fig. 15-45 Examination of the hip with the Thomas test. Response is negative in this client because the extended leg remains flat on the table.

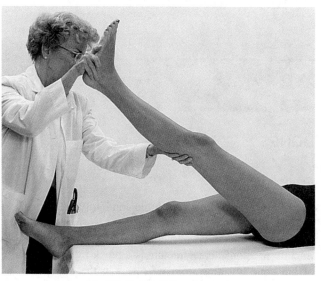

Fig. 15-46 Straight leg raising test.

★ = advanced practice

AGE-RELATED VARIATIONS

Infants, Children, and Adolescents

There are several differences in the assessment of the system for infants and young children. Infants' movement is assessed during voluntary movement and hip joints and feet are assessed for abnormalities. Children's motor development is compared with standardized tables of normal age and sequences described in Chapter 19. Musculoskeletal assessment of the older child and adolescent follows the same procedures as for adults and reveals similar expected findings. Chapter 20 presents further information regarding musculoskeletal assessment of infants, children, and adolescents.

Older Adults

Assessing the musculoskeletal system of an older adult usually follows the same procedures as for an adult. Older adults may be slower at performing range-of-motion and their muscle strength may be less than that of a younger adult. Chapter 22 presents further information regarding the musculoskeletal assessment of older adults.

Documenting Expected Findings

Musculoskeletal System
Coordinated smooth gait, complete range of motion against gravity with full resistance (5/5) in all joints without pain, muscle size symmetric bilaterally, shoulders aligned, and vertebral column straight.

CLINICAL REASONING   *Musculoskeletal System*

A 61-year-old woman presents to the emergency department complaining of severe pain to her right wrist following a 2-foot fall off of a chair. She states she is unable to move her arm.

Noticing: The nurse immediately recognizes that a fall from a chair can potentially result in significant injury—particularly with an older adult. The nurse observes the woman holding her arm against her abdomen under a pillow and recognizes this is a common protective posture with upper extremity trauma. The nurse learns from the woman that she is in good health but has a history of osteoporosis for which she takes alendronate (Fosomax). Her age and osteoporosis increase her risk for musculoskeletal injury.

Interpreting: Early in the encounter, the nurse considers several possible causes of the pain: hematoma, muscle sprain, fracture, or a combination of these. In order to deter-

mine the probability of being correct, the nurse gathers additional data.
- What is the appearance of the joint? There is moderate edema to the wrist and forearm.
- Is there evidence of joint stability? The nurse notes crepitus and increased pain to the wrist with palpation.

The experienced nurse not only recognizes a fracture by the clinical signs (edema and crepitus) and symptoms (pain, loss of motion), but interprets this information in the context of an older adult with osteoporosis who has fallen.

Responding: The nurse initiates appropriate initial interventions (protection of the joint, ice, pain relief, monitoring distal perfusion), and notifies the emergency department provider of the situation, ensuring the client receives appropriate immediate and follow-up care.

COMMON PROBLEMS & CONDITIONS

BONES

Fracture

A partial or complete break in the continuity of a bone is a fracture. The skin remains intact in a closed fracture, and the skin is broken in an open fracture (Fig. 15-47). A pathologic fracture or spontaneous fracture is a break in the continuity of the bone resulting from weakness in the bone, such as osteoporosis or a neoplasm. **Clinical Findings:** Pain caused by muscle spasm is a common symptom. Deformity and loss

of function are caused by the shortening of tissue around the bone and localized edema.

Osteoporosis

Loss of bone density (osteopenia) and decreased bone strength result in osteoporosis. Causes include factors associated with aging, such as decline of estrogen and its relationship to calcium deficit, as well as lack of weight-bearing exercise. Use of immunosuppression therapy such as glucocorticoids contributes to osteoporosis. **Clinical Findings:** Osteoporosis is

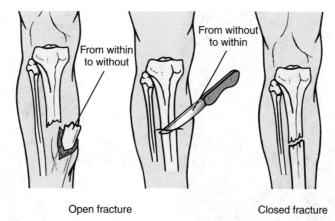

Open fracture   Closed fracture

Fig. 15-47 Open and closed fractures. *(From Lewis, Heitkemper, and Dirksen, 2007.)*

referred to as a "silent disease" because bone loss occurs without signs or symptoms. Clients may not know they have osteoporosis until they discover a loss of height, experience a spontaneous fracture (pathologic fracture) from brittle bones, or develop kyphosis (convex curvature of the thoracic spine) (Fig. 15-48).

JOINTS

Rheumatoid Arthritis

This form of arthritis is a chronic, autoimmune inflammatory disease of the connective tissue. The onset is usually gradual, with fatigue, morning stiffness lasting more than an hour, diffuse muscle ache, and weakness. Eventually the synovial lining of joints becomes inflamed, leading to deterioration of cartilage and erosion of surfaces, causing bone spurs. Ligaments and tendons around inflamed joints become fibrotic

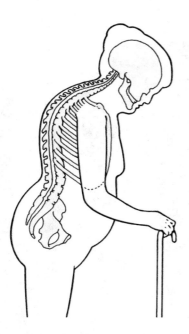

Fig. 15-48 Hallmark of osteoporosis: dowager's hump (kyphosis). *(From Seidel et al, 2003.)*

and shortened, causing contractures and subluxation (partial dislocation) of joints. **Clinical Findings:** Joint involvement usually is bilateral. Localized symptoms are pain, edema, and stiffness of the fingers, wrists, ankles, feet, and knees. Systemic symptoms caused by the autoimmune response include low-grade fever and fatigue. As the disease process continues ulnar deviation, swan-neck deformity, and boutonnière deformity may be observed (see Fig. 15-28).

Osteoarthritis

This form of arthritis is caused by degenerative changes of articular cartilage. It affects weight-bearing joints such as vertebrae, hips, knees, and ankles, but also is noted in hands and fingers. Osteoarthritis also occurs in joints with repetitive movement such as those used when playing sports on a regular basis. As the cartilage wears away, the bones move against each other, causing joint inflammation. Joint involvement may be unilateral or bilateral. **Clinical Findings:** Symptoms include joint edema and aching pain. Joint deformities of fingers develop (Heberden's nodes in distal interphalangeal (DIP) joints and Bouchard's nodes in peripheral interphangeal (PIP) joints (see Fig. 15-29).

Bursitis

This is an inflammation of a bursa, the connective tissue structure surrounding a joint. Bursa become inflamed by constant friction around joints (Fig. 15-49). Bursitis may be precipitated by arthritis, infection, injury, or excessive exercise. Common sites of bursitis are the shoulder, elbow, hip, and knee. **Clinical Findings:** Painful range of motion, edema, point tenderness, and erythema of the affected joint are common findings. Compared with arthritis, bursitis begins abruptly and causes local tenderness and edema (Hellmann and Stone, 2004).

Gout

This hereditary disorder involves an increase in serum uric acid due either to an increased production or decreased excretion of uric acid and urate salts. The disease is thought to

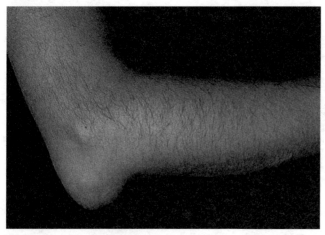

Fig. 15-49   Olecranon bursitis. *(Reprinted from the clinical slide collection of the rheumatic diseases, copyright 1991, 1995, 1997. Used by permission of the American College of Rheumatology.)*

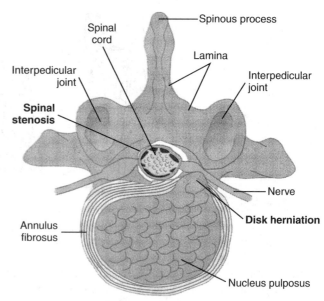

Fig. 15-51   Herniated intervertebral disk. *(From Black and Matassarin-Jacobs, 1997.)*

be caused by lack of an enzyme needed to completely metabolize purines for renal excretion. Uric acids accumulate commonly in the great toe but also in other joints such as wrists, hands, ankles, and knees. **Clinical Findings:** Manifestations include erythema and edema of joints that are very painful to move and thus limited in their range of motion. Tophi are a sign of gout; these are round, pealike deposits of uric acid in ear cartilage or large, irregularly shaped deposits in subcutaneous tissue or other joints (Fig. 15-50). Kidney stones from uric acid crystals can cause manifestations of flank pain, costovertebral angle (CVA) tenderness.

SPINE

Herniated Nucleus Pulposus (HNP)

The intervertebral disk provides a cushion between two vertebrae and contains a nucleus pulposus encased in fibrocartilage. When the fibrocartilage surrounding an intervertebral disk ruptures, the nucleus pulposus is displaced and compresses adjacent spinal nerves (Fig. 15-51). *Herniated disk*

and *slipped disk* are other names for this disorder. This rupture frequently occurs in the lumbar spine when there is increased strain on the vertebrae, such as from lifting a heavy object improperly (*www.nlm.nih.gov*, 2003). **Clinical Findings:** Manifestations depend on the location of the herniated disk. The client may complain of numbness and radiating pain in the affected extremity from a herniated lumbar disk. Straight leg raises cause pain in the involved leg by putting pressure on the spinal nerve. Cervical herniated nucleus pulposus causes arm pain and paresthesia. Deep tendon reflexes may be depressed or absent depending on the spinal nerve root involved.

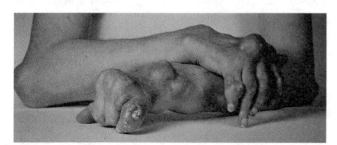

Fig. 15-50   Gout with many tophi present on the hands, on the wrists, and in both olecranon bursae. *(Reprinted from the clinical slide collection of the rheumatic diseases, copyright 1991, 1995, 1997. Used by permission of the American College of Rheumatology.)*

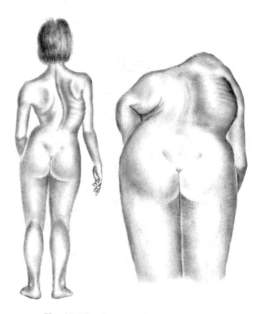

Fig. 15-52   Scoliosis. *(From Mourad, 1991.)*

Scoliosis

An S-shaped deformity of the vertebrae is called scoliosis. It is a skeletal deformity of three planes, usually involving lateral curvature, spinal rotation causing rib asymmetry, and thoracic kyphosis (Fig. 15-52). There is evidence that idiopathic scoliosis may be genetic and transmitted as an autosomal dominant trait with incomplete penetrance, or it may be multifactorial. Causes include congenital malformations of the spine, neuromuscular diseases, traumatic injury, and unequal leg length. **Clinical Findings:** Scoliosis produces uneven shoulders and hip levels. A curvature less than 10% is considered a normal variation, and curves between 10% and 20% are considered mild (Hockenberry et al, 2003). Rotation deformity also may cause a rib hump and flank asymmetry on forward flexion. Depending on the severity of the curve, physiologic function of lungs, spine, and pelvis may be compromised.

LIGAMENTS AND MUSCLES

Carpal Tunnel Syndrome

This syndrome occurs when the median nerve is compressed between the flexor retinaculum (carpal ligament) and other structures within the carpal tunnel (see Fig. 15-39). It may be caused by repetitive movements of the hands and arms, injury to the wrist, and systemic disorders such as rheumatoid arthritis, gout, and hypothyroidism. It may also occur with fluid retention that occurs with pregnancy and menopause. **Clinical Findings:** Manifestations include burning, numbness, and tingling in the hands, often at night. Clients report numbness, pain, and paresthesia during the Phalen's sign or Tinel's sign used to assess for this disorder (see Figs. 15-38 and 15-39).

CLINICAL APPLICATION & CLINICAL REASONING

See Appendix E for answers to exercises in this section.

REVIEW QUESTIONS

1 When performing a symptom analysis, the nurse determines that the client's pain may be from a bone when the pain is described as:
   1 Deep, dull, and boring.
   2 Cramping and unrelated to movement.
   3 Intermittent, sharp, and radiating.
   4 Numbness and tingling with movement.

2 "Expected findings" for the musculoskeletal system are determined by comparing:
   1 The client's function with others in the same age group.
   2 The client's function with others of the same gender.
   3 The client's function with others in the same racial group.
   4 The client's left side with the right side.

3 Biceps muscle strength is tested by applying resistance as the client:
   1 Extends the arm.
   2 Flexes the arm.
   3 Adducts the arm.
   4 Abducts the arm.

4 The nurse testing the client's muscle strength finds that the client has complete range of motion with gravity. Using Table 24-3, how would this finding be documented?
   1 Poor or 2/5.
   2 Fair or 3/5.
   3 Good or 4/5.
   4 Normal or 5/5.

5 While assessing the range of motion of the client's knee, the nurse expects the client to be able to perform which movements?
   1 Flexion, extension, and hyperextension.
   2 Circumduction, internal rotation, and external rotation.
   3 Adduction, abduction, and rotation.
   4 Flexion, pronation, and supination.

6 During an assessment of a young adult, the nurse notes that the client's shoulders are uneven. What further examination would the nurse perform for further data?
   1 Ask the client to rotate each shoulder to assess for the range of motion of each shoulder.
   2 Ask the client to push against the nurse's hands with his forearm to test triceps muscle strength.
   3 Ask the client to shrug his shoulders while the nurse pushes them down to test the trapezius muscle strength.
   4 Ask the client to bend forward at the waist while the nurse checks the alignment of the teen's vertebrae.

7 The nurse is comparing the right and left legs of a client and notices they are asymmetric. What additional data does the nurse collect at this time?
   1 Passively move each leg through range of motion and compare the findings.
   2 Observe the client's gait and legs as he walks across the room.
   3 Measure the upper and lower circumferences and length of each leg and compare the findings.
   4 Palpate the joints and muscles of each leg and compare the findings.

SAMPLE DOCUMENTATION

Review the following data obtained during an interview and examination by the nurse below:

S. C. is a 33-year-old man with a chief complaint of right wrist pain. He noticed the pain in his right wrist 1 week ago. The pain is slowly getting worse. His hand is swollen and painful on movement. He takes an aspirin and a multivitamin daily. He has no known drug allergies. There is edema over his right distal radius and medial carpals; no redness or heat is noted. There is pain on flexion and hyperextension of the radiocarpal joint. He has sensation in all fingers. He reports some pain relief after taking ibuprofen. He has history of trauma to the wrist; otherwise his history is unremarkable. He does not participate in sports. He reports that he is unable to perform his job as a computer programmer. It is painful to tie his necktie, shave his face, and button his shirt. In the right wrist his grip strength is 3/5 with pain on contraction. He is able to perform thumb opposition, but slowly and with pain. He has a negative Tinel's sign. He rates his pain as 6 on a scale of 10. In the left wrist there is no pain on range of motion. His grip strength is 5/5. His thumb opposition is brisk and without pain. His vital signs are as follows: temperature, 97.8° F (36.5° C); pulse, 76 beats/min; respiratory rate, 16; blood pressure, 128/78 mm Hg. Height, 6 feet 5 inches (196 cm); weight (measured), 200 lb (90.9 kg), body mass index 24.

Below, note how the nurse documented these same data.

S. C. is a 33-y/o ♂ c̄ CC: R wrist pain × 1 wk. He takes ASA and multivitamin daily, has NKDA.

SUBJECTIVE DATA
Pain in R wrist slowly getting worse; hand edematous, painful on movement, 6/10. Some pain relief p̄ ibuprofen. Has hx of wrist trauma; otherwise, hx is unremarkable. Does not participate in sports. Unable to perform job as computer programmer; painful to tie necktie, shave face, and button shirt.

OBJECTIVE DATA
General survey: VS: T 97.8° F (36.5° C), HR 76, RR 16, BP 128/78. Ht, 6 feet 5 inches (196 cm); wt (measured), 200 lb (90.9 kg), BMI 24.

Right wrist: Edema over R distal radius and medial carpals; Ø redness or heat. Pain on flexion and hyperextension of radiocarpal joint; grip strength 3/5 c̄ pain on contraction; able to perform thumb opposition, but slowly and c̄ pain; negative Tinel's sign; sensation present in all fingers.

Left wrist: Ø pain on ROM, grip strength 5/5, thumb opposition brisk s̄ pain; negative Tinel's sign; sensation present in all fingers.

CASE STUDY

Mrs. S. is a 46-year-old Asian woman with rheumatoid arthritis (RA). The following data are collected by the nurse during an interview and examination.

Interview Data

Mrs. S. was diagnosed with RA at age 30. Her mother and grandmother had osteoporosis. She has been taking Remicade to treat her RA. She complains of a great deal of pain in her joints, particularly in her hands, and says that she has "just learned to live with the pain because it will always be there." She states that the stiffness and pain in her joints are always worse in the morning or if she sits for too long. She denies muscle weakness other than the fact that her stiffness and soreness prevent her from doing much. Mrs. S. reports that the RA is progressing to the point where she is having difficulty doing things requiring fine motor dexterity such as changing clothes, holding eating utensils, and cutting up her food. She had different faucet handles placed in her home so she could turn the water on and off. Mrs. S. says that she rarely goes out because she feels ugly.

Examination Data

Client is able to stand, but standing erect is not possible. Gait is slow and purposeful. Significant edema and tenderness are noted on palpation of wrists, hands, knees, and ankles bilaterally. Hand grips are weak bilaterally. Subcutaneous nodules are noted at ulnar surface of elbows bilaterally.

Clinical Reasoning

1. What data deviate from normal findings, suggesting a need for further investigation?
2. What additional information should the nurse ask or assess for?
3. Based on the data, what risk factors for osteoporosis does this client have?
4. What nursing diagnoses and collaborative problems should be considered for this situation?

⚙ INTERACTIVE ACTIVITIES

Open the interactive student CD-ROM, click on Chapter 15, and choose from the following activities on the menu bar:

- **Multiple Choice Challenge.** Click on the best answer for each of these items. You will be given immediate feedback, rationale for incorrect answers, and a total score. Good luck!

- **Marvelous Matches.** Drag each word or phrase to the appropriate place on the screen. Test your ability to match clinical findings with common musculoskeletal disorders.

- **Skeleton Scramble.** Test your knowledge of anatomy by dragging bones and dropping them in their correct location.

- **Symptom Analysis.** You may select the questions you want to ask this client. Then analyze his responses to help determine the cause of his joint pain.

- **Printable Lab Guide.** Locate the Lab Guide for Chapter 15, and print and use it (as many times as needed) to help you apply your assessment skills. These guides may also be filled in electronically and then saved and e-mailed to your instructor!

- **Quick Challenge.** Use this critical thinking exercise to assess your skills through case study-style questions, then compare with expert answers!

- **Core Examination Skills Checklists.** Make sure you've got frequently-used exam skills down pat! Use these checklists to help cover all the bases for your examination.

CHAPTER 16

Neurologic System

ANATOMY & PHYSIOLOGY

The nervous system controls body functions through voluntary and autonomic responses to external and internal stimuli. Structural divisions of the nervous system are the central nervous system, which consists of the brain and spinal cord; the peripheral nervous system; and the autonomic nervous system.

CENTRAL NERVOUS SYSTEM

Protective Structures

The skull protects the brain. At the base of the skull in the occipital bone is a large oval opening termed the *foramen magnum,* through which the spinal cord extends from the medulla oblongata. There are other openings (foramina) at this base for the entrance and exit of paired cranial nerves and cerebral blood vessels.

Between the skull and the brain lie three layers termed *meninges.* The outer layer is a fibrous layer termed the *dura mater.* The middle meningeal layer, the *arachnoid,* is a two-layer, fibrous, elastic membrane that covers the folds and fissures of the brain. The inner meningeal layer, the *pia mater,* contains small vessels that supply blood to the brain. Between the arachnoid and the pia mater is the subarachnoid space, where the cerebrospinal fluid (CSF) circulates. A fold of dura mater termed the *falx cerebri* separates the two cerebral hemispheres. Another fold of dura mater, the *tentorium cerebelli,* supports the temporal and occipital lobes and separates the cerebral hemispheres from the cerebellum. Struc-

tures above the tentorium cerebelli are referred to as supratentorial and those below it as infratentorial (Fig. 16-1).

Cerebrospinal Fluid and Cerebral Ventricular System

Cerebrospinal fluid (CSF) is a colorless, odorless fluid containing glucose, electrolytes, oxygen, water, carbon dioxide, protein, and leukocytes. It circulates around the brain and spinal cord to provide a cushion, maintain normal intracranial pressure, provide nutrition, and remove metabolic wastes.

The cerebral ventricular system consists of four interconnecting chambers or ventricles that produce and circulate CSF (see Fig. 16-1). There is one lateral ventricle in each hemisphere, with a third ventricle adjacent to the thalamus and a fourth adjacent to the brainstem. The CSF circulates from the lateral ventricles through the interventricular foramen to the third ventricle, through the aqueduct of Sylvius to the fourth ventricle and into the cisterna magna, which is a small reservoir for CSF. From the cisterna magna, the CSF flows within the subarachnoid space up around the brain and down around the spinal cord. The CSF is absorbed through arachnoid villi that extend into the subarachnoid space and is returned to the venous system.

Brain

The brain, consisting of the cerebrum, diencephalon, cerebellum, and brainstem, is made up of gray matter (cell bodies)

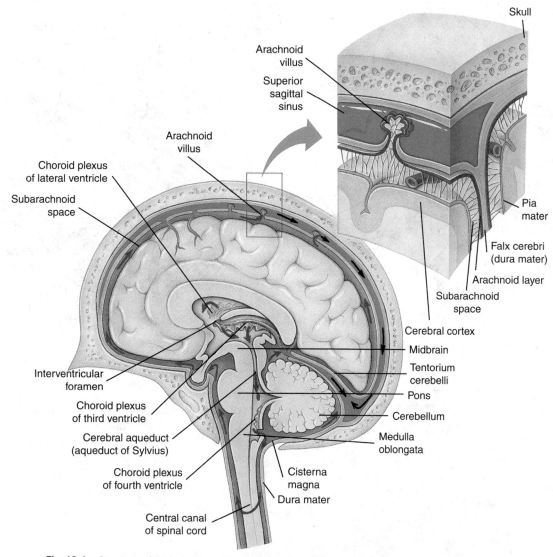

Fig. 16-1 **Structures of the brainstem and cerebrospinal fluid (CSF) circulation.** *Red arrows* represent the route of the CSF. *Black arrows* represent the route of blood flow. Cerebrospinal fluid is produced in the ventricles, exits the fourth ventricle, and returns to the venous circulation in the superior sagittal sinus. The *inset* depicts the arachnoid granulations in the superior sagittal sinus, where the CSF enters the circulation. *(Modified from Thibodeau and Patton, 1999.)*

and white matter (myelinated nerve fibers). The carotid arteries supply most of the blood to the brain and branch off into the posterior cerebral, middle cerebral, and anterior cerebral arteries (Fig. 16-2, *A*). The remaining blood flows through two vertebral arteries and into the posterior and anterior communicating arteries that supply blood through the circle of Willis (Fig. 16-2, *B*). Blood leaves the brain through venous sinuses that empty into the jugular veins.

Cerebrum

The cerebrum is the largest part of the brain and is composed of two hemispheres. Each hemisphere is divided into four lobes: frontal lobe, parietal lobe, temporal lobe, and occipital lobe (Fig. 16-3).

The frontal lobe contains the primary motor cortex and is responsible for functions related to voluntary motor activity. The distribution of the nerves that provide movement to specific parts of the body is shown in Fig. 16-4, *B*. The left

frontal lobe contains Broca's area (see Fig. 16-3), which is involved in formulation of words. The frontal lobe also controls intellectual function, awareness of self, personality, and autonomic responses related to emotion.

The parietal lobe contains the primary somesthetic (sensory) cortex. One of its major functions is to receive sensory input such as position sense, touch, shape, and texture of objects. The distribution of the nerves that receive sensations from specific parts of the body is adjacent to the motor cortex and is shown in Fig. 16-4, *A*.

The temporal lobe contains the primary auditory cortex. Wernicke's area (see Fig. 16-3), located in the left temporal lobe, is responsible for comprehension of spoken and written language. The temporal lobe also interprets auditory, visual, and somatic sensory inputs that are stored in thought and memory.

The occipital lobe contains the primary visual cortex and is responsible for receiving and interpreting visual information.

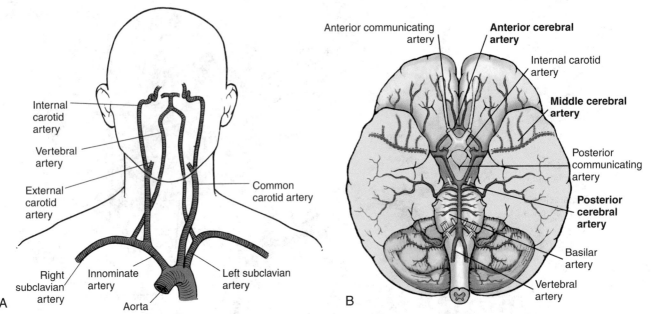

Fig. 16-2   A, Major arteries supplying blood to the brain. **B,** The circle of Willis. Note the anterior, middle, and posterior cerebral arteries, which are the major pairs of arteries supplying the cerebrum. *(From Phipps et al, 2003.)*

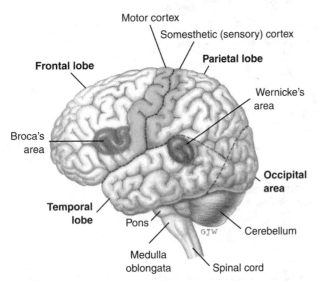

Fig. 16-3   Cerebral hemispheres. Lateral view of the brain. The motor cortex in the frontal lobe is depicted in pink, and the somesthetic cortex in the parietal lobe is depicted in blue. *(Modified from Chipps, Clanin, and Campbell, 1992.)*

Diencephalon

The thalamus, hypothalamus, epithalamus, and subthalamus make up the diencephalon (Fig. 16-5). The thalamus is a relay and integration station from the spinal cord to the cerebral cortex and other parts of the brain. The hypothalamus has several important functions in maintaining homeostasis. Some of these functions include regulation of body temperature, hunger, and thirst; formation of autonomic nervous system responses; and storage and secretion of hormones from the pituitary gland. The epithalamus contains the pineal gland, which causes sleepiness and helps regulate some endocrine function. The subthalamus is part of the basal ganglia.

Basal Ganglia

Between the cerebral cortex and midbrain and adjacent to the diencephalon lie the structures that form the basal ganglia (Fig. 16-6). The six ganglia that comprise the basal ganglia are the putamen, caudate nucleus, globus pallidus, thalamus, red nucleus, and substantia nigra. The basal ganglia's function is to create smooth, coordinated voluntary movement by balancing the production of two neurotransmitters: acetylcholine and dopamine.

Brainstem

The midbrain, pons, and medulla oblongata make up the brainstem (see Fig. 16-1). Ten of the twelve cranial nerves (CNs) originate from the brainstem (Fig. 16-7). The major function of the midbrain is to relay stimuli concerning muscle movement to other brain structures. It contains part of the motor tract pathways that control reflex motor movements in response to visual and auditory stimuli. The oculomotor nerve (CN III) and trochlear nerve (CN IV) originate in the midbrain.

The pons relays impulses to the brain centers and lower spinal nerves. The CNs that originate in the pons are trigeminal (CN V), abducens (CN VI), facial (CN VII), and acoustic (CN VIII).

The medulla oblongata contains reflex centers for controlling involuntary functions such as breathing, sneezing, swallowing, coughing, vomiting, and vasoconstriction. Motor and sensory tracts from the frontal and parietal lobes cross from one side to the other in the medulla, so that lesions on the right side of the brain create abnormal movement and sensation on the left side and vice versa. The cranial nerves that originate in the medulla are glossopharyngeal (CN IX), vagus (CN X), spinal accessory (CN XI), and hypoglossal (CN XII).

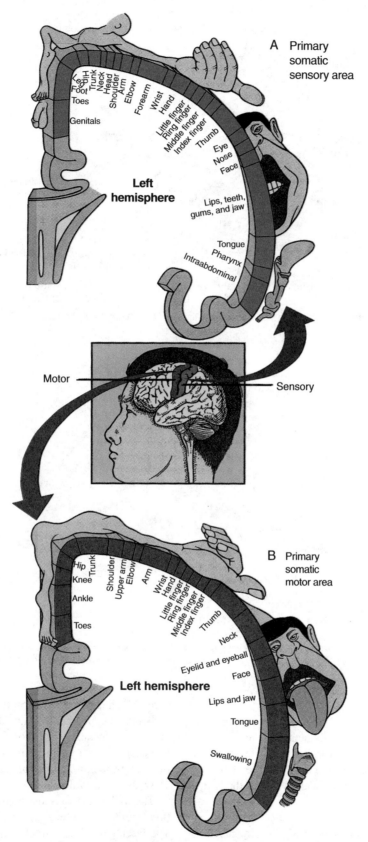

Fig. 16-4   Topography of the somesthetic and motor cortex.   Cerebral cortex seen in coronal section on the left side of the brain. The figure of the body (homunculus) depicts the relative nerve distributions; the size indicates the relative number of nerves in the distribution. Each cortex occurs on both sides of the brain but appears only on one side in this illustration. The inset shows the motor and somesthetic regions of the left hemisphere. **A,** Somesthetic cortex. **B,** Motor cortex. *(From Thibodeau and Patton, 2007.)*

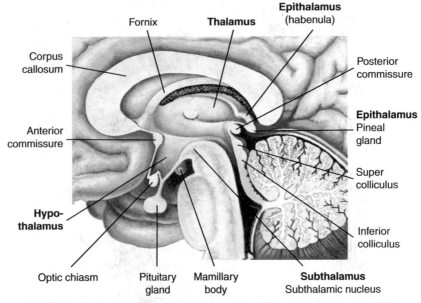

Fornix

Corpus callosum

Anterior commissure

Thalamus

Epithalamus (habenula)

Posterior commissure

Epithalamus Pineal gland

Super colliculus

Inferior colliculus

Hypo-thalamus

Optic chiasm

Pituitary gland

Mamillary body

Subthalamus Subthalamic nucleus

Fig. 16-5 **Diencephalon.** Lateral view of the brain. *(From Chipps, Clanin, and Campbell, 1992.)*

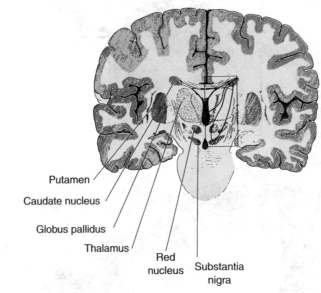

Putamen

Caudate nucleus

Globus pallidus

Thalamus

Red nucleus

Substantia nigra

Fig. 16-6 Coronal section of the brain shows six ganglia that make up the basal ganglia. *(From Cutler WP: II Neurology, IV Degenerative and Hereditary Disorders. Scientific American® Medicine, Rubenstein E, Federman DD, Eds. WebMd, New York, 1995.)*

Cerebellum

The cerebellum is separated from the cerebral cortex by the tentorium cerebelli (see Fig. 16-1). Functions of the cerebellum include coordinating movement, equilibrium, muscle tone, and proprioception. Each of the cerebellar hemispheres controls movement for the same (ipsilateral) side of the body.

Spinal Cord

The spinal cord is a continuation of the medulla oblongata that begins at the foramen magnum and ends at the first and second lumbar (L1 and L2) vertebrae. At L1 and L2 the spinal cord branches into lumbar and sacral nerve roots termed the *cauda equina.* The spinal cord consists of 31 segments, each giving rise to a pair of spinal nerves (Fig. 16-8). Nerve fibers, grouped into tracts, run through the spinal cord transmitting sensory, motor, and autonomic impulses between the brain and the

body. Myelinated nerves form the white matter of the spinal cord and contain ascending and descending tracts of nerve fibers. The descending, or motor, tracts (e.g., anterior and lateral corticospinal or pyramidal tracts) carry impulses from the frontal lobe to muscles for voluntary movement (Fig. 16-9, *A*). They also play a role in muscle tone and posture.

The ascending, or sensory, tracts carry sensory information from the body through the thalamus to the parietal lobe. The fasciculus gracilis track travels in the posterior (dorsal) column carrying sensations of touch, deep pressure, vibration, position of joints, stereognosis, and two-point discrimination (Fig. 16-9, *B*). The lateral spinothalamic tract carries fibers for sensations of light touch, pressure, temperature, and pain. The gray matter, which contains the nerve cell bodies, is arranged in a butterfly shape with anterior and posterior horns.

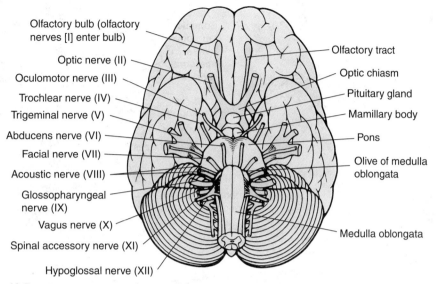

Olfactory bulb (olfactory nerves [I] enter bulb)

Optic nerve (II)

Oculomotor nerve (III)

Trochlear nerve (IV)

Trigeminal nerve (V)

Abducens nerve (VI)

Facial nerve (VII)

Acoustic nerve (VIII)

Glossopharyngeal nerve (IX)

Vagus nerve (X)

Spinal accessory nerve (XI)

Hypoglossal nerve (XII)

Olfactory tract

Optic chiasm

Pituitary gland

Mamillary body

Pons

Olive of medulla oblongata

Medulla oblongata

Fig. 16-7   Inferior surface of the brain showing the origin of the cranial nerves. *(From Seeley, Stephens, and Tate, 1995.)*

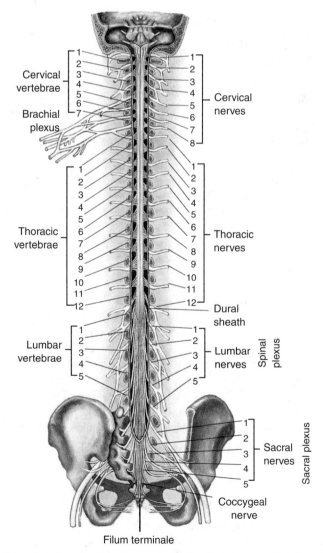

Cervical vertebrae

Brachial plexus

Thoracic vertebrae

Lumbar vertebrae

Cervical nerves

Thoracic nerves

Dural sheath

Lumbar nerves

Spinal plexus

Sacral nerves

Sacral plexus

Coccygeal nerve

Filum terminale

Fig. 16-8   View of the spinal column showing vertebrae, spinal cord, and spinal nerves exiting. *(From Chipps, Clanin, and Campbell, 1992.)*

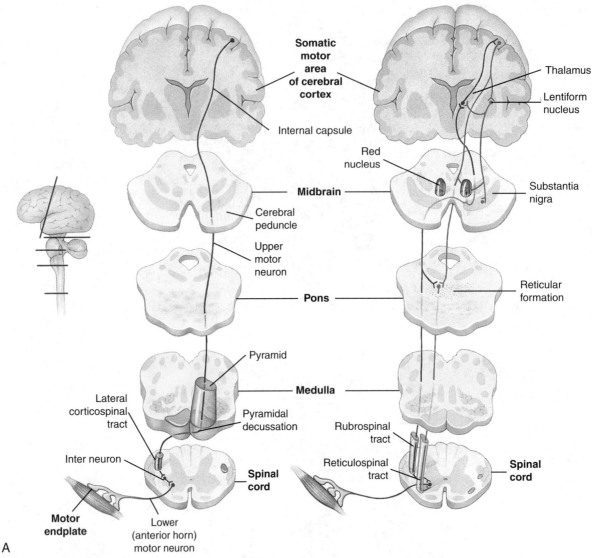

Fig. 16-9 **Examples of somatic motor and sensory pathways. A,** Motor: the pyramidal pathway through the lateral corticospinal tract and the extrapyramidal pathways through the rubrospinal and reticulospinal tracts. *(From Thibodeau and Patton, 2007.)*

PERIPHERAL NERVOUS SYSTEM

Cranial Nerves

Of the 12 pairs of cranial nerves, some have only motor fibers (five pairs) or only sensory fibers (three pairs); whereas others have both motor and sensory fibers (four pairs). Table 16-1 lists the 12 cranial nerves and their functions. Box 16-1 describes ways to remember the names and functions of the cranial nerves. Fig. 16-7 shows the location of the cranial nerves on the inferior surface of the brain.

Spinal Nerves

The 31 pairs of spinal nerves emerge from different segments of the spinal cord: 8 pairs of cervical, 12 pairs of thoracic, 5 pairs of lumbar, 5 pairs of sacral, and 1 pair of coccygeal

nerves. The first seven cervical nerves exit above their corresponding vertebrae. There are eight cervical nerves, but seven cervical vertebrae. The remaining spinal nerves exit below the corresponding vertebrae (see Fig. 16-8).

Each pair of spinal nerves is formed by the union of an efferent, or motor (ventral), root and an afferent, or sensory (dorsal), root. The motor fibers carry impulses from the brain (frontal lobe) through the spinal cord to muscles and glands, whereas sensory fibers carry impulses from the sensory receptors of the body through the spinal cord to the brain (parietal lobe). Each pair of spinal nerves and its corresponding part of the spinal cord make up a spinal segment and innervate specific body segments. The dorsal root of each spinal nerve supplies the sensory innervation to a segment of the skin known as a dermatome. Refer to the dermatome map to determine the spinal nerve that corresponds to the area where the client reports sensory alteration (Fig.

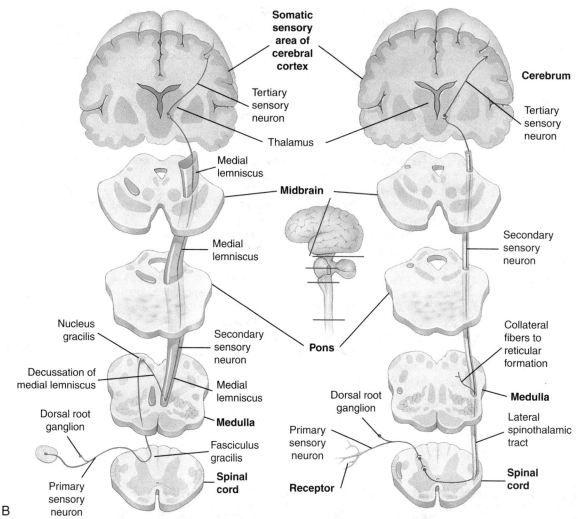

Fig. 16-9, cont'd   Examples of somatic motor and sensory pathways. **B,** Sensory: pathways of the medial lemniscal system that conducts information about discriminating touch and kinesthesis and the spinothalamic pathway that conducts information about pain and temperature. *(From Thibodeau and Patton, 2007.)*

16-10). For example, if the client complains of pain with numbness and tingling across the right knee, the nurse knows that the fourth lumbar spinal segment is involved, perhaps compressed.

Reflex Arc

Reflex arcs are tested by observing muscle movement in response to sensory stimuli. Deep tendon reflexes are responses to stimulation of a tendon that stretches the neuromuscular spindles of a muscle group. Striking a deep tendon stimulates a sensory neuron that travels to the spinal cord, where it stimulates an interneuron that stimulates a motor neuron to create movement (Fig. 16-11). Superficial reflexes are tested in the same manner. Each reflex corresponds to a specific spinal segment. Table 16-2 shows the deep tendon reflexes and superficial reflexes and the segments of the spinal cord that innervate each reflex.

AUTONOMIC NERVOUS SYSTEM

The autonomic nervous system (ANS) regulates the body's internal environment in conjunction with the endocrine system. The ANS has two components: the sympathetic nervous system and the parasympathetic nervous system (Fig. 16-12). The sympathetic nervous system (SNS) arises from the thoracolumbar segments of the spinal cord and is activated during stress (the fight-or-flight response). The SNS actions include increasing blood pressure and heart rate, vasoconstricting peripheral blood vessels, inhibiting gastrointestinal peristalsis, and dilating bronchi. By contrast, the parasympathetic nervous system (PNS) arises from craniosacral segments of the spinal cord and controls vegetative functions (breed and feed). The PNS actions are involved in functions associated with conserving energy such as decreasing heart rate and force of myocardial contraction, decreasing blood pressure and respiration, and stimulating gastrointestinal peristalsis.

Text continued on p. 371

TABLE 16-1 *The Cranial Nerves and Their Functions*

CRANIAL NERVE	FUNCTION
Olfactory (I)	Sensory: smell reception and interpretation
Optic (II)	Sensory: visual acuity and visual fields
Oculomotor (III)	Motor: raise eyelids, most extraocular movements
	Parasympathetic: pupillary constriction, change lens shape
Trochlear (IV)	Motor: downward, inward eye movement
Trigeminal (V)	Motor: jaw opening and clenching, chewing and mastication
	Sensory: sensation to cornea, iris, lacrimal glands, conjunctiva, eyelids, forehead, nose, nasal and mouth mucosa, teeth, tongue, ear, facial skin
Abducens (VI)	Motor: lateral eye movement
Facial (VII)	Motor: movement of facial expression muscles except jaw, close eyes, labial speech sounds (b, m, w, and rounded vowels)
	Sensory: taste—anterior two thirds of tongue, sensation to pharynx
	Parasympathetic: secretion of saliva and tears
Acoustic (VIII)	Sensory: hearing and equilibrium
Glossopharyngeal (IX)	Motor: voluntary muscles for swallowing and phonation
	Sensory: sensation of nasopharynx, gag reflex, taste—posterior one third of tongue
	Parasympathetic: secretion of salivary glands, carotid reflex
Vagus (X)	Motor: voluntary muscles of phonation (guttural speech sounds) and swallowing
	Sensory: sensation behind ear and part of external ear canal
	Parasympathetic: secretion of digestive enzymes; peristalsis; carotid reflex; involuntary action of heart, lungs, and digestive tract
Spinal accessory (XI)	Motor: turn head, shrug shoulders, some actions for phonation
Hypoglossal (XII)	Motor: tongue movement for speech sound articulation (l, t, n) and swallowing

From Seidel HM et al: *Mosby's guide to physical examination,* ed 6, St Louis, 2006, Mosby.

BOX 16-1 **HOW TO REMEMBER NAMES AND NERVE TYPE OF CRANIAL NERVES**

Read the words in the column on the left from top to bottom. The first letter of each word is the same as the first letter in the name of the cranial nerve. The fourth column gives the type of impulses carried by the nerve—sensory, motor, or both sensory and motor. The last column is a phrase to remember the type of nerve for each cranial nerve.

Memory Word	CN Number	CN Name	Type	Memory Word
On	CN I	Olfactory	Sensory	Some
Old	CN II	Optic	Sensory	Say
Olympic's	CN III	Oculomotor	Motor	Marry
Towering	CN IV	Trochlear	Motor	Money
Top	CN V	Trigeminal	Both	But
A	CN VI	Abducens	Motor	My
Fin	CN VII	Facial	Both	Brother
And	CN VIII	Acoustic	Sensory	Says
German	CN IX	Glossopharyngeal	Both	Bad
Viewed	CN X	Vagus	Both	Business to
Some	CN XI	Spinal accessory	Motor	Marry
Hops	CN XII	Hypoglossal	Motor	Money

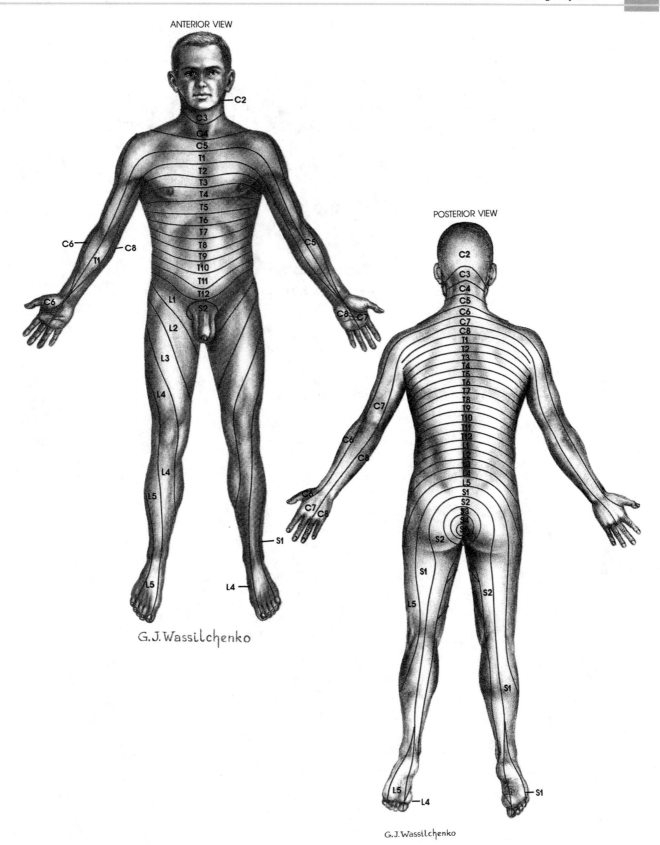

Fig. 16-10 **Dermatomal map.** Letters and numbers indicate the spinal nerves innervating a given region of skin. *(From Rudy, 1984.)*

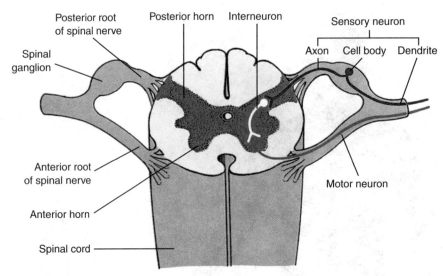

Fig. 16-11 Cross section of the spinal cord showing three-neuron reflex arc. *(From Chipps, Clanin, and Campbell, 1992.)*

TABLE 16-2 *Superficial and Deep Tendon Reflexes*	
REFLEX	**SPINAL LEVEL**
Superficial	
Upper abdominal	T7, T8, and T9
Lower abdominal	T10 and T11
Cremasteric	T12, L1, and L2
Plantar	L4, L5, S1, and S2
Deep	
Biceps	C5 and C6
Brachioradial	C5 and C6
Triceps	C6, C7, and C8
Patellar	L2, L3, and L4
Achilles	S1 and S2

Modified from Seidel HM et al: *Mosby's guide to physical examination,* ed 6, St Louis, 2006, Mosby; Rudy EB: *Advanced neurological and neurosurgical nursing,* St Louis, 1984, Mosby.

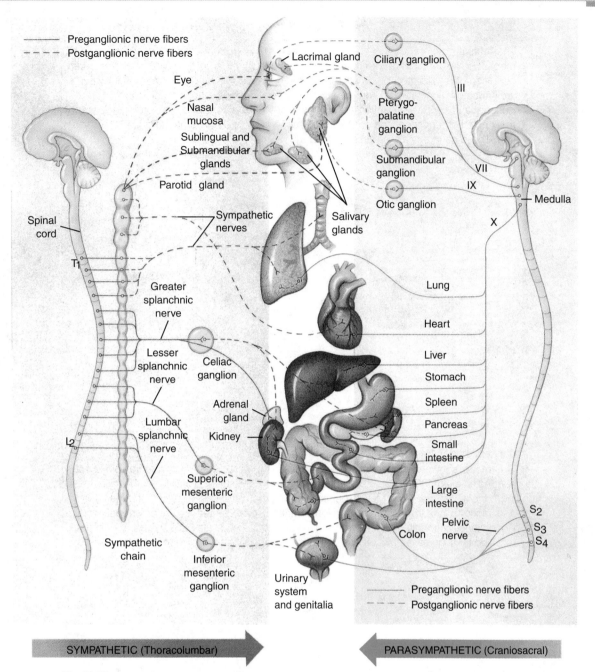

Preganglionic nerve fibers
Postganglionic nerve fibers

Lacrimal gland
Ciliary ganglion

Eye

III

Nasal mucosa
Pterygo-palatine ganglion

Sublingual and Submandibular glands

VII

Submandibular ganglion

IX

Parotid gland
Otic ganglion

Spinal cord

Medulla

Sympathetic nerves

Salivary glands

X

T1

Greater splanchnic nerve

Lung

Heart

Lesser splanchnic nerve
Celiac ganglion

Liver

Stomach

Adrenal gland

Spleen

Lumbar splanchnic nerve
Kidney

Pancreas

L2

Small intestine

Superior mesenteric ganglion

Large intestine

S2
S3
S4

Sympathetic chain

Pelvic nerve

Colon

Inferior mesenteric ganglion

Urinary system and genitalia

Preganglionic nerve fibers
Postganglionic nerve fibers

SYMPATHETIC (Thoracolumbar)

PARASYMPATHETIC (Craniosacral)

Fig. 16-12 **Innervation of organs by the autonomic nervous system.** Preganglionic fibers are indicated by *solid lines*, and postganglionic fibers are indicated by *broken lines*. *(From Thibodeau and Patton, 2007.)*

LINK TO CONCEPTS   *Intracranial Regulation*

The feature concept for this chapter is *Intracranial Regulation.* This concept represents mechanisms that facilitate or impair neurologic function. Because brain function requires perfusion of oxygenated blood and because the respiratory and cardiovascular systems are impacted by neurologic control, strong interrelationships among these concepts exist. Sensory and Tactile Perception as well as Motion are extensions of neurologic function that impact other interrelated concepts such as Nutrition, Development, Pain, and Elimination. These concepts are represented below.

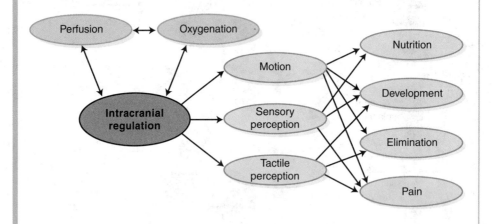

Concept Model: Intracranial Regulation

This model shows the interrelationships of concepts associated with Intracranial Regulation. As an example, a stroke results from a lack of oxygenated blood to the brain. Following a stoke, an individual may experience problems with sensory and tactile perception and motion, thus impacting elimination, nutrition, pain perception, and independence. Understanding the interrelationship of these concepts helps the nurse recognize risk factors and thus increases awareness when conducting a health assessment.

HEALTH HISTORY

RISK FACTORS *CVA, Stroke*

As you conduct a health history related to the nervous system, it is important to consider common risk factors associated with blood flow to the brain and follow up with additional questions should risk factors exist.

Cerebrovascular Accident (CVA), Stroke

- *Age:* Older adults are at greater risk.
- *Gender:* Men have a greater risk than women. However, women account for more than half of the deaths from CVAs. Women who are pregnant have higher risk than nonpregnant women as do women who take birth control pills and smoke or have hypertension.
- *Family history:* Risk is greater if parent, grandparent, or sibling had a CVA.
- *Race:* African Americans have a higher risk of death from CVA than Caucasians.
- Previous CVA or heart attack increases risk of a CVA.
- High blood pressure (greater than 120/80 mm Hg) puts undue pressure on arteries. (M)
- *Smoking:* Nicotine constricts blood vessels and carbon monoxide reduces the oxygen in the blood.(M)
- Diabetes mellitus contributes to hypertension, hypercholesterolemia, and thrombus formation. (M)
- Atherosclerosis narrows the carotid vessels, reducing the blood flow to the brain. (M)
- High serum cholesterol forms plaques in the vessels that impair blood flow to the brain. (M)
- Obesity increases workload on the heart and increases risk of high cholesterol and physical inactivity. (M)
- Excessive alcohol intake increases blood pressure. (M)
- Transient ischemic attacks (TIAs) are warning signs that there is inadequate blood flow to the brain. (M)
- Atrial fibrillation may form blood clots in the atrium that can travel to the brain. (M)
- Cocaine use increases risk of CVAs. (M)

Data from *www.americanheart.org,* 2007.
M = modifiable risk factor.

GENERAL HEALTH HISTORY

Present Health Status

Have you noticed any changes in your ability to move around or participate in your usual activities?

The client's perception of his or her functioning is the primary source of data. Difficulty moving because of weakness or spasticity may indicate a neuromuscular problem. Often clients can identify that they are having difficulty in performing their usual activities, but they may not associate it with a neurologic disorder.

Do you have any chronic diseases? High blood pressure? Myasthenia gravis? Multiple sclerosis? If yes, describe. In what ways does this chronic disease keep you from maintaining a healthy lifestyle?

Chronic diseases may affect mobility and daily living. These questions may help identify risks for injury, opportunities for teaching, and needs for additional resources.

What medications do you take? Are you taking medications as prescribed?

Both prescription and over-the-counter medications should be documented. Side effects of medications may influence the nervous system. Drugs (prescription or street drugs) or alcohol may interfere with the functioning of the nervous system. Note any anticonvulsant medications, antitremor drugs, antivertigo agents, or pain medications that could alter a client's neurologic examination.

How much alcohol do you drink per week? Do you use or have you ever used substances such as marijuana, cocaine, barbiturates, tranquilizers, or any other mood-altering drugs?

Documentation of these substances is necessary because they may alter the client's cognitive or neuromuscular function. Also the actions of these substances may interfere with medications that may be prescribed.

Past Medical History

Have you ever had injury to your head or spinal cord? If yes, describe when this happened. What residual changes have you experienced since the injury?

Previous injury to the central nervous system may leave residual deficits such as weakness or spasticity that you can anticipate during the examination. Injury to the frontal lobe can cause changes in memory and cognition.

Have you ever had surgery on your brain, spinal cord, or any of your nerves? If yes, describe? What was the outcome of the surgery?

A history of surgery may provide additional information about possible neurologic problems and the findings to anticipate during the examination.

Have you ever had a stroke? If yes, describe when and what residual changes you have as a result of the stroke.

Previous stroke (cerebrovascular accident [CVA]) may leave residual deficits such as aphasia that affect your subjective data collection or hemiparesis that you will assess further during the examination.

Do you have a seizure disorder? If yes, describe the kind of seizure, how often you had them, and what you do to prevent the seizures.

Although seizure will probably not be evident during the examination, you need to determine how the client is caring for this disorder to maintain safety and prevent recurrence of seizures.

Family History

In your family, has anyone ever had a stroke, seizures, or tumor of the brain or spinal cord?

Family history may be used to determine the client's risk for these conditions.

PROBLEM-BASED HISTORY

Commonly reported problems related to the neurologic system are headache, dizziness, seizures, loss of consciousness, changes in movement (tremors, weakness, or incoordination), changes in sensations (numbness or tingling), difficulty swallowing, or difficulty communicating such as inability to understand speech or inability to speak. As with symptoms in all areas of health assessment, a symptom analysis is completed, which includes the location, quality, quantity, chronology, setting, associated manifestations, and alleviating and aggravating factors (see Box 3-3 in Chapter 3).

Headache

Describe your headaches. What do they feel like? Where do you feel the pain? How long do they last? How often do you have them?

These questions analyze the symptoms of headaches to help determine the cause. Headaches may be related to compression from tumors or increased intracranial pressure or ischemia from impaired circulation within the brain. (Also see Chapter 11 for history of migraine, cluster, and tension headaches.)

Have you had any recent surgeries or medical procedures such as spinal anesthesia or lumbar puncture?

A transient headache can occur after some diagnostic tests, such as a lumbar puncture. When the client is in an upright position, the loss of CSF causes tension on the meninges, causing a headache.

Dizziness

What does it feel like when you are dizzy or lightheaded? Do you feel as if you may faint? How often do you experience this dizziness? What makes the dizziness worse?

The word "dizzy" can be used by clients to refer to different sensations such as lightheadedness, vertigo, or ataxia. Try to distinguish among these disorders by seeking clarification from the client. Dizziness may be sensation of lightheadedness or fainting with an inability to maintain balance caused by decreased cerebral blood flow. To others dizziness mean vertigo, a sensation of instability described below. Dizziness may refer to ataxia, which is an inability to coordinate movement or a staggering gait caused by a cerebellar disorder.

Have you ever experienced a sensation that feels like the room is spinning (objective vertigo), or do you feel that you are spinning (subjective vertigo)? Does this happen suddenly or gradually? What makes the vertigo worse? What relieves the vertigo?

Vertigo (when the room seems to be spinning) may be caused by a neurologic dysfunction (usually with a gradual onset) or a problem with the vestibule such as an inner ear infection (labyrinthitis) or Ménière's disease (usually with a sudden onset). Vertigo suggests a balance problem that may be related to equilibrium involving the cerebellum or inner ear (*www.nidcd.nih.gov/health/balance*, 2003). Chapter 11 has addition questions about vertigo related to inner ear problems.

Seizures

Have you had a seizure before? How often are you having seizures or convulsions? When was your last seizure? What are they like? Do you become unconscious?

Seizure may be caused by idiopathic epilepsy, a pathologic process, endogenous or exogenous poison, metabolic disturbances, or fever (see Common Problems and Conditions later in this chapter).

Do you have any warning signs before the seizure starts? Describe what happens.

An aura can precede a seizure; it can involve auditory, gustatory, olfactory, visual, or motor sensations. The area in the brain that corresponds to the aura provides information about seizure origin.

When the client loses consciousness during the seizure, refer these questions to persons who observed the client's seizure: Describe the seizure movements that you observed. Did you notice any other signs, such as a change in color of the face or lips; loss of consciousness (note how long)? Did the client urinate or have a bowel movement during the seizure? After the seizure, how long did it take the client to get back to normal?

Responses to these questions help identify the areas of the brain involved in the seizure activity. Figure 16-4, *B,* is helpful in understanding the path a seizure may follow. For example, if the seizure begins in the wrist and travels to the head, neck, and trunk, you can follow the path of the excessive nervous discharge of the seizure along the motor cortex. This is an example of a simple seizure in which the client maintains consciousness.

How do you feel after the seizure? Are you confused? Have a headache or aching muscles? Do you spend time sleeping?

Affirmative answers to these questions may indicate the expected recovery phase of a generalized seizure. Clients may be weak, confused, or sleepy after a seizure because the brain's glucose supply was used during the seizure and it takes time to replace it.

Are there any factors that seem to start these seizures, such as stress, fatigue, activity, or discontinuing medication? Do you take any actions to prevent hurting yourself during seizures?

Answers to these questions help plan prevention strategies for seizures or any injury experienced during the seizure.

How have the seizures affected your life? Your occupation? Do you wear any identification that indicates you have seizures?

Because seizures may be a chronic disease that affects clients' driving, personal relationships, and employment, the nurse needs to learn how seizures have affected the client's life and if the client has adapted to the seizure condition. Carrying identification about seizures helps those who may assist a client who is seizing.

Loss of Consciousness

When did you lose consciousness or have a blackout or faint or felt you were not aware of your surroundings? Did the change occur suddenly? Can you describe what happened to you just before you lost consciousness? Were there other symptoms associated with the change of consciousness?

Loss of consciousness may be due to cardiovascular disorders, which tend to cause symptoms more rapidly, or neurologic disorders. Loss of consciousness is also associated with drugs, psychiatric illness, or metabolic diseases such as hypoxia, liver or kidney failure, or diabetes mellitus.

Changes in Movement

How long have you had a change in your mobility? Describe the change. Is it continuous or intermittent?

The client's description helps guide subsequent questions for the symptom analysis.

Have you noticed any tremors or shaking of the hands or face? When did they start? Do they seem worse when you are anxious or at rest? When you focus on doing something (intention)? What relieves the tremors—rest, activity, or alcohol? Do they affect your performance of daily activities?

Answers to these questions may help identify the cause of the altered mobility. For example, Parkinson's disease causes tremor at rest, whereas cerebellar disorders cause tremor with intentional movement.

Have you felt any sense of weakness in or difficulty moving parts of your body? Is this confined to one area or generalized? Is it associated with anything in particular (e.g., activity)? Do you do anything to relieve the weakness?

Decreased circulation to the brain can cause these symptoms. Some type of TIA or CVA may have occurred.

Do you have problems with coordination? Do you have difficulty keeping your balance when you walk? Do you lean to one side or fall? Which direction? Do your legs suddenly give way?

A cerebrovascular accident may be the cause, but dysfunction of the cerebellum or inner ear should also be considered when balance is impaired. Multiple sclerosis, Parkinson's disease, or brain tumor may also be causes. If a client reports falls in one direction, such as to the right, this may indicate that muscle weakness is due to impaired nerve function on the left side of the brain.

Changes in Sensation

Where are you experiencing numbness or tingling? How does it feel? Is it associated with any activity?

These questions relate to some types of central nervous system disorder (e.g., multiple sclerosis or CVA), peripheral nerve disorder (e.g., diabetics mellitus may cause peripheral neuropathy), peripheral vascular disease, or anemia (vitamin B_{12} deficiency anemia causes paresthesia). Paresthesias often fluctuate with posture, activity, rest, edema, or underlying disease. Hypoesthesia is decreased sensation that may indicate a sensory problem from impaired circulation or nerve compression. Identifying the location of the abnormal sensation may help identify its cause.

Difficulty Swallowing (Dysphagia)

How long have you had problems swallowing? Do these problems involve liquids or solids? Both? Do you have excessive saliva or drooling? Do you cough or choke when trying to swallow?

These may be due to dysfunction of cranial nerves IX (glossopharyngeal), X (vagus), or XI (hypoglossal). Parkinsonism and myasthenia gravis may cause excessive salivation that may increase the need to swallow. A cerebrovascular accident may cause weakness of muscles involved in swallowing.

Difficulty Communicating (Dysphasia/Aphasia)

How long have you had problems speaking? Are you having difficulty forming words or finding the right words? Have you had difficulty understanding things that are said to you? When did this begin? How long did it last?

Aphasia is the term for defective or absent language function, whereas *dysphasia* is an impairment of speech not as severe as aphasia. Inability to comprehend speech of others and of oneself is termed *receptive aphasia* or *fluent aphasia* and is associated with lesions in Wernicke's area in the temporal lobe. Inability to spontaneously communicate or translate ideas into meaningful speech or writing is termed *expressive aphasia* or *nonfluent aphasia* and is associated with lesions in Broca's area in the frontal lobe. Lesions in the frontal or temporal lobe may occur following a brain tumor, head injury, or CVA. Parkinson's disease may create difficulty forming words because of bradykinesia (slow movement) of facial muscles. *Note:* These questions may need to be asked of the person accompanying the client when the client is unable to respond.

HEALTH PROMOTION   *Traumatic Brain Injury*

Traumatic brain injury (TBI) results from a blow or sudden jolt to the head. The severity of injury may range from mild to severe. An estimated 1.5 million people sustain TBI in the United States each year. Crashes (involving motor vehicles, bicycles, pedestrians, and recreational vehicles), falls, assaults, and sports-related injuries are common causes. Driving while impaired and failing to take safety precautions are two important risk factors for such injury.

Goals and Objectives—*Healthy People 2010*

Injury and violence is one of the 10 leading health indicators of *Healthy People 2010*. The *Healthy People 2010* goal for injury and violence prevention is to reduce injuries, disabilities, and deaths caused by unintentional injuries and violence. Twelve specific objectives apply to TBI, including the following: reduce hospitalization for nonfatal head and spinal cord injuries, reduce deaths and nonfatal injuries caused by motor vehicle crashes and pedestrian injuries, increase use of automobile safety belts and use of child restraints, and increase the proportion of motorcyclists and bicyclists using helmets.

Recommendations to Reduce Risk (Primary Prevention)

U.S. Preventive Services Task Force
- Counsel individuals to use lap/shoulder belts while in a car. Children should ride in an appropriate-size child safety seat in accordance with the manufacturer's instructions in the middle of the rear seat.
- Individuals should be advised against riding in the back of pickup trucks or in cargo areas of vehicles unless equipped with seat belts.
- Counsel individuals against driving while under the influence of drugs or alcohol or riding as a passenger with an impaired driver.
- Advise individuals who ride on motorcycles to wear a safety helmet.
- Discuss with individuals and parents of children and adolescents the importance of wearing approved safety helmets and not riding in motor vehicle traffic while riding bicycles and all-terrain vehicles.
- It is unknown if counseling to prevent pedestrian injuries has long-term benefits.

Centers for Disease Control and Prevention
- Encourage helmet use during recreation and sports activities.
- Recommend taking fall prevention measures for children and older adults.
- Counsel parents to place children in safety seats and seat belts.
- Recommend avoidance of drug- or alcohol-impaired driving.

Centers for Disease Control and Prevention, National Center for Injury Prevention and Control: *Traumatic brain injury in the United States—a report to Congress,* Atlanta, 1999, Centers for Disease Control and Prevention; Centers for Disease Control and Prevention, National Center for Injury Prevention and Control: Traumatic brain injury (available at *www.cdc.gov*); US Department of Health and Human Services: Leading health indicators. In *Healthy people 2010: understanding and improving health,* ed 2, Washington, DC, 2000, US Government Printing Office (available at *www.healthypeople.gov*); US Preventive Services Task Force: Counseling to prevent motor vehicle injuries. In *Guide to clinical preventive services,* ed 2, 1996 (available at *www.ahrq.gov*).

EXAMINATION

By the time you are ready to begin the neurologic exam, you have already collected data about this system that were described in Chapter 7, Mental Health Assessment, Chapter 11, Head, Eyes, Ears, Nose and Throat, and Chapter 15, Musculoskeletal System. Refer to these chapters for the procedures as needed.

ROUTINE TECHNIQUES

- ASSESS mental status and level of consciousness. ⚷
- EVALUATE speech. ⚷
- NOTICE cranial nerve functions.
- OBSERVE gait. ⚷
- EVALUATE extremities for muscle strength. ⚷

SPECIAL CIRCUMSTANCES OR ADVANCED PRACTICE

- ASSESS cranial nerves.
  - TEST nose (CN I).
  - ASSESS eyes (CN II, III, IV, & VI).
  - TEST ears (CN VIII).
  - ASSESS face (CN V).
  - TEST tongue for taste (CN VII & IX).
  - INSPECT tongue (CN XII).
  - INSPECT oropharynx (CN IX & X).
  - TEST shoulders and neck muscles (CN XI).
- ASSESS cerebellum.
  - TEST cerebellar function.
- ASSESS peripheral nerves.
  - TEST extremities for sensation.
  - TEST deep tendon reflexes.
  - TEST for plantar reflex (Babinski sign). ★
  - TEST for ankle clonus. ★
  - TEST for superficial reflexes.
- ASSESS altered level of consciousness.
  - ASSESS for consciousness.
  - ASSESS for meningeal signs.

EQUIPMENT NEEDED

Aromatic materials • Penlight • Tuning fork (200 to 400 Hz) • Cotton-tipped applicator • Tongue blade • Examination gloves • 4×4 gauge • Reshaped paper clip • Cotton ball • Percussion hammer

⚷ = core examination skill

★ = advanced practice

PROCEDURES AND TECHNIQUES WITH NORMAL FINDINGS

ABNORMAL FINDINGS

⚷ ASSESS mental status and level of consciousness.

Say the client's name and note the response. The client is expected to turn toward you and respond appropriately. While taking the client's history you gather data about his or her mental status and level of consciousness. More detail is provided on this assessment in Chapter 7, Mental Health Assessment.

Clients who do not know their name or their location are disorientated. Those who require excessive stimulation or even painful stimuli to respond have a decrease in level of consciousness and require follow-up care and close supervision to maintain safety.

PROCEDURES AND TECHNIQUES WITH NORMAL FINDINGS	ABNORMAL FINDINGS

 EVALUATE speech for articulation and voice quality and conversation for comprehension of verbal communication.

The client's voice has inflection and sufficient volume with clear speech. The client's responses indicate an understanding of what is said.

Errors in choice of words or syllables; difficulty in articulation, which could involve impaired thought processes or dysfunction of the tongue or lips; slurred speech (tone sounds slurred); poorly coordinated or irregular speech; monotone or weak voice; nasal tone, rasping, or hoarseness; whispering voice; and stuttering are abnormal responses.

NOTICE cranial nerve functions.

Assessing cranial nerves is not ordinarily performed during a routine examination. They are assessed when you suspect an abnormal finding of one or more of the cranial nerves. However, you collect data about the expected cranial nerve functions during the interview. If you notice the expected findings, then you document "CNs II–XII grossly intact."

- CN I (olfactory nerve) is frequently not tested, but if the client mentions altered taste, this may indicate a need to test for smell.
- If clients are able to move around the environment and see the chair to sit down, this indicates function of CN II (optic nerve).

Client reports of absence of smell or lack of taste of food and drink are abnormal.

The client bumping into furniture, squinting, or needing assistance to locate a chair may be an indication of a vision problem.

- Observe the client's eye movements during the interview. If the eyes move equally from side to side, up and down, and obliquely, this indicates function of CN III (oculomotor nerve), CN IV (trochlear nerve), and CN VI (abducens nerve).
- If the eyes blink, this indicates function of the ophthalmic branch of CN V (trigeminal nerve).
- If the client's face is symmetric when he or she talks, this indicates function of CN VII (facial nerve).
- If the client can hear you, this indicates function of CN VIII (acoustic nerve).

The client's eyes not moving or moving in opposite directions is abnormal.

Lack of blinking is abnormal.

The client's face appears symmetric.

Indications of hearing loss include the client asking you to repeat yourself; repeatedly misunderstanding questions asked; leaning forward, or placing the hands behind his or her ears to screen out environmental noises.

- If you observe clients swallowing their saliva, this indicates function of CN IX (glossopharyngeal nerve) and CN X (vagus nerve).
- Hearing the clients' guttural speech sounds (e.g., k or g) indicates another function of CN X (vagus nerve).

- If the clients shrug their shoulders or turn their head during the interview, this indicates function of CN XI (spinal accessory nerve).

- If clients can enunciate words, this indicates function of the tongue and CN XI (hypoglossal nerve).

Inability to swallow saliva is an abnormality.

Absence of guttural sounds or nasal speech may indicate a vagus nerve abnormality.

Absence or difficulty in turning the head may indicate a XI cranial nerve abnormality.

Speech that is not clearly articulated may indicate an abnormality with the tongue.

PROCEDURES AND TECHNIQUES WITH NORMAL FINDINGS	ABNORMAL FINDINGS

OBSERVE gait for balance and symmetry.

When clients walk into the room, notice the gait. They should be able to maintain upright posture, walk unaided, maintain balance, and use opposing arm swing. Observing equilibrium is a test of CN VIII (acoustic nerve).

Poor posturing, ataxia, unsteady gait, rigid or absent arm movements, wide-based gait, trunk and head held tight, lurching or reeling, scissors gait, or parkinsonian gait (stooped posture, flexion at hips, elbows, and knees) is abnormal.

EVALUATE extremities for muscle strength.

Muscle strength: Test muscle strength according to the procedures outlined in Chapter 15. Muscle strength may be part of the musculoskeletal or neurologic system assessment.

A fasciculation is a localized uncontrollable twitching of a single muscle group innervated by a single motor nerve fiber that may be observed or palpated. There are many causes of fasciculation, including side effects of medications, cerebral palsy, neuralgia, and poliomyelitis.

Paralysis is lack of voluntary movement that is spastic or flaccid. Spastic paralysis is the involuntary contraction of muscles and occurs with upper motor neuron damage such as the pyramidal tract injury that occurs after a spinal cord injury or CVA. Flaccid paralysis is the lack of muscle tone and deep tendon reflexes that occurs after a lower motor neuron damage such as injury to the cauda equina from spina bifida.

SPECIAL CIRCUMSTANCES AND ADVANCED PRACTICE

ASSESS individual cranial nerves.

TEST nose for smell.

Evaluate the olfactory cranial nerve (CN I). Have the client close his or her eyes and mouth. Occlude one nostril while testing the other. Ask the client to identify common aromatic substances held under the client's nose. Examples include coffee, toothpaste, orange, and oil of cloves (Fig. 16-13).

Inability to smell anything or incorrect identification of odors is abnormal. Nasal allergies can impair ability to smell. Loss of smell may be caused by an olfactory tract lesion. *Anosmia* is the term used for loss of or impaired sense of smell.

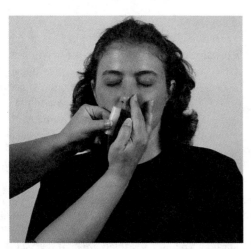

Fig. 16-13 Examination of the olfactory cranial nerve (CN I). *(From Chipps, Clanin, and Campbell, 1992.)*

= core examination skill

| PROCEDURES AND TECHNIQUES WITH NORMAL FINDINGS | ABNORMAL FINDINGS |

TEST eyes for visual acuity.

Test the optic nerve (CN II) for visual acuity using Snellen's chart and an ophthalmoscopic examination of the eye (see Chapter 11).

Refer the client to an ophthalmologist for further evaluation of vision and eye function when abnormalities are suspected. Chapter 11 provides more details.

TEST eyes for peripheral vision.

See Chapter 11 for the confrontation test. The presence of peripheral vision indicates function of the optic nerve (CN II).

If the client cannot see the pencil or finger at the same time you see it, peripheral field loss is suggested. Refer the client for further evaluation. Lesions in the central nervous system (e.g., tumors) may cause peripheral visual defects such as loss of vision in half or one quarter of the visual field, either medially or laterally.

OBSERVE eyes for extraocular muscle movement.

The oculomotor (CN III), trochlear (CN IV), and abducens (CN VI) nerves are tested together because they control muscles that provide eye movement (see Chapter 11).

Eye movements that are not parallel indicate extraocular muscle weakness or dysfunction of CN III, CN IV, or CN VI. Report nystagmus other than that noted as normal. Report ptosis (eyelid droop) that may occur with ocular myasthenia gravis.

OBSERVE eyes for pupillary size, shape, equality, constriction and accommodation.

Pupils should appear equal, round, and reactive to light and accommodation. See Chapter 11 for this assessment technique.

Increased intracranial pressure or trauma to the midbrain may exert pressure on CN III, resulting in diminished to absent pupillary constriction, ptosis of the eye, and altered superior and inferior movement of the eyeball. Pupil size can be changed by drug effects (e.g., constricted by heroin or morphine and dilated by cocaine).

EVALUATE face for movement and sensation.

Evaluate the trigeminal nerve (CN V) for facial movement and sensation. Test motor function by having the client clench his or her teeth, then palpate the temporal and masseter muscles for muscle mass and strength. There should be bilaterally strong muscle contractions (Fig. 16-14, *A*).

Inequality in muscle contractions, pain, twitching, or asymmetry is abnormal. Disorders of the pons (e.g., a tumor) may cause altered function of CN V or CN VII. A tic or mimic spasm is an involuntary movement of small muscles, usually of the face. Occasional tics may have psychogenic causes aggravated by anxiety or stress. Multiple tics and facial grimaces may occur with Gilles de la Tourette's syndrome.

To test sensation of light touch (supplied by the three branches of CN V), have the client close his or her eyes, then wipe cotton lightly over the anterior scalp (ophthalmic branch), paranasal sinuses (maxillary branch), and jaw (mandibular branch). A tickle sensation should be present equally over the three areas touched. Repeat the procedure on the other side of the face.

Decreased or unequal sensation is abnormal. Record the extent of the involved areas of the face.

PROCEDURES AND TECHNIQUES WITH NORMAL FINDINGS	ABNORMAL FINDINGS

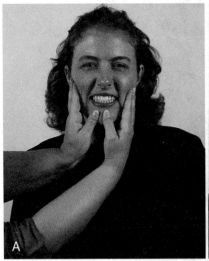
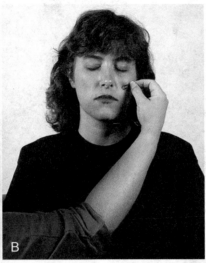

Fig. 16-14   Examination of the trigeminal nerve (CN V) for motor function, **A,** and sensory function, **B.** *(From Chipps, Clanin, and Campbell, 1992.)*

To test deep sensation, use alternating blunt and sharp ends of a paper clip over the client's forehead, paranasal sinuses, and jaw. The client should be able to feel pressure and pain equally throughout these areas and should be able to differentiate between sharp and dull (Fig. 16-14, *B*). Repeat the procedure on the other side of the face.

Test the ophthalmic branch (sensory) of CN V and motor function of CN VII by testing for the corneal reflex. *This test may be omitted when the client is alert and blinking naturally.* Ask the client to remove contact lenses if applicable and to look up and away from you. Approach the client from the side and lightly touch the cornea with a wisp of cotton. There should be a bilateral blink to corneal touch. Clients who wear contact lenses regularly may have diminished or absent reflex.

Evaluate the facial cranial nerve (CN VII) for movement. Inspect the face at rest and during conversation. Have the client raise the eyebrows, purse the lips, close the eyes tightly, show the teeth, smile, and puff put the cheeks. He or she should be able to correctly perform each request, and the movements should be smooth and symmetric (Fig 16-15).

Decreased or unequal sensation is abnormal. Trigeminal neuralgia is characterized by stablike pain radiating along the trigeminal nerve, caused by degeneration of or pressure on the nerve.

Absence of a blink is abnormal. Be sure to check that this abnormal response is not caused by the presence of contact lenses.

Asymmetry, facial weakness, drooping of one side of the face or mouth, or inability to maintain position until instructed to relax is abnormal.

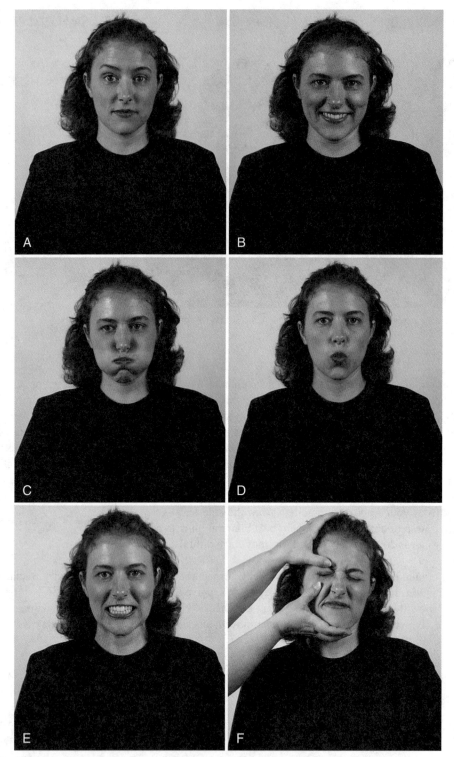

Fig. 16-15 **Examination of the facial nerve (CN VII).** Ask the client to make the following movements: **A,** Raise eyebrows and wrinkle forehead. **B,** Smile. **C,** Puff out cheeks. **D,** Purse lips and blow out. **E,** Show teeth. **F,** Squeeze eyes shut while you try to open them. *(From Chipps, Clanin, and Campbell, 1992.)*

PROCEDURES AND TECHNIQUES WITH NORMAL FINDINGS

TEST ears for hearing.

Evaluate the acoustic nerve (CN VIII) for hearing. Assessment of sensorineural hearing loss using the Rinne and Weber's test is described in Chapter 11. Tests for the vestibular function of CN VIII usually are not performed (Swartz, 2006).

TEST tongue for taste.

Evaluate taste over the anterior and posterior tongue. For the anterior two thirds of the tongue (CN VII, facial), instruct the client to stick out the tongue and leave it out during the testing process. Use a cotton applicator to place on the client's anterior tongue small quantities of salt, sugar, and lemon one at a time. The client should be able to correctly identify salty and sweet tastes (Fig. 16-16). Test the glossopharyngeal nerve for taste of the posterior one third of the tongue or pharynx (CN IX). The client should be able to taste bitter and sour tastes. Taste, the sensory component of CN VII and CN IX, usually is not tested unless the client reports a problem (O'Hanlon-Nichols, 1999).

INSPECT oropharynx for gag reflex and movement of soft palate.

Evaluate the glossopharyngeal nerve (CN IX) and the vagus nerve (CN X) together for movement of the soft palate and gag reflex. Instruct the client to say "ah" to test CN X. There should be equal upward movement of the soft palate and uvula bilaterally. To test the gag reflex, touch the posterior pharynx with the end of a tongue blade; the client should gag momentarily. Movement of the posterior pharynx and gag reflex test CN IX. See Chapter 11 for more detail.

ABNORMAL FINDINGS

Sensorineural hearing loss may be indicated using Weber's test by lateralization of sound to the unaffected ear or Rinne test when air conduction is longer than bone conduction in the affected ear, but by a less than 2:1 ratio.

Inability to identify tastes or consistently identifying a substance incorrectly is abnormal. Loss of smell and taste may occur together. Clients who are chronic smokers may have decreased taste.

Asymmetry of the soft palate or tonsillar pillar movement, any lateral deviation of the uvula, or absence of the gag reflex may indicate disorders of the medulla oblongata. For example, tumors may cause pressure on CN IX or CN X.

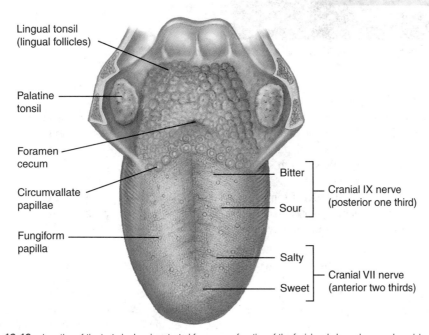

Fig. 16-16 Location of the taste bud regions tested for sensory function of the facial and glossopharyngeal cranial nerves. *(From Seidel et al, 2006.)*

PROCEDURES AND TECHNIQUES WITH NORMAL FINDINGS

ABNORMAL FINDINGS

TEST the tongue for movement, symmetry, strength, and absence of lesions; test for muscle strength.

Evaluate the hypoglossal nerve (CN XII) by observing movement and symmetry of the tongue. Ask the client to protrude his or her tongue. Note symmetry. Then ask the client to move the tongue toward the nose, the chin, and side to side (Fig. 16-17).

Wearing gloves, grasp the tongue with a 4×4 gauze pad, and palpate all sides (see Fig. 11-45). Test the tongue's muscle strength by asking the client to press the tip of the tongue inside the check, while you resist the pressure from outside of the client's cheek with your fingers. Repeat the procedure on the other side. The tongue should be moist, pink, and symmetric without lumps, nodules or ulcers. Tongue strength should be evident by resistance to outside pressure.

Asymmetric movement or weakness of the tongue may indicate impairment of the hypoglossal cranial nerve (CN XII). The tongue deviates toward the impaired side. Tumors of the tongue may develop from alcohol, tobacco, or chronic irritation.

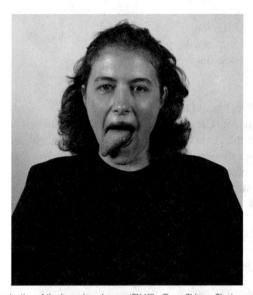

Fig. 16-17   Examination of the hypoglossal nerve (CN XII). *(From Chipps, Clanin, and Campbell, 1992.)*

TEST shoulders and neck muscles for strength and movement.

Have the client turn his or her head to the side against your hand; repeat with the other side (see Fig. 15-17, *A*). Observe the contraction of the opposite sternocleidomastoid muscle, and note the force of movement against your hand. Movement should be smooth, and muscle strength should be strong and symmetric.

Weakness or pain when pushing against your hand or asymmetry is abnormal.

Evaluate the spinal accessory nerve (CN XI) for movement. Ask the client to shrug his or her shoulders upward against your hands (see Fig. 15-22). Contraction of the trapezius muscles should be strong and symmetric.

Unilateral or bilateral muscle weakness or any pain or discomfort is abnormal.

TEST cerebellar function for balance and coordination.

To test cerebellar function, use at least two techniques for each area assessed (e.g., balance and coordination of upper and lower extremities). Choose these techniques based on the client's age and overall physical ability. For example, not every client should have to perform deep knee bends.

Abnormal findings may be due to a variety of causes, such as cerebellar tumors, stroke, Parkinson's disease, or inner ear problems.

PROCEDURES AND TECHNIQUES WITH NORMAL FINDINGS	ABNORMAL FINDINGS

Tests for Balance

- Perform the Romberg test. Have the client stand with feet together, arms resting at sides, eyes open, and then eyes closed. Stand close to the client with arms ready to "catch" client if he or she begins to fall off balance. There will be slight swaying, but the upright posture and foot position should be maintained.

- Have the client close his or her eyes and stand on one foot, then the other. He or she should be able to maintain position for at least 5 seconds.
- Have the client walk in tandem, placing the heel of one foot directly against the toes of the other foot. The client should be able to maintain this heel-toe walking pattern along a straight line (Fig. 16-18).
- Have the client hop first on one foot and then on the other. The client should be able to follow directions successfully and have enough muscle strength to accomplish the task (Fig. 16-19).
- Have the client hold one hand outward and perform several shallow or deep knee bends. The client should be able to follow directions successfully, with muscle strength adequate to accomplish the task.
- Have the client walk on toes, then heels. The client should be able to follow directions, walking several steps on the toes and then on the heels. The client may need to use the hands to maintain balance.

If the client sways with eyes closed but not open, the problem is probably proprioceptive. If the client sways with eyes open and closed, the problem is probably a cerebellar disorder and is documented as a positive Romberg sign (Seidel et al, 2006).

Inability to maintain single-foot balance for 5 seconds is abnormal.

Inability to walk heel-to-toe or using a wide-based gait to maintain the upright posture is abnormal.

Inability to hop or maintain single-leg balance is abnormal.

Inability to perform activity because of difficulty with balance or lack of muscle strength is abnormal.

Inability to retain balance, poor muscle strength, or inability to complete the activity is abnormal.

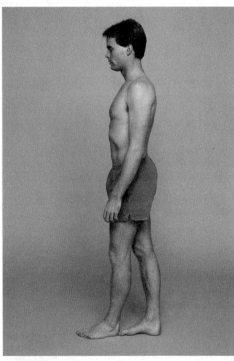

Fig. 16-18　Evaluation of balance with heel-toe walking on a straight line. *(From Seidel et al, 2003.)*

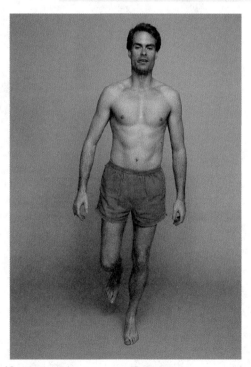

Fig. 16-19　Evaluation of balance with the client hopping in place on one foot. *(From Seidel et al, 2003.)*

PROCEDURES AND TECHNIQUES WITH NORMAL FINDINGS

Upper Extremity

Have the client alternately tap thighs with hands using rapid pronation and supination movements. Timing should be equal bilaterally and movement purposeful; the client should have no problem maintaining a rapid pace (Fig. 16-20).

Have the client close eyes and stretch arms outward. Use index fingers to alternately touch the nose rapidly. The client should be able to repeatedly touch the nose in a rhythmic pattern.

Evaluate the client's ability to perform rapid, rhythmic, alternating movement of fingers by having the client touch each finger to the thumb in rapid sequence. Test each hand separately. The client should be able to rapidly and purposefully touching each finger to thumb (Fig. 16-21).

Have the client rapidly move his or her index finger back and forth between his or her nose and your finger 18 inches (46 cm) away. Test one hand at a time. The client should be able to maintain the activity with a conscious, coordinated effort (Fig. 16-22).

ABNORMAL FINDINGS

Inability to maintain rapid pace is abnormal. An intention tremor—an involuntary muscle contraction during a purposeful movement of an extremity that disappears when the extremity is not moving—may indicate cerebellar dysfunction.

Cerebellar dysfunction may cause the client to miss touching his or her nose several times or cause the arms to drift downward.

Inability to coordinate fine, discrete, rapid movement is abnormal. An intention tremor may be observed during the movement, indicating a cerebellar dysfunction.

Inability to maintain continuous touch with both his or her own nose and the nurse's finger, inability to maintain the rapid movement, or obvious difficulty coordinating are abnormal.

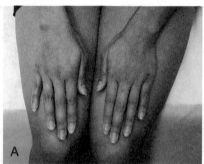 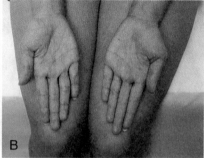

Fig. 16-20 **Examination of coordination with rapid alternating movements.** Ask client to tap top of thighs with both hands, alternately with palms down **(A)** and palms up **(B)**.

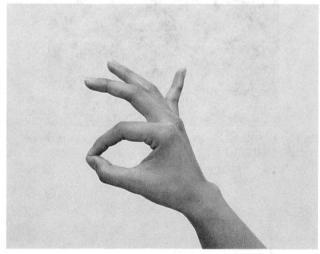

Fig. 16-21 **Examination of finger coordination.** Ask client to touch each finger to thumb in rapid sequence.

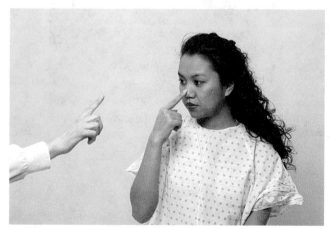

Fig. 16-22 **Examination of fine motor function.** Ask client to alternately touch own nose and the nurse's index finger with the index finger of one hand.

PROCEDURES AND TECHNIQUES WITH NORMAL FINDINGS	ABNORMAL FINDINGS

PROCEDURES AND TECHNIQUES WITH NORMAL FINDINGS

Lower Extremity

With the client lying supine, ask him or her to place the heel of one foot to the knee of the other leg, sliding it all the way down the shin (Fig. 16-23). Repeat on the other leg. The client should be able to run the heel down the opposite shin purposefully, with equal coordination.

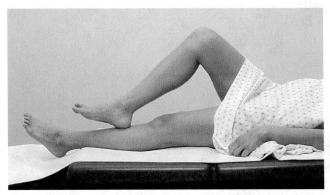

FIG. 16-23 **Examination of lower extremity coordination.** Ask client to run heel of one foot down shin of other leg. Repeat with opposite leg.

ASSESS peripheral nerves.

ASSESS for sensation.

Sensory function: Ask the client to close his or her eyes during the tests of sensory function. Areas routinely assessed are the hands, lower arms, abdomen, lower legs, and feet. If sensation is intact, no further evaluation is needed; if impaired, assess sensation systemically from digits up or from shoulder or hip down to identify the area that is without sensation. Compare bilateral responses in each sensory testing area. Try to map out the area involved using the dermatome map (see Fig. 16-10) to identify the spinal nerve providing sensation to that area of the body.

To test sensation to light touch (superficial touch), use a cotton wisp and the lightest touch possible to test each designated area (client's eyes are closed) (Fig. 16-24, *A*). The client should perceive light sensation and be able to correctly point to or name the spot touched.

★ A monofilament is used to test peripheral sensation of clients with peripheral neuropathy as may occur with diabetes mellitus (see Fig. 4-26).

Test sharp and dull sensation by using the pointed tip of a paper clip (or broken tongue blade) to lightly prick each designated area (client's eyes are closed) (Fig. 16-24, *B*). Alternate sharp and dull sensations to more accurately evaluate the client's response. The client should be able to distinguish sharp from dull and be able to identify the area touched.

Ask the client to close his or her eyes for the test of vibratory sense. Place a vibrating tuning fork on a bony area, such as the styloid process of the radius (wrist), medial or lateral malleolus (ankle), and sternum (chest) and ask the client to describe the sensation (Fig. 16-24, *C*). He or she should feel a sense of vibration. Also ask the client to report when he or she no longer feels vibration, then stop vibration of the tuning fork by touching it with your fingers but without moving it from its location on the bony prominence.

ABNORMAL FINDINGS

Clients with cerebellar disease may overshoot the knee and oscillate back and forth. With loss of position sense, the client may lift the heel too high and have to look to ensure that the heel is moving down the shin.

Impaired or absent sensation is abnormal. Absence of sensation may be due to compression of the nerve, whereas inflammation of the nerve may cause abnormal sensation. Diabetes mellitus may cause absent or abnormal sensation.

Abnormal findings include the client reporting that he or she does not feel the light touch, incorrectly identifying the area touched, or reporting an asymmetric response.

Abnormal findings include the client reporting that he or she does not feel the sharp or dull touch, being unable to distinguish between sharp and dull, or reporting an asymmetric response.

Unequal or decreased vibratory sensation is abnormal. The client may not be able to distinguish the change in sensation from vibration to nonvibration or may not feel the vibration in one or more locations. Referring to the dermatome drawing (see Fig. 16-10) will help identify the spinal nerve supplying this area. This may be found in clients with diabetes mellitus and those who have had a CVA or spinal cord injury.

★ = advanced practice

PROCEDURES AND TECHNIQUES WITH NORMAL FINDINGS	ABNORMAL FINDINGS

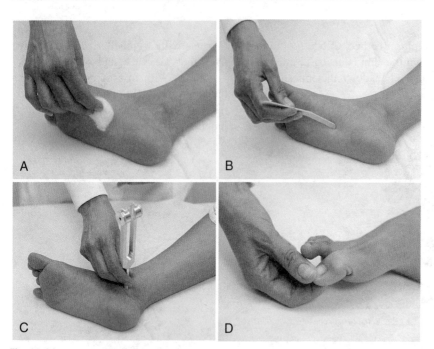

Fig. 16-24 Evaluation of peripheral nerve sensory function. **A,** Superficial tactile sensation. **B,** Superficial pain sensation. **C,** Vibratory sensation. **D,** Position sense of joints.

Test kinesthetic sensation by grasping the client's finger or toe and moving its position 1 cm up or down (client's eyes are closed) (Fig. 16-24, *D*). The client should be able to describe how the position has changed.

★ Test stereognosis by asking the client to close his or her eyes. Place a small, familiar object in the client's hand and ask him or her to identify it (Fig. 16-25, *A*). The object should be properly identified.

Test two-point discrimination by touching selected parts of the body simultaneously while the client's eyes are closed (Fig. 16-25, *B*). Use the points of two cotton-tipped applicators or reshape a paper clip so that two prongs can be lightly pressed against the client's skin simultaneously. Ask the client how many points he or she detects. The expected values for two-point discrimination are listed in Box 16-2.

Evaluate graphesthesia using a blunt instrument to draw a number or letter on the client's hand, back, or other area (client has eyes closed) (Fig. 16-25, *C*). The client should be able to recognize the number or letter drawn.

If the client cannot distinguish the change in position, it may indicate impairment of sensory (afferent nerves) or parietal lobe.

Altered stereognosis may indicate a parietal lobe or sensory nerve tract dysfunction and is documented as tactile agnosia (Seidel et al, 2006).

Inability to distinguish two-point discrimination is abnormal. Report the anatomic location of the sensory alteration.

If the client cannot distinguish the number or letter, it may indicate a parietal lobe lesion.

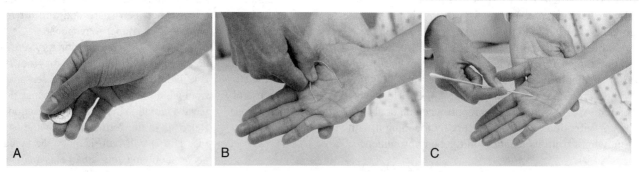

Fig. 16-25 Evaluation of cortical sensory function. **A,** Stereognosis: identification of a familiar object by touch. **B,** Two-point discrimination. **C,** Graphesthesia: draw letter or number on palm and ask client to identify by touch.

★ = advanced practice

| PROCEDURES AND TECHNIQUES WITH NORMAL FINDINGS | ABNORMAL FINDINGS |

| BOX 16-2 | **MINIMAL DISTANCES FOR DISTINGUISHING TWO POINTS** |

Location	Minimal Distance
Tongue	1 mm or $1/32$ inch*
Fingertips	2-8 mm or $2/32$* to $5/16$ inch
Toes	3-8 mm or $3/32$* to $5/16$ inch
Palm of hand	8-12 mm or $5/16$ to $1/2$ inch
Chest and forearms	40 mm or $1\frac{1}{2}$ inches
Back	40-70 mm or $1\frac{1}{2}$ to $2\frac{3}{4}$ inches
Upper arms and thighs	75 mm or 3 inches

*Too small to measure with conventional inch ruler.

EVALUATE extremities for deep tendon reflexes.

Reflexes: Test deep tendon reflexes for muscle contraction in response to direct or indirect percussion of a tendon. Box 16-3 outlines the scoring system. Hold the reflex hammer between your thumb and index finger, and briskly tap the tendon with a flick of the wrist. The client must be relaxed and sitting or lying down.

- To elicit the *triceps reflex,* ask the client to let a relaxed arm fall onto your arm. Hold his or her arm, with elbow flexed at a 90-degree angle, in one hand. Palpate and then strike the triceps tendon just above the elbow with either end of the reflex hammer (Fig. 16-26, *A*). (Some nurses prefer the flat end because of the wider striking surface.) The expected response is the contraction of the triceps muscle that causes visible or palpable extension of the elbow. An alternative arm position is to grasp the upper arm and allow the lower arm to bend at the elbow and hang freely; then strike the triceps tendon.
- The *biceps reflex* is elicited by asking the client to let his or her relaxed arm fall onto your arm. Hold the arm with elbow flexed at a 90-degree angle, and place your thumb over the biceps tendon in the antecubital fossa and your fingers over the biceps muscle. Using the pointed end of the reflex hammer, strike your thumb instead of striking the tendon directly (Fig. 16-26, *B*). The expected response is the contraction of the biceps muscle that causes visible or palpable flexion of the elbow.
- The *brachioradial reflex* is elicited by asking the client to let his or her relaxed arm fall into your hand. Hold the arm with the hand slightly pronated. Using either end of the reflex hammer, strike the brachioradialis tendon directly about 1 to 2 inches (2.5 to 5 cm) above the wrist (Fig. 16-26, *C*). The expected response is pronation of the forearm and flexion of the elbow.

Abnormal response may range from a hyperactive to a diminished response. Observe whether the abnormal reflex response is unilateral or bilateral. Table 16-2 lists the spinal level of each reflex.

| BOX 16-3 | **SCORING DEEP TENDON REFLEXES** |

Test the five deep tendon reflexes (triceps, biceps, brachioradial, patellar, and Achilles) using a reflex hammer. Compare the reflexes bilaterally. Reflexes are graded on a scale of 0 to 4, with 2 being the expected findings. Findings are recorded as follows:

0 = no response
1 + = sluggish or diminished
2 + = active or expected response
3 + = slightly hyperactive, more brisk than normal; not necessarily pathologic
4 + = brisk, hyperactive with intermittent clonus associated with disease

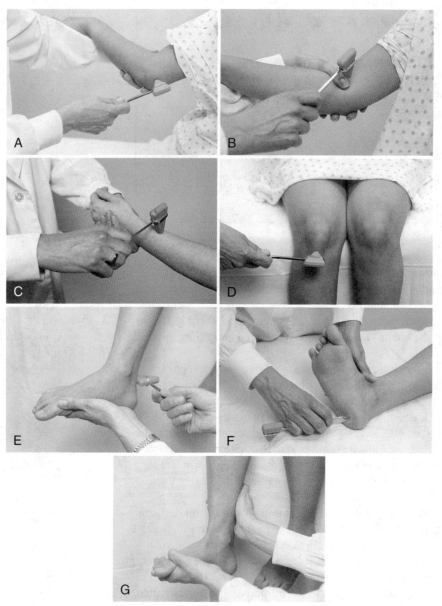

Fig. 16-26   Location of tendons for evaluation of deep tendon reflexes.   **A,** Triceps reflex. **B,** Biceps reflex. **C,** Brachioradialis reflex. **D,** Patellar reflex. **E,** Achilles reflex. **F,** Babinski's reflex. **G,** Ankle tonus.

PROCEDURES AND TECHNIQUES WITH NORMAL FINDINGS

ABNORMAL FINDINGS

- The *patellar reflex* is tested with the client sitting with legs hanging free. Flex the client's knee at a 90-degree angle and strike the patellar tendon just below the patella (Fig. 16-26, *D*). The expected response is the contraction of the quadriceps muscle, causing extension of the lower leg. When no response is found, divert the client's attention to another muscular activity by asking him or her to pull the fingers of each hand against the other. While the client is pulling, strike the patellar tendon.

- The *Achilles tendon* is tested by flexing the client's knee and dorsiflexing the ankle 90 degrees. Hold the bottom of the client's foot in one hand while you use the flat end of the reflex hammer to strike the Achilles tendon at the level of the ankle malleolus (Fig. 16-26, *E*). The expected response is the contraction of the gastrocnemius muscle, causing plantar flexion of the foot.

PROCEDURES AND TECHNIQUES WITH NORMAL FINDINGS

★ Check for the plantar reflex. Using the end of the handle on the reflex hammer, stroke the lateral aspect of the sole of the foot from heel to ball, curving medially across the ball of the foot (Fig. 16-26, *F*). The expected findings should be plantar flexion of all toes.

★ Test for ankle clonus if reflexes are hyperactive. Support the client's knee in a partly flexed position. With the other hand, sharply dorsiflex the foot and maintain it in flexion (Fig. 16-26, *G*). There should be no movement of the foot.

EVALUATE for superficial reflexes.

Testing abdominal reflexes is described in Chapter 14 (see Fig. 14-19). Elicit the reflexes by stroking the abdomen away from the umbilicus with the handle of a reflex hammer. In assessing the neurologic system, you correlate the expected response with the spinal level involved. See Table 16-2 for the spinal level of these reflexes. The testing of superficial reflexes is included here for completeness; however, there is little clinical significance to their presence or absence (Swartz, 2006).

For male clients: Check the cremasteric reflex. Lightly stroke the upper, inner aspect of the thigh with the reflex hammer or tongue blade. The ipsilateral testicle should rise slightly.

ABNORMAL FINDINGS

Dorsiflexion of the great toe with fanning of the other toes is an abnormal response termed a *positive Babinski's sign* and may indicate pyramidal (motor) tract disease.

Rhythmic oscillations between dorsiflexion and plantar flexion are abnormal responses.

Diminished to absent response is found on the side of a corticospinal tract (motor tract) lesion (Swartz, 2006).

Absence of the cremasteric reflex is seen in disorders of the pyramidal (motor) tract above the level of the first lumbar vertebrae.

★ = advanced practice

ADDITIONAL ASSESSMENT TECHNIQUES FOR SPECIAL CASES

Altered Level of Consciousness

During the history the nurse can usually determine if the client is alert and oriented by the way that questions are answered. A change in level of consciousness (LOC) is the earliest and most sensitive indicator of alterations in cerebral function. Consciousness involves awareness, arousal, and cognition. Awareness and arousal require an intact reticular activating system in the brainstem. Cognition depends in a functioning cerebral cortex.

Assessing Awareness

Mental status is an indication of awareness and is determined by orientation, memory, attention, calculation, recall, and language, as well as judgment, insight, and abstraction. Mental status is discussed in Chapter 7. When clients' orientation becomes a concern while taking a history or talking with clients, the nurse asks questions to determine if these clients are oriented to time, place, and person. For example, ask the clients if they know what year it is, where they are, and their name. Date and time are the first orientation to disappear. Healthy people often do not remember the day or time. After the nurse reorients the clients, however, they should remember the correct date and time. Loss of orientation to time is only an abnormality when clients do not remember the day and date after the nurse has reoriented them. Orientation to place is the second orientation to be lost, and again the client is expected to remember the place, town, and state after reorientation. For example, the nurse may say to the client, "You are a client in Memorial Hospital in Dallas, Texas." Orientation to person is reported when clients do not know who they are, even after reorientation. Orientation to person is the last orientation to be lost and the first to return followed by orientation to place and finally time. The documentation of "oriented × 3" (O × 3) means the client is oriented to time, place, and person; "oriented × 2" (O × 2) means the client is oriented to person and place but not time; and "oriented × 1" (O × 1) means the client is oriented to person but not to place or time.

Assessing Arousal

A modified neurologic assessment is needed for the unconscious client because he or she cannot actively participate. When interacting with an unconscious client, *always* assume that he or she can hear *everything* you say: thus you tell the client what action you are going to do before you do it. For example, tell the client, "I am going to hold your eyelid open and shine a light into your eye to check your pupils."

As with assessment of any client, inspection is used first to observe respiratory pattern. For example, Cheyne-Stokes breathing is periods of apnea alternating with hyperventilation (see Chapter 12, Fig. 12-13) and is seen in clients with brainstem compression or bilateral cerebral dysfunction. Central neurogenic hyperventilation (sustained hyperventilation) (see Chapter 12, Figure 12-13) is seen in clients with lesions of the midbrain and pons or those who have diabetes mellitus who are in ketoacidosis.

Pupillary response is assessed next. The pupillary response is controlled by CN III (oculomotor), which originates from the midbrain. Small, reactive pupils are seen in bilateral cerebral dysfunction. Bilaterally dilated pupils may indicate overdose of hallucinogenics or central nervous system stimulants (see Chapter 11, Table 11-1) or pressure in the brainstem that is compressing CN III bilaterally. A unilateral fixed and dilated pupil is suggestive of pressure on the ipsilateral CN III (Swartz, 2006).

Documenting Altered Level of Conscious Using Descriptors or a Scale

Altered levels of consciousness can be documented using descriptors that verbally explain findings or a scale that uses numbers assigned to the findings. Applying pain may be a necessary part of assessment for consciousness. You want to determine how much stimulation or pain is required to elicit a response from the client. You begin with a touch and a normal tone of voice. If this does not create a response, you shake clients on the shoulder or leg and shout at them. If this does not produce a response, you then resort to painful stimuli, beginning peripherally and moving centrally. When painful stimuli are used, they should be applied until clients respond in some way or for at least 15 seconds. Painful stimuli should be used no more than 30 seconds if there is no response. You may begin with depressing the nail at the cuticle with your fingernail or with an object such as the length of a pen or pencil. If this does not elicit a response, squeeze the trapezius muscle very hard and observe for any movement. If this does not yield a response, push upward on the supraorbital notch above the eye. Do not push inward on the eyeball, but on the bony orbit above the eyeball. Table 16-3 describes techniques for applying painful stimuli (Lower, 2003).

Descriptors of consciousness in decreasing order of awareness and arousal are lethargy, obtunded, stuporous, semicomatose, and comatose. Clients who are **lethargic** can be aroused with saying their name and touching them. Once aroused, they response appropriately but return to "sleep" as soon as the stimuli ceases. Those who are **obtunded** require louder verbal stimuli and vigorous shaking to prompt a response: they carry out requests while awake, but return to "sleep" when stimuli stops. Clients who are **stuporous** require painful stimuli to respond and the response usually is a withdrawal from the source of pain. **Semicomatose** clients require painful stimuli and respond with abnormal flex-

TABLE 16-3 *Techniques for Applying Painful Stimuli*

Assessing Peripheral Pain	Technique
Pressing on the nail plate	Apply pressure to only those extremities that did not respond to central painful stimuli. Press in the nail (at the cuticle) with the shaft of a pencil or pen. Apply pressure for 15 to 30 seconds and observe for response.

Assessing Central Pain	Technique
Squeezing the trapezius muscle	Squeeze the trapezius muscle by grasping the muscle with the thumb and two fingers, pinch 1 to 2 inches, and twist.
Applying supraorbital pressure	Avoid applying supraorbital pressure if the client has facial fractures. Palpate the orbital rim beneath the eyebrow until you locate the notch near the center where a sensory nerve is located. With your thumb, push firmly on the notch. (Do not push inward on the eye globe.)
Applying mandibular pressure	Using your index and middle fingers, push up and inward at the angle of the client's jaw (just below the earlobe).
Rubbing the sternum	This technique should be used as a last resort because it can cause bruising. Apply pressure downward with your knuckles to the midsternum and turn your knuckles to the left and right without moving them from the sternum.

ion or extension. **Comatose** clients do not response to any stimuli, even central pain.

Since there may be some overlap in the descriptors used to assess consciousness, some nurses prefer the Glasgow Coma Scale (GCS), which uses a 15-point scale to assess consciousness (Fig. 16-27). This scale is only useful to assess clients with altered consciousness. The client is assessed for the best response to eye opening, motor response, and verbal response. For example, when assessing a client who has altered consciousness and is paralyzed on one side due to a stroke, the nurse uses the motor response of the client's unaffected side for best motor response. An arbitrary number is assigned to describe the motor response. The response observed from the client may be a localization of pain (score of 5) when he or she moves as if trying to remove the stimulus, an attempt to withdraw from the stimulus (score of 4), abnormal flexion (formerly called decorticate posturing) (score of 3), abnormal extension (formerly called decerebrate posturing) (score of 2), or no response at all to any painful stimuli (score of 1). See Fig. 16-27 for examples of abnormal flexion and extension.

When the client is unable to speak because of an endotracheal or tracheostomy tube placement, the best verbal response of the Glasgow Coma Scale cannot be assessed. Each institution has its specific way of documenting this. For example, if the client is comatose, the score may be recorded as 2T, meaning 1 for best eye response, 1 for best motor response, and T for "tube," indicating that verbal response cannot be assessed. A score from 14 to 3 is considered abnormal. The lower the score, the deeper the coma.

Glasgow Coma Scale

Best eye-opening response	Spontaneously	4
	To verbal command	3
	To pain	2
	No response	1
Best verbal response	Oriented, converses	5
	Disoriented, converses	4
	Inappropriate words	3
	Incomprehensible sounds	2
	No response	1
Best motor response		
To verbal command	Obeys pain	6
To painful stimulus	Localizes	5
	Flexion—withdrawal	4
	Flexion—decorticate	3
	Extension—decerebrate	2
	No response	1
	TOTAL	(3-15)

Abnormal flexion (Decorticate) Rigid flexion; upper arms held tightly to the sides of body; elbows, wrists, and fingers flexed; feet are plantar flexed, legs extended and internally rotated; may have fine tremors or intense stiffness

Abnormal extension (Decerebrate) Rigid extension; arms fully extended; forearms pronated; wrists and fingers flexed; jaws clenched, neck extended, back may be arched; feet plantar flexed; may occur spontaneously, intermittently, or in response to a stimulus

Fig. 16-27   Glasgow Coma Scale. *(Modified from Chipps, Clanin, and Campbell, 1992.)*

Meningeal Irritation

Meningeal signs are assessed when meningitis is suspected. These include tests for Kernig's sign and Brudzinski's sign.

- Kernig's sign is tested by flexing one of the client's legs at the hip and knee, then extending the knee (Fig. 16-28, *A*). No pain reported is a negative Kernig's sign. If a client has inflammation of the meninges, he or she will report pain along the vertebral column when the leg is extended, a positive Kernig's sign indicating irritation of the meninges.
- Brudzinski's sign is tested with the client supine. The nurse flexes the client's neck (Fig. 16-28, *B*). The client should report no pain or resistance to neck flexion. A positive Brudzinski's sign occurs when the client passively flexes the hip and knee in response to head flexion and reports pain along vertebral column.

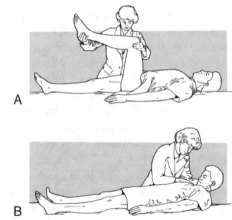

A

B

Fig. 16-28   Kernig's sign and Brudzinski's sign are tests of meningeal irritation. **A,** *Kernig's sign.* Flex one of the client's legs at the hip and knee. Note resistance or pain. **B,** *Brudzinski's sign.* With the client recumbent, place your hands behind the client's head and flex the neck forward. Note resistance or pain. Watch also for flexion of the client's hips and knees in reaction to your maneuver. *(From Chipps, Clanin, and Campbell, 1992.)*

Documenting Expected Findings

Neurologic System

Oriented to person, place and time. Speech understandable and of sufficient volume. Cranial nerves grossly intact. Balanced gait with upright posture. Muscle strength 5/5 and movement coordinated bilaterally, negative Romberg sign. Peripheral sensation intact. Deep tendon reflexes 2+ bilaterally.

AGE-RELATED VARIATIONS

INFANTS, CHILDREN, AND ADOLESCENTS

There are several differences in the assessment of the system for infants and young children. Infants' sensation and cranial nerves are assessed by observation. Unique reflexes are assessed in infants. Children's motor development is compared with standardized tables of normal age and sequences of motor development. Assessment of the older child and adolescent follows the same procedures and reveals similar expected findings. Chapter 20 presents further information regarding neurologic assessment of infants, children, and adolescents.

OLDER ADULTS

Assessing the neurologic system of an older adult usually follows the same procedures as for the younger adult. Tests for balance and gait of older adults are often assessed to identify those at risk for falls. Chapter 22 presents further information regarding the neurologic assessment of older adults.

CLINICAL REASONING   *Neurologic System*

A 19-year-old male college student is brought to the student health services with a chief complaint of headache. He is accompanied by his roommate, who explains that the client was playing football and struck the right side of his head when he collided with another player.

Noticing: The experienced nurse immediately understands that a blow to the head such as this can result in mild or significant injury, knows neurologic changes may be overt or subtle. The nurse learns that the incident took place four hours ago—since then the client has complained of a headache that has become worse. The client is alert, and oriented to time, place, and person; his vital signs are within expected parameters. Given the nature of his injury and symptom, the nurse recognizes the possibility of closed head injury (CHI); this background knowledge sets up the possibility of noticing signs of brain swelling in an individual presenting with these manifestations.

Interpreting: Early in the encounter, the nurse considers two possible causes of the headache: scalp trauma (hematoma, laceration), CHI, or both. The nurse also knows that

CHI can present in many ways, depending on the type of injury. The nurse gathers additional data.

- Is there evidence of external trauma? The nurse palpates a lump over the right temporal region of the scalp. The skin is intact.
- Was there a loss of consciousness? The client was "knocked out" for a few minutes.
- Are there any neurologic changes? The client does not recall playing football or sustaining the injury. The roommate reports he keeps asking the same questions. The nurse notes an unsteady gait with ambulation; PERRLA.

The experienced nurse not only recognizes abnormal clinical findings (loss of consciousness, headache, memory impairment, unsteady gait), but interprets this information in the context of an individual who has had a recent blow to the head.

Responding: The nurse initiates appropriate initial interventions and notifies the primary care provider of the situation, ensuring the client receives appropriate immediate and follow-up care.

COMMON PROBLEMS & CONDITIONS

DISORDERS OF THE CENTRAL NERVOUS SYSTEM

Multiple Sclerosis

Progressive demyelination of nerve fibers of the brain and spinal cord results in multiple sclerosis (MS). It is an autoimmune disorder initiated by a virus that attacks the myelin at various sites of the central nervous system. **Clinical Findings:** Manifestations vary depending on the areas of the central nervous system that are affected by the demyelination. Common symptoms are fatigue, depression, and paresthesias. Common signs are focal muscle weakness; ocular changes (diplopia, nystagmus); bowel, bladder, and sexual dysfunction; gait instability; and spasticity.

Meningitis

Inflammation of the meninges that surround the brain and spinal cord is termed *meningitis*. It may result from invasion of bacteria, viruses, fungi, parasites, or other toxins. **Clinical Findings:** Meningitis produces severe headache, fever, and generalized malaise. Signs of meningeal irritation include stiff neck and positive Brudzinski's and Kernig's signs (see Fig. 16-28). Level of consciousness may decrease with drowsiness and reduced attention span, which may progress to stupor and coma. Confusion, agitation, and irritability may occur.

Encephalitis

Inflammation of the brain tissue and meninges is termed *encephalitis*. It is caused by bacteria, viruses, fungi, and parasites. **Clinical Findings:** Manifestations of encephalitis are variable, depending on the invading organism and the part of the brain involved. The onset may be gradual or sudden with symptoms of headache and nausea and signs of fever, nuchal rigidity, lethargy, irritability, and vomiting. Over several days the client may develop decreased consciousness, motor weakness, tremors, seizures, aphasia, and positive Babinski's sign (Hickey, 2003).

Spinal Cord Injury

Any traumatic disruption of the spinal cord can result in a spinal cord injury (SCI). Common causes of SCIs are vertebral fractures and dislocations, such as those suffered by individuals involved in car accidents, sports injuries, and other violent impacts. Injury to the cervical spinal cord may result in quadriplegia, whereas injury to the thoracic and lumbar spinal cord may result in paraplegia. **Clinical Findings:**

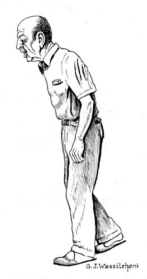

Fig. 16-29 Posture and shuffling gait associated with Parkinson's disease. *(From Rudy, 1984.)*

Manifestations of complete spinal cord transection include paresthesia or anesthesia, and signs are paralysis below the level of injury with loss of bowel and bladder control. Spinal cord injuries damage the upper motor neurons, causing a spastic paralysis. When the injury to the spinal cord is incomplete, manifestations are variable and correlate to the location and extent of injury.

Craniocerebral Injury (Head Injury)

Any injury to the scalp, skull, or brain that is sufficient to alter normal function can result in craniocerebral injury. Open head injuries result from fractures or penetrating wounds; closed head injuries result from blunt head injury producing cerebral concussion, contusion, or laceration. **Clinical Findings:** Manifestations of head injury are variable depending on the severity of the trauma and the areas of the brain involved. Residual deficits in memory, cognition, and motor and sensory abilities depend on the extent of injury on the brain.

Parkinson's Disease

Parkinson's disease develops slowly as the brain's dopamine-producing neurons in the substantia nigra of the basal ganglia degenerate. **Clinical Findings:** The disease is characterized by resting tremor, bradykinesia, and rigidity. Other manifestations include masklike facies, trunk-forward flexion, muscle weakness, shuffling gait, and finger pill-rolling tremor (Fig. 16-29; see Fig. 16-6).

Cerebrovascular Accident (Stroke)

When cerebral blood vessels become occluded by a thrombus or embolus or when intracranial hemorrhage occurs, the brain tissues become ischemic, resulting in a cerebrovascular accident or stroke. Hemorrhage can be caused by hypertension or a cerebral aneurysm (a weakened area in an artery that balloons out due to the high pressure of blood). **Clinical Findings:** Manifestations are directly related to the area of the brain involved and the extent of ischemic area. For example, ischemia to the left frontal lobe may result in paralysis of the right arm or leg. There may be sudden unilateral numbness or weakness of the face, arm, or leg. The client may complain of trouble walking, dizziness, or loss of balance or coordination. A sudden, severe headache with no known cause may be a symptom. There may be sudden confusion, difficulty swallowing (dysphagia), difficulty speaking or understanding speech (aphasia), or partial loss of vision. See the problem-based history for additional information on assessing clients with aphasia or dysphagia.

Alzheimer Disease

This is an incurable, degenerative neurologic disorder that begins with a decline in memory. Alzheimer disease is the most common cause of dementia in Western countries. The exact cause is unknown; however, theories suggest genetic tendency, altered function of neurotransmitters, or a mutation for encoding certain precursor proteins as contributing factors. **Clinical Findings:** Three stages of Alzheimer's disease have been described. The early stage lasts 2 to 4 years when the client's memory begins to fail, such as forgetting names and misplacing items. The second stage lasts from 2 to 12 years when the client experiences progressive memory loss and has difficulty with activities of daily living. Language skills deteriorate and the client becomes disoriented and confused with poor concentration. During the final stage the client requires total care and is unable to communicate (Hickey, 2003).

DISORDERS OF CRANIAL NERVES

Trigeminal Neuralgia

An intense paroxysmal pain along one or all three of the branches of the trigeminal nerve (CN V) is termed *trigeminal neuralgia* or *tic douloureux.* Although the etiology is unknown, trauma to the face or head and infection of the teeth or jaw are contributing factors. Many clients can identify trigger points in small areas on the cheek, lip, gum, or forehead that initiate pain when stimulated. **Clinical Findings:** Clients report an abrupt, intense unilateral pain along the tissue innervated by the trigeminal nerve that lasts a few seconds (Hickey, 2003).

Bell's Palsy

This is an acute unilateral paralysis of the facial nerve. About 80% of clients recover fully after a few weeks to months. **Clinical Findings:** Clients report a history of pain behind the ear or on the face a few hours or days before the onset of paralysis. On the affected side the eye does not close, the forehead does not wrinkle, and the client is unable to whistle or smile (Hickey, 2003).

DISORDERS OF PERIPHERAL NERVES

Myasthenia Gravis

This neuromuscular disease is characterized by weakness of voluntary muscles that improves with rest and administration of anticholinesterase drugs. In myasthenia gravis acetylcholine receptor sites are destroyed by autoantibodies causing muscle weakness. In some cases myasthenia gravis is associated with tumors of the thymus gland. There are three types of myasthenia: (1) ocular, which affects only the eyes; (2) bulbar, which involves the nerves that innervate the muscles needed for swallowing (CNs IX, X, XI, and XII); and (3) generalized, which affects skeletal muscles of the arms, legs, and trunk. **Clinical Findings:** Manifestations vary with the type of myasthenia. Ocular myasthenia produces muscle weakness confined to the muscles of the eye, causing ptosis and diplopia. Clients with bulbar myasthenia often aspirate saliva and other fluids because of impaired swallowing. Generalized myasthenia produces weakness of the face, limbs, and trunk, including the muscles of breathing.

Guillain-Barré Syndrome

This acute syndrome is characterized by widespread demyelinization of nerves of the peripheral nervous system. Guillain-Barré syndrome affects the motor component of peripheral nerves and is believed to be caused by a cell-mediated autoimmune response to a viral infection. Clients usually have a respiratory or gastrointestinal viral infection weeks before the onset. Between 80% and 90% of clients recover from this syndrome with few or no residual deficits; however, clients may die when respiratory depression develops rapidly. **Clinical Findings:** The usual manifestation is an ascending paralysis that begins with weakness and paresthesia in the lower extremities that ascends to the upper extremities and face. There is a descending variation of Guillain-Barré syndrome that begins with the facial, glossopharyngeal, vagus, and hypoglossal cranial nerves and moves downward more commonly to the hand, but it can reach the feet. Deep tendon reflexes are absent. If ascending paralysis reaches the thorax, respiratory depression may result (Hickey, 2003).

CLINICAL APPLICATION & CLINICAL REASONING

See Appendix E for answers to exercises in this section.

REVIEW QUESTIONS

1 The nurse gives a key to a client with a tumor in the cerebrum and asks the client to close her eyes and identify the object. The client manipulates the key, but she cannot identify what it is. From this finding the nurses suspects that the client's tumor is located in which lobe of the cerebrum?
   1 Frontal lobe.
   2 Parietal lobe.
   3 Temporal lobe.
   4 Occipital lobe.

2 During a symptom analysis the client reports a pain that radiates from the right lateral thigh, over the knee, and around to the right medial ankle. The nurse refers to the dermatomal map (see Fig. 16-10) to determine that the client's description of pain is consistent with dysfunction of which spinal nerve?
1 Second lumbar (L2).
2 Third lumbar (L3).
3 Fourth lumbar (L4).
4 Fifth lumbar (L5).

3 The nurse is checking the deep tendon reflexes of a client who has compression of the fifth and sixth cervical nerves on the right. Which deep tendon reflex will be diminished?
1 Right biceps reflex.
2 Left brachioradialis reflex.
3 Right triceps reflex.
4 Left patellar reflex.

4 When assessing a client with a tumor within the medulla oblongata, the nurse notes which abnormal finding?
1 Absent gag reflex.
2 Inability to smile and raise eyebrows.
3 Loss of sensation to the face.
4 Hearing deficit with unsteady gait.

5 What techniques does the nurse use to test the triceps reflex?
1 Hold the knee in a slightly flexed position while the nurse strokes the end of the foot with a dull object.
2 The nurse holds the client's relaxed forearm with the hand slightly pronated while striking the appropriate tendon with a reflex hammer.
3 The nurse holds the client's relaxed arm with elbow flexed at a 90-degree angle, places a thumb over the appropriate tendon, and strikes the thumb with the pointed end of the reflex hammer.
4 Hold the client's relaxed arm, with elbow flexed at a 90-degree angle, in one hand. Strike the appropriate tendon just above the elbow with either end of the reflex hammer.

6 The nurse is assessing a client who is unconscious and notices no response to calling the client's name, shouting, and gently shaking. Which technique should the nurse use next to assess for central pain as an indicator of consciousness?
1 Apply pressure to the client's nail plate at the cuticle with the shaft of a pencil.
2 Apply pressure downward with the knuckles on the midsternum.
3 Squeeze the trapezius muscle by grasping the muscle, pinching, and twisting.
4 Apply firm pressure to the supraorbital rim beneath the eyebrow.

7 Which techniques are used to assess the cerebellum?
1 Apply a pointed tip of a paper clip to lightly prick various areas of the upper and lower extremities to test for sensation.
2 Have the client walk on the heels and then on the toes to test for balance.
3 With the client's eyes closed, grasp the client's finger or toe and move its position 1 cm up or down to determine if the client perceives that the digit has moved.
4 Have the client lie supine and flex the hips and knees to test for mobility and range of motion.

SAMPLE DOCUMENTATION

Review the following data obtained during an interview and examination by the nurse below:

H. S. is a 48-year-old woman with a foot injury. She states that she dropped a hammer on her left foot yesterday helping her husband with repairs to their one-story home. Her vital signs are as follows: blood pressure, 138/88 mm Hg; pulse, 88 beats/min; respiratory rate, 14; temperature, 98.8° F (37° C). H. S. has no allergies to any medications. She takes aspirin 81 mg daily and captopril 50 mg twice a day. H. S. is a cooperative, alert woman in a wheelchair accompanied by her husband. Cranial nerves II through XII are intact. She applied ice to and elevated her left foot after dropping the hammer on it. She states that her height is 5 feet 7 inches (159 cm) and her weight is 160 lb (72.7 kg). Examination of her upper extremity (UE) revealed voluntary, symmetric, coordinated movement with full range of motion and sensation to vibration, cotton, and sharp object bilaterally. She communicates and dresses appropriately. She had a CVA 18 months ago leaving her with a residual paralysis of her left leg. She has a history of multiple accidents in the last year. Examination of her lower extremity (LE) reveals that the right leg has voluntary, symmetric, coordinated movement with full range of motion and sensation to vibration, cotton, and sharp object. The left leg has no voluntary movement with anesthesia; the dorsum of the left foot is edematous with erythema. Her deep tendon reflexes are 2+ bilaterally in the upper extremities and right leg and 0 in the left leg. H. S. states that she will not give up her independence. Her muscle strength is 5 in arms and right leg, 0 in left leg. She has a history of hypertension and a family history of CVA (both parents).

Below, note how the nurse documented these same data.

48-y/o ♀. CC: "dropped hammer on left foot yesterday." Medical hx: HTN, CVA 18 mo ago c̄ LLE paralysis. Family hx: CVA, both parents. Allergies: NKDA. Medications: ASA 81 mg qd, captopril 50 mg bid.

SUBJECTIVE DATA

Injured (L) foot yesterday helping make repairs to one-story home. Applied ice and elevated (L) foot. Hx of accidents since CVA, states she will not give up her independence.

OBJECTIVE DATA

General survey: BP 138/88 mm Hg; P 88 beats/min; RR 14; T 98.8° F (37° C). Ht 5 feet 7 inches (159 cm); wt 160 lb (72.7 kg) stated. Cooperative ♀ in WC accompanied by husband.

Mental status: Communicates and dresses appropriately. Alert, 0 × 3.

Cranial nerves: CNs II–XII intact.

Motor and sensory: UE: voluntary, symmetric, coordinated movement c̄ full ROM, muscle strength 5, sensation to vibration, cotton, sharp object bil; DTR 2+ bil. LE: (R), voluntary, symmetric, coordinated movement c̄ full ROM, muscle strength 5, sensation to vibration, cotton, sharp object; DTR 2+. (L) muscle strength 0, no voluntary movement c̄ anesthesia; DTR 0; dorsum of foot edematous, erythematous, c̄ no sensation.

CASE STUDY

L. T. is a 54-year-old African American man admitted to the hospital with a diagnosis of acute CVA. The following data are collected by the nurse during an interview and examination.

Interview Data

Mr. T.'s wife tells the nurse that he was fine until this morning, when he suddenly had a headache, fell to the floor, and could not get up. Mrs. T. adds that her husband made only mumbling noises, and she could not understand him. He has type 2 diabetes mellitus and hypertension. He stopped smoking last year.

Examination Data

- *Neurologic examination:* Awake, alert man. Unable to talk, but able to follow commands. Client cries and avoids eye contact with his wife and nurse.

- Cranial nerves III, IV, V, VI, and VIII are intact bilaterally. Client has asymmetry and unequal movements of face, with a drooping of the left side of face. Has asymmetry of shoulder shrug, with weakness noted on left side. Supination and pronation of right hand, unable to perform with left hand. Light touch with sharp and dull sensation present on right arm and leg, no sensation on left arm or leg. Right arm and leg muscle strength 5, left arm muscle tone 0, left leg 1. Unable to move around in bed unassisted at this time. Assessment of balance deferred.

Clinical Reasoning

1. What data deviate from normal findings, suggesting a need for further investigation?
2. What additional information should the nurse ask or assess for?
3. Based on the data, what risk factors for cerebrovascular accident does this client have?
4. What nursing diagnoses and collaborative problems should be considered for this situation?

INTERACTIVE ACTIVITIES

Open the interactive student CD-ROM, click on Chapter 16, and choose from the following activities on the menu bar:

- **Multiple Choice Challenge.** Click on the best answer for each of these items. You will be given immediate feedback, rationale for incorrect answers, and a total score. Good luck!

- **Marvelous Matches.** Drag each word or phrase and place it below the appropriate cranial nerve on the screen. Test your ability to match cranial nerves with the techniques for testing their functions.

- **Name Game.** Identify each of the anatomic parts of the figure shown. Watch out where you place your answer—it won't stick if it is in the wrong place!

- **Printable Lab Guide.** Locate the Lab Guide for Chapter 16, and print and use it (as many times as needed) to help you apply your assessment skills. These guides may also be filled in electronically and then saved and e-mailed to your instructor!

- **Quick Challenge.** Use this critical thinking exercise to assess your skills through case study-style questions, then compare with expert answers!

- **Core Examination Skills Checklists.** Make sure you've got frequently-used exam skills down pat! Use these checklists to help cover all the bases for your examination.

CHAPTER 17

Breasts and Axillae

ANATOMY & PHYSIOLOGY

The breasts are paired mammary glands located within the superficial fascia of the anterior chest wall. Breasts are a feature of all mammals, evolving as milk-producing organs to provide nourishment for offspring. During embryologic development, these glands develop along paired "milk lines," an embryonic ridge that extends between the limb buds of what will become the axillae and the inguinal regions. Normally, only one gland develops on each side in the pectoral region. After birth, the glands undergo little additional development in the male. In the female, however, the breasts undergo considerable development during adolescence, under the influence of estrogen and progesterone.

FEMALE BREAST

The breast of the mature female has a distinctive shape; however, there is great variation in "normal" breast size. The breasts extend vertically from the second to the sixth ribs and laterally from the sternal margin to the midaxillary line and are divided into four quadrants by imaginary vertical and horizontal lines intersecting at the nipple (Fig. 17-1).

The female breast is composed of three types of tissue: glandular tissue, fibrous tissue, and subcutaneous and retromammary fat tissue. The glandular tissue is arranged into 15 to 20 lobes per breast, radiating around the nipple in a spoke-like pattern (Fig. 17-2). Each lobe is composed of 20 to 40 lobules, or alveoli, containing the milk-producing acini cells.

During lactation, milk produced by acini cells empties into the lactiferous ducts. These ducts drain milk from the lobes to the surface of the nipple. The largest amount of glandular tissue lies in the upper outer quadrant of each breast. From this quadrant, the breast tissue extends into the axilla, forming the axillary tail of Spence.

The breast is supported by a layer of subcutaneous fibrous tissue and by multiple fibrous bands termed *Cooper's ligaments.* These suspensory ligaments extend from the connective tissue layer and run through the breast, attaching to the underlying muscle fascia. Subcutaneous and retromammary fat surrounds the glandular tissue and composes most of the breast.

Centrally located on the breast, the nipple is surrounded by the pigmented areola. The nipples are composed of epithelium intertwined with circular and longitudinal smooth muscle fibers. These muscles contract in response to sensory, tactile, or autonomic stimuli, producing erection of the nipple and causing the lactiferous ducts to empty. A number of sebaceous glands, termed *Montgomery's glands,* are located within the areolar surface, aiding in lubrication of the nipple during lactation.

Throughout the reproductive years, the breasts undergo a cyclic pattern of size change, nodularity, and tenderness during the menstrual cycle. The breasts are smallest during days 4 through 7 of the menstrual cycle. Three to four days before the onset of menses, many women experience breast tenseness, fullness, tenderness, and pain because of hormonal changes and fluid retention.

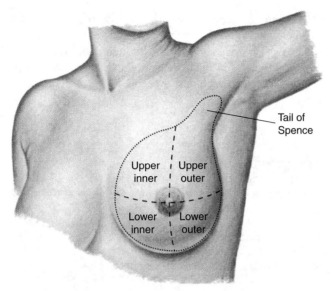

Fig. 17-1 Quadrants of the left breast and axillary tail of Spence. *(From Seidel et al, 2006.)*

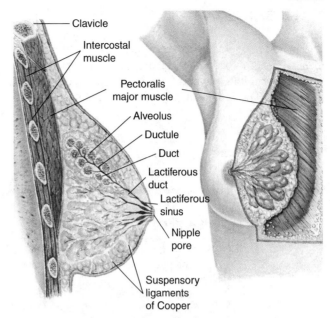

Fig. 17-2 Anatomy of the breast, showing position and major structures. *(From Seidel et al, 2006.)*

The breasts undergo a dramatic change during pregnancy and lactation in response to luteal and placental hormones. These changes include an increase in the number of lactiferous ducts and an increase in the size and number of alveoli. See Chapter 21 for further information.

Lymphatic Network

Each breast contains an extensive lymphatic network, which drains into lymph nodes in several areas. As blood flows through the capillary bed, fluid is forced out into the interstitial space, then into the cells. Most of the fluid is reabsorbed into the capillaries; however, fluid left in the interstitial spaces is absorbed by the lymph system and carried through the lymph nodes. More than 75% of lymph drainage from the breast flows outward toward the axillary lymph node groups and then upward to the subclavicular and supraclavicular nodes (Bennett et al, 2001). Other routes for lymph drainage include flow through the anterior axillae (pectoral) nodes (above the breast), internal mammary nodes (in the thorax), and subdiaphragmatic nodes (toward the abdomen), and through cross-mammary pathways to the opposite breast (Fig. 17-3).

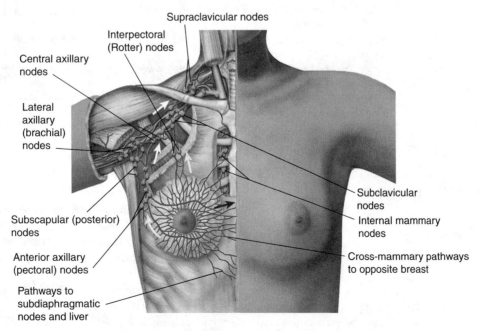

Fig. 17-3 Lymphatic drainage of the breast. *(From Seidel et al, 2006.)*

MALE BREAST

The male breast undergoes very little additional development after birth, and the gland remains rudimentary. It consists of a thin layer of undeveloped tissue beneath the nipple. The areola of the nipple is small when compared with the female. During puberty, the male breast may become slightly enlarged, producing a temporary condition termed *gynecomastia*. Although gynecomastia is usually unilateral, it may occur bilaterally. The older male may also have gynecomastia secondary to a decrease in testosterone.

HEALTH HISTORY

RISK FACTORS   *Breast Cancer*

As you conduct a health history related to the breasts, it is important to consider common risk factors associated with breast cancer and follow up with additional questions should they exist.

- *Gender:* Females account for 99% of breast cancer cases.
- *Age:* Risk increases with age; 18% of cases are diagnosed in women between ages 40 and 50, and 77% are older than age 50.
- *Race/ethnicity:* White women have the highest incidence of breast cancer.
- *Genetic:* 10% of breast cancer cases are associated with a genetic mutation of BRCA-1 or BRCA-2.
- *Family history:* Breast cancer in a first-degree family relative (on either maternal or paternal side) especially before age 50 increases risk; risk is highest if relative is mother or sister.
- *Personal medical history:*
  Those with a history of breast cancer have increased risk of subsequent episodes.
  Those with a history of proliferative breast disease with a biopsy-confirmed atypical hyperplasia have increased risk.
  Exposure to ionizing radiation to chest area as child or young adult (for treatment of other cancer such as Hodgkin's disease) increases risk.
- *Reproductive history:*
  Long menstrual history (menarche before age 12; menopause after age 50) increases risk.
  Nulliparity increases risk.
  First full-term pregnancy after age 30 increases risk.
- *Breast density:* Increased breast density is associated with higher risk of breast cancer.
- *Estrogen replacement:* Hormone replacement therapy for more than 5 years after menopause increases risk. (M)
- *Alcohol intake:* Increased alcohol intake (two to five drinks a day) is associated with increased risk. (M)
- *Obesity:* Obesity, especially after age 50, or increased weight gain as an adult increases breast cancer risk. (M)

From American Cancer Society: *Cancer facts and figures, 2007,* Atlanta, 2007, American Cancer Society; American Cancer Society: What are risk factors for breast cancer? American Cancer Society website (available at *www.cancer.org*).
M = modifiable risk factor.

GENERAL HEALTH HISTORY

Present Health Status

Do you perform breast self-examination (BSE)? If so, how often?

Evaluating self-care behaviors helps guide further education and encourages health-enhancing behaviors. Women should know how their breasts normally feel and be encouraged to report any breast change promptly to their health care providers.

Do you have regular examination of your breasts by a health care professional? If so, how often? Have you ever had a mammogram? If so, when was your last mammogram? How frequently do you have a mammogram?

Clinical breast examination (CBE) is recommended every 3 years for women between ages 20 and 39 and annually for women starting at age 40 (Smith, 2003). Because mammography is considered an effective method for breast cancer screening, it is important to determine if and when last mammography was done in women over 40.

What medications do you currently take? Do you take vitamin supplements? If so, which vitamins?
Some medications such as oral contraceptives can cause cyclic breast discomfort or nipple discharge. Some individuals take vitamin E supplementation to reduce symptoms of breast edema and tenderness.

How much chocolate and caffeine do you consume each day or each week?
A diet high in methylxanthines (found in foods containing caffeine) may cause benign breast disease such as fibrocystic changes.

Past Medical History

Have you ever had a breast problem such as fibrocystic breast changes, fibroadenomas, or breast cancer? If so, describe. When did it occur? How was it diagnosed? How was it treated?
A history of breast cancer increases the risk of recurrence. Fibrocystic disease and fibroadenoma complicate the evaluation of the breasts because the presence of cysts makes it difficult to detect new masses or lumps.

Do you have a past medical history involving ovarian cancer, endometrial cancer, or colon cancer?
A personal history of ovarian, endometrial, or colon cancer increases the risk of breast cancer.

Have you ever had surgery on a breast (e.g., biopsy, mastectomy, lumpectomy, or breast reduction or augmentation)? If so, when was it, and what was it for?
This is helpful background information: it may affect findings noted with examination.

How old were you when you began menstruating? How old were you at menopause (if appropriate)?
Menarche before age 12 or menopause after age 50 increases the risk for breast cancer.

Have you ever been pregnant? If so, at what age did you have your children?
Nulliparous or first child born after age 30 is a risk factor for breast cancer.

Family History

Is there a history of breast cancer or breast disease in your family? If so, in whom? At what age did this relative have breast cancer or disease? Did it affect one or both breasts?
Family history is a risk factor for breast cancer, particularly if it involves first-degree relatives. A premenopausal onset and bilateral disease increases the risk further.

PROBLEM-BASED HISTORY

The most commonly reported problems related to the breasts are pain or tenderness, breast lump, nipple discharge, and pain or lumps in the axillae. As with symptoms in all areas of health assessment, a symptom analysis is completed, which includes the onset, location, duration, characteristics, aggravating and alleviating factors, related symptoms, and treatments (see Box 3-3 in Chapter 3).

Breast Pain or Tenderness

Where does it hurt? Is it in one breast or both? Is there a specific location, or is the pain generalized? When did the pain in your breasts first begin?
Determine the onset and location of the breast pain. Pain occurring bilaterally is more likely attributed to hormonal effects; pain in one breast could suggest a pathologic condition.

Describe the pain. Rate the severity of the pain on a scale from 0 to 10. Does the pain or tenderness prevent you from carrying out routine activities?
Determine the characteristics of the pain. Some women with breast cancer report a burning or pulling sensation in addition to a vague pain. Rapidly growing cysts may be very painful. Limitations in activity may also help the nurse understand how the pain affects the client.

Have you noticed any specific activities that bring on the pain? For example, do you experience pain during sexual activity? When you exercise? When wearing a certain bra, or when not wearing a bra?
Determine any aggravating factors for the pain. Strenuous activity can bring on pain, as can the other specific causes noted.

Have you noted any recent changes in your breasts, such as changes in size, shape, tenderness, lumps, or discharge?
Question the client for associated symptoms with the breast pain.

Is the breast tenderness associated with a swollen feeling to the breasts? If yes, when do you notice the swelling? Is the swelling related to your menstrual cycle?
Cyclic bilateral breast edema or fullness is a normal occurrence caused by hormonal fluctuations associated with the menstrual cycle. Significant edema should be further evaluated, especially if it is unilateral, has other associated findings, or influences the woman's ability to participate in normal activities.

Breast Lump

Where is the breast lump? When did you first notice the lump?

Establish the onset and location of all breast lumps. Some lumps may be present over a period of several years. If such lumps do not undergo change, they may be insignificant but still should be examined. Any new lumps or changes in a previously identified lump should be of particular concern.

Is the lump always present, or does it seem to come and go? Is there a relationship between the lumps and your menstrual cycle?

Lumps that change in size in relation to the menstrual cycle may be influenced by hormonal fluctuations.

Is the lump tender to the touch? If yes, does the severity of the tenderness change related to menstruation?

Determine the characteristics of the lump. Some lumps are tender whereas others are painless. The degree of pain or tenderness may be affected by hormonal fluctuations.

Have you recently experienced injury to the breasts? If yes, did the lump develop after the injury?

Lumps resulting from an injury may be associated with a hematoma. Typically these resolve in a short period of time.

Have you noticed any other symptoms such as redness, swelling, or dimpling associated with this lump?

Determine associated changes to the breast—redness, edema, localized heat, rash, and dimpling are all symptoms requiring further evaluation.

Nipple Discharge

When did you first notice the discharge from your nipple? Have you ever noticed this before? Does it affect one or both nipples?

Determine onset, location, and duration of nipple discharge. Unilateral nipple discharge is concerning because it is more commonly associated with a pathologic condition than is bilateral nipple discharge (Hussain, Policarpio, & 2006).

Describe the discharge. Color? Is it thick or thin? Is there an odor associated with the discharge? Does the discharge occur at specific times, such as always before your menstrual period or with breast manipulation?

Nipple discharge may indicate a pathologic condition. A bloody or blood-tinged discharge is alarming and must be investigated.

Does the discharge occur spontaneously, or does it occur only when expressed?

If the discharge is spontaneous, it is helpful to know if this occurs intermittently or constantly. Spontaneous discharge is considered an abnormal finding. Discharge that is not spontaneous may result from medications or from endocrine disorders.

Have you noticed other symptoms such as breast pain or a breast lump?

Determine if there are any other associated breast symptoms or onset of other symptoms. Headaches or changes in vision along with nipple discharge may suggest a pituitary tumor or mass (Hussain, Policarpio, & Vincent, 2006).

Axillary Lumps or Tenderness

When did you first notice the lumps or tenderness under your arms?

Because the tail of Spence extends up into the axilla and because most lymphatic drainage flows toward the axillary nodes, a symptom analysis for lumps and tenderness is needed. Determine the onset of symptoms.

Where is the lump or tenderness located? Under one arm or both arms? Does this come and go, or is it always present? Has the tenderness or lump gotten worse?

Determine the location and characteristics of the lump or tenderness.

Do you shave your underarms? If so, how often? Do you notice a relationship to shaving your arms and the tenderness? Do you use deodorant or antiperspirant under your arms?

Shaving and use of deodorants and antiperspirants can cause discomfort and a mild inflammation to the axilla.

What have you done to treat this, if anything?

Explore self-care practices; this may be helpful to guide future treatment strategies.

Breast Swelling or Enlargement (Men)

Describe the change to your breast you have been experiencing. When did you first notice it? Have the changes occurred on one or both sides?

Gynecomastia is the enlargement of one or both breasts in the male. Although it may occur at any time, it is most prevalent during puberty and in the older adult man. Although breast cancer in men is rare, the most common initial symptom is a breast mass.

Have you experienced any other symptoms such as pain or discharge?

Nipple discharge is an uncommon associated symptom of breast cancer in the male, but when it occurs, it is usually serosanguineous.

HEALTH PROMOTION   *Breast Cancer*

It is estimated that 180,510 women were diagnosed with breast cancer in 2007, making it the most frequently diagnosed nonskin cancer in women. Additionally, breast cancer is the second leading cancer-related cause of death in women; an estimated 40,460 women were expected to die from breast cancer in 2007.

Goals and Objectives—*Healthy People 2010*
The overall *Healthy People 2010* goal related to cancer is to reduce the number of new cancer cases, as well as illness, disability, and death caused by cancer. Two specific objectives relate to breast cancer: (1) reduce the breast cancer death rate and (2) increase the proportion of women age 40 or over who have received a mammogram within the preceding 2 years.

Recommendations to Reduce Risk (Primary Prevention)
U.S. Preventive Services Task Force
- Tamoxifen and raloxifen should not be used for the primary prevention of breast cancer in women at low or average risk for breast cancer.

Screening Recommendations (Secondary Prevention)
American Cancer Society
- Annual screening mammography should be done for women of average risk at age 40. Women should have the opportunity to become informed about the benefits, limitations, and potential harm associated with regular screening.
- CBE is recommended as part of a periodic health examination at least every 3 years for average-risk, asymptomatic women in their twenties and thirties, and annually for asymptomatic women age 40 and over.
- Women in their twenties should be informed about the benefits and limitations of BSE. Women who choose to do BSE should be instructed and have their technique reviewed during periodic health examinations. It is acceptable for women to choose not to perform BSE or to perform BSE on an irregular basis.

From American Cancer Society: *Cancer facts and figures, 2007*, Atlanta, 2007, American Cancer Society; Smith RA et al: American Cancer Society guidelines for breast cancer screening: update 2003, *CA Cancer J Clin* 53:141-169, 2003; US Department of Health and Human Services: Cancer. In *Healthy People 2010: understanding and improving health*, ed 2, Washington, DC, 2000, US Government Printing Office (available at *www.healthypeople.gov*).
BSE, Breast self-examination; *CBE,* clinical breast examination.

EXAMINATION

ROUTINE TECHNIQUES

- INSPECT both breasts.
- INSPECT the skin of the breasts.
- INSPECT the areolae.
- INSPECT the nipples.
- INSPECT the axillae.

SPECIAL CIRCUMSTANCES OR ADVANCED PRACTICE

- INSPECT the breasts in various postures.
- PALPATE the breasts and axillae.
- PALPATE the nipples.

EQUIPMENT NEEDED
Gloves in presence of nipple drainage or open lesions

PROCEDURES AND TECHNIQUES WITH NORMAL FINDINGS

ABNORMAL FINDINGS

FEMALE BREAST EXAMINATION

ROUTINE TECHNIQUES

Always explain the procedure to the client before you begin. Let her know that you will be touching her breasts, and be sure to obtain her permission before you begin the examination. Initially, position the client so that she is sitting on the examination table facing you. She should be sitting erect with her gown dropped to the waist.

PROCEDURES AND TECHNIQUES WITH NORMAL FINDINGS

INSPECT the breasts, noting size, shape, contour, and symmetry.

Start by inspecting the breasts with the client sitting with her arms at her sides. It is common for the breasts to be slightly unequal in size. Breast size may vary significantly, but symmetry or only slight asymmetry should be considered normal. The breast contour should be smooth, convex, and even (Fig. 17-4). Gently lift each breast with your fingers and inspect the lower and outer aspects of each breast for dimpling, retraction, or bulging.

INSPECT the skin of the breasts for color, pigmentation, vascularity, surface characteristics, and lesions.

The skin of the breast should appear smooth and evenly pigmented. The skin color should be similar to skin on the rest of the body, although it may be lighter in color compared with sun-exposed skin surfaces. The venous patterns should be bilaterally similar. The venous pattern may be pronounced in obese or pregnant females.

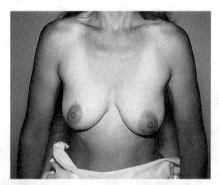

Fig. 17-4   Breasts should appear bilaterally symmetric.

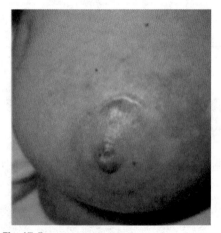

Fig. 17-5   Erythema of the breast. *(From Swartz, 2002.)*

ABNORMAL FINDINGS

Note evidence of marked asymmetry of size or shape of the breasts. Significant and rapid changes in the size of one breast could indicate an inflammatory process or a growth. Dimpling, retraction, or bulging could indicate a malignancy.

Note any localized or generalized areas of discoloration. Inflammation, e.g., cellulitis, or breast abscess in the breast tissue may cause surface erythema and heat (Fig. 17-5).

A rash on both breasts is likely caused by a dermatitis; unilateral breast rash, especially surrounding the areola, could be associated with Paget's disease of the breast.

Unilateral hyperpigmentation is also considered an abnormal finding. Obese women, or women with large breasts, may have a red rash with demarcated borders from candidiasis due to excessive moisture.

Unilateral venous patterns on the breast may occur secondary to dilated superficial veins from an increased blood flow to a malignancy. Roughened, tough, or thickened skin is considered abnormal. Edema may give the skin an orange-like texture termed *peau d'orange* (Fig. 17-6). Note any lesions or newly developed moles or those that have changed or are tender.

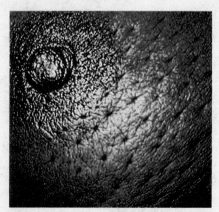

Fig. 17-6   Peau d'orange appearance caused by edema. *(From Gallager et al, 1978.)*

PROCEDURES AND TECHNIQUES WITH NORMAL FINDINGS

INSPECT the areolae for color and surface characteristics.

The color of the areola may vary depending on the client's skin color. Figure 17-7 shows the variations of areola color, ranging from pink to black. The areola should be round or oval and appear bilaterally similar. Montgomery's tubercles (Fig. 17-7, *B*) may appear as slightly raised bumps on the areola tissue. Hairs on the nipple may also be seen. These are all normal variations.

INSPECT the nipples for position, symmetry, surface characteristics, lesions, bleeding, and discharge.

Most women's nipples protrude, although some may appear to be flat or actually inverted. All should be considered normal if they have remained unchanged throughout adult life, and the nipples are symmetric bilaterally. Nipple *inversion* (a nipple that is recessed as opposed to protruding) can be a normal or an abnormal finding. Consider it normal if it is not a new finding and if it can be everted with manipulation.

ABNORMAL FINDINGS

Abnormal findings include areolae that are unequal bilaterally, have an irregular shape, or have lesions or changes in pigmentation.

Nipples that point in different directions, or those that are not symmetric, should be considered abnormal. Recent nipple inversion or nipple *retraction* (a nipple that is pointing or pulled in a different direction) is suggestive of malignancy, and the client should be referred for further evaluation (Fig. 17-8).

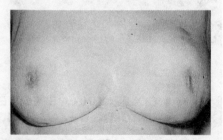

Fig. 17-8 Nipple retraction. *(From Mansel and Bundred, 1995.)*

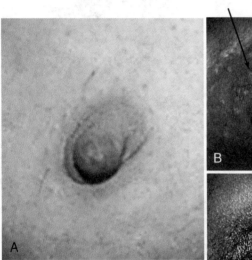
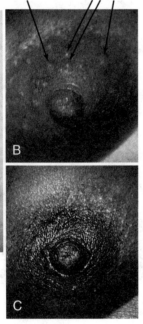

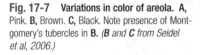

Fig. 17-7 Variations in color of areola. **A,** Pink. **B,** Brown. **C,** Black. Note presence of Montgomery's tubercles in **B.** *(B and C from Seidel et al, 2006.)*

PROCEDURES AND TECHNIQUES WITH NORMAL FINDINGS

Nipples are normally smooth and intact without evidence of crusting, bleeding, or discharge. Note presence of supernumerary nipples. Supernumerary nipples are considered a normal variation, although they are uncommon. These nipples look similar to pink or brown moles and generally appear along the embryonic "milk line" (Fig. 17-9).

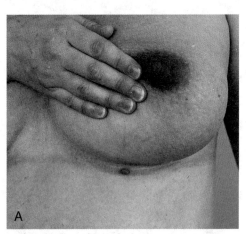 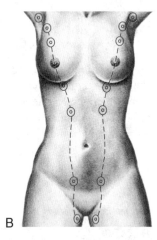

Fig. 17-9 **A,** Supernumerary nipple. **B,** Supernumerary nipples may arise along the "milk line." **(A,** From Mansel Bundred, 1995. **B,** From Thompson et al, 2002.)

<table>
<tr><td>**BOX 17-1**</td><td>**COLLECTING A SPECIMEN FOR CYTOLOGIC EXAMINATION**</td></tr>
</table>

Cytologic examination of nipple discharge requires proper specimen collection and management. Wearing gloves, express a small amount of nipple discharge. Use a cotton-tipped applicator to collect a small sample of the discharge. Using a rolling technique, smear the discharge from the cotton-tipped applicator on a clear microscopic slide and spray with cytologic fixative. Be sure to label the specimen with the client's name, the date, and the source (right or left breast).

ABNORMAL FINDINGS

Deviations from normal include nipple edema, redness, pigment changes, ulceration or crusting, erosion or scaling, and wrinkling or cracking. A red, scaly nipple with discharge and crusting that lasts more than a few weeks could indicate *Paget's disease,* a rare type of breast cancer (Fig. 17-10). Nipple discharge is usually considered an abnormal finding. If a client has nipple discharge, a specimen should be collected for possible cytologic examination (Box 17-1). Table 17-1 presents various types of discharge and possible causes.

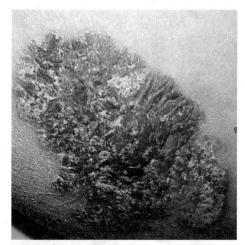

Fig. 17-10 Paget's disease. *(From Habif, 1996.)*

TABLE 17-1 *Nipple Discharge*

COLOR OF DISCHARGE	POSSIBLE CAUSE
Serous (yellow)	Usually normal
Serosanguineous (straw colored)	Carcinoma
	Ductal ectasia
Sanguineous (bloody)	Carcinoma
	Intraductal papilloma
	Ductal ectasia
	Prepartum women from vascular engorgement
Clear (watery)	Pharmacologic causes
	Carcinoma
Milky	Pituitary adenoma
	Pharmacologic causes
	Galactorrhea
Purulent	Infectious process
	Ductal ectasia
Multicolored (green, gray, brown)	Fibrocystic changes
	Carcinoma
	Infectious process
	Ductal ectasia

PROCEDURES AND TECHNIQUES WITH NORMAL FINDINGS	ABNORMAL FINDINGS

SPECIAL CIRCUMSTANCES OR ADVANCED PRACTICE

INSPECT the breasts in various positions for bilateral pull, symmetry, and contour.

Ask the client to remain seated and raise her arms over her head (Fig. 17-11, *A*). This position adds tension to the suspensory ligaments and will accentuate dimpling or retractions. Observe and compare the breasts, areola, and nipples. Then evaluate for any bilateral pull on the suspensory ligaments. The breasts should appear equal on both sides (bilaterally symmetric).

With her arms still raised, have the client lean forward (Fig. 17-11, *B*). It may be helpful for the nurse to hold onto the client's hands to provide balance.

Inspect the breasts for symmetry and bilateral pull, as previously described. The breasts should hang equally with a smooth contour, and pull should be symmetric. This is an especially useful technique if the client has large and pendulous breasts, because the breasts fall away from the chest wall and hang freely. Next, inspect the breasts while the seated client pushes her hands onto her hips or pushes her palms together, thus contracting the pectoral muscles (Fig. 17-11, *C*). There should be no deviations in contour and symmetry of the breasts.

Note any asymmetry or appearance of attachment (fixation), bulging, or retraction of either breast.

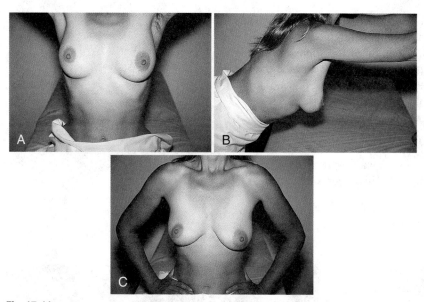

Fig. 17-11 **A,** Client with arms extended overhead. **B,** Client with arms raised and leaning forward. **C,** Client sitting and pressing her hands on hips.

PROCEDURES AND TECHNIQUES WITH NORMAL FINDINGS

INSPECT and PALPATE the axillae for evidence of rash, lesions, or masses.

Procedure. Instruct the client to relax both arms at her sides. Using your left hand (if you are right-handed), lift one of the client's arms and support it so that her muscles are loose and relaxed (Fig. 17-12). While in this position, use your right hand to palpate each axilla. (If the client has a rash or an open lesion in the axilla, wear examination gloves.) You must have short fingernails to prevent injury to the client.

Reach your fingers deep into the axilla, and slowly and firmly slide your fingers along the client's chest wall, first down the middle of the axilla, then along the anterior border of the axilla, and finally along the posterior border. Then turn your hand over and examine the inner aspect of the client's upper arm. During all maneuvers, position the client's arm with your other hand to maximize the examining area. In all positions, palpate for areas of enlargement, masses, lymph nodes, or isolated areas of tenderness. Palpation of lymph nodes in the axilla is included with CBE because lymph nodes are accessible and may provide clues regarding the presence of inflammation or lesions.

Findings. The nurse should not expect to palpate lymph nodes of the breast.

PALPATE the breasts for tissue characteristics.

Position. The preferred position for breast palpation is supine with a small pillow or towel placed under the shoulder of the breast to be examined. Instruct the client to place her arm over her head. The combination of the slight shoulder elevation and the arm positioning flattens the breast tissue evenly over the chest wall. A sitting position may be used if the client has difficulty lying down, if the client is young and has very small breasts, or if the client has very large breasts making palpation difficult in a supine position.

Technique. Using the finger pads of the first two or three fingers of your examining hand, gently, firmly, and systematically palpate all four quadrants of the breast and the tail of Spence (Fig. 17-13). Use a systematic approach to breast palpation that begins and ends at a designated point. This ensures that all areas of the breast are examined.

ABNORMAL FINDINGS

Infections in the breast, arm, and even the hand may cause lymphatic drainage into the axillary area. Enlargement and tenderness of lymph nodes in the axilla may indicate such an infection. Hard, fixed nodules or masses may suggest metastatic carcinoma or lymphoma.

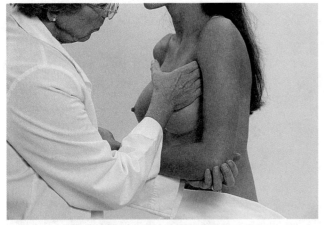

Fig. 17-12 Raise and support client's arm while palpating axilla.

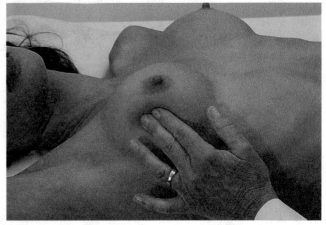

Fig. 17-13 Palpate the breasts using your finger pads.

PROCEDURES AND TECHNIQUES WITH NORMAL FINDINGS

Several motions may be used for breast palpation (Table 17-2). Press firmly enough to get a feel of the underlying tissue, but not so firmly that the tissue is compressed against the rib cage. Do not lift your fingers from the chest wall during the palpation because this breaks the continuity of the palpation. Instead, gently slide your fingers over the breast tissue, moving along the designated pattern of palpation.

If the sitting position is used for a woman with very large breasts, ask the client to lean slightly forward, and position your hands between the breasts as shown in Fig. 17-14. While supporting the inferior side of the breast with one hand, palpate the breast with the other hand starting at the top of the breast and slowly slide the finger pads down the breast. Repeat the technique until all breast tissue is examined. If a mass is identified, specifically palpate the mass for characteristics, including its location, size, shape, consistency, tenderness, mobility, delineation of borders, and retraction (Fig. 17-15). Characteristics that should be included when assessing a mass are presented in Box 17-2. Transillumination may be used to confirm the presence of fluid in superficial masses.

ABNORMAL FINDINGS

Abnormal findings during the breast palpation include masses or isolated areas of tenderness or pain. Conditions that may cause lumps or masses include breast cancer, fibroadenoma, and fibrocystic breast disease. These are discussed in greater detail in the common problems and conditions later in this chapter. Breast engorgement (in clients who are not pregnant or premenstrual) is also an abnormal finding.

TABLE 17-2 *Methods for Breast Palpation*

Circular Method

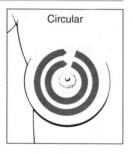

This is the most common palpation technique. Place the finger pads of your middle three fingers against the outer edge of the breast. Press gently in small circles around the breast until you reach the nipple. Try not to lift your fingers off the breast as you move from one point to another.

Wedge Method

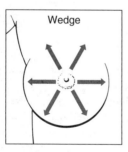

Place the finger pads of your middle three fingers on the areola, and palpate from the center of the breast outward. Return your fingers to the areola and again palpate from center outward covering another section of the breast (in a spokelike fashion). Repeat this until the entire breast has been covered.

Vertical Strip Method

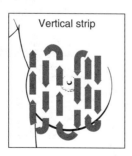

Place the finger pads of your middle three fingers against the top outer edge of the breast. Palpate downward, then upward, working your way across the entire breast.

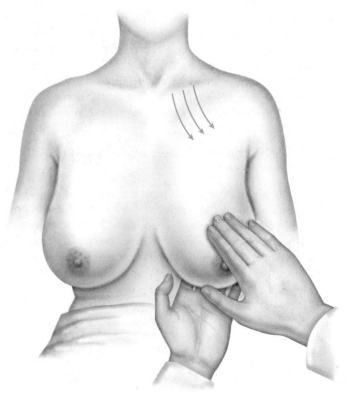

Fig. 17-14 Manual palpation of large breasts. *(From Seidel et al, 2003.)*

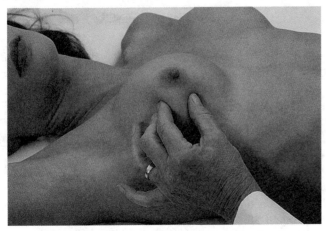

Fig. 17-15   Palpate the borders and mobility of a breast mass.

| BOX 17-2 | **BREAST MASS CHARACTERISTICS** |

Note and record the following:
- *Location:* Which breast; which quadrant (may describe as position on the clock or draw on chart to show location).
- *Size:* Measure the width, length, and thickness in centimeters.
- *Shape:* Is the mass oval, round, lobed, irregularly shaped, or indistinct?
- *Consistency:* Is the mass hard, soft, firm, or rubbery?
- *Tenderness:* Is the mass tender during palpation?
- *Mobility:* Does the lump move during palpation or is it fixed to the overlying skin or the underlying chest wall?
- *Borders:* Are the edges of the mass discrete or poorly defined?
- *Retractions:* Is there any dimpling of the tissue around the mass?

Modified from Seidel HM et al: *Mosby's guide to physical examination,* ed 6, St Louis, 2006, Mosby.

PROCEDURES AND TECHNIQUES WITH NORMAL FINDINGS

Findings. The breast should feel firm, smooth, and elastic, without the presence of lumps or nodules. Typically the breast should be nontender on palpation. After pregnancy or menopause, the breast tissue may feel softer and looser. During the premenstrual period, the client's breasts may be engorged, may be slightly tender, and may have generalized nodularity. Most women have a firm transverse ridge along the lower edge of the breast termed the *inframammary ridge.* This firm ridge is normal and should not be mistaken for a breast mass.

PALPATE the nipples for surface characteristics and discharge.

With the client in the supine position, palpate the nipples. The nipples should be soft and pliable with no masses or discharge. If a discharge is present, note the color, consistency, quantity, and odor. Try to determine the origin of the discharge by gently palpating the areola completely around the nipple with your index finger (Fig. 17-16). Observe for the appearance of discharge through one of the duct openings. NOTE: Wear examination gloves if there is a history of nipple discharge or if discharge is observed.

ABNORMAL FINDINGS

Thickening of the nipple tissue, a mass, and loss of elasticity are signs consistent with malignancy. Nipple discharge is considered an abnormal finding except during pregnancy or lactation (see Table 17-1). Discharge may occur secondary to fluid retention of the ducts, infection, hormonal flux, or carcinoma. If a nipple discharge is present, a specimen should be collected for possible cytologic evaluation (see Box 17-1).

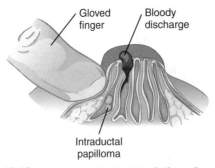

Gloved finger

Bloody discharge

Intraductal papilloma

Fig. 17-16   Express nipple discharge by palpating on the areola.

PROCEDURES AND TECHNIQUES WITH NORMAL FINDINGS

ABNORMAL FINDINGS

MALE BREAST EXAMINATION

As part of a comprehensive examination, it is essential to examine the male client's breasts. Inspect the male breast while the client is seated with his arms at his sides.

INSPECT the breasts and nipples.

With the client in a seated position, inspect both breasts, looking for breast symmetry, color, skin lesions, and enlargement. The breasts should be flat and without rashes or lesions. Men who are overweight often have a thicker fatty layer of tissue on the chest, giving the appearance of breast enlargement. If this is noted, it is important to determine if there has been a history of weight gain. If the client reports that his breasts became full as he gained weight, the condition is most likely within normal limits. The nipple and areolar areas should be intact, smooth, and of equal color, size, and shape bilaterally.

Note any asymmetry or distinct differences between the two sides. Note any ulcerations, masses, or swelling. If the client reports a sudden bilateral or unilateral breast enlargement with associated tenderness, the nurse should consider the situation abnormal and should refer the client for further evaluation.

PALPATE the breasts and nipples

With the client in the same position, palpate the breasts and areolar areas. The tissue should feel smooth, intact, and nontender. Note evidence of tenderness, unilateral enlargement, or masses.

Unilateral or bilateral breast enlargement in men is termed *gynecomastia*. Breast cancer can occur in men. It commonly manifests as a hard, painless, irregular nodule often fixed to the area under the nipple. These conditions are discussed in greater detail later in this chapter.

PALPATE the axilla.

If not already done as part of the lymphatic assessment, palpate the client's axillary area for tenderness or lymphatic enlargement. Palpation of the axilla of a male client provides information about the lymphatic system. Lymph nodes should not be palpable, or they should be small, soft, mobile, and nontender.

The presence of a lump is considered abnormal. See abnormal findings of axilla previously described in the female exam.

FREQUENTLY ASKED QUESTIONS

It is embarrassing to think about performing a breast examination on a client. What can be done to get over this?
This is not an uncommon feeling for a beginner to have. Probably the most important thing to consider first are your own feelings about breast examination in general. Are you uncomfortable about the thought of touching someone else's breasts? Is the discomfort associated with your own perceived inability or lack of experience? Another key point is to consider the therapeutic purpose for the exam; remember this is simply a process of data collection and an opportunity for client teaching. Like most other skills, you will become less nervous with experience. As you gain experience, you will also gain confidence. You will also feel more confident about performing a breast examination if you have established a solid rapport with your client. Typically, you will perform less invasive examination procedures first, so by the time you get to the breast examination, you and the client will feel more at ease with one another.

FREQUENTLY ASKED QUESTIONS

What is the difference between a clinical breast examination and a breast self-examination?

A *clinical breast examination* (CBE) is performed by a health care professional, usually as part of an annual examination. It involves inspection and palpation of the breasts and axilla. Although this examination can be performed by any nurse, most often it is performed by nurse practitioners. The primary goal of the CBE is to detect breast cancer. A *breast self-examination* (BSE) is performed by women on themselves. Until recently it was strongly recommended that all women perform BSE; it is now considered optional. Women who choose to do this are taught to inspect their breasts in the mirror and palpate their breasts and axillae on a monthly basis. The primary goal of BSE is to increase women's self-awareness regarding how their breasts normally feel so that any changes will be detected. For further information, see the Health Promotion box regarding breast examination in this chapter.

Documenting Expected Findings

Breast

Female breast exam

Breasts moderate size, evenly pigmented, bilaterally symmetric, and hang equally with smooth contour. Venous patterns bilaterally similar. Breasts firm, smooth, elastic without tenderness, lumps, or nodules. Areola round, nipples protruding, symmetric, soft, pliable, smooth, and intact without discharge. Axillary lymph nodes are not palpated.

Male breast exam

Nipples and areola intact, smooth, evenly pigmented and of equal color, size and shape bilaterally. Tissue feels smooth, intact and nontender. Axillary lymph nodes are not palpated.

AGE-RELATED VARIATIONS

INFANTS AND CHILDREN

The breast assessment among infants and children requires only inspection. Neonates of both genders may have slightly enlarged breast secondary to the mother's estrogen. Maternal hormones are also responsible for a small, watery, whitish discharge referred to as "witch's milk" seen in small percent of newborns during the first few weeks of life. Chapter 20 presents further information regarding the assessment of the breasts in these age groups.

ADOLESCENTS

Breast development (known as *thelarche*) initially begins in preadolescence and continues through adolescence. Girls are often sensitive about having their breasts exposed for examination; thus the nurse must take the time to reassure them and ensure privacy. Males may experience an unexpected enlargement of the breasts (known as gynecomastia) as a result of obesity or body change transition during early puberty. Chapter 20 presents further information regarding breast assessment among adolescent clients.

OLDER ADULTS

Atrophic changes to the female breast begin by age 40 and continue through menopause. As the glandular tissue atrophies, the breast tissue is gradually replaced with fat and connective tissue. Postmenopausal women should continue to have regular breast examinations because of the increased risk of breast cancer with age. Chapter 22 presents further information regarding breast assessment among older adults.

CLIENTS WITH SITUATIONAL VARIATIONS

CLIENTS WITH A MASTECTOMY

Women who have had a mastectomy require the same breast assessment as all other women. Many women experience anxiety or fear as they worry about the recurrence of cancer or metastasis. Some women may also have personal issues regarding body image and may feel self-conscious about exposing the chest. The nurse should be sensitive to this but also reassure the client that it is necessary to perform a comprehensive examination. In addition to examining the remaining breast in the usual manner, the nurse should assess the mastectomy site and the scar because malignancy recurrence is possible at the scar site (Fig. 17-17, A). The mastectomy site and axilla should be inspected for color changes, redness, rash, irritation, and visible signs of edema, thicken-

ing, or lumps. Note areas that may have had muscle resection. Also note any signs of lymphedema in the affected upper extremity. Lymphedema is a localized accumulation of lymph fluid in the interstitial spaces caused by removal of the lymph nodes.

Using the finger pads of your examining hand, palpate the side with the mastectomy, especially around the area of the scar. Use a small circular motion, assessing for thickening, lumps, edema, or tenderness; then use a sweeping motion to palpate the entire chest area on the affected side to ensure that nothing has been missed. Finally, palpate the axillary and supraclavicular areas for lymph nodes. If the client has had breast reconstruction or augmentation, perform the breast examination in the usual manner, paying particular attention to scars (Fig. 17-17, B and C).

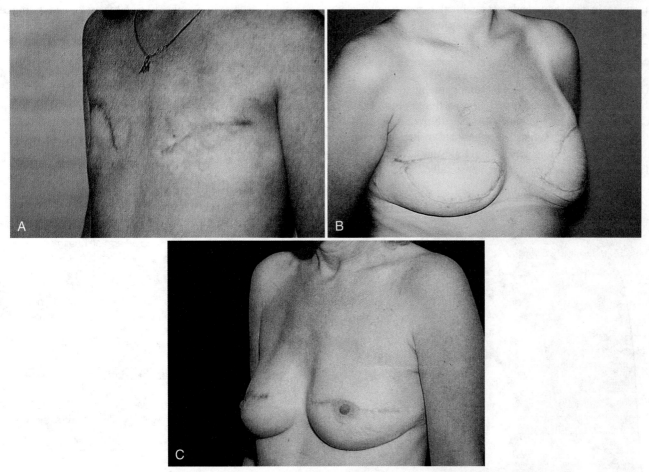

Fig. 17-17   **A,** Appearance of chest following bilateral mastectomy. Postoperative breast reconstruction before, **B,** and after, **C,** nipple-areolar reconstruction. *(Courtesy Brian W. Davies. From Fortunato and McCullough, 1998.)*

COMMON PROBLEMS & CONDITIONS

BENIGN BREAST DISEASE

Noncancerous breast conditions account for 90% of clinical breast problems. *Benign breast disease* is a term that represents a number of breast-related problems, including breast pain or tenderness, swelling, lumps, discharge, and inflammation.

Fibrocystic Changes to the Breast

The term *fibrocystic changes to the breast* refers to a variety of conditions associated with multiple benign masses within the breast caused by ductal enlargement and the formation of fluid-filled cysts, commonly seen among middle aged women (Fig. 17-18). **Clinical Findings:** Typically, cysts manifest as one or more palpable masses that are round, well delineated, mobile, and tender. The degree of discomfort experienced can range from slightly tender to very painful; the cysts often fluctuate in size and tenderness with the menstrual cycle. Symptoms tend to subside after menopause (Table 19-3).

Fibroadenoma

This is a common benign breast tumor among young women that consists of glandular and fibrous tissue (Fig. 17-19). **Clinical Findings:** Fibroadenoma usually manifests unilaterally as a small, solitary, firm, rubbery, nontender lump (Marchant, 2002). It is generally mobile and well delineated. This tumor does not change premenstrually.

Ductal Ectasia

Ductal ectasia is a benign breast disease characterized by inflammation and dilation involving one or multiple subareolar ducts. It affects perimenopausal and postmenopausal women. **Clinical Findings:** The initial symptom is a sticky nipple discharge that is commonly dark green or black (Rahal et al., 2005). As the disease progresses, inflammatory signs and symptoms occur. The woman may experience burning or itching of the nipple and edema in the areolar area. The discharge may become purulent or sanguineous. A complication that can occur is a breast abscess.

Intraductal Papilloma

An intraductal papilloma is a small, benign, wartlike tumor growth in the major ducts usually within 1 to 2 cm of the areolar edge. One or more ducts may be affected. This most commonly occurs in women 40 to 60 years of age. **Clinical Findings:** The clinical presentation usually associated with intraductal papilloma is a spontaneous bloody discharge from the nipple; occasionally a mass is palpated.

BREAST CANCER

Breast cancer is a major health problem for women. It is the most common non–skin-related malignancy in American women.

ETHNIC & CULTURAL VARIATIONS

Healthy People 2010 is designed to achieve two overarching goals: increase quality and years of healthy life and eliminate health disparities. Eliminating racial and ethnic disparities in health requires enhanced efforts at preventing disease, promoting health, and delivering appropriate care. One of the focus areas in which racial and ethnic minorities experience disparity related to health access and outcome is cancer screening and management.
- White women have a higher incidence of breast cancer than nonwhites.
- Hispanic women have the lowest rate of cancer screening of any ethnic group.
- African American women are more likely to die from breast cancer than are women of any other racial or ethnic group.

Invasive Breast Cancer

The most common type of breast cancer is an invasive malignancy arising from the ducts or the lobules. Breast cancer is most prevalent in women ages 40 to 60 years (see Table 17-3).

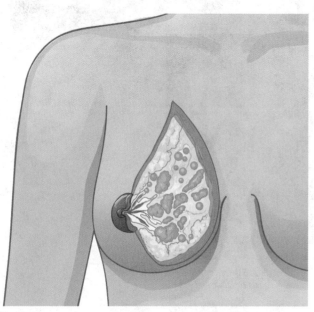

Fig. 17-18   Fibrocystic changes to the breast. The cysts are depicted as green masses.

TABLE 17-3 *Differentiation of Breast Masses*

	FIBROCYSTIC CHANGES TO BREAST	FIBROADENOMA	CANCER
Age range	20-49	15-55	30-80
Occurrence	Usually bilateral	Usually bilateral	Usually unilateral
Location	Upper outer quadrant	No specific location	48% occur in the upper outer quadrant, but may occur in any part of the breast or axillary tail
Nipple discharge	No	No	If present, may be bloody or clear
Pain	Yes	No	Usually none
Number	Multiple or single	Single; may be multiple	Single
Shape	Rounded	Rounded or discoid	Irregular or stellate
Consistency	Soft to firm; tense	Firm, rubbery	Hard, stonelike
Mobility	Mobile	Mobile	Fixed
Retraction signs	Absent	Absent	Often present
Tenderness	Usually tender	Usually nontender	Usually nontender
Borders	Well delineated	Well delineated	Poorly delineated; irregular
Variations with menses	Yes	No	No

Modified from Seidel HM et al: *Mosby's guide to physical examination,* ed 6, St Louis, 2006, Mosby; Fogel CI, Woods NF: *Health care of women: a nursing perspective,* St Louis, 1981, Mosby.

Clinical Findings: A breast malignancy usually manifests as a solitary, unilateral, nontender lump, thickening, or mass (Fig. 17-20). As the mass grows, there may be breast asymmetry, discoloration (erythema or ecchymosis), unilateral vein prominence, peau d'orange, ulceration, dimpling, puckering, or retraction of the skin. The lesion is sometimes fixed to underlying tissue. Its borders are irregular and poorly delineated. The nipple may be inverted or diverted to one side. A serosanguineous or clear nipple discharge may be present. There may be crusting around the nipple or erosion of the nipple or areola. Lymph nodes may be palpable in the axilla.

Noninvasive Breast Cancer

Two types of cancers categorized as noninvasive are ductal carcinoma in situ (DCIS) and lobular carcinoma in situ (LCIS). The term *in situ* is used to describe an early, noninvasive stage of cancer. DCIS is a true precursor of invasive ductal carcinoma and is considered the more important of the two. LCIS is a risk factor for subsequent development of breast cancer. **Clinical Findings:** The most common manifestation of DCIS or LCIS is an abnormal mammogram. Occasionally, DCIS is clinically detected as a lump with well-defined margins or nipple discharge.

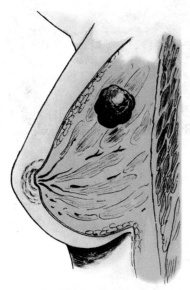

Fig. 17-19 Fibroadenoma.

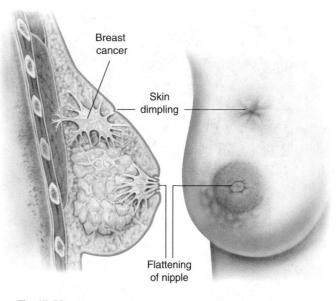

Fig. 17-20 Clinical signs of breast cancer: nipple retraction and dimpling of skin. *(From Seidel et al, 2006.)*

OTHER BREAST CONDITIONS

Mastitis

Mastitis is an inflammatory condition of the breast usually caused by a bacterial infection. The condition occurs most frequently in lactating women secondary to milk stasis or a plugged duct. The incidence is highest in the first few weeks postpartum and decreases thereafter (Barbosa-Cesnik et al, 2003). In nonlactating women, mastitis may also result from foreign bodies (such as nipple rings and breast implants) or from trauma. **Clinical Findings:** The infection generally occurs in one area of the breast, which appears as red, edematous, tender, warm to the touch, and hard. Axillary lymph nodes are often enlarged and tender. The client usually has an associated fever and chills, and often experiences general malaise (Fig. 17-21).

Galactorrhea

The term *galactorrhea* means inappropriate lactation. Causes include endocrine-related disorders (such as a pituitary tumor), systemic diseases (such as renal failure), and side effects of many medications (especially those that interfere or suppress dopamine—i.e., codeine, morphine, metoclopramide, phenothiazines, reserpine). **Clinical Findings:** The manifestation is milky-appearing nipple discharge (Fig. 17-22). There are no other specific symptoms because any additional signs or symptoms are likely based on the underlying cause (e.g., headache or change in vision if caused by a pituitary tumor).

Gynecomastia

Gynecomastia is a noninflammatory enlargement of one or both male breasts representing the most common breast problem in men. It can occur at any age. In neonates, the cause is typically associated with maternal hormones. At puberty the condition is idiopathic and transient. Common causes in adult men include side effect of medications, adrenal or testicular tumors, liver disease, or renal disease. **Clinical Findings:** Gynecomastia may be unilateral or bilateral and manifests as enlargement of the male breast (Fig. 17-23).

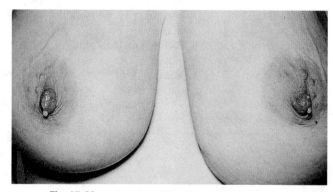

Fig. 17-22   Galactorrhea. *(From Mansel and Bundred, 1995.)*

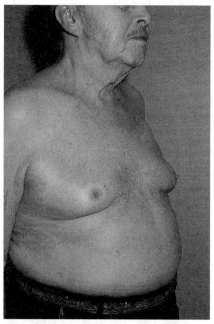

Fig. 17-23   Gynecomastia in an adult male. *(From Swartz, 2006.)*

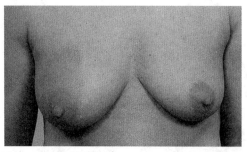

Fig. 17-21   Clinical signs of acute mastitis. *(From Mansel and Bundred, 1995.)*

CLINICAL APPLICATION & CLINICAL REASONING

See Appendix E for answers to exercises in this section.

REVIEW QUESTIONS

1 Which of the following findings is considered abnormal when conducting an exam on a 68-year-old woman?
  1 Dark pink areola.
  2 Pendulous breasts.
  3 Serous nipple drainage.
  4 Granular feeling when palpating the breast.

2 During a routine health examination, a 47-year-old female client tells the nurse that she performs breast self-examination "once in a while." The nurse should base his or her response on which of the following facts?
  1 Those who routinely perform BSE are more likely to survive breast cancer.
  2 Because breast cancer is always found by health care professionals, BSE is no longer indicated.
  3 Performance of BSE is an important indication of a client's compliance with health care.
  4 BSE is now considered optional; it is a personal choice.

3 A 58-year-old woman has found a small lump in her breast. Which of the following data from her history are risk factors for breast cancer?
  1 Her husband's mother died from breast cancer at age 43.
  2 She drinks a glass of wine each night with dinner.
  3 Menarche occurred at age 14; menopause occurred at age 46.
  4 She underwent radiation treatment for Hodgkin's disease at age 17.

4 A clinical breast examination includes palpation of the axillary lymph nodes for which of the following reasons?
  1 Axillary nodes fluctuate during the month in response to the menstrual cycle.
  2 Axillary node tenderness is the most common initial symptom of breast cancer.
  3 The lymph network in the breast primarily drains toward the axillary lymph nodes.
  4 This is a matter of convenience because of the close proximity of the axilla to the breasts.

5 A 19-year-old college student comes to the student health center because she discovered a small, nontender lump in her right breast. The nurse recognizes that the most common cause of breast lumps in women her age is:
  1 Breast cancer.
  2 Fibroadenoma.
  3 Ductal ectasia.
  4 Breast abscess.

6 A 58-year-old man seeks treatment for "recent breast enlargement." On examination, the nurse notes bilateral enlargement of the breasts. Which of the following questions asked by the nurse is most appropriate based on this finding?
  1 "What medications are you currently taking?"
  2 "Have you recently been lifting weights?"
  3 "Did your mother have large breasts?"
  4 "Have you ever had cancer before?"

SAMPLE DOCUMENTATION

Review the data obtained during an interview and examination by the nurse below:

Kelli Marquez is a 23-year-old Hispanic woman with a primary complaint of breast pain. Her vital signs are: temperature, 101.6° F (38.7° C); pulse, 116 beats/min; respirations, 24; blood pressure, 114/76 mm Hg. She delivered a baby 10 days ago and has been breast-feeding. About 2 days ago, she noticed that her left breast was becoming tender, and it has been getting continually worse. Her pain is constant and right now her pain is rated at 6 out of 10. She stopped using her left breast for breast-feeding because the pain was too much and now the right nipple is becoming sore. Kelli states that she has also been feeling "run down" and has no energy to take care of her baby. She has asked her mother to help her with the baby; she states, "I feel horrible about not meeting my baby's needs." She is also concerned about the baby's health and if the baby is getting enough to eat. She is taking no medications at this time. She states that she is not allergic to any medications. Her left breast is very swollen with erythema around the nipple that extends upward toward the sternum. The skin overlying the area is warm to touch. No pus or drainage is seen. Kelli is extremely sensitive to pain with even slight manipulation and palpation of the breast. The lymph nodes in her left axilla are slightly enlarged and are tender. Her right breast is soft and nontender. The left nipple is slightly red with a crack, but no inflammation is noted. No masses are palpated. Kelli states that she is in perfect health and has never been sick except for surgery to remove her appendix in college at age 19.

Below, note how the nurse documented these same data.

23 y/o Hispanic ♂. CC: L breast pain. Medical Hx: 10 days postpartum; appendectomy age 19. Medications: none. Allergies: NKDA.

Subjective Data

K. M. states that she is breast-feeding; tenderness in L breast ×2 days; getting progressively worse. Pain is constant; rated 6/10; continues breast-feeding using only R breast; states R nipple sore. Also reports fatigue and expresses concern about health and nutrition of baby; feels "horrible" about not being able to meet baby's needs; mother helping with infant care.

Objective Data

General survey: Vital signs: 101.6° F (38.7° C); HR 116; RR, 24; BP 114/76. Alert female, appears fatigued.

Left breast: Edema with erythema around nipple extending upward medially; skin warm to touch; no exudate. Extreme pain reported with slight manipulation of L breast.

Right breast: No erythema or edema noted; nipple is slightly red with crack; no nipple discharge. Breast is soft, nontender, no masses.

Axillae: Lymph nodes in L axilla slightly enlarged, tender; R axilla nodes not palpable.

CASE STUDY

Julie Fisher is a 46-year-old woman who came to the clinic because she had discovered a lump in her left breast. The following data are collected during an interview and examination.

Interview Data

Julie tells the nurse that she first noticed the lump about 9 months ago. Because it seemed small and did not hurt, she did not feel that it was much to worry about. Recently, Julie began noticing that the lump felt bigger and decided she better have someone look at it. Julie tells the nurse, "I just know it is not cancer because I am much too young and healthy. And if it is, I am not about to let some doctor mutilate me with a knife. I'd rather die than have my breast cut off." The nurse asks her if she has noticed any redness or dimpling of the breast. Julie tells the nurse, "No, not really, but I don't pay attention to those sorts of things." Julie tells the nurse that she started having regular menstrual cycles at age 11 and has not reached menopause. She has never been married and has no children.

Examination Data

- *General survey:* Alert, well-nourished female; hesitant to expose her breast for examination.
- *Breast examination:* Inspection reveals breasts of typical size with right and left breast symmetry. The skin of both breasts is smooth, with even pigmentation. The nipples protrude slightly with no drainage noted. The left nipple is slightly retracted. Significant dimpling is noted on left breast in upper outer quadrant when arms are raised over her head. Right breast is firm, smooth, elastic, without lumps or tenderness. Palpation of the left breast reveals a large, hard lump in the upper outer quadrant. No lumps or masses are noted in right breast. The left nipple produces a serosanguineous discharge when squeezed; the right nipple is unremarkable.

Clinical Reasoning

1. What data deviate from normal findings, suggesting a need for further investigation?
2. What additional information should the nurse ask or assess for?
3. Based on the data, what recommendations for health promotion should be considered for Julie?
4. What nursing diagnoses and collaborative problems should be considered for this situation?

⊙ INTERACTIVE ACTIVITIES

Open the interactive student CD-ROM, click on Chapter 17, and choose from the following activities on the menu bar:

- **Multiple Choice Challenge.** Click on the best answer for each question. You will be given immediate feedback, rationale for incorrect answers, and a total score. Good luck!

- **Marvelous Matches.** Drag each word or phrase to the appropriate place on the screen. Test your ability to match a clinical finding to the clue provided.

- **Risk Factors.** Review this client's history and identify risk factors. Complete your assessment by deciding which risks are modifiable or nonmodifiable. You only get one shot, so choose carefully!

- **Printable Lab Guide.** Click on the "Lab Guides" tab at the top of your screen. Locate the Lab Guide for Chapter 17, and print and use it (as many times as needed) to help you apply your assessment skills. These guides may also be filled in electronically and then saved and e-mailed to your instructor!

- **Quick Challenge.** Use this critical thinking exercise to assess your skills through case study-style questions, then compare with expert answers!

CHAPTER 18

Reproductive System and the Perineum

ANATOMY & PHYSIOLOGY

FEMALE REPRODUCTIVE SYSTEM

The anatomy of the female reproductive system can be categorized into external genitalia and internal structures and organs. Physiologic function discussed in the chapter is limited to menstrual cycle and menopause. The process of pregnancy is discussed in Chapter 21.

External Genitalia

The external female genitalia are collectively referred to as the *vulva*. The vulva includes the mons pubis, labia majora, labia minora, clitoris, prepuce, vaginal vestibule, ducts of the Skene's and Bartholin's glands, vaginal orifice, urethral meatus, and perineum (Fig. 18-1).

The mons pubis is a layer of adipose tissue that lies over the symphysis pubis. After puberty, this surface is covered with coarse hair that extends down over the outer labia to the perineal and anal areas. The labia majora are folds of tissue that extend downward from the mons pubis, surround the vestibule, and meet at the perineum. The outer surfaces are covered with hair, whereas the inner surfaces are hairless and smooth.

Lying inside the labia majora are darker, smooth folds called the labia minora. In some women, the labia minora are completely enclosed within the labia majora; in others the labia minora protrude between the labia majora. Each of the labia minora divides into a medial and lateral aspect. The medial aspects join superior to the clitoris to form the clitoral hood (prepuce), and the lateral aspects join inferior to the clitoris to form the frenulum. The clitoris is a small, cylindric bud of erectile tissue that is a primary center of sexual stimulation. The fourchette is a tense band or fold of mucous membrane connecting the posterior ends of the labia minora, just behind (posterior to) the vagina.

The vaginal vestibule is the area that lies between the labia minora and contains the urethral (urinary) meatus, the introitus (vaginal opening), hymenal tissue, and Bartholin's and Skene's glands. The urethral meatus is located just below the clitoris and appears as an irregularly shaped slit. The vaginal introitus lies immediately below the urethral meatus and varies in size and shape. The hymen is a fold of mucous membrane at the vaginal opening separating the external genitalia from the vagina and appears as small, fleshy tags of skin (sometimes referred to as hymenal remnants or hymenal tags).

The ducts of Skene's glands and Bartholin's glands open within the vestibule. The tiny Skene's glands are numerous and are located in the paraurethral area. During sexual intercourse, they secrete a lubricating fluid. The ducts are not usually visible. Bartholin's glands are small and round, located on either side of the introitus, at approximately the 5 and 7 o'clock posi-

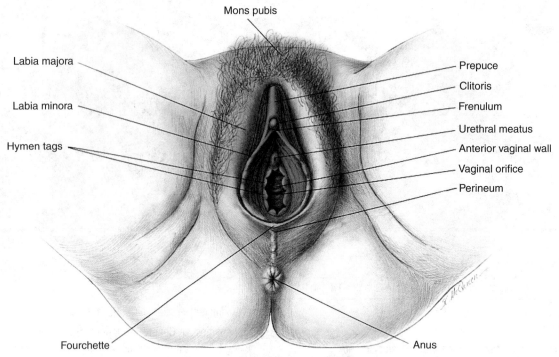

Fig. 18-1 Female external genitalia. *(From Stenchever, 2001.)*

tions. The ducts of the Bartholin's glands open onto the sides of the vestibule in the space between the hymen and the labia minora. The ductal openings are usually not visible. During sexual excitement, Bartholin's glands secrete a mucoid material into the vaginal orifice for lubrication.

The perineal surface is the triangular-shaped area between the vaginal opening and the anus. The pelvic floor consists of a group of muscles that form a suspended sling supporting the pelvic contents. These muscles attach to various points on the bony pelvis and form functional sphincters for the vagina, rectum, and urethra.

Internal Structures and Organs

The internal structures include the vagina, uterus, fallopian tubes, and ovaries (Fig. 18-2). They are supported by four pairs of ligaments: cardinal, uterosacral, round, and broad ligaments.

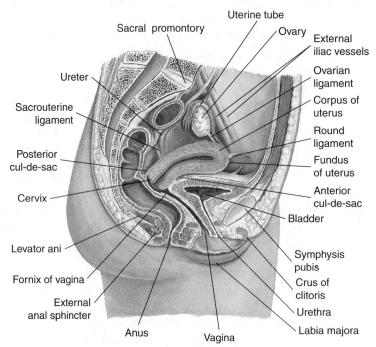

Fig. 18-2 Midsagittal view of female pelvic organs. *(From Seidel et al, 2006.)*

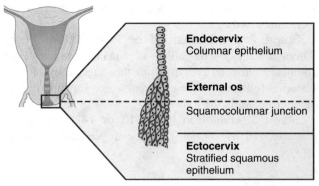

Fig. 18-3   Types of cervical cells: endocervical, external os, and ectocervix. *(Used with permission from Mashburn J, Scharbo-DeHaan M: A clinician's guide to Pap smear interpretation, Nurse Pract 22(4):115-8, 124, 126-7, 1997. Springhouse Corporation.)*

Vagina

The vagina is a canal composed of smooth muscle and is lined with mucous membrane that extends posteriorly from the vestibule to the uterus. It inclines posteriorly at an angle of approximately 45 degrees to the vertical plane of the body. The canal has transverse ridges of mucous membrane lining the vagina in the reproductive years. The uterine cervix enters superiorly and anteriorly into the vaginal cavity to form a recess, or fornix, around the cervix. The fornix is divided into anterior, posterior, and lateral fornices, through which the internal pelvic walls can be palpated. The vagina carries menstrual flow from the uterus and is the receptive organ for the penis during sexual intercourse. During birth, the vagina becomes the terminal portion of the birth canal.

Uterus

The uterus is a hollow, thick, pear-shaped, muscular organ. It is suspended and stabilized in the pelvic cavity by the four pairs of ligaments (listed previously). It is fairly mobile, usually loosely suspended between the bladder and rectum. The cervix is a mucus-producing gland that is the lowest portion of the uterus. It is visible (during a speculum ex-

amination) and palpable in the upper vagina. The cervical opening, or the os, is visible on the surface of the cervix. It appears as a small, round opening in a nulliparous woman (never having borne a child) or as an irregular slit in parous women. The outer surface of the cervix (known as the ectocervix) is layered with squamous cells, and the cervical canal is layered with columnar cells. In some women the juncture of these two types of cells (the squamocolumnar junction) can be observed as a circumscribed red circle around the os (Fig. 18-3).

The portion of the uterus above the cervix is known as the corpus. The corpus is composed of three sections: the isthmus (the narrow neck from which the cervix extends into the vagina); the main body of the uterus; and the fundus, which is the bulbous top portion of the uterus (Fig. 18-4). The fundus maintains its anterior position by the attached round ligaments, which are occasionally palpable on either side of the uterus.

Fallopian Tubes

The fallopian tubes extend from the fundus laterally 3 to 5 inches to the ovaries. The fimbriated ends of the fallopian tubes partially project around the ovary to capture and draw ova into the tube for fertilization (Fig. 18-4). The ova are transported to the uterus by rhythmic contractions of the tubal musculature. The inner tube is lined with cilia that further assist in transport of the ova.

Ovaries

The almond-shaped ovaries are connected to the uterine body by the ovarian ligaments. The primary functions of the ovaries include ovulation and secretion of reproductive hormones. Ovulation is the release of an ovum (egg), which usually occurs monthly as part of the menstrual cycle. The two dominant female sex hormones produced by the ovaries are estrogen and progesterone. These hormones have several functions, including triggering sexual maturation at puberty, development of secondary sex characteristics, and regulation of the menstrual cycle.

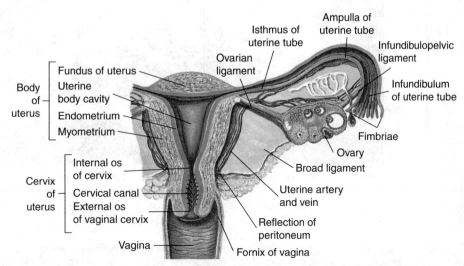

Fig. 18-4   Cross-sectional view of internal female genitalia and pelvic contents. *(From Seidel et al, 2006.)*

Menstrual Cycle

The hypothalamus, the anterior pituitary, and the ovaries together regulate the menstrual cycle. The menstrual cycle follows a predictable 28-day cycle. The five stages are described below and illustrated in Fig. 18-5.

Stage 1: Menstrual Phase (Days 1 to 4). The menstrual cycle begins with the menstrual phase. During this phase, estrogen and progesterone levels have decreased, trig-

gering a shedding of the upper layers of endometrium and menstrual bleeding.

Stage 2: Postmenstrual or Preovulatory Phase (Days 5 to 12). The follicle-stimulating hormone (FSH) stimulates follicular growth during this stage. The ovary and maturing follicle produce estrogen, which supports egg development within the follicle.

Stage 3: Ovulation (Days 13 or 14). Ovulation is characterized by a steep rise in estrogen and luteinizing

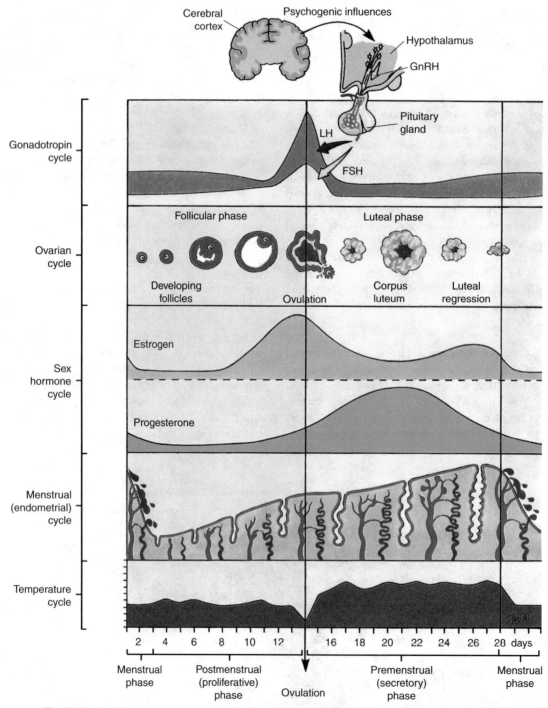

Fig. 18-5   Female menstrual cycle. Diagram shows the interrelationship of the cerebral, hypothalamic, pituitary, and uterine functions throughout a standard 28-day menstrual cycle. The variations in basal body temperature are also shown. *(From Thibodeau and Patton, 2007.)*

hormone (LH). The egg is expelled from the follicle and drawn into the fallopian tube by the fimbriae and cilia. A subsequent rise in progesterone causes thickening of the uterine wall.

Stage 4: Secretory Phase (Days 15-20). After ovulation, the FSH and LH hormones decline. The egg moves into the uterus and the follicle becomes a corpus luteum. Secretion of progesterone rises and predominates while estrogen declines. The uterine wall continues to thicken in anticipation of receiving a fertilized egg.

Stage 5: Premenstrual Phase (Days 21 to 28). If fertilization of the egg and subsequent implantation does not occur, the corpus luteum degenerates and progesterone production decreases. Estrogen levels begin to rise again as a new follicle develops. When the thickened uterine wall begins to shed, menstruation starts, which marks the beginning of another menstrual cycle.

Menopause

Women undergo a period of decreased hormonal function starting between ages 35 and 40. This period is termed the *climacteric,* a long transition phase extending many years. It includes endocrine, somatic, and psychologic changes involving a complex relationship between the ovarian and hypothalamic-pituitary factors. During this period, the woman undergoes a series of changes associated with aging and estrogen depletion. *Menopause* is defined as the permanent cessation of menses and is considered complete after the woman has experienced an

entire year with no menses. Ovulation usually ceases 1 to 2 years before menopause. The age at which women reach menopause varies greatly, but the mean age is 50.

MALE REPRODUCTIVE SYSTEM

The anatomy of the male reproductive system can be categorized into internal structures (testes, ducts, and glands) and external genitalia (penis, scrotum) (Fig. 18-6).

Internal Structures

Testes

The testes are paired sex organs located within the scrotum. They are oval shaped, with a smooth surface and rubbery texture. The primary function of the testes is the production of sperm (spermatogenesis). Each testicle contains a series of coiled ducts (seminiferous tubules), where spermatogenesis occurs. As sperm are produced, they move toward the center of the testis, traveling into the efferent tubules adjacent to the epididymis (see Fig. 18-6).

Ducts

The ducts are responsible for the transportation of sperm. Sperm travel from the epididymides to the vas deferens, to the ejaculatory duct, and out the urethra.

Once formed in the testes, sperm move into the comma-shaped *epididymis*—a long and elaborately coiled duct that

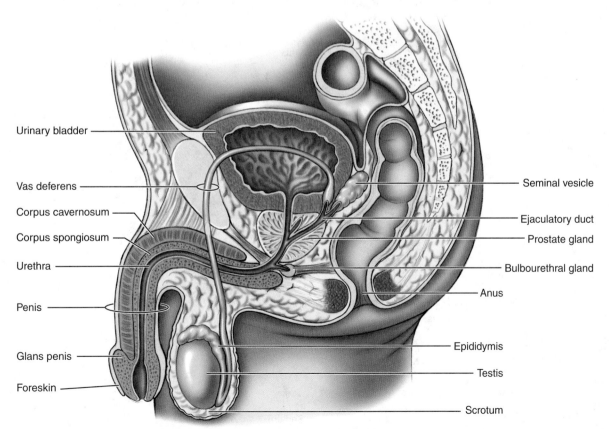

Urinary bladder

Vas deferens

Corpus cavernosum

Corpus spongiosum

Urethra

Penis

Glans penis

Foreskin

Seminal vesicle

Ejaculatory duct

Prostate gland

Bulbourethral gland

Anus

Epididymis

Testis

Scrotum

Fig. 18-6 Male reproductive organs. *(From Herlihy et al, 2007.)*

lies on the posterolateral surface of each testis (Fig. 18-7). As sperm move through the epididymis, they receive nutrients and mature. Eventually sperm exit the epididymis through the vas deferens.

The *vas deferens* (also known as the ductus deferens) transport sperm from the epididymis to the ejaculatory duct. It is enclosed within the spermatic cord (a connective tissue sheath) along with arteries, veins, and nerves as it ascends through the inguinal canal (see Figs. 18-6 and 18-7). The cord enters the inguinal canal through the external inguinal ring; this ring is vulnerable to hernias, or protrusion of the abdominal contents. In the abdominal cavity, the vas deferens travels up and around to the posterior aspect of the bladder, where it unites with the seminal vesicle. The union of the seminal vesicles with the vas deferens forms the *ejaculatory duct* just before the entrance into the prostate gland. Within the ejaculatory duct, sperm are transported downward through the prostate gland and into the prostatic portion of the urethra.

The innermost tube of the penis, the *urethra,* is usually about 7 to 8 inches (18 to 20 cm) from bladder to meatus. It extends out of the base of the bladder, traveling through the prostate gland into the pelvic floor and through the penile shaft (see Fig. 18-6). The urethral orifice is a small slit at the tip of the glans. The urethra is the terminal passageway for both urine and sperm. During ejaculation, sperm travel from the ejaculatory duct through the urethra and out of the body.

Glands

Three glands (seminal vesicles, prostate gland, and bulbourethral glands) produce and secrete fluid that makes up most of the fluid in the ejaculate (semen). These secretions serve as a medium for the transport of sperm and also provide an alkaline environment that promotes sperm motility and survival.

The *seminal vesicles* (small pouches lying between the rectum and the posterior bladder wall) join the ejaculatory duct at the base of the prostate (see Fig. 18-6). The *prostate gland* lies beneath the urinary bladder and surrounds the upper portion of the urethra. The posterior surface of the prostate lies adjacent to the anterior rectal wall. Two of the three prostate lobes are palpable through the rectum (right and left lateral lobes). These lobes are divided by a slight groove known as the median sulcus. The third lobe (median lobe) is anterior to the urethra and cannot be palpated. *Bulbourethral glands,* located on either side of the urethra just below the prostate, also secrete fluid that contributes to the semen, providing a medium for transport of the sperm.

External Genitalia

Scrotum

The scrotum is a pouch covered with thin, darkly pigmented, rugous (wrinkled) skin. A septum divides the scrotum into two pendulous compartments, or sacs. Each sac contains a testis and an epididymis, which is suspended by the *spermatic cord,* a network of nerves, blood vessels, and the vas deferens discussed previously (see Fig. 18-7). Because sperm production requires a temperature slightly below body temperature, the testes are suspended outside the body cavity; the temperature of the scrotum is controlled by a layer of muscle under the scrotal skin that contracts or relaxes in response to the outside temperature. When the temperature is cold, the scrotal sac and its contents move close to the body;

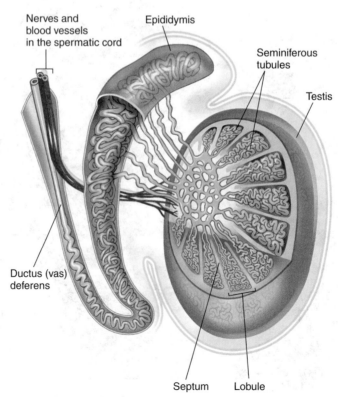

Fig. 18-7   Scrotum and its contents. *(From Thibodeau and Patton, 2007.)*

conversely, when the temperature rises, the scrotal sac relaxes and the testes drop downward.

Penis

The penis serves two functions: It is the final excretory organ in urination, and during intercourse it introduces sperm into the vagina. The body of the penis contains two layers of tissue, the corpora cavernosa and the corpus spongiosum, that encase the urethra (see Fig. 18-6). This smooth, spongy tissue becomes firm when engorged with blood, forming an erection. The corpus spongiosum expands at its distal end to form the glans penis.

The glans penis is lighter pink in color than the rest of the penis. It is exposed when the prepuce (the foreskin) is either pulled back or surgically removed (circumcision). The corona is the ridge that separates the glans from the shaft of the penis. The skin covering the penis is thin, hairless, and a little darker than the rest of the body; it adheres loosely to the shaft to allow for expansion with erection.

Erection is a neurovascular reflex that occurs when increased arterial dilation and decreased venous outflow cause the two corpora cavernosa to become engorged with blood. This reflex can be induced by psychogenic and local reflex mechanisms, both under the control of the autonomic nervous system. The psychogenic erection can be initiated by any type of sensory input (auditory, visual, tactile, or imaginative) whereas local reflex mechanisms are initiated by tactile stimuli. Ejaculation—the emission of semen from the vas deferens, epididymides, prostate, and seminal vesicles—is followed by constriction of the vessels supplying blood to the corpora cavernosa and gradual return of the penis to its relaxed, flaccid state.

RECTUM AND ANUS

The rectum and anus are the terminal structures of the gastrointestinal (GI) tract. They are presented in this chapter because these structures make up the posterior portion of the perineum in the male and female and because these structures are usually examined in conjunction with examination of the reproductive system.

Rectum

The proximal end of the rectum lies at the distal end of the sigmoid colon and extends down for approximately 5 inches (12 cm) to the anorectal junction (Fig. 18-8). Three semilunar folds of tissue called rectal valves (superior, middle, and inferior rectal valves) lie within the rectal wall and extend across half the circumference of the rectal lumen. The function of these valves is not well understood but is thought to support feces while allowing flatus to pass. The most distal of these valves (the inferior rectal valve) can be palpated with digital examination.

Anal Canal and Anus

The anal canal extends from the anorectal junction to the anus (see Fig. 18-8). The anal canal is lined with mucous

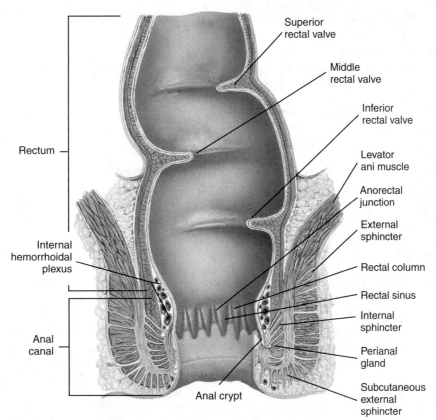

Fig. 18-8   Anatomy of the anus and rectum. *(From Seidel et al, 2006.)*

membranes arranged in longitudinal folds called rectal columns that contain a network of arteries and veins (frequently referred to as the internal hemorrhoidal plexus). Between each of the columns is a recessed area called the anal crypt into which the perianal glands empty. Surrounding the anal canal are two concentric rings of muscle, the internal and external sphincters. The internal sphincter consists of smooth muscle and is under involuntary control. The external sphincter, consisting of skeletal muscle, is under voluntary control, allowing for control of defecation. The lower portion of the anal canal is sensitive to painful stimuli, whereas the upper portion is relatively insensitive.

The anus is the terminal portion of the rectum, located on the perineum. It is hairless, moist mucosal tissue surrounded by hyperpigmented perianal skin. Normally the anus is closed except during defecation.

HEALTH HISTORY

RISK FACTORS　*Reproductive Cancer*

As you conduct a health history related to the reproductive system, it is important to consider common risk factors associated with reproductive cancers and follow up with additional questions should they exist.

FEMALE REPRODUCTIVE CANCERS
Cervical Cancer
- Highest incidence in women ages 40 to 50
- Sexual history: sexual intercourse at early age; lifetime history of multiple sex partners or partners with multiple sexual partners
- Infection with human papillomavirus (HPV) or human immunodeficiency virus (HIV)
- Cigarette smoking (M)

Ovarian Cancer
- Risk increases with age; median age is 63
- Nulliparity
- Use of infertility drugs or hormone replacement therapy (M)
- Personal history of breast cancer or hereditary nonpolyposis colon cancer
- Family history of ovarian and breast cancer
- BRCA-1 and BRCA-2 gene mutations
- Elevated tumor marker CA 125

Endometrial Cancer
- High cumulative exposure to estrogen; this includes the following:
- Early menarche and late onset of menopause (increased number of ovulatory cycles)
- Nulliparity
- Estrogen replacement therapy (M)
- Infertility
- Nonpolyposis colon cancer
- Obesity (M)
- Family history of endometrial, breast, colon, or ovarian cancer

MALE REPRODUCTIVE CANCERS
Testicular Cancer
- Age (highest incidence in young men ages 20 to 34)
- Cryptorchidism (undescended testicle at birth)
- Family history (increased risk if brother has had testicular cancer)
- History of testicular cancer in other testicle
- Ethnicity and culture (highest incidence among Caucasian men in the United States and the United Kingdom)

Prostate Cancer
- *Age:* Highest incidence is in older men; 75% of new cases occur in men over age 65.
- *Family history:* First-degree relative with prostate cancer increases risk.
- *Ethnicity:* African American men have the highest incidence of prostate cancer—two times higher than white men. Worldwide, the highest prevalence is in North America and northwestern Europe.

Data from American Cancer Society: *Cancer facts and figures 2007,* Atlanta, 2007, American Cancer Society; National Cancer Institute website (available at *www.nci.nih.gov*).
M = modifiable risk factor.

RISK FACTORS   *Sexually Transmitted Disease (STD)*

As you conduct a health history, it is important to consider common risk factors associated with reproductive infections and follow up with additional questions should they exist. STDs can occur with oral, vaginal, or rectal sex, and between heterosexual or homosexual partners.

- Sexual activity with new or multiple sex partners, including prostitutes who trade sex for money or drugs; two or more sex partners in last year (M)
- Sexual activity with individual who has multiple partners (M)
- Sexual activity with individual with history of STD (M)
- Failure to consistently and correctly use protective barrier* (M)

*Latex condoms are effective in preventing infections transmitted via mucosal surfaces (e.g., gonorrhea, chlamydia, HIV), but may not be as effective in preventing infections transmitted by skin-to-skin contact (HSV, HPV, syphilis, etc.).
M = modifiable risk factor.

GENERAL HEALTH HISTORY

Present Health Status

Do you have any chronic illnesses? If so, describe.

Many chronic illnesses may affect the reproductive functioning in women and men. For example, endocrine disorders may impact a woman's menstrual cycle; diabetes mellitus, vascular insufficiency, cardiac, and respiratory disease can contribute to erectile dysfunction (Albaugh, 2002).

Do you take any medications? If so, what do you take, and how often?

Both prescription and over-the-counter medications should be noted. Ask if the medications are taken as prescribed. Many medications can affect reproductive system functioning or libido. For example, medications such as oral contraceptives and broad-spectrum antibiotics can alter the balance of the normal vaginal flora in women. In men, some medications, such as diuretics and antihypertensives, can cause impotence.

Do you ever perform self-examination of your genitalia?

Assess the self-examination behaviors of all men and women. In one study, the majority of adolescent males were aware of testicular cancer, but only 10% performed testicular self-examination regularly (Ward et al, 2005). Health care awareness does not necessarily translate to health practice; the need to teach self-examination is of great importance.

How often do you have an examination of your genitalia by a health care professional? What were the results?

Assess self-care behaviors. Ideally, women should have a pelvic examination and Pap smear regularly. Men should have an examination of their genitalia and prostate on a regular basis, depending on their age.

Have you received the Hepatitis A or B vaccine? Females: Have you received the human papillomavirus (HPV) vaccine?

Assess self-care behaviors. Preexposure vaccination is one of the most effective methods for preventing some sexually transmitted infections. Hepatitis B vaccination is recommended for all unimmunized individuals at risk for STD. Hepatitis A vaccine is recommended for unimmunized men who have sex with men. HPV vaccine is now available and recommended for females ages 9 to 26 (CDC, 2006).

Past Medical History

Have you had any reproductive problems in the past? If so, describe.

Identify previous problems with the reproductive system because this information may be helpful when documenting current problems or risk factors for other medical problems. For example, women with endometriosis have been shown to have an increased risk of ovarian cancer (Modugno et al, 2004).

Have you ever had surgery on your reproductive organs or rectum? If so, when? How did you feel about having the surgery? How has it affected you?

If a women reports that she has had a hysterectomy, ask if it was an abdominal or vaginal approach, and ask if she had a total (uterus, fallopian tubes, and ovaries removed) or a partial (uterus removed; tubes and ovaries not removed) hysterectomy. Additionally, ask the client why she had the hysterectomy, when it was performed, if she had any accompanying bowel or bladder repairs, and what problems or concerns she has had since the surgery.

Men may have had surgery to treat an enlarged prostate, prostate cancer, hydrocele, varicocele, or testicular cancer.

Both men and women may have had surgical procedures to prevent pregnancy (vasectomy or a tubal ligation) or surgical procedures involving the anus or rectum (such as hemorroidectomy).

Do you have a history of cancer? If so, what type of cancer? How was it treated?

In women, a history of breast cancer or nonpolyposis colon cancer is a risk factor for some types of female reproductive cancers. In men, a history of testicular cancer increases risk of reoccurrence in other testicle (ACS, 2007).

Family History

Women: Has any woman in your family ever had cancer of the cervix, ovary, uterus, breast, or colon? If so, who? When?

A family history of these cancers (particularly in a first-degree relative) increases risk for certain female reproductive cancers (ACS, 2007).

Men: Has any man in your family ever had cancer of the prostate or testicle? If so, who? When?

A family history of these cancers (particularly in a first-degree relative) increases risk for certain prostate and testicular cancers (ACS, 2007).

Sexual History

Are you currently in a sexual relationship? If yes, do you prefer relationships with men, women, or both? What type of sex do you engage in (penile-vaginal, penile-rectal, recipient rectal, oral)?

The type of sex one participates in may provide useful information for risk assessment of sexually transmitted infections. Cross infections from mouth, anus, and genitalia can occur. Men and women need to feel accepted when discussing their health concerns. If the nurse seems genuinely interested and concerned, the client may appreciate the opportunity to discuss sexuality issues or problems.

How frequently do you engage in sexual activities? Are you and your partner(s) satisfied with the sexual relationship? Do you communicate comfortably about sexual activity?

It is important to determine the frequency of sexual activity, as well as the client's satisfaction. Questions related to sexual activities and satisfaction are found on health history forms; health care practitioners, however, have been found to offer little discussion related to sexuality unless an issue is raised by the client (Lewis & Black, 2006).

Do you or your partner(s) have multiple partners? How many sexual partners have you had in the past 3 months?

The rationale for this type of questioning is to determine the numbers and types of sexual encounters. This information may be used to determine the client's risk for STD.

How do you protect yourself from sexually transmitted disease (STD)? Do you use a protective barrier such as a condom every time you have intercourse?

Determine level of understanding and practice regarding safe sex and STD. Individuals may not have accurate information. When used correctly and consistently, condoms are highly effective in preventing sexual transmission of HIV, Chlamydia, gonorrhea, and trichomoniasis. The effectiveness of preventing transmission of Herpes simplex virus-2 is less well established (CDC, 2006).

Are you currently using any birth control measures? If so, what type? How effective do you feel this has been? Do you have any difficulty with the measures? Do you use birth control measures every time you have intercourse?

All women who have the potential to become pregnant or men who have the potential to create a pregnancy should be questioned about contraceptive practices. Information should be gathered about appropriate use of the contraception, length of use, and satisfaction with the product.

How old were you when you first had intercourse? Was it by choice? Have you ever been forced into sexual acts as a child or an adult? If so, how has this impacted you and your partner?

Inquire about current or past sexual abuse. Research has shown that women may wait years before disclosing sexual abuse or assault; delay in disclosure is even more likely when the perpetrator is a family member (Monroe et al, 2005). Sexual abuse or assault often causes ongoing sexual difficulties for the victims and their partners. Smith (2005) found male partners of women who were sexually assaulted were left feeling angry, guilty, and helpless. Men can also be victims of physical and sexual abuse, but it is often very difficult for them to admit to such abuse.

Do you or your partner(s) frequently use drugs or alcohol before you engage in sexual activity?

Drug and alcohol use leads to high-risk sexual behavior.

OBSTETRIC HISTORY

Menstruation

What was the date of the first day of your last menstrual period (LMP)? How often do you have periods? How long do they usually last?

A menstrual history consists of the LMP, usual menstrual interval, and the duration of menses. Women who are menopausal should be asked at what age menopause occurred.

How would you describe your usual amount of flow—light, moderate, heavy? How many pads or tampons do you use over the course of a day? An hour?

Normal flow is difficult to determine, but any change from what is "normal" for the client should be noted.

Have you noted any change in your periods recently?

Change in menstruation could reflect hormonal imbalance. Menstruation that is irregular or of frequently long or short intervals may indicate a lack of ovulation (Katz et al, 2007).

How old were you when you started having periods?

Menarche typically occurs between ages 12 and 14 years, although the range spans ages 8 to 16. Onset between ages 16 and 17 suggests an endocrine problem. Early onset of menarche (before age 11) is a risk factor for endometrial cancer (ACS, 2007).

Pregnancy

Have you ever been pregnant? If so, how many times? How many babies have you had? Have you had any miscarriages, abortions, or infants who died before they were born? If so, how many?

Gravida refers to the number of pregnancies; *para* refers to the number of pregnancies that reached 20 weeks or longer. See Chapter 21 for more information regarding documentation of obstetric history.

Do you think you may be pregnant now? What symptoms have you noticed?

Symptoms may include missed or abnormal periods, nausea or vomiting, breast changes or tenderness, and fatigue.

Have you ever had difficulty becoming pregnant? If so, have you seen a health care practitioner? What have you tried to do to become pregnant? How do you feel about not being able to become pregnant?

It is as important to inquire about difficulty becoming pregnant as it is to inquire about actual pregnancy. It is often highly distressing for the couple trying unsuccessfully to become pregnant, and the nurse may need to provide referral for counseling or encourage them to discuss their feelings.

FREQUENTLY ASKED QUESTIONS

Early menarche, late menopause, and nulliparity are all considered risk factors for endometrial cancer and breast cancer. What is the connection, and why are these risk factors important?
The key concept is the total number of ovulatory cycles a woman has. The greater the number of ovulatory cycles, the greater the risk of endometrial and breast cancer due to hormonal stimulation. For example, a woman with a history of menarche at age 10, menopause at age 55, and no pregnancies has had approximately 45 years of ovulatory cycles, or approximately 540 ovulatory cycles. Compare this with a woman with a history of menarche at age 14, menopause at age 50, and three full-term pregnancies. This represents 36 years minus 27 months (while pregnant), or approximately 405 ovulatory cycles. The difference between the two scenarios is 135 ovulatory cycles.

PROBLEM-BASED HISTORY

The most commonly reported problems related to the reproductive system and perineum for men and women include pain, genital lesions and discharge, problems with urination, and rectal bleeding. Common problems unique to women include problems or changes with menstrual cycle and menopausal symptoms. As with symptoms in all areas of health assessment, a symptom analysis is completed, which includes the onset, location, duration, characteristics, aggravating and alleviating factors, related symptoms, and treatments (see Box 3-3 in Chapter 3).

Pain

When did the pain begin? Where is the pain located? Describe the characteristics of the pain. On a scale of 0 to 10, how would you rate the intensity of the pain? Is the pain aggravated by other activity or function (such as menstrual cycle)?

Men and women may experience lower abdominal, pelvic, or rectal pain from a number of problems involving the reproductive system, urinary tract (urethra, bladder, ureters), or the rectum and anus. Women with unexplained pelvic pain should be screened for Chlamydia (Loyd et al, 2006).

Rectal discomfort may be associated with a number of factors, including poor hygiene, infection, hemorrhoids, and abscess (Box 18-1). Symptoms such as burning with urination suggest urinary tract infection (UTI).

Among men, pain in the groin or scrotum may occur from hernia or problems in the spermatic cord, testicles, or prostate gland. Testicular pain can occur secondary to almost any problem of the testis or epididymis, including epididymitis, orchitis, hydrocele, spermatic cord torsion, and testicular cancer.

Do you have associated symptoms such as discharge or bleeding, abdominal distention or tenderness, or pelvic fullness?

Determine if there are any associated symptoms with the pain.

What have you done, if anything, to treat the pain? How effective was the treatment?

Knowledge of previous self-treatment measures may be helpful in identifying appropriate treatment strategies.

Lesion

When did you first become aware of the lesion? Where exactly is the lesion located? What does it look like? Is it tender?

A lesion or sore on the genitalia is often caused by STD or cancer, but may also be associated with other problems. Establish when the lesion was first noticed because this may be important in identifying the cause.

Do you have any other symptoms, such as pain, bleeding, discharge, burning pain with urination, pelvic fullness, or abdominal pain?

These are symptoms commonly associated with STD.

BOX 18-1 FOCUS ON PAIN *Anus and Rectum*

Rectal fistula, fissure, and perianal abscess are among the most painful problems associated with the anus and rectum. When these problems are acute, walking is very painful, and the client has trouble finding a position of comfort. Oftentimes the client will be observed sitting to the side or will frequently shift uncomfortably. The client may prefer to lie prone, avoiding any pressure to the area.

Have you had a sexual relationship with someone who has an STD? If so, when? Have you ever been treated for any of these infections? If so, was the treatment successful?

Sexual contact with a partner with untreated STD increases a person's risk for STD.

Vaginal or Penile Discharge

When did the discharge begin? What color is the discharge? Describe its odor and consistency.

Identify onset of the symptom. Penile discharge suggests infection. Among women, normal discharge is clear or cloudy, with minimal odor. A change may suggest a vaginal infection. Specific appearance or odor of the discharge may help identify the causative organism.

Do you have other symptoms such as pain or itching?

These are associated symptoms. Irritation from the discharge can cause itching, rash, or pain with intercourse. Pelvic, abdominal, or urinary pain associated with discharge suggests infection.

If sexually active, does your partner have a discharge? Have you or your partner had a recent change or addition in sex partners?

A common cause of penile and vaginal discharge is STD.

Problems with Menstruation

What kinds of problems with menstruation are you experiencing? Have you noticed clotted blood during your periods? If so, when did this begin? Is it becoming worse over time?

Menorrhagia is a term for heavy menses. Clotting of blood indicates a heavy flow or vaginal pooling.

Do you have cramps or other pains associated with your period? Does this occur each month? What relieves the discomfort? Do the cramps or pains interfere with your normal activities?

Dysmenorrhea is a term for painful or difficult menses. It is often associated with hormonal imbalance.

Do you ever have spotting between periods?

Spotting between periods or midcycle bleeding may indicate hormonal imbalance or a need for dose adjustment if the client is taking hormonal contraceptives or hormonal replacement.

Do you have any other problems or symptoms before menses, such as headaches, bloated feeling, weight gain, breast tenderness, irritability, or moodiness? Does this seem to be associated with all of your periods or just occasionally? Does it interfere with your routine activities?

Hormonal fluctuation associated with the menstrual cycle may cause the client to have symptoms that are frequently referred to as premenstrual syndrome (PMS). Asking how routine activities are affected by symptoms helps the nurse gain a better understanding of the significance of the symptoms.

Menopausal Symptoms

When did your menstrual periods slow down or stop? Describe the symptoms you are experiencing.

Amenorrhea means absent menses. The perimenopausal period for most women occurs between ages 42 and 58. Common symptoms experienced during menopause include hot flashes, excessive sweating, back pain, palpitations, headaches, vaginal dryness, painful intercourse, changes in sexual desire, or mood swings (Katz et al, 2007).

Are you being treated for any symptoms associated with menopause? Are you taking hormonal replacement? If so, what are you taking and how much? Have you noted any side effects?

Estrogen replacement therapy (ERT) may cause fluid retention, breast pain or enlargement, and vaginal bleeding. A link between cardiovascular disease and ERT has also been found.

How do you feel about going through menopause?

Although this is a normal life stage, psychologic reactions range from a sense of loss to positive acceptance.

ETHNIC & CULTURAL VARIATIONS

Differences in attitudes and beliefs regarding menopause are found among women from various ethnic backgrounds. African American women are more positive in attitude toward menopause than other ethnic groups. Interestingly, African American women are also more likely to experience hot flashes than white women.

Data from Sommer et al, 1999; Grisso, 1999.

Difficulty with Erection

When did you first notice problems with attaining or maintaining an erection? Did this problem develop suddenly, or over a period of time? Do you have this problem consistently, or does the problem come and go?

Erectile dysfunction (ED) is a common problem, yet a very delicate topic. It is highly age dependent; some degree of ED affects 22% of men by age 40, and 49% by age 70 (Albaugh, 2002).

Do you have an idea about what might be contributing to the problem?

ED may be associated with medications, chronic illness (e.g., diabetes, hypertension, or treatment for prostate cancer), sexual dissatisfaction, or emotional problems. ED may also be an indicator for underlying complications among men with diabetes (Zheng et al, 2006). If you identify a client who has difficulty with erection, it is generally best to refer him to a health care professional who specializes in this area.

Problems with Urination

What kind of problem or change with urination are you experiencing? Is it hard to urinate? Do you have to urinate more frequently than normal?

Infection is the most common problem among men and women. A common problem among older men is urinary obstruction.

Have you experienced any pain or burning with urination? Is the urine clear or cloudy? Discolored? Bloody? Foul smelling? If so, do you have other symptoms such as frequent urination in small amounts? Feeling that you cannot wait to urinate?

These symptoms may accompany problems such as infection or acute cystitis among men and women and prostatitis among men. Urethritis in the young, sexually active male

may indicate STD such as Chlamydia or gonorrhea (CDC, 2007).

Do you think you are urinating more frequently than you consider normal? Do you awaken at night because you have to urinate?

Medications, especially those for cardiovascular problems, diuretics, and antihistamines, may cause increased urination. When the client has a urinary tract disorder or prostate problem, there is usually an increase in nocturia (awakening at night to urinate), urinary frequency, and urgency.

Men: Do you have any trouble initiating or maintaining a urine stream? Is the stream narrower or weaker than usual? Afterward, do you feel that you still have to urinate?

Hesitancy, straining, loss of force or decreased caliber of the stream, terminal dribbling, sensation of residual urine, and recurrent episodes of acute cystitis may be symptoms of a progressive prostate obstruction. Prostate enlargement, a common condition among older men, gradually obstructs the urethra, impeding urinary flow. Determine onset of the prob-

---

HEALTH PROMOTION *Sexually Transmitted Disease*

Background

There are an estimated 19 million new STD cases each year in the United States; nearly 50% of these involve young people aged 15 to 24 years. Women tend to suffer more serious consequences of STD than do men; ethnic groups with the highest incidence of STD are African Americans and Hispanics.

Goals and Objectives—*Healthy People 2010*

Responsible sexual behavior is one of the 10 leading health indicators identified by *Healthy People 2010*. Nineteen specific goals are related to STD, which include measures to promote abstinence or barrier protection, reduce number of adolescents and young adults with STDs, and increase STD screenings.

Recommendations to Reduce Risk (Primary Prevention)
Centers for Disease Control and Prevention (CDC)

- Safe Sex Practices: Abstain from sexual intercourses or be in a long-term, mutually monogamous relationship with an uninfected partner. Before initiating sexual activity with a new partner, both should be tested for STDs including HIV.
- Preexposure Vaccinations: HAV is given with childhood immunizations; unimmunized men who have sex with men (MSM) should be encouraged to receive vaccination. HBV is given with childhood immunizations; unimmunized adults who have more than one sex partner or MSM should be encouraged to receive vaccination. HPV vaccine is recommended for girls age 11 to 12 and for girls and young women age 13 to 26 who did not receive the vaccination when they were younger.

- Barrier Protection: A male condom should be used if sexual activity will involve an individual whose infection status is unknown or who is infected with an STD. Use of a spermicide alone is not effective in preventing sexually transmitted infection.

Screening Recommendations (Secondary Prevention)
Centers for Disease Control and Prevention

- *HIV:* HIV screening for all persons seeking evaluation and treatment for STDs; HIV testing should be offered for all pregnant women at the first prenatal visit or at delivery if they did not receive prenatal care.
- *Chlamydia:* Annual screening for all sexually active women under age 20; sexually active women age 20 to 24 who meet *either* of the following criteria: inconsistent use of a barrier contraceptive or more than one sexual partner during the last 3 months; and sexually active women older than age 24 who meet *both* above stated criteria. Pregnant women should be screened at the first prenatal visit and again during the third trimester if they have high-risk behaviors.
- *Gonorrhea:* Annual screening for all sexually active women under age 25 and all high-risk sexually active women over age 25. Screening should be done on all pregnant women with high-risk behaviors at the first prenatal visit.
- *Syphilis:* All high-risk individuals should be screened. Screening should be performed on all pregnant women at the first prenatal visit and again during the third trimester or at delivery if they have high-risk behaviors.

From Centers for Disease Control and Prevention: Sexually transmitted diseases treatment guidelines 2006, *MMWR* 55(RR-11), 2006; US Department of Health and Human Services: Centers for Disease Control and Prevention. *Sexually Transmitted Disease Surveillance, 2005.* Atlanta, GA: U.S. Department of Health and Human Services, November 2006; *Healthy People 2010: understanding and improving health,* ed 2, Washington, DC, 2000, US Government Printing Office (available at *www.healthypeople.com*).

lem. If benign prostatic hyperplasia is suspected, use the symptom index tool (Table 18-1).

Rectal Bleeding

When did the rectal bleeding first start? Is the problem constant, or does the problem come and go? Describe the color and amount of blood.
Determine onset and duration of the problem. Determine characteristics of the bleeding. Bleeding from high in the intestinal tract produces black, tarry stools, whereas bleeding near the rectum is associated with bright red bleeding. Black

or dark, nontarry stools may occur with certain medications such as iron supplements.

Have you had accompanying abdominal cramping or pain? Have you been constipated? Have you felt fatigued?
Identify associated symptoms. Some conditions such as ulcerative colitis can cause rectal bleeding accompanied by abdominal cramping. The passage of hard, dry stools can contribute to rectal bleeding. Fatigue is a significant finding in clients who develop anemia secondary to rectal bleeding.

TABLE 18-1   *The American Urological Association Symptom Index for Benign Prostatic Hyperplasia*

QUESTIONS	NOT AT ALL	LESS THAN 1 TIME IN 5	LESS THAN HALF THE TIME	ABOUT HALF THE TIME	MORE THAN HALF THE TIME	ALMOST ALWAYS
1. During the last month or so, how often have you had a sensation of not emptying your bladder completely after you finished urinating?	0	1	2	3	4	5
2. During the last month or so, how often have you had to urinate again less than 2 hours after you finished urinating?	0	1	2	3	4	5
3. During the last month or so, how often have you found you stopped and started again several times when you urinated?	0	1	2	3	4	5
4. During the last month or so, how often have you found it difficult to postpone urination?	0	1	2	3	4	5
5. During the last month or so, how often have you had a weak urinary stream?	0	1	2	3	4	5
6. During the last month or so, how often have you had to push or strain to begin urination?	0	1	2	3	4	5
	NONE	1 TIME	2 TIMES	3 TIMES	4 TIMES	5 OR MORE TIMES
7. During the last month, how many times did you most typically get up to urinate from the time you went to bed at night until the time you got up in the morning?	0	1	2	3	4	5

Score:
   7 or below indicates mild symptoms
   8-19 = moderate symptoms
   Above 20 = severe symptoms
From Barry MJ et al: The American Urologic Association symptom index for benign prostatic hyperplasia, *J Urol* 148(11):1549-1557, 1992.

HEALTH PROMOTION   *Reproductive Cancers*

Background

Reproductive cancers accounted for 306,380 new cases and 55,740 deaths in the United States in 2007. The large majority of new cases and deaths involve prostate cancer (218,890 and 27,050 respectively). Among women nearly half of new cancer cases (39,080) were caused by endometrial cancer, and over half of the deaths (15,280) were caused by ovarian cancer. Despite these facts, cancer of the cervix receives the most attention in health promotion literature, because effective screening through cytologic testing exists only for cervical cancer.

Goals and Objectives—*Healthy People 2010*

The overall *Healthy People 2010* goal related to cancer is to reduce the number of new cancer cases, as well as illness, disability, and death caused by cancer.

Recommendations to Reduce Risk (Primary Prevention)
U.S. Preventive Services Task Force

- It is unknown if counseling women about measures for primary prevention of gynecologic cancers is effective in reducing long-term morbidity and mortality rates.
- There are no specific recommendations for prevention of prostate or testicular cancers.
- Clinicians are encouraged to promote the practice of certain healthy behaviors (e.g., smoking cessation, safe sex practices, and maintaining healthy body weight) because these may reduce the incidence of certain cancers.

Screening Recommendations (Secondary Prevention)

Cervical Cancer:
- The U.S. Preventive Services Task Force (USPSTF) and American Cancer Society (ACS) recommend routine screening for cervical cancer. USPSTF recommends screening in all sexually active women at least every 3 years after onset of sexual activity or age 21 (whichever comes first) through age 65.

Endometrial Cancer:
- ACS recommends annual screening with biopsy for women age 35 who have or are at risk for hereditary non-polyposis colon cancer (HNCC).

Prostate Cancer:
- Because longer-term outcomes are unclear, USPSTF reports there is insufficient evidence to recommend for or against routine screening for prostate cancer using PSA or DRE.
- The ACS recommends that PSA and DRE screening tests be done annually for men, starting at age 50, or at age 45 for men with increased risk factors (African American men or men with a first-degree relative who had prostate cancer at a young age).

Ovarian Cancer:
- Routine screening for ovarian cancer is not recommended by USPSTF or ACS.

Testicular Cancer:
- Routine screening for testicular cancer is not recommended by USPSTF or ACS.

From American Cancer Society: *Cancer facts and figures 2007,* Atlanta, 2007, American Cancer Society; US Department of Health and Human Services: Cancer. In *Healthy People 2010: understanding and improving health,* ed 2, Washington, DC, 2000, US Government Printing Office (available at *www.healthypeople.gov*); US Preventive Services Task Force: *Guide to clinical preventive services* (available at *www.ahrq. gov*).

Note: PSA = Prostate Specific Antigen; DRE = Digital Rectal Exam.

EXAMINATION

FEMALE EXAM

ROUTINE TECHNIQUES	SPECIAL CIRCUMSTANCES OR ADVANCED PRACTICE
• INSPECT the pubic hair and skin over the mons ☞ pubis and inguinal area. • INSPECT the labia majora, labia minora, and clitoris. ☞ • INSPECT the urethral meatus, vaginal introitus, and perineum. • INSPECT the perianal area and anus.	• PALPATE the Skene's and Bartholin's glands. ★ • INSPECT and PALPATE for vaginal wall tone. ★ **Speculum Examination** • INSPECT the cervix. ★ • OBTAIN cervical cell smear and cultures. ★ • INSPECT the vaginal walls. ★ **Bimanual Examination** • PALPATE the vagina. ★ • PALPATE the cervix and uterus. ★ • PALPATE the adnexa and ovaries. ★ • PALPATE the uterus and ovaries using a ★ recto-vaginal approach. **Rectal Examination** • PALPATE the rectum. ★ • PALPATE the anal sphincter. ★ • EXAMINE the stool.

EQUIPMENT NEEDED
Examination gloves • Light source • Speculum • Swabs • Lubricating gel

☞ = core examination skill   ★ = advanced practice

PREPARING FOR THE FEMALE EXAMINATION

Before you begin this procedure, prepare the room. Assemble the equipment, obtain a sheet, pillow, and gown, and be sure the room temperature is warm. Women may feel apprehensive about having their genitalia examined, especially if the nurse is male. If necessary, arrange for a female assistant.

Before bringing the woman to the examination room, ask her to empty her bladder. Next, ask the woman to undress and put on a gown. Some women may be more comfortable with their socks on. Allow for privacy while she prepares. Once the woman is ready for the examination, help her into the lithotomy position, with body supine, feet in the stirrups, and knees apart. Provide adequate draping with a sheet. Position the client with her buttocks at the edge of the examination table. Ask the woman to place her arms at her sides or across her chest, but not over her head (this tightens the abdominal muscles). Position the sheet completely over the client's lower abdomen and upper legs, exposing only the vulva for your examination. Push the sheet down so that you can see the woman's face as you proceed. Sit on a stool at the end of the table between the client's legs.

Help the woman to relax. The lithotomy position may make the woman feel embarrassed and vulnerable. If the client seems uncomfortable or embarrassed, you may ask her if she would like her head elevated so that she can see you better. It may help to readjust the stirrups either outward or inward to reduce the stress on the pelvis and legs. In addition, make sure that the client is adequately covered and that you are in a private location where others may not walk in during the examination.

As you start the examination, reassure her that you will tell her everything that you are going to do before you actually do it. Assure her that if she becomes too uncomfortable, you will stop what you are doing and reassess what is happening. Always remember to touch the inner aspect of her thigh before you touch the external genitalia. (Don't be tentative with your touch—once you make physical contact, maintain it throughout the procedure.) Be sure to talk to the woman throughout the examination to tell her what you are doing, what you are seeing or feeling, and how long it will be until you are finished.

PROCEDURES AND TECHNIQUES WITH NORMAL FINDINGS	ABNORMAL FINDINGS

ROUTINE TECHNIQUES: FEMALE EXAM

INSPECT the pubic hair and skin over the mons pubis and inguinal area for distribution and surface characteristics.

Hair distribution varies but usually covers an inverse triangle with the base over the mons pubis; some hair may extend up midline toward the umbilicus. The skin should be smooth and clear (Fig. 18-9).

Note any male hair distribution (diamond-shaped pattern), patchy loss of hair, or absence of hair in any client over 16 years of age. Observe for presence of skin lesions or infestations (nits or lice) of skin or pubic hair.

INSPECT and **PALPATE** the labia majora, labia minora, and clitoris for pigmentation and surface characteristics.

The skin pigmentation of the labia should be darker than the client's general skin tone, and the tissues may appear shriveled or full, gaping or closed, usually symmetric, with a smooth skin surface and a dry or moist texture. Gently touch the client on the inner thigh and tell her that you are going to spread the labia apart. Spread the labia majora to view the inner surface of the labia majora, labia minora, and the surface of the vestibule (Fig. 18-10). Pigmentation should be dark pink. The area should appear moist, and the tissue should appear symmetric and without drainage, lesions, or sores.

Palpate the labia minora between your thumb and the second fingers of your other hand. The tissue should feel smooth and soft, without nodules or masses, and the palpation should elicit no statements of discomfort from the client.

The clitoris is located midline between the labia minora. It is normally a smooth, pink, and moist cylindric structure about the size of an eraser head.

Observe for signs of inflammation, edema, excoriation, leukoplakia (white patches), ulceration, drainage, lesions, nodules, and marked asymmetry.

Inflammation, irritation, excoriation, vaginal discharge, and pain are abnormal findings. Discoloration or tenderness may be the result of traumatic bruising.

Note any enlargement, atrophy, inflammation, lesions, or discharge.

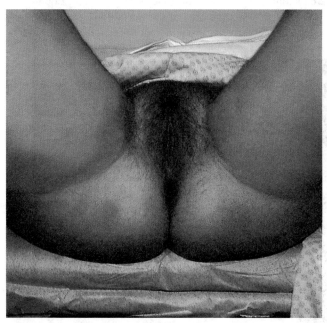

Fig. 18-9   Inspection of the external genitalia.

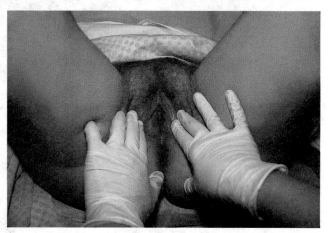

Fig. 18-10   Inspection of the labia.

= core examination skill

PROCEDURES AND TECHNIQUES WITH NORMAL FINDINGS	ABNORMAL FINDINGS

INSPECT the urethral meatus, vaginal introitus, and perineum for positioning and surface characteristics.

Inspect the urethral meatus and the tissues immediately surrounding it. There should be a midline location of an irregular opening or slit close to or slightly within the vaginal introitus. The vaginal introitus may appear as a thin vertical slit or a large orifice with irregular edges from the hymenal remnants; the tissues should appear moist. The posterior skin surface of the perineum between the vaginal introitus and the anus should appear smooth and without lesions or discoloration. If the client has had an episiotomy, a scar (midline or mediolateral) may be visible.

Note any discharge from the surrounding (Skene's) glands or the urethral opening, polyps, inflammation, or a lateral position of the meatus. Note any surrounding inflammation, discolored or foul-smelling vaginal discharge, bleeding or blood clots, edema, skin discoloration indicative of tissue bruising, or lesions. Note scars, skin tags, lesions, inflammation, fissures, lumps, or excoriation.

INSPECT the perianal area and anus for color and surface characteristics.

The anus should exhibit increased pigmentation and coarse skin; no lesions should be present, the skin should be intact. The anus should be tightly closed. Hemorrhoids may be seen in the adult; differentiate hemorrhoids from other lesions.

Note lesions or fissures around the anus. Lesions associated with sexually transmitted disease frequently appear on or around the anus.

SPECIAL CIRCUMSTANCES OR ADVANCED PRACTICE: FEMALE EXAM

★ **PALPATE the Skene's and Bartholin's glands for surface characteristics, discharge, and pain or discomfort.**

With the labia still spread apart, insert the index finger of your dominant hand (palm surface up) into the vagina as far as possible. Exert upward pressure on the anterior vaginal wall surface and milk the Skene's glands by moving your finger outward toward the vaginal opening (Fig. 18-11). The glands are located in the paraurethral area and are not usually visible. The glands area should be nontender and without discharge.

Note any tenderness or discharge; collect a sample of any discharge that is present for culture. Discharge from the Skene's and Bartholin's glands is usually indicative of an infection. Edema in the area of the Bartholin's glands that is painful and "hot to the touch" may indicate an abscess of the Bartholin's gland. The abscess is generally pus filled and is gonococcal or staphylococcal in origin. A nontender mass, which is the result of chronic inflammation of the gland, is usually indicative of a Bartholin's cyst.

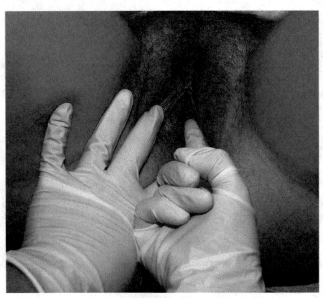

Fig. 18-11 Palpation of Skene's gland.

★ = advanced practice

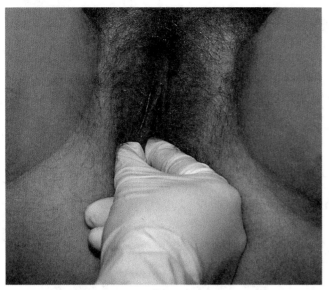

Fig. 18-12 Palpation of Bartholin's gland.

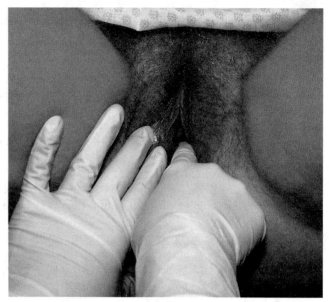

Fig. 18-13 Assessing vaginal tone.

PROCEDURES AND TECHNIQUES WITH NORMAL FINDINGS

Next, palpate the lateral tissue of the vagina bilaterally. Use your thumb and index finger to palpate the entire area, paying attention to the posterolateral portion of the labia majora where the Bartholin's glands are located (Fig. 18-12). The glands are not usually visible. The surface should appear smooth, pink, and shiny, and it should be nontender, without discharge.

★ **INSPECT and PALPATE for vaginal wall tone.**

With your examining finger still in the vagina, instruct the client to squeeze the vaginal orifice around your finger. The nulliparous client is usually able to squeeze tightly, so that you will feel the vaginal wall tissue firmly around your examining finger (Fig. 18-13). If the woman has had children (vaginal delivery), she may not squeeze as tightly. NOTE: Vaginal wall tone is not routinely assessed unless there is a specific indication such as a history of incontinence or discomfort.

Remove your finger from the vagina. Holding the labia apart, ask the client to bear down as you watch for vaginal wall bulging and urinary incontinence. Ask the client to cough and again inspect for bulging and incontinence.

ABNORMAL FINDINGS

Note inability of client to constrict the vaginal orifice around your finger.

Bulging of the anterior wall may indicate a cystocele. Bulging of the posterior vaginal wall may indicate a rectocele. If the cervix is visible at the opening of the vagina, it may indicate signs of a uterine prolapse. The presence of urine during either bearing down or coughing may be indicative of stress incontinence.

★ = advanced practice

PROCEDURES AND TECHNIQUES WITH NORMAL FINDINGS

ABNORMAL FINDINGS

★ SPECULUM EXAMINATION

Tell the client that you will now use a speculum to do the internal examination (Box 18-2). Using a speculum of appropriate size, follow these steps:

1. Locate the cervix using the middle finger on your nondominant hand; visualize the location in your "mind's eye"—this helps you to locate the cervix with the speculum.
2. Place the index and middle fingers of your nondominant hand inside the vaginal introitus and spread it apart about 1 inch (2.5 cm). Exert downward pressure against the posterior wall; wait for the vaginal wall muscles to relax (Fig. 18-14).
3. As downward pressure is exerted, simultaneously insert the speculum (with blades closed) over your fingers, holding the speculum at an oblique angle (Fig. 18-15). After the blades pass over your fingers, the speculum must be rotated to a horizontal position as it is inserted.

BOX 18-2 **CLINICAL NOTES**

- Make sure that you know how to use the speculum before you start, including how to lock the blades open in place and how to release the lock.
- Make sure that the speculum is warm (especially if it is metal). If necessary, run it under warm water to warm it up. The speculum may also be kept warm by wrapping it in a heating pad or placing it under a warming light.
- Pick the correct size speculum for the client. Do not assume that a wide-blade Graves' speculum will be comfortable for all women. If the client is not sexually active, she will most likely need a narrower-blade speculum.
- Lubricate the speculum with warm water. Do not use lubricant. This will interfere with cytologic analysis.
- Make sure that you have all of the necessary supplies within reach before you start (e.g., slides, applicators, test tubes with KOH, and saline).

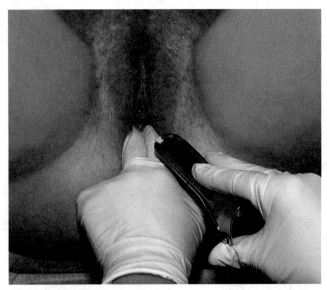

Fig. 18-14   Apply downward pressure on vagina before inserting the speculum.

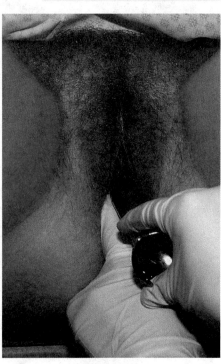

Fig. 18-15   Insertion of closed speculum blades with oblique angle.

★ = advanced practice

4. After the blades have passed the introitus, remove your fingers while exerting downward pressure. Maintain downward and posterior pressure on the blades directed at a 45-degree angle until the speculum is completely inserted (Fig. 18-16).

5. With speculum fully inserted and blades horizontal, open the blades of the speculum and look for the cervix. If you see a smooth, shiny wall, you are probably below the cervix; if you see rough or rugated wall, you are probably above the cervix. Reposition the speculum if necessary to visualize the cervix; once visualized, lock the blades in the open position (Fig. 18-17).

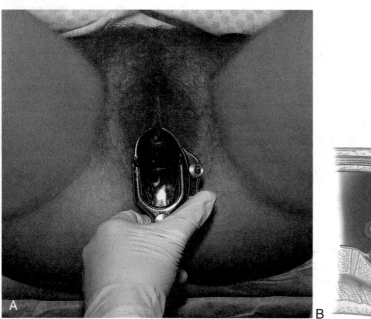
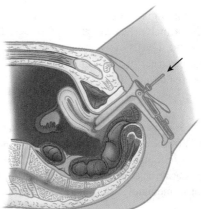

Fig. 18-16   **A,** Direct the speculum downward at a 45-degree angle. **B,** Cross-sectional view. *(**B,** From Seidel et al, 2006.)*

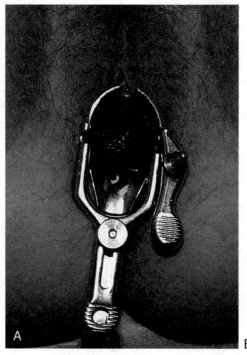
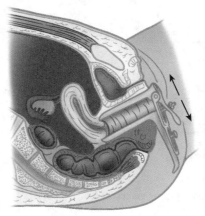

Fig. 18-17   **A,** Open speculum blades. **B,** Cross-sectional view. *(**B,** From Seidel et al, 2006.)*

PROCEDURES AND TECHNIQUES WITH NORMAL FINDINGS

★ **INSPECT the cervix for color, surface characteristics, position, size and shape, and discharge.**

The cervix should appear smooth, and it should be an evenly distributed pink color (except during pregnancy, when it is a bluish color secondary to increased vascularity). A symmetric, circumscribed erythema surrounding the os (the opening) may indicate the normal condition of exposed columnar epithelium, known as the squamocolumnar junction. You may see nabothian cysts, which appear as smooth, round, small, yellow, raised areas (Fig. 18-18). Absence of a cervix is an expected finding for a woman who has had a hysterectomy (Box 18-3).

The cervix should be midline and point in a direction related to the position of the uterus. An anterior-pointing cervix indicates a retroverted uterus. A posterior-pointing cervix indicates an anteverted uterus. A midline cervix indicates a midposition uterus (see Table 18-3).

The cervix should be about 1 inch (2.5 cm) in diameter and project into the vagina slightly (1 inch or less), forming fornices. The os of a nulliparous client is small and round. The os of a parous client is generally slit shaped and may be irregular. An everted cervix (a normal variant) is manifested by a circular, raised erythematous area around the os (see Fig. 18-18).

If discharge is present, determine whether it is coming from the cervix itself or whether it is from the vagina and has only pooled near the cervix. A mucous plug may be present at the os of the cervix. If a discharge is present, it should be odorless, creamy or clear, thin, thick, or stringy. At the middle of the menstrual cycle or immediately after menstruation, the discharge may be heavier.

ABNORMAL FINDINGS

Note any reddened granular area around the os (especially if asymmetric), friable tissue (tissue that readily bleeds), red patches or lesions, strawberry spots, or white patches. A pale-appearing cervix may be associated with menopause or anemia. Reddened, irregular color, or patchy appearance with irregular borders can be an abnormal finding and requires further investigation.

The cervix deviating to either the right or left from a midline position may indicate a pelvic mass, uterine adhesions, or pregnancy and requires further investigation.

Note if the cervix is over 1.75 inches (4 cm) in diameter. A projection of more than 1 inch (2.5 cm) into the vaginal canal is an abnormal finding and may indicate a pelvic or uterine mass. A lacerated cervix has a torn slit appearance, indicating injury.

A discharge with an odor or a discharge that is colored, such as yellow, green, or gray, usually indicates a bacterial or fungal infection.

BOX 18-3 **CLINICAL NOTE**

Performing a speculum examination on a client who has had a *hysterectomy* is essentially the same as examining any other client. The most obvious finding during the assessment will be the absence of a cervix and uterus. If the client has had her ovaries removed and is not taking hormone replacement therapy, many findings are consistent with findings present in older, postmenopausal women.

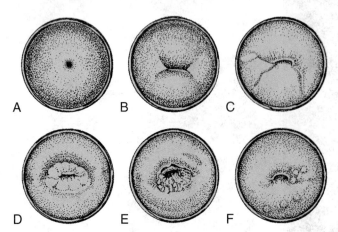

Fig. 18-18 **Common appearances of the cervix. A,** Nulliparous cervix. Note rounded os. **B,** Parous cervix. Note slit appearance of os. **C,** Multigravidous, lacerated. **D,** Everted. **E,** Eroded. **F,** Nabothian cysts. *(From Seidel et al, 2006.)*

★ = advanced practice

PROCEDURES AND TECHNIQUES WITH NORMAL FINDINGS

★ **OBTAIN smears and cultures.**

Often during the speculum examination, a culture or smear is indicated. These specimens should be collected while the speculum is still in place, but after the cervix and surrounding tissue have been inspected.

Papanicolaou (Pap) smear: The Pap smear should always be the first specimen collected. It is used as a screening test to detect cervical and endometrial dysplasia and cancer. Follow the guidelines in Table 18-2 for specimen collection. Box 18-4 presents newer screening technology.

TABLE 18-2 *Procedure for Collecting Pap Smear Specimen*

	PROCEDURE	RATIONALE	
Ectocervical specimen	Insert vertical projection of spatula into os until lateral projection is against cervix. Rotate 360 degrees, maintaining contact with cervix, scraping the entire cervical surface. Remove and spread the material from both sides of the spatula thinly on a glass slide; immediately spray slide with cytologic fixative; label slide "ectocervical specimen."	Avoid applying a thick sample on the slide—this will make it difficult to visualize cells.	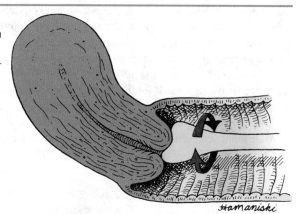
Endocervical specimen	Insert a cytobrush into cervical os. Rotate 360 degrees. Remove and place sample on slide using a rolling or twisting motion on the slide. Immediately spray slide with cytologic fixative; label slide "endocervical specimen."	Use of brush as opposed to cotton-tipped applicator has improved the quality of the sample of endocervical cells.	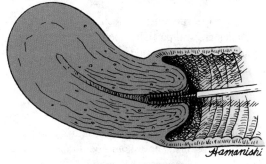
Ectocervical/ endocervical specimen	Use a Cervex-brush. (It collects both ectocervical and endocervical specimens of the same time.) Insert the central long bristles into the os until the lateral bristles bend against the ectocervix. Apply gentle pressure and rotate the brush 3 to 5 times to the left and right. Withdraw brush and paint the glass slide with two single strokes in the same place on the slide applying the first stroke with one side to the brush, the second stroke with the other side of the brush. Apply a fixative; label slide "ectocervical and endocervical specimen."	Use of a Cervex-brush reportedly causes less spotting after the examination, yet provides a quality sample of ectocervical and endocervical cells.	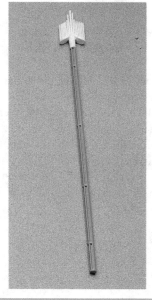

★ = advanced practice

BOX 18-4   TESTING FOR CERVICAL CANCER

Liquid-based cytology (e.g., ThinPrep) permits testing of specimens for human papillomavirus (HPV). Although liquid-based cytology may have improved sensitivity over conventional Pap smear screening, it is considerably more costly and may possibly be associated with lower specificity. Studies suggest that this method is not likely to be cost-effective unless used with screening intervals of 3 years or longer.

PROCEDURES AND TECHNIQUES WITH NORMAL FINDINGS

It is important that specimens are not collected while the client is menstruating, or if the client took a bath, used a vaginal douche, or inserted topical vaginal inserts or lubrications within the last 48 hours. Also, do not use lubrication jelly on the speculum if specimens are to be collected. These will affect the quality of samples taken and could result in false negative results. In women who have undergone a hysterectomy in which the cervix was removed, Pap testing is not required unless the hysterectomy was performed because of cervical cancer or its precursors. If a routine Pap smear is indicated, the sample should be collected from along the suture line, using the blunt end of a spatula. Label the specimen as vaginal cells taken from the suture line.

Additional screening tests or cultures may be collected at this time; the decision to do this is based on risk factors, the history, or clinical findings.

★ INSPECT the vaginal walls for color and surface characteristics.

Following the specimen collection, carefully unlock the speculum and, while the blades are still partially open, begin to remove the speculum gently from the vagina. The blades of the speculum tend to close by themselves. As the speculum is being removed, slowly rotate the blades of the speculum and inspect the walls of the vagina. Apply posterior, downward pressure to avoid causing discomfort to the sensitive urethra with blade removal.

The walls should be pink, moist, with transverse rugae (which diminish after vaginal deliveries and with age), and homogeneous in consistency. Note any vaginal secretions. They should be thin, clear or cloudy, odorless, and minimal to moderate in amount.

★ BIMANUAL EXAMINATION

It is important to first tell the client that you are going to perform an internal examination with your fingers and hand. Next, move to a standing position at the end of the examination table between the client's legs. If your gloves have become soiled or contaminated, put on a clean pair of gloves. Lubricate the index and middle fingers of the hand that will be placed internally. Gently insert the middle and index fingers into the vaginal opening. Insert downward pressure on the posterior vaginal wall. Wait a moment for the vaginal opening to relax. Then gradually insert your fingers their full length into the vagina.

ABNORMAL FINDINGS

Note if the wall is red or pale; if there are lesions, leukoplakia, cracks, a dried surface, or bleeding; or if it appears nodular or edematous. Report any secretions that are thick, curdy, frothy, gray, green, yellow, foul smelling, or profuse.

★ = advanced practice

| PROCEDURES AND TECHNIQUES WITH NORMAL FINDINGS | ABNORMAL FINDINGS |

★ **PALPATE the vagina for surface characteristics and discomfort.**

Palpate the vaginal wall as you insert your fingers. The wall should feel smooth and should be nontender. Once your fingers are fully extended into the vaginal wall, position your thumb (which is outside the vagina and near but not on the urethra and clitoris) out of the way so that it is not uncomfortable for the client.

Abnormalities of the vaginal wall include nodules, cysts, discomfort, and unusual tissue growths.

★ **PALPATE the cervix and uterus for position, size, surface characteristics, mobility, and discomfort.**

Procedure: Locate the cervix with the fingers of your internal hand. Place the palmar surface of the fingers of your other hand on the lower abdomen midway between the umbilicus and the pubis (Fig. 18-19). The hand on the abdomen should gently hold the uterus downward against the internal examination hand so that the cervix can be evaluated. Palpate the cervix and vaginal fornices with the palmar surfaces of the fingers of your internal hand.

Findings: The cervix should feel evenly rounded or slightly ovoid, firm (like the tip of a nose), and smooth. The cervix should be slightly mobile in each direction without causing discomfort (documented as no cervical motion tenderness [CMT] noted). It should be located in the midline position; the fornices (pockets surrounding the cervical protrusion) should be pliable and smooth, and there should be no tenderness.

Note if the cervix is enlarged, irregular, soft or nodular, hard, immobile or associated with discomfort as it moves, and laterally displaced (not in the midline). Painful cervical movement suggests an inflammatory process such as acute pelvic inflammatory disease (PID) or a ruptured tubal pregnancy.

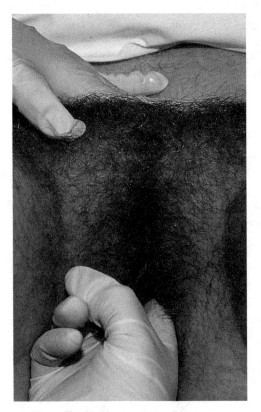

Fig. 18-19   Bimanual palpation.

★ = advanced practice

PROCEDURES AND TECHNIQUES WITH NORMAL FINDINGS

Procedure: Move the fingers from the cervical os into the anterior fornix of the vagina. Slowly slide the hand that is on the abdomen toward the pubis with the palmar surface of your fingers pressing downward to push the pelvic organs closer for your internal fingers to palpate. It may be helpful to visualize the hands working together to "trap" the uterus between the two hands. The uterus is generally assessed with the *internal fingers;* it is not normally palpable abdominally by the external hand. Determine the uterine size and position.

Findings: The nonpregnant uterus is small and usually lies under the symphysis pubis in the pelvis. In a parous client, the uterus may feel larger. Various uterine positions include anteverted, anteflexed, midposition, retroverted, and retroflexed (Table 18-3). Most women have an anteverted uterus.

Determine surface characteristics by palpating the uterine wall with the internal fingers in the vaginal fornices. Normally, it feels smooth and firm. Gently move the uterus between your external hand and internal fingers. It should move freely and be nontender.

★ **PALPATE the adnexa and ovaries for size, shape, and tenderness.**

Procedure: Place the abdominal hand on the left lower abdominal quadrant and the intravaginal hand in the left fornix of the vagina. Lift the internal fingers upward as the external fingers press down and inward to "trap" the ovary between the hands (Fig. 18-20). You will know if you have located the ovary when you reach a slight bulging area in the lower quadrant and when the client complains of a "twinge" sensation of slight tenderness.

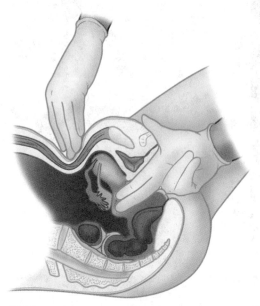

Fig. 18-20   Bimanual palpation of the adnexa. *(From Seidel et al, 2003.)*

ABNORMAL FINDINGS

An enlarged uterus in a nonpregnant woman is abnormal and requires further evaluation. An enlarged uterus may be caused by fibroid tumor, adenomyosis, or carcinoma.

Report any irregular contour, soft, nodular consistency, or masses. A uterus that feels irregular or nonsmooth is abnormal and requires further evaluation. A soft uterus is usually associated with pregnancy; an irregular surface suggests fibroids. Note if the uterus is fixed or tender during this maneuver. A fixed uterus may indicate adhesions. Tenderness may indicate pelvic inflammation or a ruptured tubal pregnancy.

An ovary larger than 2 inches (5 cm) is considered abnormal and requires further evaluation. If any masses are noted in the adnexa, evaluate their characteristics: size, shape, location, tenderness, and consistency.

★ = advanced practice

TABLE 18-3 *Positions of the Uterus*

Anteverted

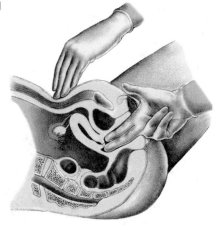

The uterus is palpated at the level of the pubis between the external and internal hands; the uterus points anteriorly, the cervix will be aimed posteriorly.

Anteflexed

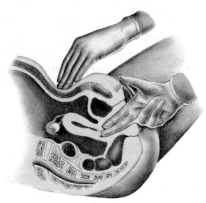

The uterus is palpable at the level of the pubis between the external and the internal hands; the uterus points anteriorly, the cervix points along the axis of the vaginal canal.

Midposition

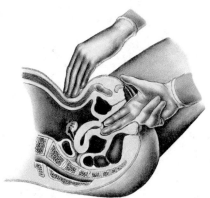

The uterus may not be palpable between the external and internal hands; the uterus points upward, the cervix is pointed along the axis of the vaginal canal.

Retroverted

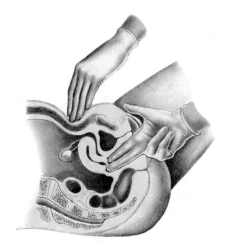

The uterus is positioned posteriorly and is not palpable between the external and internal hands. The cervix is pointed anteriorly.

Retroflexed

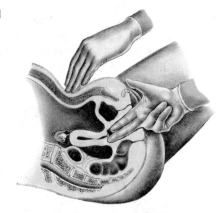

The uterus is positioned posteriorly and is not palpable between the external and internal hands. The cervix is directed along the axis of the vaginal canal.

PROCEDURES AND TECHNIQUES WITH NORMAL FINDINGS

ABNORMAL FINDINGS

Findings: The ovary may not always be palpable, but if it is, it should feel smooth, firm, and ovoid. The ovaries are approximately walnut sized and should be mobile. Fallopian tubes have a very small diameter and normally are not palpable or sensitive. In thin women, the only other structure that may be palpable is the round ligament. Move the hands to the right side and use the same techniques to evaluate the right ovary and adnexa.

★ **PALPATE the uterus and ovaries using the rectovaginal approach.**

Procedure: The rectovaginal examination allows for a more complete evaluation of the posterior side of the uterus. To prepare for rectovaginal examination, change the intravaginal glove. (This prevents transfer of organisms from the vagina to the rectum.) Tell the client what you will be doing and that the procedure will be uncomfortable; she may feel the pressure of a bowel movement. Lubricate the first two fingers of the newly gloved hand. Place your middle finger, palm side up, over the anus. Ask the client to bear down; while she is doing so, gently insert your middle finger into the rectum. Insert your index finger into the vagina and locate the cervix.

Place the external hand on the lower abdomen and apply downward pressure. Repeat the steps as described in the bimanual examination (Fig. 18-21). Keep the index finger of the internal hand under the cervix as a landmark.

Findings: The findings should be the same as previously described in the bimanual examination procedure section.

Note marked tenderness, nodularity, enlargement, and masses that seem immobile. All of these findings should be considered abnormal. If a mass is detected in the adnexa, evaluate its characteristics, including size, shape, location, tenderness, and consistency.

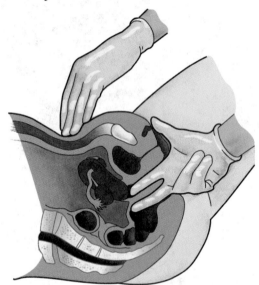

Fig. 18-21 Rectovaginal examination. *(From Lowdermilk and Perry, 2004.)*

RECTAL EXAMINATION

NOTE: The female rectal examination may be done in conjunction with the pelvic examination or independent of a pelvic examination. The female client should remain in a lithotomy position (if the examination is being done in conjunction with the pelvic examination). If the examination is independent of a pelvic exam, the client should assume the left lateral position. Before the exam, tell the client what you will be doing and that the procedure will be uncomfortable; she may feel the pressure of a bowel movement. Lubricate the first

★ = advanced practice

PROCEDURES AND TECHNIQUES WITH NORMAL FINDINGS	**ABNORMAL FINDINGS**

two fingers of a gloved hand. Place your middle finger, palm side up, over the anus. Ask the client to bear down; while she is doing so, gently insert your middle finger into the rectum. Insert your index finger into the vagina and locate the cervix.

★ **PALPATE the rectal wall for surface characteristics.**

Procedure: With the index and middle fingers inserted as far as possible, instruct the client to bear down. This brings more rectal wall into the range of palpation. Gently rotate the finger in the rectum (middle finger) to evaluate the characteristics of the rectal wall.

    Findings: The wall should feel smooth and be without any areas of masses, fistulas, fissures, or tenderness. The septum between the vagina and the rectum should be thin, smooth, and intact. Occasionally the cervix may be palpable on the anterior wall; this could be mistaken for a mass.

Note any areas of masses, polyps, nodules, irregularities, and tenderness.

★ **PALPATE the anal sphincter for muscle tone.**

Withdraw your fingers slowly and evaluate the characteristics of the anal tone with the middle finger. The anus should tighten evenly around the examination finger.

Note the presence of rectal stricture.

EXAMINE stool for characteristics and presence of occult blood.

Slowly remove the gloved finger from the client's rectum. Inspect the gloved finger for color and consistency of stool. It should be brown and soft. Use a guaiac test to evaluate for occult blood (Box 18-5). A negative response is expected.

Note the presence of blood, pus, mucus, or abnormal color of stool (Box 18-6). A positive guaiac test indicates the presence of blood.

BOX 18-5 **GUAIAC TESTING**

If stool is present on your gloved finger, use the guaiac test to check the stool for occult blood.
1. Obtain a guaiac slide and developer (*A*).
2. Open the flap of the cardboard guaiac slide.
3. Dab the gloved finger containing stool on the paper in the boxes of the slide (*B*).
4. Close the flap and remove soiled gloves. Don clean examination gloves.
5. Turn the slide to the reverse side and open the cardboard flap.
6. Apply 2 drops of developing solution on each box of guaiac paper (*C*).
7. Wait 30 to 60 seconds and note the color of the paper. A bluish discoloration of the paper indicates presence of occult blood and is documented as guaiac positive.

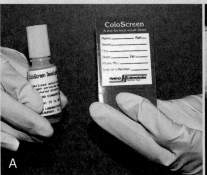
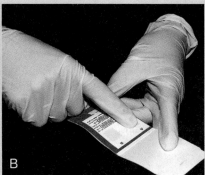
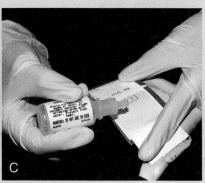

★ = advanced practice

BOX 18-6	**STOOL COLORS AND SIGNIFICANCE**
COLOR	**SIGNIFICANCE**
Bright red	Hemorrhoidal or lower rectal bleeding
Tarry black	Upper intestinal tract bleeding or excessive iron or bismuth ingestion
Light tan or gray	Obstruction of the biliary tract (obstructive jaundice)
Pale yellow	Malabsorption syndrome

Documenting Expected Findings

Female Examination

Pubic hair inverse triangle pattern with smooth, clear, and intact skin. Labia symmetric, smooth, soft, and moist with pigment darker than general skin tone. Clitoris midline between labia minora with smooth, pink, moist cylindric structure. Urinary meatus midline with an irregular opening. Vaginal introitus moist and appears as a thin vertical slit. No tenderness or discharge noted in the areas of Skene's or Bartholin's glands.

Cervix smooth, pink, midline, posterior pointing, round, about 1 inch in diameter, nulliparous, easily movable and without discharge or tenderness. Uterus smooth, firm, anteverted, and freely movable. Ovaries size of walnut, oval, smooth, firm, and mobile bilaterally. Vaginal walls smooth, pink, moist with transverse rugae and minimal thin, clear, and odorless discharge. Skin of the perineum intact and smooth. Anus darker pigmented and coarse skin and tightly closed. Rectal wall smooth and intact. Septum between vagina and rectum thin, smooth, and intact. Anal sphincter tone tight and stool soft and brown.

PROCEDURES AND TECHNIQUES WITH NORMAL FINDINGS	**ABNORMAL FINDINGS**

MALE EXAM

ROUTINE TECHNIQUES	**SPECIAL CIRCUMSTANCES OR ADVANCED PRACTICE**
• INSPECT the pubic hair. • INSPECT and PALPATE the penis. 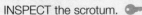 • INSPECT the scrotum. 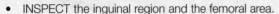 • INSPECT the inguinal region and the femoral area. • INSPECT and PALPATE the sacrococcygeal areas. • INSPECT the perianal area and anus.	**Scrotum and Testes** • PALPATE the scrotum. • PALPATE the testes, epididymides, and vas deferens. • TRANSILLUMINATE the scrotum. ★ **Inguinal Region** • Palpate the inguinal canal. ★ **Rectal Examination** • PALPATE the anus. • PALPATE the anal canal. • PALPATE the prostate. ★ • EXAMINE stool.

EQUIPMENT NEEDED

Examination gloves • Lubricating gel • Light source (if transillumination is needed)

 = core examination skill   ★ = advanced practice

PREPARING FOR THE MALE EXAMINATION

The client is positioned in one of two ways, either standing or lying down. (The client needs to stand to evaluate for a hernia.) If the client is standing, the nurse should be seated facing the client and wearing gloves.

Men may feel apprehensive about having their genitalia examined, especially if the examiner is female. This may be seen as an invasion of privacy rather than accepted as a necessary component of examination. As a nurse, you must be aware of these concerns and approach the genitalia examination in a professional, matter-of-fact way, projecting confidence throughout the examination (Box 18-7).

BOX 18-7	CLINICAL NOTE

When examining male genitalia, use a firm, deliberate touch. If an erection occurs, reassure the client that this is a normal physiologic response to touch and that he could not have prevented it. Do not stop the evaluation; this will focus further on the erection and reinforce the client's embarrassment.

PROCEDURES AND TECHNIQUES WITH NORMAL FINDINGS	ABNORMAL FINDINGS

ROUTINE TECHNIQUES: MALE EXAM

INSPECT pubic hair for distribution and general characteristics.

Hair distribution varies widely but is normally in a diamond-shaped pattern that may extend to the umbilicus. The hair should appear coarser than scalp hair. The hair should be free of parasites, and the skin should be intact, smooth, and clear.

Note patchy growth, loss, or absence of hair; distribution of hair in a female pattern (triangular, with the base over the pubis); nits or pubic lice; scars; lower abdominal or inguinal lesions; or a rash. *Tinea cruris* ("jock itch") is a common fungal infection found in the groin that appears as large, clearly marginated, red patches that are pruritic. *Monilial infections* are red, eroded patches with scaling and pustules and are associated with immobility, systemic antibiotics, and immunologic deficits.

INSPECT and PALPATE the penis for surface characteristics, color, tenderness, and discharge.

The dorsal vein should be apparent on the dorsal surface of the shaft of the penis. The skin is usually dark and hairless, with a wrinkled surface and frequently apparent vascularity. In uncircumcised men, the prepuce is present and folded over the glans (Fig. 18-22, *A*); in circumcised men the amount of prepuce is variable (Fig. 18-22, *B*). If the client has not been circumcised, ask him to retract the foreskin. The foreskin should retract easily and completely over the glans.

Failure of the ability to retract the foreskin, discomfort on retraction, or difficulty returning the foreskin to the original position should be considered abnormal. *Phimosis* is a very tight foreskin that cannot be retracted over the glans (Fig. 18-23). *Paraphimosis* is the inability to return the foreskin over the glans (Fig. 18-24).

= core examination skill

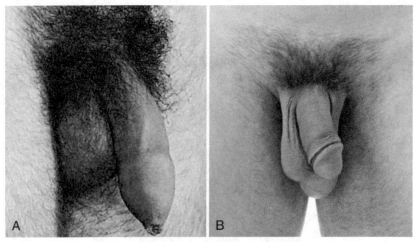

Fig. 18-22   A, Uncircumcised penis. **B,** Circumcised penis.

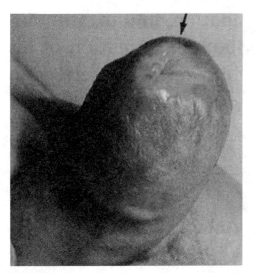

Fig. 18-23   Phimosis. *(From* 400 Self-assessment picture tests in clinical medicine, *1984. By permission of Mosby International.)*

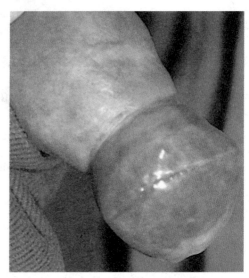

Fig. 18-24   Paraphimosis. *(From Lloyd-Davies et al, 1994.)*

PROCEDURES AND TECHNIQUES WITH NORMAL FINDINGS

Inspect the glans and under the fold of the prepuce. The glans should be smooth, pink, and bulbous. Note any erythema, lesions, edema, nodules, or presence of discharge. (If discharge or smegma is present, obtain a specimen on a slide for microscopic examination.) The prepuce fold is wrinkled and loosely attached to the underlying glans; it is darker than the glans. NOTE: Circumcised penises have varying lengths of foreskin remaining; some have multiple folds, and others have none.

Inspect the urethral meatus. It should be located centrally at the distal tip of the glans, and no discharge should be present. The meatus should appear as a slitlike opening.

ABNORMAL FINDINGS

Balanitis is inflammation of the glans that commonly occurs in clients with phimosis (Fig. 18-25).

Note if the meatus is located either on the upper surface of the penis (epispadias) or on the bottom of the penis (hypospadias) and if there is a discharge present. The discharge may be yellow-green or milky-white or have a foul odor (Fig. 18-26).

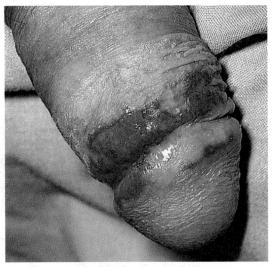

Fig. 18-25   Balanitis. *(From Swartz, 2006.)*

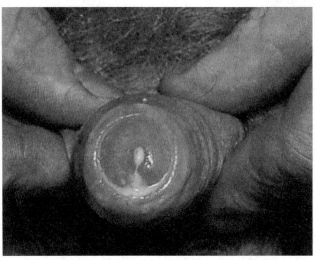

Fig. 18-26   Purulent penile discharge. *(From Swartz, 2006.)*

PROCEDURES AND TECHNIQUES WITH NORMAL FINDINGS

Palpate the glans anteroposteriorly to open the distal end of the urethra (Fig. 18-27). The surface should be pink and smooth, and no discharge should be present.

Palpate the entire shaft of the penis between the thumb and first two fingers. The penis shaft should be nontender and smooth, with a semifirm consistency.

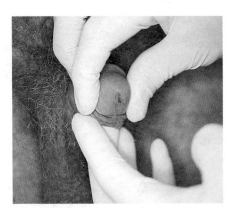

Fig. 18-27   Examination of urethral meatus.

INSPECT and PALPATE the sacrococcygeal areas for surface characteristics and tenderness.

The skin surface should be smooth and clear, and there should be no tenderness on palpation.

ABNORMAL FINDINGS

Report any erythema, edema, discharge, or crusting.

Note tenderness, edema, nodules, or induration.

A dimple with an inflamed tuft of hair or a tender palpable cyst in the sacrococcygeal area suggests a pilonidal cyst or sinus (see Common Problems and Conditions later in this chapter).

PROCEDURES AND TECHNIQUES WITH NORMAL FINDINGS	ABNORMAL FINDINGS

INSPECT the perianal area and anus for pigmentation and surface characteristics.

The buttocks are spread with both hands to inspect this area. The anus should exhibit increased pigmentation and coarse, intact skin. The anus should be tightly closed. No lesions or inflammation should be present. Ask the client to bear down while you inspect the anal area. Again, no lesions should be observed.

Note the presence and location of inflammation and lesions. Identify the location of the abnormality in terms of the position of a clock, with the 12 o'clock position being toward the symphysis pubis and the 6 o'clock position toward the sacrococcygeal area. Lesions that may be seen include external hemorrhoids, ulcerations, warty growths (condylomata acuminta), skin tags, inflammation, fissures, and fistulas. While the client is straining, note the presence of internal hemorrhoids, polyps, tumors, and rectal prolapse (see Common Problems and Conditions later in this chapter).

INSPECT the scrotum for color, texture, surface characteristics, and position.

Hold the penis out of the way with the back of your hand (or ask the client to hold the penis out of the way) while you inspect the scrotum (Fig. 18-28). The scrotal sac is divided in half by the septum; the two sides often appear asymmetric—the left side tends to hang lower than the right because of a longer spermatic cord (see Fig. 18-22, *B*). The scrotal skin is usually more deeply pigmented than the body skin, with a coarse-appearing surface. Small bumps on the scrotal skin are known as sebaceous cysts or sebaceous glands; these are considered a normal finding. The scrotal surface should be a consistent color without lesions. Be sure to lift the scrotum to examine the underside as well. This area is deeply pigmented, hairless, and has a rugous surface.

   Temperature affects the appearance of the scrotum. When the environmental temperature is very cold, the testes retract slightly upward, causing the scrotum to become smaller and tighter in appearance. Conversely, when the temperature is hot, the testes extend downward and the scrotal sac hangs loosely. A client who has a fever may have a pendulous-appearing scrotum.

Scrotal lesions, or scrotal redness (either generalized or isolated), are considered abnormal and may indicate an infection. Excessive differences between the right and left sides are an abnormal finding.

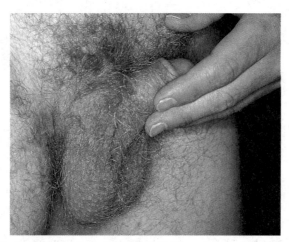

Fig. 18-28   Inspect the scrotum and ventral surface of the penis as the client positions his penis.

⚷➤ = core examination skill

PROCEDURES AND TECHNIQUES WITH NORMAL FINDINGS	ABNORMAL FINDINGS

INSPECT the inguinal region and the femoral area for bulges.

The client should assume a standing position for this part of the examination. Ask the client to bear down. While he is straining, inspect the inguinal canal and femoral area (area just above where the femoral artery is palpated) for presence of a bulge. There should be no bulges.

NOTE: If a bulge is seen, palpate the inguinal ring (described in the Special Circumstances or Advanced Practice section that follows).

Note any bulges in the area of the external ring or the femoral area. Presence of bulges suggests a hernia. See Table 18-4 and Common Problems and Conditions later in this chapter.

SPECIAL CIRCUMSTANCES OR ADVANCED PRACTICE: MALE EXAM

PALPATE the scrotum for surface characteristics and tenderness.

Palpate each half of the scrotum (Fig. 18-29). The surface should feel coarse, with the skin intact and loose over a muscle layer. The thickness of the skin of the scrotum changes with temperature and age. In cold or cool temperatures, the scrotal skin feels thickened. As the individual ages, the skin thins. The scrotum should be nontender.

Note any marked tenderness or edema.

PALPATE the testes, epididymides, and vas deferens for location, consistency, tenderness, and nodules.

Palpate the testes simultaneously with both hands, using the thumb and the first two fingers. Note that the testes are present in each sac; they should be equal in size, mildly sensitive but nontender to moderate compression, smooth and ovoid, and movable.

On the posterolateral surface of each testis, palpate the epididymis—it will feel like a tubular, comma-shaped structure, which collapses when gently compressed between your fingers and thumb. This area should be smooth and nontender.

Note if the testes have not distended into the sac or are enlarged (unilaterally or bilaterally), atrophied, markedly tender, nodular or irregular, or fixed.

If a problem is noted with the epididymides, determine its position in relation to the testes (i.e., proximal or distal); whether it can be moved with your fingers; and if it disappears when the client lies down. Report any tenderness, irregular placement, enlargement, induration, or nodules.

Report any tenderness, tortuosity, thickened or beaded area, or induration.

The vas deferens lies within the spermatic cord. To palpate, grasp both spermatic cords between the thumb and forefinger and palpate, starting at the base of the epididymides, moving upward to the inguinal ring. Because the vas deferens lies within the spermatic cord along with arteries and veins, it is difficult to specifically identify with palpation. The vas deferens feels like a smooth, cordlike structure. It should be nontender and palpable from the epididymis to the external inguinal ring.

PROCEDURES AND TECHNIQUES WITH NORMAL FINDINGS	ABNORMAL FINDINGS

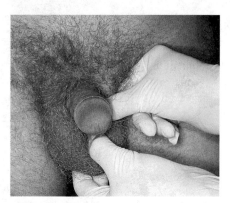

Fig. 18-29   Palpating the scrotum and testes.

★ **TRANSILLUMINATE the scrotum for evidence of fluid and masses.**

If a mass, fluid, or irregularity is suspected, transilluminate each scrotal sac. This technique is performed by using a bright penlight or transilluminator and pressing the light source up against the scrotal sac (Fig. 18-30). There should be no additional contents or fluid. The testes and epididymides do not transilluminate.

Note any mass that is distal or proximal to the testis. It may or may not be tender. Hydroceles and spermatoceles are fluid-filled masses and therefore transilluminate; tumors, hernias, and epididymitis do not.

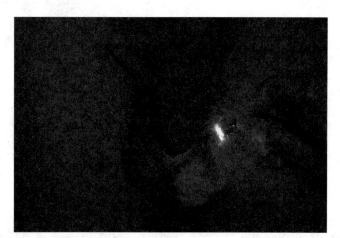

Fig. 18-30   Transillumination of the scrotum. *(From Swartz, 2006.)*

INGUINAL REGION

★ **PALPATE the inguinal canal for evidence of indirect hernia or direct hernia.**

With the client in a standing position, palpate both the right and left inguinal rings. Use your index finger or middle finger of the hand corresponding to the client's side (Fig. 18-31) (e.g., right hand for right side). Insert your finger into the lower aspect of the scrotum. The finger should follow the spermatic cord upward through the triangular, slitlike opening of the inguinal ring into the inguinal canal. Ask the client to bear down or cough. You should not feel any bulging against your fingertip.

Note any palpable mass that touches your fingertip or pushes against the side of your finger.

★ = advanced practice

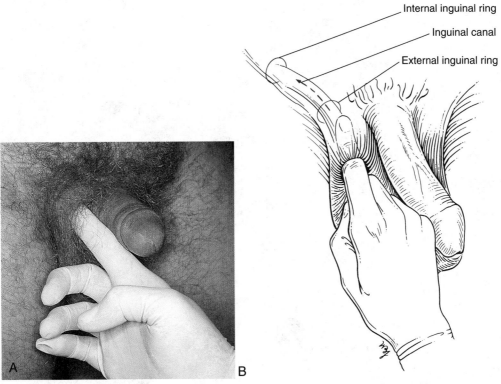

Internal inguinal ring

Inguinal canal

External inguinal ring

A

B

Fig. 18-31 **A,** Palpating for inguinal hernia. **B,** Position of gloved finger inserted through inguinal canal. *(B, From Swartz, 2006.)*

PROCEDURES AND TECHNIQUES WITH NORMAL FINDINGS

ABNORMAL FINDINGS

RECTAL EXAMINATION

The male client should assume either the left lateral position with the hips and knees flexed, a knee-chest position, or the standing position with the hips flexed and the client bending over the examination table with feet pointed together (Fig. 18-32).

PALPATE the anus for sphincter tone.

Ask the client to bear down. Place the finger pad surface of a gloved and lubricated index finger at the anal opening; as the sphincter relaxes, slowly insert the finger, pointing toward the client's umbilicus (Fig. 18-33). Ask the client to tighten the anus around your examining finger. The sphincter should tighten evenly around your finger with minimum discomfort to the client.

A hypotonic sphincter can occur with neurologic deficits, following rectal surgery, or with anal/rectal trauma (especially trauma associated with frequent anal sex). Hypertonic sphincter may be associated with lesions, inflammation, scarring, or anxiety related to the examination. Extreme pain with anal palpation almost always indicates a local inflammation such as a fissure, fistula, or cyst.

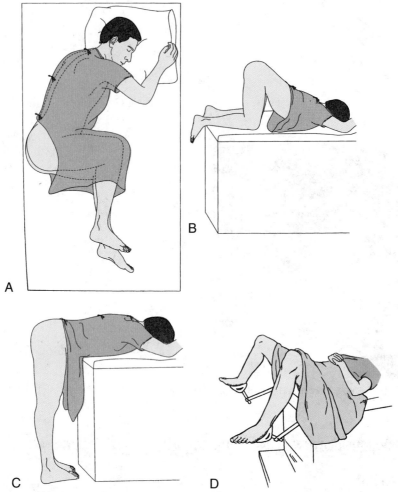

Fig. 18-32   Positions for rectal examination. A, Left lateral or Sims' position. **B,** Knee-chest position. **C,** Standing position. **D,** Lithotomy position. *(From Barkauskus et al, 2002.)*

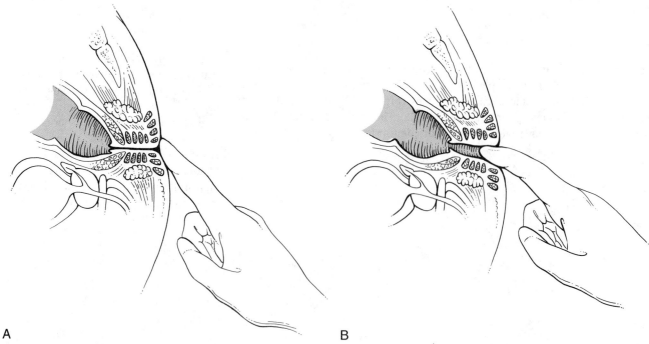

Fig. 18-33   Rectal examination. A, Relax sphincter with gentle pressure with the palmar surface of the finger. **B,** Insert the finger into the anal canal. *(From Swartz, 2006.)*

| **PROCEDURES AND TECHNIQUES WITH NORMAL FINDINGS** | **ABNORMAL FINDINGS** |

★ **PALPATE the anal canal and rectum for surface characteristics.**

Rotate the finger around the musculature of the anal ring to palpate the surface characteristics. The area should be smooth, with even pressure on your finger. Insert the finger as far as possible into the rectum to palpate all four rectal walls. There should be a continuous smooth surface, and the client should experience only minimal discomfort.

Note any nodules, irregularities, masses, presence of hard stool, or tenderness.

★ **PALPATE the prostate (through the anterior rectal surface) for size, contour, consistency, mobility, and tenderness.**

Palpate the posterior surface of the prostate gland by palpating the anterior surface of the rectum (Fig. 18-34). (*NOTE:* The client may state that he has the urge to urinate during the prostate examination. Reassure him that this is a normal sensation.) Note the size, contour, consistency, and mobility of the gland. It should be about 1.5 inches (3.8 cm) in diameter and project less than 0.5 inch (1 cm) into the rectum. The contour is symmetric and bilobed, with a palpable vertical groove in the center (referred to as the sulcus). The prostate should feel firm, smooth, and slightly mobile. Palpation should not produce tenderness.

Note if the prostate projects more than 0.5 inch (1 cm) into the rectum. Estimate classification of prostate enlargement (Box 18-8). Note if there is asymmetry or if the median sulcus is obliterated; also note any tenderness, a boggy feeling, irregularity, or nodules. A rubbery or boggy consistency may indicate benign hyperplasia. A stony-hard or nodular prostate may indicate carcinoma, prostate calculi, or fibrosis.

BOX 18-8	**CLASSIFICATIONS OF PROSTATE ENLARGEMENT**

Grade	Protrusion Into Rectum
Grade I	⅜ to ¾ inch (1 to 2 cm)
Grade II	¾ to 1⅛ inches (2 to 3 cm)
Grade III	1⅛ to 1¾ inches (3 to 4 cm)
Grade IV	Greater than 1¾ inches (4 cm)

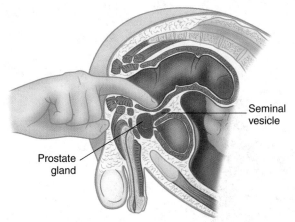

Fig. 18-34   Palpation of the anterior surface of the prostate gland. Feel for the lateral lobes and median sulcus. *(From Seidel et al, 2006.)*

Seminal vesicle

Prostate gland

★ = advanced practice

PROCEDURES AND TECHNIQUES WITH NORMAL FINDINGS

ABNORMAL FINDINGS

EXAMINE stool for characteristics and presence of occult blood.

Slowly remove the gloved finger from the client's rectum. Inspect the gloved finger for color and consistency of stool. It should be brown and soft. Use a guaiac test to evaluate for occult blood (see Box 18-5). A negative response is the expected finding.

Note the presence of blood, pus, mucus, or abnormal color of stool (see Box 18-6). A positive guaiac test indicates the presence of blood.

Documenting Expected Findings

Male Examination

Pubic hair diamond pattern with smooth, clear, and intact skin. Penis is uncircumsized, hairless, wrinkled surface and dorsal vein noted. Shaft smooth and nontender. Glans smooth, pink, and bulbous. Urinary meatus slitlike opening in center of glans with pink, smooth urethra without discharge. Sacrococcygeal area smooth, clear, and nontender. Scrotum deeply pigmented, hairless. coarse with rugous surface and intact skin. Testicles smooth, ovoid, and movable bilaterally, epididymis smooth and nontender bilaterally. No bulges or hernia detects in inguinal area.

Skin of the perineum intact and smooth. Anus darker pigmented and coarse skin and tightly closed. Rectal wall smooth and intact. Prostate symmetric, firm, smooth, slightly mobile. Anal sphincter tone tight and stool soft and brown.

FREQUENTLY ASKED QUESTIONS

In what situations will a nurse perform a rectal examination? It seems like this is something a physician would do.
It is important to remember that a rectal examination includes both an inspection of the anus and an internal examination. Inspection of the anus is done routinely by nurses in a number of situations. For example, when a client has rectal bleeding or pain, the nurse will inspect the anus; the nurse also inspects the anus before inserting a suppository or administering an enema. A common indication for a nurse to palpate the rectum is with a client who is suspected of having a fecal impaction. Most nurses do not routinely perform a prostate examination unless it is a part of their regular practice, such as a nurse in advanced practice.

ETHNIC & CULTURAL VARIATIONS

Circumcision has been a common practice of the dominant American culture. Rationales for circumcision include prevention of phimosis and decreased incidence of glans penis inflammation, cancer of the penis, urinary tract infections in infants, and sexually transmitted disease (particularly syphilis, gonorrhea, and warts). However, the decision to circumcise a newborn infant is based largely on cultural practice. Judaism and Islam incorporate circumcision as part of their belief systems. Most Native Americans, Alaskan Natives, and Hispanics, on the other hand, may be uncircumcised because of their belief system.

AGE-RELATED VARIATIONS

INFANTS AND CHILDREN

Infants and children have functionally immature reproductive systems. For this reason, examination is usually limited to inspection of external genitalia. Further examination may be warranted if parents, caregivers, or the nurse notice a problem. The nurse should always maintain an awareness of the potential for sexual abuse among infants and children. Chapter 20 presents further information regarding reproductive assessment for this age group.

ADOLESCENTS

The onset of puberty (pubescence) marks the beginning of sexual development for boys and girls. A focus for this age group is assessing sexual maturity and the client's response. Adolescents are often self-conscious about the changes; for this reason, the nurse must provide privacy, assure confidentiality, and be reassuring. Chapter 20 presents further information regarding assessment of the reproductive system among adolescents.

OLDER ADULTS

The history and examination of older adults is similar to what has been previously described for the younger adult. Sexual response and physical changes to the genitalia occur as a result of the aging process. Chapter 22 presents further information related to assessment of the older adult.

COMMON PROBLEMS & CONDITIONS

INFECTIONS

Bacterial Vaginosis

Bacterial vaginosis (BV) is caused by an alteration of the normal vaginal flora with other bacteria; a number of bacteria can cause BV, including *Gardnerella vaginalis, Mobiluncus,* and *Mycoplasma hominis.* **Clinical Findings:** The typical signs and symptoms of BV include malodorous vaginal discharge and vulvar itching and irritation.

Candida Vaginitis

Candidiasis is a fungal (yeast) infection usually caused by *Candida albicans.* It has been estimated that 75% of all women have at least one fungal infection; 40% to 45% will have two or more infections at some point during their lifetime (CDC, 2007). *Candida* infections are more prevalent in women who have diabetes mellitus or who are pregnant. **Clinical Findings:** Some women have asymptomatic infections. Those who have symptoms frequently experience vulvar pruritus associated with a thick, cheesy, white vaginal discharge. Vaginal soreness and external dysuria (caused by splash of urine on inflamed tissue) may occur. Erythema and edema to the labia and vulvar skin may be visible.

Sexually Transmitted Disease

Sexually transmitted diseases (STDs; also commonly referred to as sexually transmitted infections [STIs]) represent a large number of infections that are transmitted through sexual activity. There are well over 50 different STDs. Listed here are those the nurse may observe in conjunction with examination of the genitalia.

Chlamydia

Chlamydia is the most common STD in the United States, occurring most frequently among sexually active adolescents and young adults under the age of 25 (CDC, 2007). **Clinical Findings, Women:** Chlamydia infection is asymptomatic in up to 75% of women because it often does not cause enough inflammation to produce symptoms (CDC, 2007). When symptoms occur, the most common are urinary symptoms (such as dysuria, frequency, or urgency) and vaginal symptoms (such as spotting or bleeding after sex, or purulent cervical discharge). The most important examination findings in a Chlamydia infection include purulent or mucopurulent cervical discharge, cervical motion tenderness, or cervical bleeding on introduction of a cotton swab (friability). **Clinical Findings, Men:** This infection usually occurs in the urethra, but it can also affect the rectum. The most common symptoms associated with urethral infection include dysuria, discharge, and urethral itch. If untreated, urethral infection can spread to the epididymis and cause epididymitis.

Gonorrhea

Caused by the aerobic, gram-negative diplococcus *Neisseria gonorrhoeae,* this is currently the second most frequently reported STD in the United States. It is transmitted from genital-genital, oral-genital, and rectal-genital contact. **Clinical Findings, Women:** In most women gonorrhea causes a yellow or green vaginal discharge, dysuria, pelvic or abdominal pain, and abnormal menses. Vaginal itching and burning may be severe. **Clinical Findings, Men:** The most common clinical manifestation of gonorrhea is urethritis. Specific clinical findings include mucopurulent or purulent discharge and dysuria (CDC, 2007). If untreated, gonorrhea can lead to epididymitis.

Syphilis

Syphilis is a chronic systemic disease caused by *Treponema pallidum* that is transmitted congenitally or by sexual contact. Syphilis infection progresses through four stages if left untreated: primary phase, secondary phase, latent phase, and tertiary phase. Primary and secondary phases occur within months of exposure; latent and tertiary syphilis occur over a number of years (Katz, 2007). Fetal exposure (from an infected mother) results in congenital syphilis. **Clinical Findings, Adults:** The clinical manifestations of syphilis vary depending on the phase of infection. Primary syphilis produces a single, firm, painless open sore or chancre with indurated borders at the site of entry on the genitals or mouth (Fig. 18-35, *A*). In men the most common location is on the shaft of the penis (Fig. 18-35, *B*). This ulcer typically appears about 21 days after infection and usually heals within 3 to 6 weeks. Secondary syphilis occurs 6 to 12 weeks after the initial lesion. Individuals develop a rash characterized by red macules and papules over the palms of the hands and soles of the feet. Round or oval, flat grayish lesions known as condyloma latum develop in the anogenital area (Fig. 18-35, *C*). Latent

syphilis follows the secondary stage and can last from 2 to 20 years; during this period the clients are asymptomatic. Tertiary infection has destructive effects on the neurologic, cardiovascular, ophthalmic, and musculoskeletal systems. **Clinical Findings, Neonates:** Infected neonates are often premature with intrauterine growth retardation. Manifestations include retinal inflammation, glaucoma, destructive bone and skin lesions, and central nervous system involvement.

Trichomonas

Trichomonas is a highly contagious STD caused by the protozoan *Trichomonas vaginalis,* which inhabits the vagina and lower urinary tract, particularly the Skene's ducts. **Clinical Findings:** Although some women are asymptomatic, the primary symptom is a malodorous greenish-yellow vaginal discharge often accompanied by vulvar irritation (CDC, 2006). The walls of the vagina and the cervix may have petechial "strawberry patches" (Fig. 18-36).

Herpes Genitalis

Herpes is a sexually transmitted viral infection caused by the herpes simplex virus. Herpes simplex virus type 1 (HSV1) and herpes simplex virus type 2 (HSV2) are two different antigen subtypes of the herpes simplex virus. HSV1 is more commonly associated with gingivostomatitis and oral ulcers (fever blisters), whereas HSV2 is usually associated with genital lesions. However, both types can be transmitted to both sites through genital-oral contact (Box 18-9).

Clinical Findings, Women: Herpes genitalis is far more common among women than in men, and women usually have a more severe clinical course. Typical early symptoms

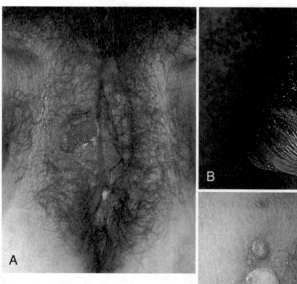
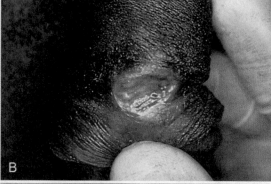
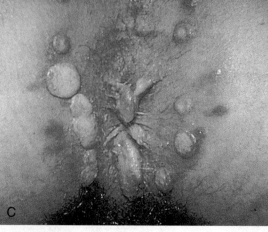

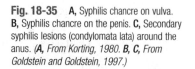

Fig. 18-35   **A,** Syphilis chancre on vulva. **B,** Syphilis chancre on the penis. **C,** Secondary syphilis lesions (condylomata lata) around the anus. (*A, From Korting, 1980. **B, C,** From Goldstein and Goldstein, 1997.*)

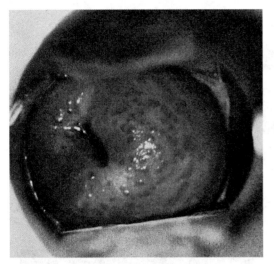

Fig. 18-36 **Trichomoniasis.** The vaginal mucosa and cervix are inflamed and speckled with petechial lesions. *(From Seidel et al, 2006.)*

include burning or pain with urination, pain in the genital area, and fever. Examination findings reveal single or multiple vesicles that can be found on the genital area or the inner thigh. After vesicles rupture, small, painful ulcers are observed (Fig. 18-37, *A*). **Clinical Findings, Men:** The typical clinical manifestations for males include lesions that appear anywhere along the shaft of the penis or near the glans (Fig.

> **BOX 18-9** **CLINICAL NOTE**
>
> Sexually transmitted disease (STD) can occur on the genitalia, on the anus, and in the oral cavity. Furthermore, STD can be present concurrently in more than one location. Therefore, if STD is suspected, examination of other areas is warranted.

18-37, *B*). The lesion is identified because of the red superficial vesicles, which are frequently quite painful. It is important to note that many men with HSV2 are unaware that they have an infection because the symptoms may be mild.

Human Papillomavirus (Genital Warts, Condylomata Acuminatum)

One of the most common STDs is human papillomavirus (HPV) because it is highly contagious and because these infections are often asymptomatic or unrecognized (CDC, 2006). HPV infection is associated with early onset of sexual activity, multiple sex partners, and infrequent use of barrier protection. Although it previously was considered benign, HPV has been linked to malignancies of the cervix and penis. **Clinical Findings:** HPV can cause wartlike growths that are termed *condylomata acuminata* (Fig. 18-38). The warts typically appear as soft, papillary, pink to brown, elongated le-

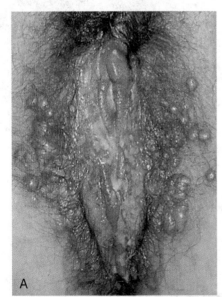

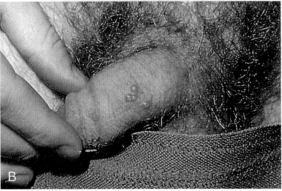

Fig. 18-37 **Herpes lesions. A,** Female. **B,** Male. *(A, From Swartz, 2006. B, From Goldstein and Goldstein, 1997.)*

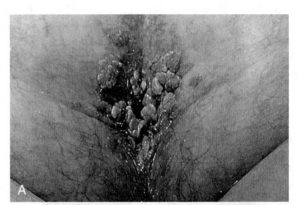

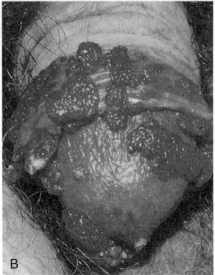

Fig. 18-38 **Condyloma acuminatum. A,** Female. **B,** Male. *(A, From Goldstein and Goldstein, 1997. B, From* Diagnostic picture tests in clinical medicine, *1984.)*

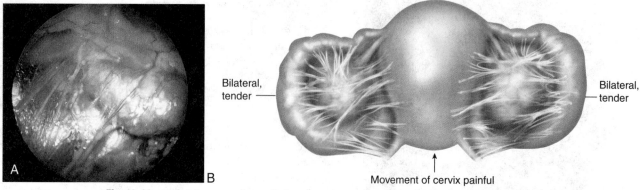

Fig. 18-39 Pelvic inflammatory disease. (*A, From Symonds and MacPherson, 1994. B, From Seidel et al, 2006.*)

sions that may occur singularly or in clusters on the internal genitalia, the external genitalia, and the anal-rectal region. When in clusters, they take on a cauliflower-like appearance.

Pediculosis Pubis (Crabs, Pubic Lice)

Pediculosis pubis is a parasitic infection usually transmitted by sexual contact. **Clinical Findings:** The primary symptom of pubic lice infestation is severe pruritus in the perineal area. Clients may also notice the lice or nits (eggs) in the pubic hair. Examination findings include excoriation and an area of erythema; on close inspection the lice and nits can be seen. Nits are tiny, yellow-white eggs that are attached to the hair shaft. The adult lice are larger, tan to grayish-white in color, and have a crablike appearance when viewed under a magnifying glass. Lice feces appear as tiny dark spots (resembling pepper) and may be seen adjacent to the hair shafts.

Pelvic Inflammatory Disease (Women)

Pelvic inflammatory disease (PID) is a polymicrobial infection of the upper reproductive tract affecting any or all of the following structures: endometrium, fallopian tubes, ovaries, uterine wall, or broad ligaments. It usually is caused by untreated gonococcal and Chlamydia infections. PID is a leading cause of infertility in the United States (Katz, 2007). **Clinical Findings:** PID can occur as an acute or chronic disease; thus symptoms may vary. Acute PID is associated with very tender adnexal areas (ovaries and fallopian tubes). Typically, the pain is so severe that the client is unable to tolerate bimanual pelvic examination. Other symptoms include fever, chills, dyspareunia, and abnormal vaginal discharge. Chronic PID is associated with tender, irregular, and fixed adnexal areas (Fig. 18-39).

Epididymitis

An inflammation of the epididymis and vas deferens is referred to as epididymitis. It is usually caused by the spread of infection from the urethra or bladder. Among sexually active men under the age of 35, it is most often associated with STDs involving *C. trachomatisa* and gonorrhea (CDC, 2006). **Clinical Findings:** Classic symptoms include dull, unilateral

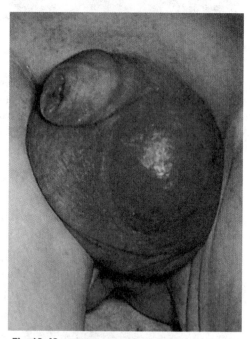

Fig. 18-40 Epididymitis. (*From Lloyd-Davies et al, 1994.*)

scrotal pain that develops over a period of hours to days. The scrotum becomes erythematous and edematous (Fig. 18-40). Associated symptoms may include fever and dysuria. A hydrocele may be seen with transillumination.

BENIGN REPRODUCTIVE CONDITIONS AFFECTING WOMEN

Premenstrual Syndrome

Premenstrual syndrome (PMS) is a group or cluster of recurrent symptoms experienced by women associated with their menstrual cycle. It is thought to be associated with fluctuations in hormone levels as well as changes in altered sensitivity of the neurotransmitter serotonin (Clayton et al, 2006). A history of sexual abuse as an adolescent is also associated with PMS in adulthood (Koci & Strickland, 2007). **Clinical Findings:** A combination of emotional, cognitive, and physical symptoms begin during the last half of the menstrual cycle and diminish after menstruation begins. Common emotional symptoms include mood swings, depression or sadness, irritability, tension, anxiety, restlessness, and anger. Common cognitive symptoms include difficulty concentrating, confusion, forgetfulness, and being accident prone. Physical symptoms may include excessive energy or fatigue, nausea or changes in appetite, insomnia, back pain, headaches, general muscular pain, breast tenderness, and fluid retention.

Endometriosis

Endometriosis is a benign, progressive disease process characterized by the presence and growth of uterine tissue outside the uterus (Fig. 18-41). It is found primarily in women of reproductive age in all ethnic and social groups (Katz et al, 2007). **Clinical Findings:** Common symptoms include pelvic pain, dysmenorrhea, and heavy or prolonged menstrual flow. In some women clinical examination findings include small, firm, nodular-like masses palpable along the uterosacral ligaments. The uterus may be tender. However, in many women with endometriosis, a clinical examination will not detect any abnormality.

Uterine Leiomyomas

Leiomyomas (also called fibroids) are common benign uterine tumors that most commonly affect women over age 35 (March, 2002). The tumors can occur singly or in multiples, and can range in size from microscopic lesions to large tumors that fill the entire abdominal cavity. Leiomyomas are most prominent during reproductive years and tend to shrink after menopause. **Clinical Findings:** The majority of women with leiomyomas are asymptomatic. Those who have symp-

toms often report pelvic pressure and heaviness, urinary frequency, dysmenorrhea, pelvic or back pain, and abdominal enlargement. If large enough, the leiomyomas can be detected by palpation during a pelvic examination. The tumors typically feel firm, smooth, and irregular in shape (Fig. 18-42).

Ovarian Cysts

Ovarian cysts are benign cystic growths within the ovary. Cysts may be solitary or multiple; they can occur unilaterally or bilaterally. Ovarian cysts occur most commonly in young, menstruating women (Katz et al, 2007). **Clinical Findings:** Most ovarian cysts are asymptomatic. When symptoms occur they often include tenderness and a dull sensation or feeling of heaviness in the pelvis. If a cyst ruptures, a sudden onset of abdominal pain occurs. Examination findings for an ovarian cyst include a nontender, fluctuant, mobile, and smooth mass on the ovary (Fig. 18-43).

MALIGNANT REPRODUCTIVE CONDITIONS AFFECTING WOMEN

Cervical Cancer

Cancer of the cervix is usually caused by HPV infection. **Clinical Findings:** The most common symptom is abnormal vaginal bleeding such as bleeding between normal menstrual periods, bleeding after intercourse, or menstrual bleeding that is heavier or lasts longer than normal. On examination a lesion may be visible; the lesion usually has

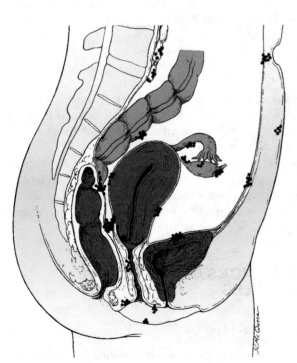

Fig. 18-41 Common sites of endometriosis. *(From Herbst et al, 1992.)*

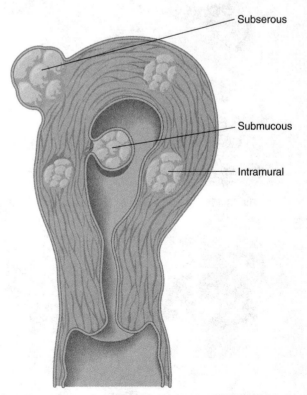

Fig. 18-42 Uterine leiomyomas (fibroids). *(From McCance, 2002.)*

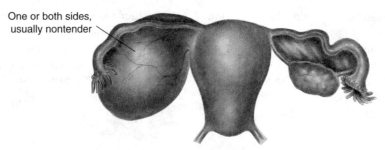

Fig. 18-43 Ovarian cyst. *(From Seidel et al, 2006.)*

One or both sides, usually nontender

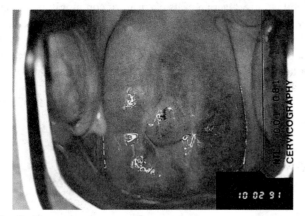

Fig. 18-44 Cervical cancer. The lesion is seen on the cervical os. *(From Symonds and Macpherson, 1994.)*

ETHNIC & CULTURAL VARIATIONS

Healthy People 2010 is designed to achieve two overarching goals: increase quality and years of healthy life and eliminate health disparities. Eliminating racial and ethnic disparities in health requires enhanced efforts at preventing disease, promoting health, and delivering appropriate care. One of the focus areas in which racial and ethnic minorities experience disparity in health access and outcome is cancer screening and management. African American women are more than twice as likely to die of cervical cancer than are white women (*www.cdc.gov/omh*, 2003).

a hard granular surface that bleeds easily and has irregular borders (Fig. 18-44).

Endometrial Cancer

The most common gynecologic malignancy is endometrial cancer. It occurs most often in postmenopausal women, especially those women taking estrogen. **Clinical Findings:** The cardinal symptom is abnormal uterine bleeding or spotting, although a watery vaginal discharge is frequently noted several weeks to months before the bleeding (Fig. 18-45).

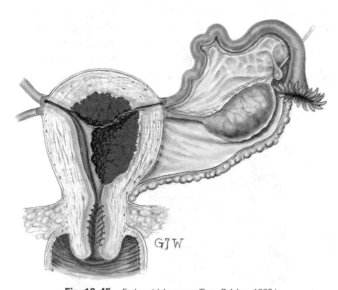

Fig. 18-45 Endometrial cancer. *(From Belcher, 1992.)*

Ovarian Cancer

Ovarian cancer has the highest mortality rate of the gynecologic cancers because it is typically undetected; thus it is known as the "whispering disease." It most commonly occurs among white women over age 50 who live in Western, industrialized nations. **Clinical Findings:** There are usually no symptoms until advanced stages of the disease. The most common symptom of ovarian cancer is abdominal distention or fullness. By the time ovarian malignancies are palpable, the disease is usually advanced (Fig. 18-46).

CONDITIONS OF THE SCROTUM/ TESTICLES

Testicular Torsion

This condition is caused by the twisting of the testicle and spermatic cord, cutting off blood supply; it is considered a surgical emergency. It may occur at any age, but the preva-

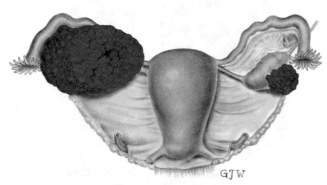

Fig. 18-46 Cancer of the ovaries. *(From Belcher, 1992.)*

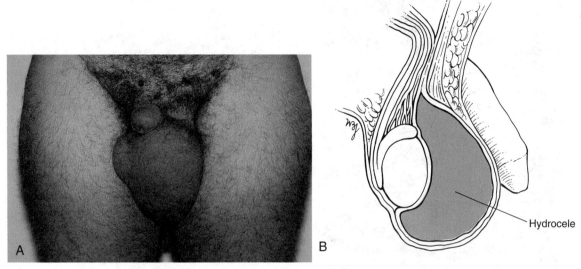

Fig. 18-47 **A,** Hydrocele. **B,** Cross section of hydrocele. *(From Korting, 1980.)*

lence is highest during adolescence. **Clinical Findings:** The hallmark finding of testicular torsion is a history of sudden onset of severe pain and scrotal swelling. The testicle becomes very tender, and the scrotum becomes edematous and often slightly discolored. It is not associated with physical activity or trauma.

Hydrocele

A hydrocele is an accumulation of fluid within the scrotum. In infants, hydroceles often resolve on their own, but occasionally surgical intervention is required (Schneck & Bellinger, 2007). In adults, the cause of hydrocele is often unknown, but may result from infection or a malignancy. **Clinical Findings:** Gradual scrotal enlargement is the most common symptom. The scrotum appears enlarged; edema appears on the anterior surface of the testis, but may also extend up into the spermatic cord area (Fig. 18-47). Transillumination of the scrotum is indicated when a hydrocele is suspected. A light red glow indicates the presence of fluid; failure to glow suggests a mass.

Spermatocele

A spermatocele is a cystic mass that occurs within the epididymis or spermatic cord. It is filled with sperm and seminal fluid. **Clinical Findings:** This condition is usually painless, but is characterized by significant testicular edema in the involved testicle. A separate mass is palpated within the testis adjacent to the epididymis or spermatic cord. Because the lesion is a cyst, it transilluminates (Fig. 18-48).

Varicocele

This condition is caused by an abnormal dilation and tortuosity of the veins along the spermatic cord (Fig. 18-49). The cause is often multifactorial; the dilation is thought to be caused by differences in venous drainage between the right and left sides. Varicocele is a condition primarily affecting boys and young men; most often it affects the left side. **Clinical Findings:** The client may describe a pulling sensation or a dull ache or have scrotal pain. The veins above the testis tend to feel thickened; a palpable mass is usually detected in the scrotum. 90% of varicoceles occur on the left side (Schneck & Bellinger, 2007).

Testicular Cancer

The most common malignancy in men ages 20 to 34 is testicular cancer. **Clinical Findings:** The classic manifestation is a painless testicular mass that is usually discovered by the client or his sexual partner. When pain is an initial symptom, this is usually an indication that the mass has caused bleeding within the testicle or has caused testicular torsion. On examination, a hard and irregular mass is felt within the testis. If the mass is large enough, deformity of the scrotum may be observable (Fig. 18-50).

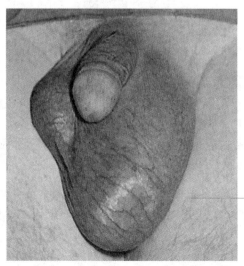

Fig. 18-48 Spermatocele. *(From Lloyd-Davies et al, 1994.)*

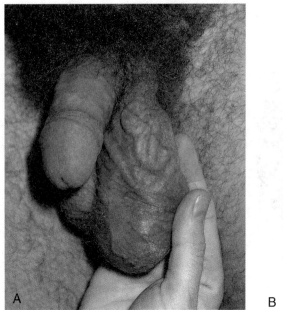
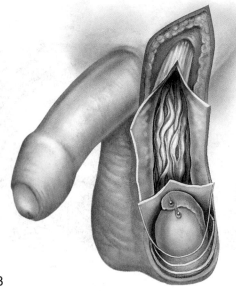

Fig. 18-49   Varicocele. (**A,** *From Swartz, 2006.* **B,** *From Seidel et al, 2006.*)

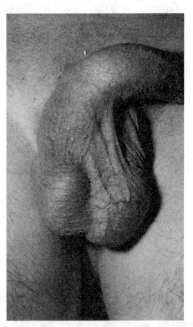

Fig. 18-50   Scrotal asymmetry caused by testicular cancer. *(From* 400 Self-assessment picture tests in clinical medicine, *1984.)*

CONDITIONS OF THE PROSTATE

Benign Prostatic Hyperplasia

Benign prostatic hyperplasia (BPH) is an enlargement of the prostate gland that usually affects older men (Fig. 18-51). At least some degree of BPH will eventually develop in all men with advanced age, causing minor to moderate symptoms. **Clinical Findings:** The American Urological Association symptom index is a tool used to assess voiding symptoms associated with obstruction of the urethra by the prostate (see Table 18-1). The higher the score, the more likely BPH is

present. In addition to symptoms, prostate examination may reveal hyperplasia. When palpated, the prostate feels smooth, firm, and rubbery, and the prostate projects more than 1 cm into the rectum.

Prostatitis

An inflammation of the prostate gland is termed *prostatitis* (Fig. 18-52). It is the most common urologic diagnosis in men under age 50 and the third most common in men over age 50 (Nickel, 2007). There are four recognized categories of prostatitis: acute bacterial prostatitis (ABP); chronic bacterial prostatitis (CBP); chronic pelvic pain syndrome (CPPS); and asymptomatic inflammatory prostatitis. **Clinical Findings:** The clinical manifestation of prostatitis is variable. The client with ABP classically has fever, chills,

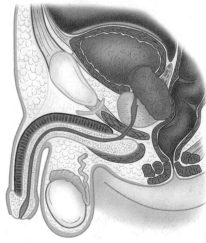

Fig. 18-51   Benign prostatic hyperplasia. *(From Seidel et al, 2006.)*

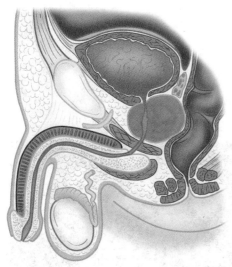

Fig. 18-52 Prostatitis. *(From Seidel et al, 2006.)*

pain in the back and rectal or perineal area, and obstructive symptoms; examination reveals an enlarged prostate that is usually tender with induration. CBP commonly causes recurrent urinary tract infection, pain, dysuria, and scrotal or penile pain; examination findings may be nonspecific or may reveal an enlarged, tender, and boggy prostate. CPPS is characterized by urinary urgency, frequency, nocturia, dysuria, and pain or discomfort; examination findings may be normal or may include a soft and boggy prostate.

Prostate Cancer

Cancer of the prostate is the leading site of cancer in men. Approximately 80% of men who reach age 80 have evidence of prostate cancer at autopsy (Bostwick et al, 2003). **Clinical Findings:** The client is usually asymptomatic until the cancer begins causing urinary obstruction resulting in difficulty urinating. On palpation, the prostate feels hard and irregular. The median sulcus is obliterated as the prostate tumor grows (Fig. 18-53).

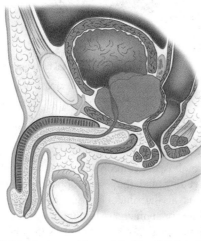

Fig. 18-53 Carcinoma of the prostate. *(From Seidel et al, 2006.)*

CONDITIONS OF THE ANUS AND RECTUM

Pilonidal Sinus

A pilonidal sinus is a small sinus tract under the skin in the sacrococcygeal region. The sinus is lined with epithelium and hair. If the hair penetrates the skin and becomes infected, a pilonidal cyst or abscess results. Nearly 80% of those affected are males; the peak ages are between 15 and 24 years. **Clinical Findings:** A pilonidal cyst or sinus is usually seen as a dimpled area with a small sinus opening that may contain a tuft of hair in the sacrococcygeal area. It is usually diagnosed in young adulthood, although occasionally it is recognized at birth by a depression in the sacral area. Generally, the individual is asymptomatic unless the area becomes infected. Once infected, the area becomes red and tender and a cyst may be palpable. The cyst often drains a mucoid or purulent discharge. The client may complain of pain and swelling at the base of the spine (Fig. 18-54).

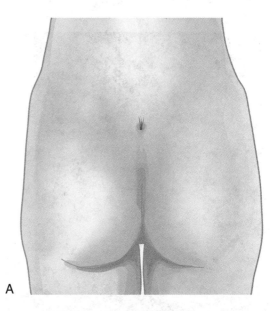

A

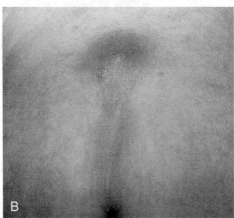

B

Fig. 18-54 **A,** Pilonidal sinus. **B,** Inflamed pilonidal cyst. *(B, From Zitelli and Davis, 1997.)*

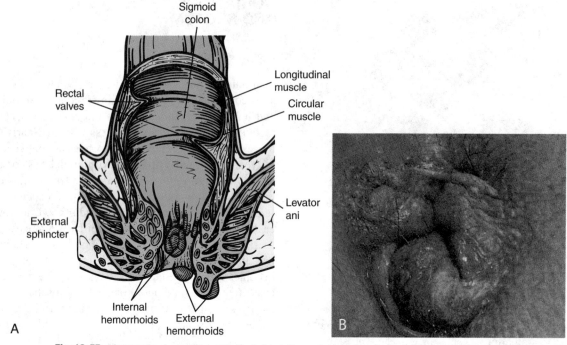

Fig. 18-55 A, Internal and external hemorrhoids. B, External hemorrhoid. (A, From Lewis, Heitkemper, and Dirksen, 2004. B, From Seidel et al, 2006. Courtesy Gershon Efron, MD, Sinai Hospital of Baltimore.)

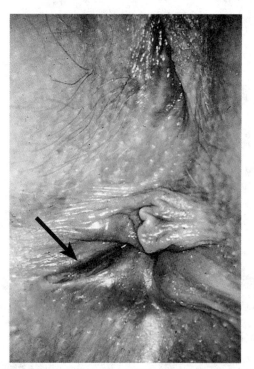

Fig. 18-56 Lateral anal fissure. (From Seidel et al, 2006. Courtesy Gershon Efron, MD, Sinai Hospital of Baltimore.)

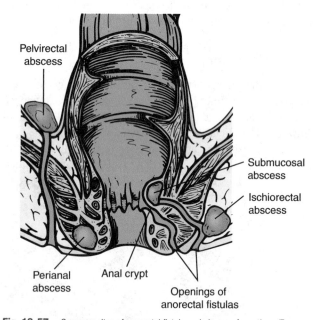

Fig. 18-57 Common sites of anorectal fistula and abscess formation. (From Lewis, Heitkemper, and Dirksen, 2004.)

Hemorrhoids

Hemorrhoids are dilated veins of the hemorrhoidal plexus resulting from increased portal venous pressure. It is thought that both genders are affected equally. **Clinical Findings:** External hemorrhoids originate outside the external rectal sphincter and appear as flaps of tissue. If they become irri-

tated or thrombosed, symptoms include localized itching and perhaps bleeding and they may appear as blue or purple shiny masses at the anus. Internal hemorrhoids originate above the interior sphincter. Although they may be present in the rectum, they may not be seen unless they become thrombosed, prolapsed, or infected (Fig. 18-55).

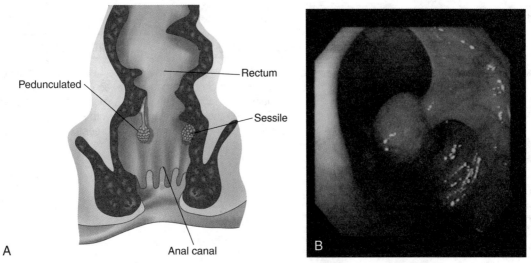

Fig. 18-58   **A,** Types of rectal polyps. **B,** Endoscopic image of a pedunculated polyp. (**B,** *From McCance and Huether, 2002. Courtesy David Bjorkman, MD, University of Utah School of Medicine, Department of Gastroenterology.*)

Anorectal Fissure

An anorectal fissure is a tear of the anal mucosa causing intense pain. It occurs in all age groups, but is seen most often in young healthy adults; the incidence is similar between genders. **Clinical Findings:** The fissure appears as a crack within the anus usually located midline in the posterior wall of the rectum (Fig. 18-56). The client experiences severe rectal pain, itching, and rectal bleeding.

Anorectal Abscess and Fistula

A pus-filled cavity in the anal or rectal area is referred to as an anorectal abscess. A fistula is an inflamed tract that forms an abnormal passage from within the anus or the rectum to the outside skin surface—usually in the perianal area. Typically, the fistula is caused by the drainage of an abscess. These conditions affect men twice as frequently as women (Nelson, 2002). **Clinical Findings:** The principal symptom of an abscess is rectal pain; frequently the client also has a fever. An area of inflammation adjacent to or within the anus is observed with edema, erythema, and induration. Often the pain is so severe that the client cannot tolerate palpation of the area. If a fistula is present, the opening on the skin usually appears as red, raised granulation tissue and the drainage is serosanguineous or purulent (Fig. 18-57).

Rectal Polyp

A rectal polyp is a protruding growth from the rectal mucosa. It may grow outward, as on a stalk (pedunculated), or may grow adhering to the mucosa (sessile) (Fig. 18-58). Most colorectal cancers arise from mutated adenomatous polyps (Jass, 2002). **Clinical Findings:** A common symptom is rectal bleeding, although often the client is unaware that a polyp exists. Occasionally, a polyp may protrude from the anus and appear as small, soft nodules. Polyps are often difficult to palpate and are most often identified during a colonoscopy exam.

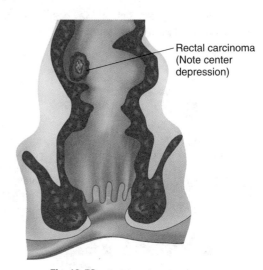

Fig. 18-59   Rectal carcinoma.

Carcinoma of the Rectum and Anus

Rectal and anal cancer occurs when a malignant tumor grows within the rectal mucosa, anal canal, or anus. **Clinical Findings:** Clients may or may not have symptoms; however, the most common symptom is rectal bleeding. If palpable, a malignant rectal tumor manifests as an irregular mass on the rectal wall with nodular, raised edges (Fig. 18-59).

PROLAPSE OR HERNIATION

Hernia

A hernia is a protrusion of part of the peritoneal-lined sac through the abdominal wall. The three most common types of hernias seen when examining the inguinal area are indirect inguinal hernia, direct inguinal hernia, and femoral hernia. **Clinical Findings:** Signs and symptoms of the various types of hernias are presented in Table 18-4.

TABLE 18-4   *Comparisons of Hernias*

	DESCRIPTION	CLINICAL SIGNS
Indirect Hernia 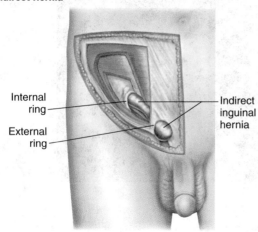 Internal ring External ring Indirect inguinal hernia The most frequent type of hernia. May occur in both sexes and in children (mostly males).	The sac herniates through the internal inguinal ring. It can remain in the inguinal canal, exit through the external canal, or actually pass into the scrotum.	The hernia feels like a soft swelling against the nurse's fingertips. The client usually complains of pain with straining. The hernia may decrease when the client lies down.
Direct Hernia 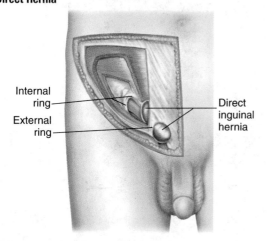 Internal ring External ring Direct inguinal hernia Less common. Occurs most frequently in males over age 40; uncommon in women.	The sac herniates through the external inguinal ring. The hernia is located in the Hesselbach triangle region. It rarely enters the scrotum.	The client has a bulge in the Hesselbach triangle area that is usually painless. The hernia pushes against the nurse's fingertips when the client bears down. May decrease when the client lies down.
Femoral Hernia 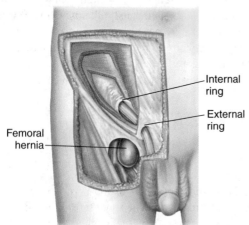 Internal ring External ring Femoral hernia The least common type of hernia. Occurs most frequently in women.	The sac extends through the femoral ring, canal, and below the inguinal ligament.	Pain in the inguinal area. The right side is more frequently affected than the left side. Pain may be severe.

Illustrations from Seidel et al, 2006.

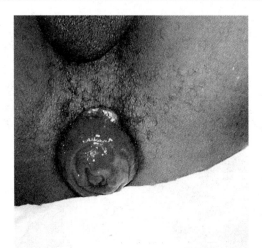

Fig. 18-60   Prolapse of the rectum. *(From Seidel et al, 2006. Courtesy Gershon Efron, MD, Sinai Hospital of Baltimore.)*

Rectal Prolapse

Rectal prolapse is a full-thickness protrusion of the rectal wall though the anus (turning inside out). The incidence is hard to determine, because many people have mild forms of this condition and never seek treatment. It can occur at any age, but most cases involve women over age 60. **Clinical Findings:** Symptoms of rectal prolapse include rectal bleeding, a mass, and change in bowel habits (such as fecal incontinence or soiling with mucous discharge). The client may report that an intestine or a hemorrhoid is hanging out of the anus. The prolapsed rectum appears as a pink mucosal bulge that is described as a "doughnut" or "rosette" (Fig. 18-60).

Uterine Prolapse

Uterine prolapse is associated with a retroverted uterus that descends into the vagina. In first-degree prolapse the cervix remains within the vagina (Fig. 18-61, *A*). In second-degree prolapse the cervix is in the introitus (Fig. 18-61, *B*). In third-degree prolapse, the cervix and vagina drop outside the introitus (Fig. 18-61, *C*). **Clinical Findings:** The primary symptoms described by individuals with uterine prolapse include a feeling of heaviness, fullness, or the sensation of "falling out" in the perineal area. The cervix is visualized low within the vagina, at the vaginal opening, or protruding from the vaginal opening.

Cystocele

Cystocele is a protrusion of the urinary bladder against the anterior wall of the vagina. **Clinical Findings:** The woman may experience a sensation of fullness or pressure, stress incontinence, occasional urgency, and a feeling of incomplete emptying after voiding. A soft bulging mass of the anterior vaginal wall is usually seen and felt as the woman bears down (Fig. 18-62, *A, B*).

Rectocele

Rectocele is a hernia-type protrusion of the rectum against the posterior wall of the vagina. **Clinical Findings:** The woman often complains of a heavy feeling within the vagina. Other commonly reported symptoms include constipation, a feeling of incomplete emptying of the rectum after a bowel movement, and a feeling of something "falling out" in the vagina. Bulging of the posterior vagina is observed as the woman bears down (Fig. 18-62, *C*).

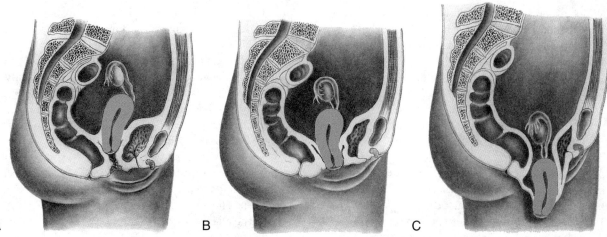

A   B   C

Fig. 18-61   Uterine prolapse. A, First-degree prolapse of the uterus. **B,** Second-degree prolapse of the uterus. **C,** Third-degree prolapse of the uterus. *(From Seidel et al, 2006.)*

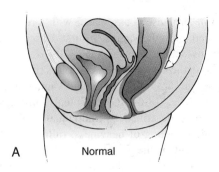

A   Normal

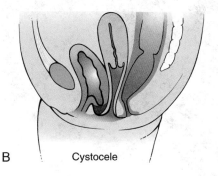

B   Cystocele

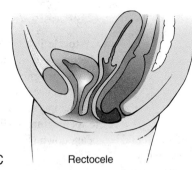

C   Rectocele

Fig. 18-62   A, Normal anatomical position. **B,** Cystocele, protrusion of the wall of urinary bladder through the vagina. **C,** Rectocele, protrusion of the rectal wall through the vagina. *(From Swartz, 2006.)*

CLINICAL APPLICATION & CLINICAL REASONING

See Appendix E for answers to exercises in this section.

REVIEW QUESTIONS

1 Which of the following findings does the nurse recognize as abnormal when examining a male client?
  1 Testes that are palpable and firm within the scrotal sac bilaterally.
  2 Discharge from the penis when the glans is compressed.
  3 Foreskin that lies loosely over the penis.
  4 The glans is a lighter skin tone than the rest of the penis.

2 A 22-year-old white male comes to the emergency department with a concern about a mass in his testicle. In addition to his age and race, which of the following is a known risk factor for testicular cancer?
  1 He had an undescended testicle at birth.
  2 His mother had breast cancer.
  3 He was treated for gonorrhea 18 months ago.
  4 He had a hydrocele during infancy.

3 What instructions should the nurse provide to the client before a visit for a pelvic examination and Pap smear?
  1 Avoid sexual intercourse for 2 days before the examination.

2 If menstruating, avoid using tampons before the examination.
3 Take a tub bath shortly before the examination.
4 Avoid douching for 24 hours before the examination.

4 While taking the health history of a 23-year-old female client, the nurse considers risk factors for sexually transmitted disease. Which of the following suggests a need for client education?
  1 The client states that she has been in a monogamous sexual relationship for 2 years.
  2 The client states that she has been sexually involved with one man for the last 2 weeks; she uses spermicidal gel to prevent pregnancy.
  3 The client has a Pap smear each year.
  4 The client uses oral contraceptives to prevent pregnancy.

5 A client has a herpes lesion on her vulva. While examining this client, the nurse should take which of the following measures?
  1 Wear examination gloves while in contact with the genitalia.
  2 Place the client in an isolation room.

3 Wash the genitalia with alcohol or betadine before the examination.

4 Inspect the genitalia only; reschedule the client for a full examination after the lesion has healed.

6 To inspect the glans penis of the uncircumcised male, the nurse retracts the foreskin. After inspection, the nurse is unable to replace the foreskin over the glans. The nurse recognizes that this situation could potentially lead to:

1 Decreased sperm production.

2 Urinary tract infection.

3 Tissue necrosis of the penis.

4 Testicular cancer.

7 Examination of the ovaries is performed by which assessment technique?

1 Inspection while a speculum is in place.

2 Palpation while the speculum is in place.

3 Percussion of the abdomen directly over the ovaries.

4 Palpation of the ovaries using a bimanual palpation technique.

8 Because of the location of the prostate gland, the nurse recognizes which of the following symptoms is commonly associated with prostate enlargement?

1 Constipation.

2 Rectal bleeding.

3 A weak urinary stream.

4 Penile discharge.

9 During an examination, the nurse palpates the Skene's glands. Which of the following best describes this process?

1 Exerting pressure over the clitoris, slide the finger downward (posteriorly) toward the vaginal opening.

2 Palpate the fourchette and slide the finger forward (anteriorly) toward the vaginal opening.

3 Exert pressure on the anterior vaginal wall and slide the finger outward toward the vaginal opening.

4 Grasp the labia majora between the index finger and thumb, and milk the labia outward.

10 A client tells the nurse that her stools are a gray to light tan color. The nurse suspects which of the following problems?

1 Gallbladder disease.

2 Hemorrhoids.

3 Rectal polyps.

4 Upper intestinal bleeding.

SAMPLE DOCUMENTATION

Review the following data obtained during an interview and examination by the nurse below:

L. T., a 48-year-old black single woman, presents with a primary symptom of "hot flashes." The client thinks she is "going through the change." She wants an examination to determine if this is the case and wants to know what she can do about it. She states that her periods have become very irregular, sometimes lasting only 1 day. The times between periods has also become irregular and range anywhere from 3 to 7 weeks. L. T. reports that her last period was a couple months ago. She states she has also been having problems sleeping and reports that she awak-

ens frequently during the night "in a sweat." She states that she has not slept well for several months. L. T. states that she is sexually active with her boyfriend of 5 years. She verbalizes concern about the effect of "the change" on the way she looks and on her ability to have sex. L. T. states that she last had a Pap smear 10 months ago during routine examination. She states that the results were normal. L. T. states that she was about 14 when she started menstruating. Vital signs for L. T. are as follows: temperature, 97.5° F (36.4° C); blood pressure, 144/86; pulse, 92; respiratory rate, 16. L. T. states that she currently takes nisoldipine 20 mg every day for the treatment of hypertension. She says that she has had high blood pressure for only 2 years and has been taking the nisoldipine for about a year. She states that she has an allergy to sulfa drugs; when she takes them she develops hives. L. T. has never been pregnant. On examination, her external genitalia are moist and pink without any lesions or drainage. Pelvic examination reveals a pink, midline cervix without lesions; vaginal discharge is clear, odorless, and scant. Bimanual palpation reveals an anteverted uterus that is small, firm, mobile, and nontender. No masses are palpable. The ovaries are also palpable bilaterally; they are small, smooth, and slightly tender to deep palpation; no masses. The rectovaginal examination reveals no tenderness, masses, fissures, or fistulas. L. T. has a small cystocele visible.

Below, note how the nurse recorded these same data in a documentation format.

---

48 y/o black ♂ CC: hot flashes. Medical Hx: HTN × 2 yr. Medications: nisoldipine 20 mg PO qd × 1 yr. Allergies: sulfa; hives. Pap smear: 10 mo ago; reports "normal" findings.

SUBJECTIVE DATA

Client believes she is "going through the change"; requests examination and wants information regarding menopause. Describes irregular periods sometimes lasting only 1 day; time between periods 3 to 7 weeks. LMP a couple of months ago. Other Sx: difficulty sleeping; night sweats. Menarche at age 14; has never been pregnant. Sexually active with male partner of 5 yr; concerned about the effect of changes on appearance and sexual function.

OBJECTIVE DATA

General survey: Vital signs: T 97.5° F (36.4° C), HR 92, RR 16, BP 144/86. Alert female, no distress.

External genitalia: Hair distribution, female pattern; no lesions or discoloration to vulva; small cystocele noted; no rectocele. No lesions noted.

Pelvic examination: Cervix pink, midline, parous, no lesions; vaginal discharge clear, odorless, and scant.

Bimanual examination: Uterus anteverted, small, firm, mobile, nontender, no masses. Ovaries bilaterally small, smooth, mild tenderness with deep palpation; no masses. Rectum without hemorrhoids, fissures, or fistulas.

CASE STUDY

Mia Richards is a 33-year-old woman who comes to the urgent care center. The following data are collected by the nurse.

Interview Data

Mia tells the nurse, "I have a really bad pain in front of my butt. It hurts so much that I can't even wipe with a tissue after I go to the bathroom. There is no way I could have a bowel movement right now." Mia states that the pain started 2 days ago and is "much worse now." When asked about her sexual activity she says, "I'm with a guy, but it's not exclusive or anything. We see other people and try not to be real serious."

Examination Data

- *External examination:* Typical hair distribution, urethral meatus intact, no redness or discharge. Perineum intact. Extreme pain response to palpation of vaginal opening; edema, redness, and mass detected on right side. Spontaneous, foul-smelling, dark yellow discharge noted with palpation over Bartholin's glands.
- *Internal examination:* Deferred because of extreme pain associated with inflammation.

Clinical Reasoning

1. What data deviate from normal findings, suggesting a need for further investigation?
2. What additional information should the nurse ask or assess for?
3. Based on the data, what risk factors for STD does Mia have?
4. What nursing diagnoses and collaborative problems should be considered for this situation?

INTERACTIVE ACTIVITIES

Open the interactive student CD-ROM, click on Chapter 18, and choose from the following activities on the menu bar:

- **Multiple Choice Challenge.** Click on the best answer for each question. You will be given immediate feedback, rationale for incorrect answers, and a total score. Good luck!

- **Crossword Wizard.** Complete a crossword puzzle using the clues associated with health assessment concepts. It's a whiz!

- **Marvelous Matches.** Drag each word or phrase to the appropriate place on the screen. Test your ability to match reproductive and perineum conditions with their descriptions.

- **The Name Game.** Identify each of the anatomic parts on the figure shown. Watch out where you place your answer—it won't stick if it's in the wrong place.

- **Symptom Analysis.** Review this client's case study. Choose from the list of questions to ask your client, practice your clinical skills by taking notes, and then rule out possible causes. See why your analysis is correct or incorrect. Good luck!

- **Printable Lab Guide.** Locate the Lab Guide for Chapter 18, and print and use it (as many times as needed) to help you apply your assessment skills. These guides may also be filled in electronically and then saved and e-mailed to your instructor!

- **Quick Challenge.** Use this critical thinking exercise to assess your skills through case study-style questions, then compare with expert answers!

- **Core Examination Skills Checklists.** Make sure you've got frequently-used exam skills down pat! Use these checklists to help cover all the bases for your examination.

CHAPTER 19

Developmental Assessment Throughout the Life Span

Physical, behavioral, and cognitive development of clients are a vital part of assessment. Nurses compare and contrast a client's actual characteristics with those described in standardized norms. For example, the growth of infants is assessed to determine if their bones and muscles are developing as expected for a specific age. Deviations from these expectations or the norm may indicate a health problem that nurses can address with the parents or caregivers. Clients are asked about actions they take to prevent illness. The client's responses are compared with recommendations such as those by the U.S. Preventive Services Task Force and the immunization schedule found in Table 19-6. Nurses also collect data related to behavioral and cognitive development from clients and compare these data with the developmental tasks that have been identified for those age groups. When deviations from the norm are found, nurses discuss the findings with clients, parents, or caregivers.

This chapter is organized by chronologic age divisions that correlate with developmental periods. Each division discusses physical, behavioral, and cognitive development, as well as developmental tasks for that age group. During the first 6 years, however, physical growth and development are so dramatic that additional data are used to describe motor development, social-adaptive behaviors, and language development.

- *Motor development* has two components: gross and fine motor behavior. Gross motor behavior refers to postural reactions such as head balance, sitting, creeping, standing, and walking. Fine motor behavior refers to the use of hands and fingers in the prehensile approach to grasping and manipulating an object.
- *Social-adaptive behavior* refers to the interactions of the infant or child with other persons, as well as the ability to organize stimuli, to perceive relationships between objects, to dissect a whole into its component parts, to reintegrate these parts in a meaningful fashion, and to solve practical problems. Examples are smiling at other persons and learning to feed self.
- *Language behavior* is used broadly to include visible and audible forms of communication, whether facial expression, gesture, postural movements, or vocalizations (words, phrases, or sentences). Language also includes the comprehension of communication by others.

THEORIES OF DEVELOPMENT

By using theories of development, nurses can describe and predict the growth and development of clients throughout the life span. Two widely used theories of behavioral and cognitive development are described briefly. These theories were developed by Erik Erikson and Jean Piaget.

Personality Development: Erikson's Theory

Erik Erikson (1902–1994) believed that the ego was the primary seat of personality functioning (Erikson, 1963). In addition to the ego, he believed that society and culture influenced behavior. Erikson believed that people developed through a predetermined unfolding of their personalities in eight stages. An analogy of a rosebud unfolding may be useful in thinking about development. Each petal opens at a certain time in a certain order, which is predetermined. If the natural order is disturbed by pulling off a petal prematurely or out of order, the development of the mature rose is affected (Boeree, 1997). Each stage involves certain developmental tasks that are psychosocial in nature and described as

TABLE 19-1 Erikson's Eight Stages of Human Development

STAGE (APPROXIMATE)	PSYCHOSOCIAL STAGE	LASTING OUTCOMES
Infancy	Basic trust versus basic mistrust	Drive and hope
Toddlerhood	Autonomy versus shame and doubt	Self-control and will power
Preschool	Initiative versus guilt	Direction and purpose
Middle childhood (school age)	Industry versus inferiority	Method and competence
Adolescence	Identity versus role confusion	Devotion and fidelity
Young adulthood	Intimacy versus isolation	Affiliation and love
Middle adulthood	Generativity versus stagnation	Production and care
Older adulthood	Ego integrity versus despair	Renunciation and wisdom

Modified from Erikson EH: *Childhood and society,* ed 2, New York, 1963, Norton.

polar opposites or conflicts (Table 19-1). For example, in the first stage, during infancy, the conflict is trust versus mistrust. Infants learn that they can depend on their caregivers to meet their needs for food, protection, comfort, and affection. When the infant develops trusting relationships with others, usually the mother, the lasting outcome tends to be ambition, enthusiasm, and motivation. By contrast, when trust is not developed, that person tends to develop apathy and indifference. However, Erikson believed that a balance was needed at each stage. For example, infants need to learn to trust, but they also need to learn a little mistrust so that they do not grow up to become gullible (Boeree, 1997). Accomplishing each successive task provides the foundation for a healthy self-identity. Each stage builds on the previous stages and must be accomplished for the person to successfully complete the next one. People with whom a person interacts, as well as environmental factors, influence the accomplishment of these tasks; however, the motivation to achieve a healthy identity arises from within each person. Although each conflict is described at a particular developmental stage, all of the conflicts exist in each person to some extent throughout life. Even though the conflict may be resolved at one time in a person's life, it may recur in similar circumstances (Erikson, 1963).

Cognitive Development: Piaget's Theory

Jean Piaget (1896–1980) described stages of cognitive development from birth to about 15 years of age. *Cognition* is defined as how a person perceives and processes information. He believed the child's main goal was to establish equilibrium between self and environment.

Piaget believed that the child's view of the world developed from simple reflex behavior to complex logical and abstract thought. To fully develop cognition, the child needs a functioning neurologic system and sufficient environmental stimuli. Piaget described four distinct, sequential levels of cognitive development (Table 19-2). Each stage represents a change in how children understand and organize their environment, and each stage is characterized by more sophisticated types of reasoning. All children move through the stages in sequential order but not necessarily at the same age (Piaget and Inhelder, 1969).

TABLE 19-2 Piaget's Levels of Cognitive Development

STAGE	AGE	CHARACTERISTICS
Sensorimotor	0-2 yr	Thought dominated by physical manipulation of objects and events.
Preoperational	2-7 yr	Functions symbolically using language as major tool.
Concrete operations	7-11 yr	Mental reasoning processes assume logical approaches to solving concrete problems.
Formal operations	11-15 yr	True logical thought and manipulation of abstract concepts emerge.

Modified from Schuster C, Ashburn S: The process of human development: a holistic life-span approach, Boston, 1992, Lippincott.

Adult Intelligence

Though Piaget's work represents the most complete work in cognitive development, it does not progress through adulthood. Theorists of adult intelligence suggest assessing the "practical" intelligence of adults. They believe intelligence develops through an interaction of biologic and environmental factors. Intellectual abilities of adults can be sustained or improved until late adulthood. Two types of adult intelligence have been described: fluid and crystallized. Fluid intelligence represents the ability to perceive complex situations and engage in short-term memory, concept formation, reasoning, and abstraction. This type of intelligence develops through central nervous system function and declines with age and physiologic change. Crystallized intelligence is associated with those skills and knowledge learned as a part of growing up in a given culture, such as verbal comprehension, vocabulary, and ability to evaluate life experiences. This type of intelligence develops through life experiences and education and remains stable or increases with maturity (Shaie, 1996). While fluid intelligence begins to decline at about age 35 to 40, crystallized intelligence is maintained longer (Merriam and Caffarella, 1999). In addition to innate ability, adult intelligence is also affected by other factors such as social class, illness, personality, and motivation. For example, adults of average intelligence who have the opportunities for education and are sufficiently motivated reveal greater increases in intelligence throughout adulthood.

Several theorists believe that the academic type of testing used to assess intelligence in children is not appropriate for adults. Intelligence in adults is gained from "real world" experiences that are difficult to measure by standardized tests. Sternberg is a theorist who proposed a three-pronged theory of intelligence. The first prong (componential subtheory) was described as the internal analytic mental mechanisms. The second (experiential subtheory) focused on how a person's learning through life experiences, combined with insight and creativity, affects the person's thinking. The third (contextual subtheory) focused on the role of the external environment in determining what constitutes intelligence in a particular situation (Sternberg, 1988). Diminished vision and slower response time may contribute to an intellectual decline in older adults.

DEVELOPMENTAL TASKS

Developmental tasks evolve from physical growth and cultural influences. As individuals grow, they are able to perform more complex tasks. For example, as infants' bones, muscles, and nervous systems mature, they progress from sitting to standing to walking. This progression increases the tasks they are able to accomplish. Likewise, as their nervous system matures, they are able to interact with family members to develop communication skills. Infants who live in an environment with several generations may have more opportunity to develop communication skills earlier because of the increased number of people with whom they interact. Families, peers, and associates expect individuals in their spheres of influence to conform in certain ways. These expectations are culturally appropriate and influence individuals' functioning in various roles and statuses for their age and gender (Duvall and Miller, 1985). For example, the developmental task of working toward a vocation may be expected of adolescent males in some cultures, but in young male adults in other cultures.

Each culture has its own developmental tasks and expectations. These tasks also vary from region to region in the United States, and even from one socioeconomic class to another within one geographic area, which may account for differences among people of various ethnic and cultural backgrounds. A developmental task is a drive from within the individual to develop in such a way as to attain a goal. The thrust to change usually comes from within the person, but it may be motivated by the demands and expectations of others (Duvall and Miller, 1985). A conflict may arise in families who move to the United States from foreign countries. Their children are expected to follow the culture of the parents' country of origin, but they also are influenced by the American culture. The developmental tasks presented in this chapter are intended to be used as a guide because there are many normal variations based on ethnic and cultural influences. The boxes in this chapter describe developmental tasks throughout the life span, including the tasks of infants, toddlers, preschoolers, school-age children, adolescents, young adults, middle adults, older adults, and young-old and old-old adults.

INFANTS

Infancy refers to the first year of life. The rapid growth and development that occur during these first 12 months are evident from the data given in Table 19-3, which lists changes in the infant by month, whereas subsequent tables document changes by intervals of 6 months to 1 year. During this time extensive neurologic and physical development occur in addition to the acquisition of psychosocial skills.

Physical Growth

Height, weight, and head circumference are measured to assess infant growth. Growth proceeds from head to toe (cephalocaudal) as evidenced by the infant's development of head control before sitting and mastery of sitting before standing. Healthy newborns weigh between 5 lb 8 oz and 8 lb 13 oz (between 2500 and 4000 g). The newborn period is the first 28 days of life. Commonly newborns lose 10% of their birth weight in the first week but regain it in 10 to 14 days. In general they double their birth weight by 4 to 5 months of age and triple it by 12 months of age. The infant grows 1 inch (2.5 cm) each month for the first 6 months, followed by 0.5 inch (1.3 cm) a month from age 6 months to 12 months. Expected head circumference for term newborns averages from 13 to 14 inches (33 to 36 cm) and increases 0.5 inch (1.3 cm) monthly for the first 6 months. By 6 months teeth begin to erupt, with a total of six to eight teeth by the end of the first year.

Behavioral and Cognitive Development

A summary of the expected developmental milestones of infants is found in Table 19-3. Erikson's developmental task of the first stage, infancy or the oral-sensory stage, is to develop trust without completely eliminating the capacity for mistrust (Boeree, 1997). Infants develop trust relationships with the mother or primary caregiver. Important criteria are the quality and consistency of the mother-child relationship. Infants who receive consistent, loving care learn that they can depend on people around them to meet their needs. By contrast, care that is inconsistent, abusive, or undependable may result in mistrust of people.

Piaget identifies sensorimotor development as the primary task at this age. Infants use their sensorimotor abilities to master motor milestones and to launch relationships with others. Not only can infants advance from crawling to walking and eating some foods, but they also have the ability to win the hearts and attention of others with an intentional smile and showing preference for familiar caregivers. Bond-

TABLE 19-3 *Expected Development of Infants*

AGE	FINE MOTOR	GROSS MOTOR	SOCIAL-ADAPTIVE	LANGUAGE
1 mo	Follows with eyes to midline Hands predominantly closed Strong grasp reflex	Turns head to side Keeps knees tucked under abdomen When pulled to sitting position, has gross head lag and rounded, swayed back	Regards face	Responds to bell Cries in response to displeasure Makes sounds during feeding
2 mo	Follows objects well; may not follow past midline Hands frequently open	Holds head in same plane as rest of body Can raise head and maintain position; looks downward	Smiles responsively	Vocalizes (not crying) Cries become differentiated Coos
3 mo	Follows past midline When in supine position puts hands together; will hold hands in front of face Pulls at blanket and clothes	Raises head to 45-degree angle Maintains posture Looks around with head May turn from prone to side position When pulled into sitting position, shows only slight head lag	Shows interest in surroundings	Laughs Coos, babbles, chuckles
4 mo	Grasps rattle Plays with hands together Inspects hands Carries objects to mouth	Actively lifts head up and looks around (Fig. 19-1) Will roll from prone to supine position When pulled to sitting position, no longer has head lag When held in standing position, attempts to maintain some weight support	Becomes bored when left alone Begins to show memory	Squeals Vocalizations change with mood
5 mo	Can reach and pick up object May play with toes	Able to push up from prone position and maintain weight on forearms Rolls from prone to supine and back to prone Maintains straight back when in sitting position	Smiles spontaneously Playful, with rapid mood changes Distinguishes family	Uses vowel-like cooing sounds with consonantal sounds (e.g., *ah-goo*)
6 mo	Will hold spoon or rattle Will drop object and reach for second offered object Holds bottle	Begins to raise abdomen off table Sits, but posture still shaky May sit with legs apart; holds arms straight as prop between legs Supports almost full weight when pulled to standing position	Recognizes parents Holds out arms to be picked up	Begins to imitate sounds Uses one-syllable sounds (e.g., *ma, mu, da, di*)
7 mo	Can transfer object from one hand to other Grasps objects in each hand Bangs cube on table	Sits alone; still uses hands for support When held in standing position, bounces Puts feet to mouth	Fearful of strangers Plays peekaboo Keeps lips closed when dislikes food	Says four distinct vowel sounds "Talks" when others are talking
8 mo	Beginning thumbfinger grasping Releases object at will Grasps for toys out of reach	Sits securely without support Bears weight on legs when supported May stand holding on	Responds to word *no* Dislikes diaper changes	Makes consonant sounds *t, d, w* Uses two syllables such as *da-da*, but does not ascribe meaning to them

TABLE 19-3   *Expected Development of Infants—cont'd*

AGE	FINE MOTOR	GROSS MOTOR	SOCIAL-ADAPTIVE	LANGUAGE
9 mo	Continued development of thumbfinger grasp May bang objects together Use of dominant hand evident	Steady sitting; can lean forward and still maintain position Begins creeping (abdomen off floor) Can stand holding onto established object when placed in that position	Seems interested in pleasing parent Shows fears of going to bed and being left alone	Responds to simple commands Comprehends *no-no*
10 mo	Practices picking up small objects Points with one finger Will offer toys to people but unable to let go of objects	Can pull self into sitting position; unable to let self down again Stands while holding on to furniture	Inhibits behavior in response to command *no-no* Repeats actions that attract attention Plays interactive games such as pat-a-cake Cries when scolded	Says *da-da, ma-ma* with meaning Comprehends *bye-bye*
11 mo	Holds crayon to mark on paper Drops object deliberately for it to be picked up	Moves about room holding onto objects Preparing to walk independently; wide-base stance Stands securely holding on with one hand	Experiences satisfaction when task is accomplished Reacts to restrictions with frustration Rolls a ball to another on request	Imitates speech sounds
12 mo (1 yr)	May hold cup and spoon and feed self fairly well with practice Can offer toys and release them Releases cube in cup	Able to twist and turn and maintain posture Able to sit from standing position May stand alone, at least momentarily	Shows emotions of jealousy, affection, anger, fear May develop habit of "security blanket" or favorite toy	*Da-da* or *ma-ma* specific Recognizes objects by name Imitates animal sounds Understands simple verbal commands (e.g., "Give it to me")

*Requires training to use.

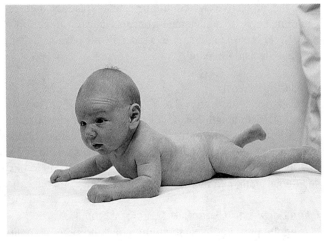

Fig. 19-1   At 4 months, infant actively lifts head and looks about.

ing takes place with caregivers; at about 1 month different cries can be identified as being related to different needs, expressive language progresses to the first word, and receptive language is developed enough to understand and briefly respond to simple disciplinary commands. Learning at the sensorimotor level of cognitive development occurs through the five senses as infants interact with the environment. Infants learn object permanence, which means that objects and people still exist when they are out of sight. The developmental tasks of infancy according to Duvall and Miller (1985) are listed in Box 19-1.

Assessment tools for the infant focus on physical growth and psychosocial development, as well as determining the mother's and father's interactions with the infant. A tool used frequently by nurses to assess development is the Denver II, used for children ages 1 month to 6 years. The Denver II form, shown in Fig. 19-2, provides assessment for gross motor movement, language, fine motor movement,

- Achieving physiologic equilibrium following birth
  - Learning to take food satisfactorily
- Learning to adjust to other persons
  - Reacting positively to both familiar and strange persons
- Learning to love and be loved
  - Responding affectionately to others through cuddling, smiling, and loving
  - Beginning to give self spontaneously and trustingly to others
- Developing system of communication
  - Learning patterns of recognition and responses
  - Establishing nonverbal, preverbal, and verbal communication
- Learning to express and to control feelings
  - Developing a sense of trust and confidence with the world
- Laying a foundation for self-awareness
  - Seeing oneself as a separate entity
  - Finding personal fulfillment with and without others

Data from Duvall EM, Miller BC: *Marriage and family development,* ed 6, New York, 1985, Harper & Row.

and personal-social. A tool that surveys parents about their child's development is Ages and Stages Questionnaire (ASQ), which identifies developmental delays in children from 4 to 60 months. The ASQ has 19 age-specific questionnaires that gather data from parents about their child's communication, fine motor movement, gross motor movement, problem solving and personal-social skills. The ASQ is available from www.brookespublishing.com by typing "ASQ" in the Search box. Preventive services recommended for infants are in Table 19-6 in the column labeled "Birth to 10 years."

CHILDREN

Toddlers

Toddlerhood is the period of growth and development from 12 to 36 months. During this period the child becomes more independent in moving about. Toddlers have a strong need to explore and master their environment. Parents who want to encourage their children's exploratory and inquiring spirit, along with the mastery of motor skills, often feel overwhelmed and exhausted at the end of the day. This exhaustion may occur when parents try to keep up with the toddlers to encourage exploration while keeping them safe.

Physical Growth

A slower but steady growth in height and weight occurs during toddlerhood. By 24 months, chest circumference exceeds head circumference. Children are half their adult height by age 2. By 30 months the birth weight is quadrupled. The usual appearance of a toddler includes a potbelly, swayback,

and short legs. The toddler may be ready for daytime control of bowel and bladder function by age 24 months. Teeth continue to erupt, with 20 teeth expected by 30 months.

Behavioral and Cognitive Development

The developmental task for toddlers is to achieve a degree of autonomy while minimizing shame and doubt. The terms *holding on* and *letting go* are used to describe this stage. Now that toddlers are walking and talking, they yearn for independence; however, they lack judgment to maintain their safety. They learn when it is safe to hold on to furniture and when to let go. The parents or caregivers try to balance their control between allowing independent exploration of the environment and keeping the toddlers safe from injury. Holding on and letting go also apply to bowel control established at this time. In their attempts to be independent, toddlers may fail to achieve their goals. Repeated failures may lead to feelings of shame and doubt in their abilities, particularly when parents try to help them do what the children should learn to do independently. When parents do not have enough patience to allow children to accomplish tasks alone, such as tying shoes, the children may doubt their ability to accomplish tasks (Boeree, 1997).

Cognitive development of the toddler remains in the sensorimotor level. Piaget's preoperational stage begins at about 2 years, when toddlers learn by trial and error and by exploration. Using their motor skills, they move around the environment and pick up objects, and, using their senses, they see, feel, smell, taste, and hear what they find.

Developmental tasks of toddlers are listed in Box 19-2. A summary of the expected development milestones, including fine and gross motor, social-adaptive, and language behaviors, is found in Table 19-4 (Fig. 19-3). The Denver II and Ages and Stages Questionnaire may be used with toddlers to assess development. Preventive services recommended for toddlers are in Table 19-6 in the column labeled "Birth to 10 years."

Preschoolers

The preschooler ranges in age from 3 to 5 years. As children's locomotion and language mature, they move away from the protective yet confining care of parental figures. Children begin to understand concepts and meanings in a more "real" sense and begin increased forms of independent play and decision making.

Physical Growth

Typical preschoolers grow 2 to 2.75 inches (5 to 7 cm) a year. By age 4, birth length has doubled, and weight increases by 3 to 5 lb (1.4 to 2.3 kg) a year. Appearance changes as the long bones grow more than the trunk, and preschoolers lose their baby fat and potbellies. By age 5, children begin to lose deciduous teeth, and the first permanent teeth erupt.

Behavioral and Cognitive Development

During the preschool years, children have become more autonomous, can communicate easily, achieve bowel and blad-

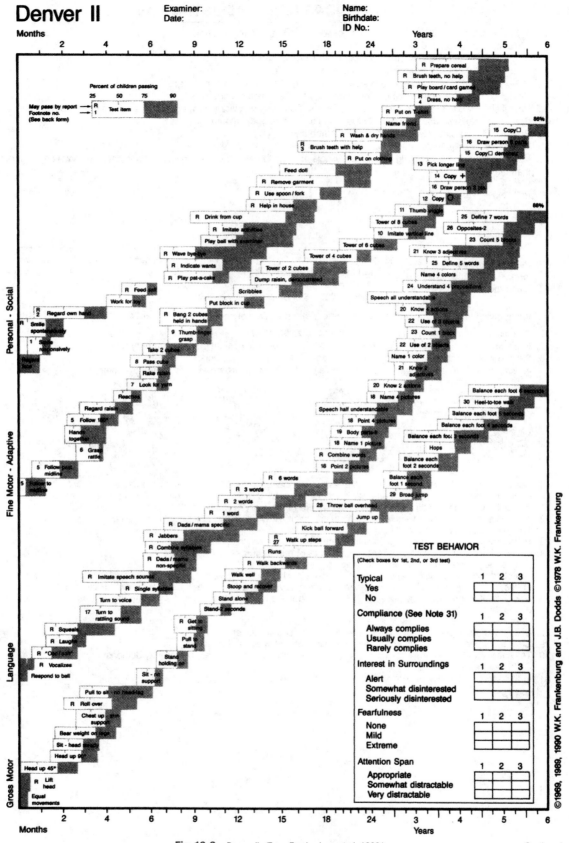

Fig. 19-2 Denver II. *(From Frankenburg et al, 1992.)*

Continued

DIRECTIONS FOR ADMINISTRATION

1. Try to get child to smile by smiling, talking or waving. Do not touch him/her.
2. Child must stare at hand several seconds.
3. Parent may help guide toothbrush and put toothpaste on brush.
4. Child does not have to be able to tie shoes or button/zip in the back.
5. Move yarn slowly in an arc from one side to the other, about 8" above child's face.
6. Pass if child grasps rattle when it is touched to the backs or tips of fingers.
7. Pass if child tries to see where yarn went. Yarn should be dropped quickly from sight from tester's hand without arm movement.
8. Child must transfer cube from hand to hand without help of body, mouth, or table.
9. Pass if child picks up raisin with any part of thumb and finger.
10. Line can vary only 30 degrees or less from tester's line. /
11. Make a fist with thumb pointing upward and wiggle only the thumb. Pass if child imitates and does not move any fingers other than the thumb.

   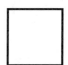

12. Pass any enclosed form. Fail continuous round motions.
13. Which line is longer? (Not bigger.) Turn paper upside down and repeat. (pass 3 of 3 or 5 of 6)
14. Pass any lines crossing near midpoint.
15. Have child copy first. If failed, demonstrate.

When giving items 12, 14, and 15, do not name the forms. Do not demonstrate 12 and 14.

16. When scoring, each pair (2 arms, 2 legs, etc.) counts as one part.
17. Place one cube in cup and shake gently near child's ear, but out of sight. Repeat for other ear.
18. Point to picture and have child name it. (No credit is given for sounds only.)
    If less than 4 pictures are named correctly, have child point to picture as each is named by tester.

 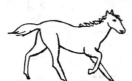  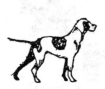 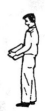

19. Using doll, tell child: Show me the nose, eyes, ears, mouth, hands, feet, tummy, hair. Pass 6 of 8.
20. Using pictures, ask child: Which one flies?... says meow?... talks?... barks?... gallops? Pass 2 of 5, 4 of 5.
21. Ask child: What do you do when you are cold?... tired?... hungry? Pass 2 of 3, 3 of 3.
22. Ask child: What do you do with a cup? What is a chair used for? What is a pencil used for?
    Action words must be included in answers.
23. Pass if child correctly places <u>and</u> says how many blocks are on paper. (1, 5).
24. Tell child: Put block **on** table; **under** table; **in front of** me, **behind** me. Pass 4 of 4.
    (Do not help child by pointing, moving head or eyes.)
25. Ask child: What is a ball?... lake?... desk?... house?... banana?... curtain?... fence?... ceiling? Pass if defined in terms of use, shape, what it is made of, or general category (such as banana is fruit, not just yellow). Pass 5 of 8, 7 of 8.
26. Ask child: If a horse is big, a mouse is __? If fire is hot, ice is __? If the sun shines during the day, the moon shines during the __? Pass 2 of 3.
27. Child may use wall or rail only, not person. May not crawl.
28. Child must throw ball overhand 3 feet to within arm's reach of tester.
29. Child must perform standing broad jump over width of test sheet (8 1/2 inches).
30. Tell child to walk forward, ⚬⚬⚬⚬⚬⚬⟶ heel within 1 inch of toe. Tester may demonstrate.
    Child must walk 4 consecutive steps.
31. In the second year, half of normal children are non-compliant.

OBSERVATIONS:

Fig. 19-2, cont'd   Denver II. *(From Frankenburg et al, 1992.)*

ETHNIC & CULTURAL VARIATIONS

Mexican American children tend to have higher weight-for-height ratio than the average American child. By contrast, Chinese and Southeast Asian children often are in the 10th percentile on the National Center for Health Statistics (NCHS) growth curves.

Body weight variations may be due to differences in bone density and musculature of the race rather than body fat. Asian and African American children usually are the lightest, followed by white children, Native American children, and then Mexican American children (Ryan et al, 1990; Strauss, 1993; in Seidel et al, 2003).

BOX 19-2 **DEVELOPMENTAL TASKS OF TODDLERS**

- Achieving physiologic equilibrium following birth
  - Learning the know-how and the where-when of elimination
  - Learning to manage one's body effectively
- Learning to adjust to other persons
  - Responding to others' expectations
  - Recognizing parental authority and controls
  - Learning the do's and don'ts of the immediate world
- Learning to love and be loved
  - Meeting emotional needs through widening spheres and variety of contacts
- Developing system of communication
  - Acquiring basic concepts such as yes/no
  - Mastering basic language fundamentals
- Learning to express and to control feelings
  - Healthy management of feelings of fear and anxiety
  - Handling feelings of frustration, disappointment, and anger appropriately for age
  - Moderating demanding attitudes
- Laying a foundation for self-awareness
  - Exploring the rights and privileges of being an individual

Data from Duvall EM, Miller BC: *Marriage and family development,* ed 6, New York, 1985, Harper & Row.

TABLE 19-4 *Expected Development of Toddlers*

AGE	FINE MOTOR	GROSS MOTOR	SOCIAL-ADAPTIVE	LANGUAGE
15 mo	Can put raisins into bottle Will take off shoes and pull toys Builds tower of two cubes Scribbles spontaneously Uses cup well, but rotates spoon	Walks alone well Able to seat self in chair Creeps up stairs Cannot throw ball without falling	Tolerates some separation from parents Begins to imitate parents' activities (e.g., sweeping, mowing lawn)	Says 10 or more words "Asks" for objects by pointing Uses *no* even when agreeing with request
18 mo	Builds tower of three to four cubes Turns pages in book two or three at a time Manages spoon without rotating	May walk up and down stairs holding hand May show running ability	Imitates housework Temper tantrums may be more evident Has beginning awareness of ownership (e.g., *my toy*)	Says 10 or more words Points to two or three body parts
24 mo (2 yr)	Able to turn doorknob Able to take off shoes and socks Able to build seven- to eight-block tower (see Fig. 19-3) Dumps raisins from bottle following demonstration Turns pages in book one at a time	May walk up stairs by self, two feet on each step Able to walk backward Able to kick ball	Parallel play demonstrated Pulls people to show them something Increased independence from mother	Has vocabulary of 300 words Uses two- or three-word phrases Uses pronouns *I, you* Uses first name Refers to self by name
30 mo (2½ yr)	Able to build eight-block tower Scribbling techniques continue Feeding self with increased neatness Dumps raisins from bottle spontaneously	Able to jump from object Walking becomes more stable; wide-base gait decreases Throws ball overhanded	Separates easily from mother In play, helps put things away In toileting, only needs help to wipe Begins to notice sex differences	Gives first and last name Uses plurals Refers to self by appropriate pronoun Names one color

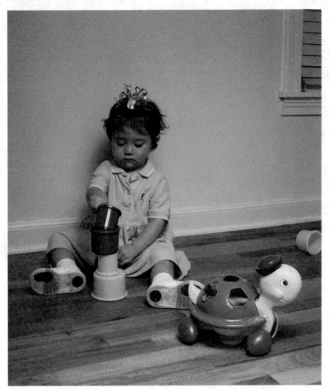

Fig. 19-3 The toddler takes great pleasure in building a tower of four blocks.

continue to explore their environments with greater skills and a new enthusiasm and motivation. When children are praised for their activities, they learn that they are meeting others' expectations and become independent and self-sufficient. At this stage their conscience develops, that inner voice that provides a sense of right and wrong.

Cognitive development continues at the preoperational level. Children begin the symbolic function, in which they develop concepts and classifications to associate one event, object, or person with a similar one. Children demonstrate this when they act out an event they have seen or experienced, but they emphasize only one aspect of the event. At this level children become egocentric, when they are self-centered and unable to understand others' viewpoints.

The developmental tasks for preschoolers as described by Duvall and Miller are listed in Box 19-3. A summary of the expected development of preschoolers, including fine and gross motor, social-adaptive, and language behaviors, is found in Table 19-5. The Denver II and Ages and Stages Questionnaire may be used with preschoolers to assess development. Preventive services recommended for preschoolers are in Table 19-6 in the column labeled "Birth to 10 years."

der continence, have an active imagination, can demonstrate basic social skills, can delay gratification, use more acceptable outlets to express frustration, and can expand their environment beyond home. The task of this age group is to learn initiative without an overabundance of guilt. Preschoolers

School-Age Children

The beginning of school is a developmental landmark for children. Entering school brings a new influential environment into children's lives. Information about concepts, life, and interpersonal relationships expands beyond the confines of the home. Teacher and peer influences may be noticed in school-age children's reactions and behavior. The school-age period lasts from approximately 6 to 12 years of age.

BOX 19-3 **DEVELOPMENTAL TASKS OF PRESCHOOLERS**

- Settling into healthy daily routines
  - Enjoying a variety of active play
  - Being more flexible and capable of accepting change
  - Mastering good eating habits
  - Mastering the basics of toilet training
  - Developing physical skills
- Becoming a participating member of the family
  - Assuming responsibility within the family
  - Giving and receiving affection and gifts freely
  - Identifying with the parent of the same sex
  - Developing an ability to share parents with others
  - Recognizing the family's unique ways
- Beginning to master impulses and to conform to expectations of others
  - Outgrowing impulsivity
  - Learning to share, take turns, enjoy companionship
  - Developing sympathy and cooperation
  - Adopting situationally appropriate behavior
- Developing healthy emotional expressions
  - Acting out feelings during play
  - Delaying gratification
  - Expressing hostility/making up
  - Discriminating between a variety of emotions, feelings

- Learning to communicate effectively with others
  - Developing a vocabulary and speech ability
  - Learning to listen, follow directions, increase attention span
  - Acquiring social skills that allow more comfortable interactions with others
- Developing ability to handle potentially dangerous situations
  - Respecting potential hazards
  - Effectively using caution and safety practices
  - Being able to accept assistance when needed
- Learning to be autonomous with initiative and a conscience of his or her own
  - Becoming increasingly responsible
  - Taking initiative to be involved in situations
  - Internalizing expectations, demands of family and culture
  - Being self-sufficient for stage of development
- Laying foundation for understanding the meaning of life
  - Developing gender awareness
  - Trying to understand the nature of the physical world
  - Accepting religious faith of parents, learning about spirituality

Data from Duvall EM, Miller BC: *Marriage and family development,* ed 6, New York, 1985, Harper & Row.

TABLE 19-5   Expected Development of Preschoolers

AGE	FINE MOTOR	GROSS MOTOR	SOCIAL-ADAPTIVE	LANGUAGE
36 mo (3 yr)	Can unbutton front buttons (Fig. 19-4) Copies vertical lines within 30 degrees Copies zero Begins to use fork	Walks up stairs, alternating feet on steps Walks down stairs, two feet on each step Pedals tricycle Jumps in place Able to perform broad jump	Dresses self with help with back buttons Pulls on shoes Parallel play Able to share toys	Vocabulary of 900 words Uses complete sentences Constantly asks questions
48 mo (4 yr)	Able to copy plus sign (+) Picks longer line three out of three times Uses scissors Can lace shoes	Walks down stairs, alternating feet on steps Able to button large front buttons Able to balance on one foot for approximately 5 seconds Catches ball	Play is associative Imaginary friend is common Boasts and tattles Selfish, impatient, rebellious	Gives first and last name Has 1500-word vocabulary Uses words without knowing meaning Questioning is at a peak
60 mo (5 yr)	Able to dress self with minimal assistance Able to draw three-part human figure Draws square (■) following demonstration Colors within lines	Hops on one foot Catches ball bounced to him or her two out of three times Able to demonstrate heel-toe walking Jumps rope	Eager to follow rules Less rebellious Relies on outside authority to control the world	Has 2100-word vocabulary Recognizes three colors Asks meanings of words Uses sentences of six to eight words

Physical Growth

The growth continues at a slow pace, with about a 5-pound weight gain and 2-inch height increase per year. Growth rates for boys and girls are similar until the growth spurt starts between 10 and 12 years of age. By age 8 or 9 there is increased smoothness and speed in motor control, making the child more agile and graceful. Bone replaces cartilage and continues to harden. Bones of the face and jaw grow at a faster rate than they have in previous years. The school-age child is slimmer, with less body fat and a lower center of gravity. Eyes and hands are well coordinated, and muscles are stronger and more developed. These changes in growth improve fine motor activities, such as drawing, needlework, and playing musical instruments, as well as gross motor activities, such as jumping, biking, and swimming. By age 12 the rest of the teeth (except the wisdom teeth) erupt.

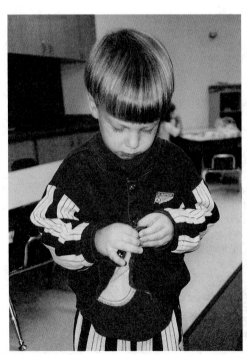

Fig. 19-4   Preschooler develops the ability to help dress self.

ETHNIC & CULTURAL VARIATIONS

Height variations exist among children of different races. Asian children are the shortest, with Hispanic children being the next taller group. African Americans and whites are the tallest group, with Native Americans being as tall or a little shorter.

- African American children achieve their growth earlier than whites. White boys match with their African American counterparts by age 9 or 10 years, whereas white girls match by age 14 or 15 years.
- Within the same racial group, obese children tend to be taller than slim children. Children from lower socioeconomic status tend to be shorter than children from high socioeconomic status (Dewey et al, 1986; Hamill et al, 1973; Lin, 1992; Malina et al, 1987; Seidel et al, 2003).

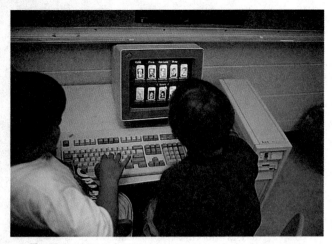

Fig. 19-5 School-age children learn the basic skills required for school.

Behavioral and Cognitive Development

The task for this age group is to develop a capacity for industry while avoiding an undue sense of inferiority. Interactions with children and teachers at school broaden children's social contacts. Industry influences a desire to achieve. Children learn how to compete and how to cooperate with others. School relationships provide social support outside the home environment, and peer approval becomes important. A sense of inferiority develops when the child is allowed little success because of interactions with rejecting teachers, peers, or parents. Feelings of racism, sexism, and other forms of discrimination contribute to feelings of inferiority. A maladaptation that may occur is inertia, in which the child feels so inferior that he or she stops making the effort to achieve goals or accomplish tasks (Boeree, 1997).

The cognitive development described by Piaget for this age is concrete operations, when children learn inductive reasoning and logical operations. In school they learn to use numbers, to read, and to classify. By the time children enter school, their development of fine and gross motor, social-adaptive, and language skills change more gradually (Fig. 19-5). Tasks for the school-age child are listed in Box 19-4. Assessment tools for school-age children focus on mental abilities and social and emotional behaviors. Preventive services recommended for school-age children are in Table 19-6 in the columns labeled "Birth to 10 years" and "11 to 24 years."

ADOLESCENTS

The hallmark of adolescence is puberty, which marks the end of childhood and the onset of adulthood. Adolescence occurs from approximately 12 years of age to 18 years of age.

Physical Growth

The growth spurt that occurs during puberty is highly variable and accounts for 20% to 25% of the final adult height. Growth frequently occurs during spring and summer months. The normal girl grows from 2 to 4.5 inches (5.1 to 11.4 cm), and the normal boy grows from 2 to 5 inches (5.1 to 12.7 cm). This height is accompanied by an increase in weight. The normal girl increases in weight by 10 to 23 lb (4.5 kg to 10.4 kg), whereas the weight of the normal boy increases from 12.5 to 29 lb (5.7 to 13.2 kg). The growth in girls occurs 18 to 24 months before that in boys, but the average weight gain for boys is 4.5 lb (2 kg) per year more than for girls (Neinstein, 1991).

BOX 19-4 **DEVELOPMENTAL TASKS OF SCHOOL-AGE CHILDREN**

- Learning the basic skills required for school (see Fig. 19-5)
  - Mastering reading and writing
  - Developing reflective thinking
  - Mastering physical skills
- Mastering money management
  - Obtaining money through socially acceptable ways
  - Buying wisely
  - Saving
  - Delaying gratification
  - Understanding role of money and place in life
- Becoming an active and cooperative member of the family
  - Participating in family discussions
  - Joining in family decision making
  - Being responsible for household chores
  - Participating in reciprocal gift giving
- Extending abilities to relate to others
  - Asserting rights
  - Developing leadership skills
  - Following social mores and customs

- Cooperating in group situations
- Maintaining close friendships
- Managing feelings and impulses
  - Coping with frustrations
  - Managing anger appropriately
  - Expressing feelings in the right time, place, and manner and to the right person
- Identifying the sex and gender role
  - Differentiating expectations based on gender
  - Understanding reproduction and gender-specific physical development
  - Managing physical growth spurts
  - Conceptualizing life as a mature man or woman
- Identifying self as worthy individual
  - Gaining status and respect
  - Growing in self-esteem and self-confidence
  - Establishing unique identity
- Developing conscience and morality
  - Determining right from wrong
  - Developing moral-guided control over behavior
  - Learning to live according to identified values

Data from Duvall EM, Miller BC: *Marriage and family development,* ed 6, New York, 1985, Harper & Row.

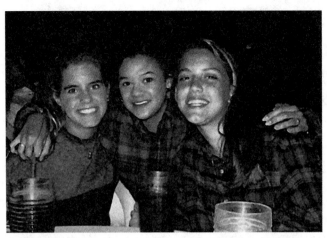

Fig. 19-6 The peer group is a major influence in adolescent development.

Behavioral and Cognitive Development

The task during adolescence is to achieve ego identity and avoid role confusion. The adolescent reviews the learning, the experiences, and the values that he or she accepted in earlier stages and modifies them into a unique and personalized identity. During this identity clarification process, adolescents may decide that previously accepted ideas and beliefs need to be changed. They may behave in new and different ways, much to the chagrin of their parents, as they "try on" differing roles and values. Adolescents begin testing and evaluating previously accepted notions about life, living, spirituality, relating, and being. Some influences to change may come from peers (Fig. 19-6). The early values of the child often are the accepted values from the parental authority in the family. Role confusion develops for adolescents who are unsuccessful in developing their own identity. They

may develop low self-esteem, have poor to no direction in their lives, and have difficulty making career choices.

Formal operations is the term Piaget gave to the adolescent years. Adolescents are able to perform abstract reasoning and form logical conclusions. They are able to form hypotheses and devise ways to test them. They use analytic skills in making judgments about their actions and future lives. Advanced intellectual skills allow them to reexamine accepted ideas, which can be a strain within the family but leads to a stronger sense of self and independence. Developmental tasks for the teen years include those listed in Box 19-5.

Assessment tools for this age group focus on social and emotional behaviors, in addition to identifying and reducing stress. Preventive services recommended for adolescents are in Table 19-6 in the column labeled "11 to 24 years."

ADULTS

Early Adulthood

Young adults (approximately 20 to 35 years of age) move away from the dependent role in the family of origin to establishing their own lifestyle. The task of young adults is to achieve some degree of intimacy as opposed to remaining isolated. These individuals begin to express their identity through work, recreation, and interpersonal relationships. Productivity, self-sufficiency, and intimacy in love relationships are driving tasks for young adults, even though they may shift back and forth in career choices, commitment, and goals as they continually redefine themselves. The young adult is ready to enter the adult world and assume a position as a responsible citizen. Achievements are the result of self-

---

BOX 19-5	**DEVELOPMENTAL TASKS OF ADOLESCENTS**

- Accepting physical changes
  - Coming to terms with physical maturation
  - Accepting one's own body
- Achieving a satisfying and socially accepted role
  - Learning masculine/feminine role
  - Realistic understanding of gender role
  - Adopting acceptable practices
- Developing more mature peer relationships
  - Being accepted by peer group (see Fig. 19-6)
  - Making and keeping friends of both sexes
  - Dating
  - Loving and being loved
  - Adapting to variety of peer associations
  - Developing skills in managing and evaluating peer relationships
- Achieving emotional independence
  - Outgrowing childish parental dependence
  - Developing mature affection for parents
  - Being autonomous
  - Developing mature interdependence

- Getting an education
  - Acquiring basic knowledge and skills
  - Clarifying sex-role attitudes toward work and family roles
- Preparing for marriage and family life
  - Formulating sex-role attitudes
  - Enjoying responsibilities
  - Developing responsible attitudes
  - Distinguishing between infatuation and mature love
  - Developing mutually satisfying personal relationships
- Developing knowledge and skills for civic competence
  - Communicating as a citizen
  - Becoming involved in causes outside oneself
  - Acquiring problem-solving skills
  - Developing social concepts
- Establishing one's identity as a socially responsible person
  - Developing philosophy of life
  - Implementing worthy ideals and standards
  - Assuming social obligations
  - Adopting mature sense of values and ethics
  - Dealing effectively with emotional responses

Data from Duvall EM, Miller BC: *Marriage and family development,* ed 6, New York, 1985, Harper & Row.

direction, with goals that may change as an outcome of re-evaluation. Mature relationships with others are important in both the work and home environments. Many young adults choose to marry and start a family. Role confusion may develop when young adults have difficulty moving from adolescence and their dependence on parents or family to developing their own identity and adult role responsibilities. Developmental tasks listed in Box 19-6 are those usually accomplished during this stage. Preventive services recommended for young adults are in Table 19-6 in the column labeled "11 to 24 years."

The focus of assessment for young adults is on career choice and mate selection.

Career Choice

Many assessment tool inventories have been developed for young adults contemplating career choices. In these inventories, basic interest areas are compared with occupational themes. The inventory responses cluster similar interest areas and relate them to an occupation or vocational choice. Stability in interest areas is important to the predictive power of these inventories. If an individual has many, varied interests, the inventory scores may be less reliable and less valid.

Mate Selection

Along with career choice, mate selection is a primary interest area for many individuals in early adulthood. The field of premarital and couple counseling has rapidly expanded since the 1940s, along with the increasing divorce rate in America. Various tools and internet services are used to match couples based on compatibilities.

Middle Adulthood

Entry into the middle years, between ages 35 and 65, may be met with the feeling that one's best years have passed, especially in light of today's emphasis on youth.

Physical Growth

There are obvious physical signs of aging, such as wrinkling of the skin, graying or loss of hair, and changes in muscle tone and mass. Changes in vision and hearing may affect social relationships and learning unless corrective actions are taken.

Behavioral and Cognitive Development

During this time many decisions have been made concerning career, partner, children, lifestyle, and living arrangements. The task is to reach a balance between generativity and stagnation. Generativity involves showing concern for the generations to follow. This may be accomplished by raising children and grandchildren or may be in the form of writing, teaching, inventing, or performing community service projects to contribute to the welfare of those who follow. Stagnation develops when the person is so self-absorbed that he or she ceases to be a productive member of society. For persons who have successfully met the developmental tasks of earlier stages, this can be a period of stability, self-understanding, and self-actualization. For others this is the time of the midlife crisis, when they feel that life is stagnant or incomplete. Frustration drives them to search for new directions and goals in life. During middle age one reaps the benefits of career success, support of family and friends, and experiences of earlier years. Developmental tasks for this stage are listed in Box 19-7. Preventive services recommended for middle adults are in Table 19-6 in the column labeled "25 to 64 years."

Older Adulthood

The later years, beginning with age 65, are for most adults productive years met with a sense of pleasure and enjoyment. Older adults represent the fastest-growing population in the United States, and probably the least understood. They are a highly diverse group.

Physical Growth

Though many physical changes accompany aging, most older adults are active members of society and have independent lifestyles. Chronic health problems are common but usually can be managed.

BOX 19-6 DEVELOPMENTAL TASKS OF YOUNG ADULTS

- Establishing one's autonomy as an individual
- Planning a direction for one's life
- Getting an appropriate education
- Working toward a vocation
- Appraising love and sexual feelings
- Becoming involved in love relationships
- Selecting a mate
- Getting engaged
- Being married

Data from Duvall EM, Miller BC: *Marriage and family development,* ed 6, New York, 1985, Harper & Row.

BOX 19-7 DEVELOPMENTAL TASKS OF MIDDLE ADULTS

- Providing a comfortable and healthful home
- Allocating resources to provide security in later years
- Division of household responsibilities
- Encouragement of both husband and wife roles within and beyond the family
- Maintaining emotional and sexual intimacy
- Incorporating all family members into family circle as family enlarges, and caring for extended family
- Participating in activities outside the home
- Developing competencies that maintain family functioning during crises and encourage achievement

Data from Duvall EM, Miller BC: *Marriage and family development,* ed 6, New York, 1985, Harper & Row.

BOX 19-8   DEVELOPMENTAL TASKS OF OLDER ADULTS

- Making satisfying living arrangements
- Adjusting to retirement
- Establishing comfortable routines
- Maintaining physical and mental health
- Maintaining love, sex, and marital relations
- Remaining in touch with other family members
- Keeping active
- Finding the meaning in life

Data from Duvall EM, Miller BC: *Marriage and family development*, ed 6, New York, 1985, Harper & Row.

Behavioral and Cognitive Development

The task of development is to achieve ego integrity with a minimal amount of despair. Ego integrity is achieved when older adults can look back at their lives and accept the course of events and the choices they made as being necessary. Despair may develop with the death of one's spouse and friends or the adjustment related to retirement. Society is becoming more aware of the presence of ageism and stereotyping against a person due to age. Older adults are encouraging positive attitudes about aging and making society aware of the developmental tasks they experience and the barriers to leading a healthy, happy life in a society that values youth. Ego integrity develops as older adults give back to society and as they interact with grandchildren.

Cognitive development in the old-old adult was reported in a longitudinal study of subjects ranging from 73 to 99 years of age. Researchers found that although many subjects reported some decline in abilities, more than half displayed no decline. A study of 18 people ages 100 to 106 found that these centenarians reported rich late-life learning experiences, the majority of which occurred through social interaction (Merriam and Caffarella, 1999). Developmental tasks for older adults are summarized in Box 19-8.

The lengthy time span for this age group is divided in several ways. Lueckenotte (2000) describes young-old from ages 65 to 74, middle-old from ages 75 to 84, and old-old as 85 years and older. Separate tasks with different age groupings are identified in Box 19-9. Preventive services recommended for older adults are in Table 19-6 in the column labeled "Over 65 years."

FAMILY DEVELOPMENT AND ASSESSMENT

Most individuals in America grow up within the social unit of a family. However, the definition and composition of family structures have changed over the years. Families are no longer traditionally two married heterosexual parents with children who live under one roof. Blended families are composed of stepchildren and children from the current unit. Homosexual couples join as family units, some of which include children. There are single-parent families: some from divorce, some never married, and some formed because of adoption or artificial fertilization. There are also intergenerational families in which multiple generations live together under one roof or in which grandparents or even great-grandparents raise and care for their grandchildren. An Ethnic and Cultural Variations box describes some cultures in which extended families may be main-

BOX 19-9   DEVELOPMENTAL TASKS OF YOUNG-OLD AND OLD-OLD ADULTS

Young-Old (Approximately 65 to 85 Years)
- Preparing for and adjusting to retirement
- Adjusting to lower and fixed income of retirement
- Establishing physical living arrangements
- Adjusting to new relationships with adult children and their offspring
- Managing leisure time
- Adjusting to slower physical and intellectual responses
- Dealing with death of parents, spouse, and friends

Old-Old (Approximately over 85 Years)
- Learning to combine new dependency needs with continued need for independence
- Adapting to living alone
- Accepting and adjusting to possible institutional living
- Establishing affiliation with age group
- Adjusting to increased vulnerability to physical and emotional stress
- Adjusting to loss of physical strength, illness, and approach of one's own death
- Adjusting to losses of spouse, home, and friends

Data from Brown M: *Readings in gerontology,* St Louis, 1984, Mosby.

ETHNIC & CULTURAL VARIATIONS

In many cultures the extended family is important in the care of children. In African American families, when mothers are unable to provide emotional and physical support for their children, grandmothers, aunts, and extended family members readily provide assistance or take responsibility for the children. About 44% of all children living with grandparents today are African American. Of these, 66% of these children have grandparents as the primary caregivers.

Chinese family members emphasize loyalty to the family and tradition. Personal independence is not valued. Often children live with grandparents or aunts and uncles so that individual family members can obtain a better education or reduce financial burden.

Mexican American families are patriarchal, with some evidence of a slow change to a more egalitarian pattern in recent years. Children are highly valued because they ensure the continuation of the family and cultural values.

Navajo families have separate dwellings, but are grouped together by family relationships. The Navajo family unit consists of the nuclear family and relatives such as sisters, aunts, and their female descendants. The elderly play an important role in keeping rituals and instructing children and grandchildren (Purnell and Paulanka, 2003).

TABLE 19-6 *Preventive Services Throughout the Life Span**

	BIRTH TO 10 YEARS	11 TO 24 YEARS	25 TO 64 YEARS	OVER 65 YEARS
Screening	Height and weight Hemoglobinopathy at birth Phenylalanine level at birth Blood pressure after age 3 Vision screen by age 3	Height and weight Blood pressure Papanicolaou (Pap) test/ *Chlamydia* screening Rubella serologic tests Vision screening	Height and weight Blood pressure Cholesterol screening Pap test (women) Mammogram (women) Vision screening Fecal occult blood test or sigmoidoscopy (or both; men and women over 50) Rubella serologic tests or vaccination history (women of childbear- ing age)	Height and weight Blood pressure Cholesterol screening Pap test (women) Fecal occult blood test or sigmoidoscopy (or both) Mammogram and clinical breast examination Vision screening Hearing screening
Counseling	**Injury prevention:** Infant/child safety seats for children <5 years Lap-shoulder belt for chil- dren >5 years Smoke detector in home Bicycle helmet; bicycle safety Hot water heater tempera- ture <120°-130° F (49°-54° C) Window and stair guards; pool fences Safe storage of drugs, toxic substances, fire- arms, and matches Syrup of ipecac, poison control numbers Cardiopulmonary resusci- tation (CPR) training for parents and caretakers **Substance abuse:** Effects of passive smoke Anti-tobacco message **Diet and exercise:** Breast-feeding, iron- enriched formula and foods (infants and toddlers) Limit fat and cholesterol, maintain caloric bal- ance; emphasize grain, fruits, vegetables (ages 2-10); regular physical activity	**Injury prevention:** Lap-shoulder seat belts Helmet use Smoke detector in home Safe storage of firearms **Substance abuse:** Avoid tobacco use Avoid underage drinking Avoid alcohol and drug use while driving, swimming, boating, etc. **Sexual behavior:** Sexually transmitted infec- tion prevention: absti- nence, avoid high-risk behavior; use con- doms or female barrier with spermicide Unintended pregnancy: contraception **Diet and exercise:** Limit fat and cholesterol, maintain caloric bal- ance; emphasize grain, fruits, vegetables; reg- ular calcium intake; regular physical activity	**Injury prevention:** Lap-shoulder seat belts Helmet use Smoke detector in home Safe storage of firearms **Substance abuse:** Tobacco cessation Avoid alcohol and drug use while driving, swimming, boating, etc. **Sexual behavior:** Sexually transmitted in- fection prevention: abstinence, avoid high-risk behavior; use condoms or fe- male barrier with spermicide Contraception **Diet and exercise:** Limit fat and cholesterol, maintain caloric bal- ance; emphasize grain, fruits, vegeta- bles; regular calcium intake (women) Regular physical activity	**Injury prevention:** Lap-shoulder seat belts Helmet use Fall prevention Smoke detector in home Safe storage of firearms Hot water heater temper- ature <120°-130° F (49°-54° C) **Substance abuse:** Tobacco cessation Avoid alcohol and drug use while driving, swimming, boating, etc. **Sexual behavior:** Sexually transmitted in- fection prevention: abstinence, avoid high-risk behavior; use condoms **Diet and exercise:** Limit fat and cholesterol, maintain caloric bal- ance; emphasize grain, fruits, vegeta- bles; regular calcium intake (women) Regular physical activity

Data from Report of the US Preventive Services Task Force: *Guide to clinical preventive services,* ed 2, Baltimore, MD, 1996, Williams & Wilkins, *www. cdc.gov/vaccines/recs/schedules,* 2007.

*The U.S. Preventive Services Task Force–recommended interventions—screening tests, counseling interventions, immunizations, and chemoprophylactic regimens—for the prevention of more than 80 target conditions. The clients who receive these services are asymptomatic individuals of all age groups and risk categories. The recommendations are based on a standardized review of current scientific evidence.

[a]Vaccine abbreviations: *DTaP,* diphtheria and tetanus toxoids and acellular pertussis vaccine; *Hep A,* hepatitis A virus vaccine; *Hep B,* hepatitis B virus vaccine; *Hib, Haemophilus influenzae* type b conjugate vaccine; *HPV,* human papilloma virus; *IPV,* inactivated poliovirus vaccine; *MCV4,* meningococcal vaccine; *MMR,* measles, mumps, and rubella virus vaccine live; *Td,* adult tetanus toxoid (full dose) and diphtheria toxoid (reduced dose) for children older than 7 years and adults; *PCV,* pneumococcal conjugate vaccine; *rota,* rotavirus vaccine.

TABLE 19-6   *Preventive Services Throughout the Life Span—cont'd*

	BIRTH TO 10 YEARS	11 TO 24 YEARS	25 TO 64 YEARS	OVER 65 YEARS
Dental health	Regular visits to dental care provider Floss daily; brush with fluoride toothpaste daily Advice about baby bottle tooth decay	Regular visits to dental care provider Floss daily; brush with fluoride toothpaste daily	Regular visits to dental care provider Floss daily; brush with fluoride toothpaste daily	Regular visits to dental care provider Floss daily; brush with fluoride toothpaste daily
Immunizations[a]	Hep B, Rota, DTaP, Hib, PCV, IPV, MMR, varicella, Hep A See *www.cdc.gov* for schedule	DTap, HPV, MCV4, tetanus See *www.cdc.gov* for schedule	Tetanus, varicella, influenza See *www.cdc.gov* for schedule	Tetanus, varicella, influenza, pneumococcal, zoster See *www.cdc.gov* for schedule
Chemoprophylaxis	Ocular antibiotic prophylaxis at birth Multivitamin	Multivitamin with folic acid (females planning or capable of pregnancy)	Multivitamin with folic acid (women planning or capable of pregnancy)	

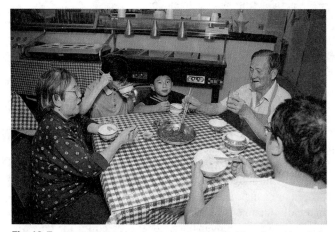

Fig. 19-7   The family unit typically shares some degree of time, financial, and physical resources and responsibilities for the unit maintenance.

TABLE 19-7   *Developmental Tasks of the Family*

STAGES	THEMES
Married couple	Without children; establishing satisfying marriage; adjusting to pregnancy; fitting into kin network
Childbearing	Oldest child birth to 30 months; nurturing infants; establishing home
Family with preschoolers	Oldest child 2½ to 6; adapting to needs of children; decreased energy and privacy as parents
Family with school-age children	Oldest child 6 to 13; being part of community of school-age families; encouraging educational achievement of children
Family with teenagers	Oldest child 13 to 20; balancing freedom and responsibility; establishing postparental interests
Family launching young adults	First child gone until last child's leaving home; maintaining supportive home base
Middle-age parents	Empty nest to retirement; refocusing on marriage; maintaining kin ties
Aging family members	Retirement to death of both spouses; coping with bereavement; adapting home for aging; adjusting to retirement; living alone

Data from Duvall EM, Miller BC: *Marriage and family development,* ed 6, New York, 1985, Harper & Row.

tained. For our purposes, a *family* is defined as two or more individuals who share bonds of commitment, loyalty, and affection. The family unit typically shares some degree of time, financial, and physical resources, as well as responsibilities for the unit maintenance (Fig. 19-7). Duvall and Miller (1985) define the functions and tasks of the family unit through stages for the traditional family of the past, that is, the two-parent, married, heterosexual couple with children, in Table 19-7.

In stepfamilies, a biologic parent lives elsewhere, and the children commonly move between the homes of two biologic families. Virtually all members of a stepfamily sustain primary relationship loss. The parent and stepparents must repeatedly deal with a part-time relationship with the stepchild if the stepchild is involved with the other biologic parent. The relationship between the adult parents outside of the stepfamily predates the new marriage and the relationship with the stepparent. This can create conflicts and loyalty divisions in parenting strategies and with the child. Children within a

stepfamily struggle with being members of more than one household, while stepparents cope with parenting a child to whom they are not related.

Single-parent families are rising in number because of the increasing divorce rate in America and the decreasing social stigma related to unwed mothers. In single-parent families the child lives with one biologic parent. Both the child and the single parent sustain a loss from the absent biologic parent of the child. There is great variation in the involvement of the absent parent of the child; some are actively involved with the child, whereas others have minimal to no involvement. Other children may be added to the single-parent family from the same or different biologic parentage. Financial difficulties are a common stressor for single-parent families because only one adult is present to care for the children, maintain the home, and provide for the family.

CLINICAL APPLICATION & CLINICAL REASONING

See Appendix E for answers to exercises in this section.

REVIEW QUESTIONS

1 Which immunizations does the nurse ask about when interviewing a 75-year-old client?
 1 Measles, mumps, and rubella.
 2 Tetanus and influenza.
 3 Hepatitis B and varicella.
 4 Inactivated polio vaccine.
2 Which statement reflects an expected developmental task of a 40-year-old man?
 1 "I'll be completing my degree this year and then I plan to marry my fiancée."
 2 "I am staying active with plenty of volunteer activities every day of the week."
 3 "My wife and I have divided up the chores with the children since we are both working."
 4 "My life is going to be different now that dad has died and the care of mom is my responsibility."
3 Which of the following are expected assessment findings related to the 11-year-old child?
 1 Five-pound weight gain and beginning of a growth spurt.
 2 Loss of deciduous teeth and eruption of permanent teeth.
 3 Development of mature relationships and beginning of dating.
 4 Acting out of feelings during play and sports.
4 A nurse is assessing an infant who is able to pull up to a sitting position, turn from prone to side position, laugh and babble, and show interest in her surroundings. These behaviors are consistent with an infant of what age?
 1 7 months old.
 2 5 months old.
 3 3 months old.
 4 1 month old.
5 A 15-year-old boy approaches the school nurse and describes how uncomfortable he is around the girls because most of them are taller than he is. The nurse counsels the boy that:
 1 She will evaluate his diet to determine if he is eating enough nutrients.

2 Genetics play an important part in height and that if his parents are short, he may be short as well.
3 Sleep is necessary for growth and he should make sure he is getting adequate sleep.
4 The growth spurt during adolescence occurs in girls 18 to 24 months before it occurs in boys.

CASE STUDY

Mrs. C. is a 78-year-old woman who is brought to the geriatric clinic by her son and daughter-in-law. Mrs. C.'s son tells the nurse that his father died 5 months ago, and ever since then his mother has "gone downhill." Mr. C. indicates that his mother is no longer keeping her house clean or cooking appropriate meals. Also, her personal hygiene habits have dramatically changed. She has lost interest in getting her hair done, and she no longer likes to get dressed for the day. Mr. C. tells the nurse, "When I suggest a retirement home, she becomes very angry and tells me to mind my own business. I am just worried about Mom, and I want to make sure she is well cared for." During this conversation Mrs. C. sits quietly. She interjects only to say, "I have taken care of you, your brother, and your father. Now all of a sudden you think I am helpless and want to lock me away." Mrs. C. appears clean, although her hair is matted and her clothes are badly wrinkled and do not match. Her speech is clear, but her overall affect is very dull. She does not make eye contact with her son or the nurse. A physical examination demonstrates normal bodily functioning consistent with her age.

Clinical Reasoning

1. List the subjective data described in the case study.
2. List the objective data described in the case study.
3. Which of Erikson's developmental stages is Mrs. C. experiencing?
4. Based on what is known from the interview, which developmental tasks of older adults may Mrs. C. be struggling with?
5. What additional assessment data are needed?

INTERACTIVE ACTIVITIES

Open the interactive student CD-ROM, click on Chapter 19, and choose from the following activities on the menu bar:

- **Multiple Choice Challenge.** Click the best answer for each question. You will be given immediate feedback, rationale for incorrect answers, and a total score. Good luck!

- **Marvelous Matches.** Drag each word or phrase and drop it below the appropriate place on the screen. Test your ability to match the age group with the specific focus of developmental assessment for that age. Then test your ability to match the developmental milestones to the appropriate age—from 1 month to 4 years.

- **Quick Challenge.** Use this critical thinking exercise to assess your skills through case study-style questions, then compare with expert answers!

CHAPTER 20

Assessment of the Infant and Child

Pediatric nursing encompasses a wide range of ages, from birth through adolescence, making health assessment a challenge. In order to adequately assess children, the nurse considers differences in anatomy and physiology that occur with growth, developmental milestones specific to age, as well as the psychosocial issues unique to infants, toddlers, preschoolers, school-age children, and adolescents. Adding to this complexity is the fact that the children are assessed in the context of their family; thus, nurses performing pediatric assessments must be skilled at interviewing and observing both families and children. In performing the physical exam, the nurse adjusts examination components and techniques to meet the unique needs of each age group. Table 20-1 presents definitions for these age groups.

ANATOMY & PHYSIOLOGY

Children differ anatomically and physiologically from adults in many important ways; generally, the younger the child, the greater these differences. Of particular importance are differences that exist at birth, including immaturities of the central nervous system, in respiratory and cardiovascular function, and in immune functions. These immaturities are evident in such things as heart and respiratory rate, reflexes, and pain response. Differences in anatomy and physiology also place young children at unique risk for certain illnesses such as otitis media. Even the adolescent, who may be adult-like in size and appearance, is still undergoing maturation of body systems, including the reproductive system and the central nervous system, and of cognitive function. Box 20-1 summarizes basic variations in anatomy and physiology in infants and children.

TABLE 20-1 *Pediatric Age Groups*

Newborn (Neonate)	Birth-28 days
Infant	1-12 months
Toddler	1-3 years
Preschool	3-6 years
School Age	6-12 years
Adolescent	12-18 years

BOX 20-1 **SELECTED ANATOMIC AND PHYSIOLOGIC DIFFERENCES IN CHILDREN**

Skin
- Newborns, especially preterms, have thinner, more permeable skin than older children and adults.
- Newborns and young infants have decreased subcutaneous fat and a large body surface area, which can lead to thermoregulation problems.
- Apocrine sweat glands and sebaceous gland activity increase in adolescents resulting in more oily skin and acne.

Head
- The cranial bones are soft and not fused at birth. The anterior and posterior fontanels remain open until 2-3 months and 9-18 months, respectively. This allows for continuing head growth.
- Infants' and small children's heads are larger in proportion to their body.
- The brain and CNS are immature at birth; major development occurs during the first year of life and continues throughout childhood. The immature brain is particularly vulnerable to injury.

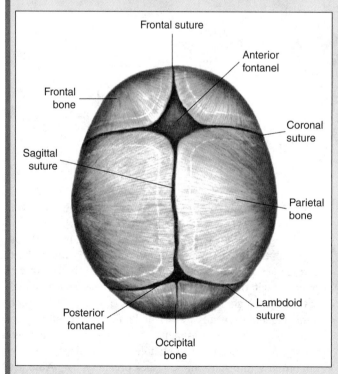

Frontal suture
Anterior fontanel
Frontal bone
Coronal suture
Sagittal suture
Parietal bone
Posterior fontanel
Lambdoid suture
Occipital bone

Ears, Nose, Throat, Mouth
- The Eustachian tubes are shorter and straighter in infants and young children, increasing their susceptibility to ear infections.
- Newborns and young infants are obligate nose breathers.

- The airway is vulnerable to obstruction because the nasal passages are small, the trachea narrower and less rigid, and the tongue large.
- 20 deciduous teeth appear between 6 and 24 months of age, permanent teeth begin to erupt at about age 6.

Lungs
- Young infants rely on the diaphragm and abdominal muscles for breathing; the chest wall is thinner and more flexible.
- The respiratory rate is faster in newborns, infants, and young children.

Heart
- Several anatomic shunts are present in the newborn heart, closing shortly after birth.
- The heart rate is faster in infants and young children; the rate frequently increases on inspiration (sinus arrhythmia).
- The heart lies more horizontally in the chest; the PMI is higher (4th ICS) and more lateral in young infants and toddlers.
- Innocent murmurs are common throughout childhood.

Musculoskeletal
- Bones are softer in children, making them more vulnerable to fractures.
- Infants and young toddlers are usually bowlegged; preschoolers and young school aged children are often "knock-kneed."
- Scoliosis commonly presents in early adolescence.

Lymph System
- Lymph tissue increases during childhood, reaching a peak between 6 and 9 years. Children at this age often have large tonsils.

Neurologic
- Major growth of the nervous system occurs during the first year of life; motor control develops in a cephalocaudal direction, from head to trunk to extremities.
- Primitive reflexes are present at birth and disappear in a predictable pattern throughout early infancy.
- Infants, including preterm infants, perceive and react to pain. This pain response in manifested primarily by physiologic changes (HR, BP, oxygen saturation).

Breasts
- Breasts remain undeveloped until the onset of puberty.

Reproductive System
- Genitalia of males and females do not undergo development until the onset of puberty.

Note: CNS = central nervous system; ICS = intercosal space; PMI = point of maximum impulse.

HEALTH HISTORY

RISK FACTORS　*Ears and Auditory System (Neonates/Infants)*

As you conduct a health history for infants and children related to the ears and auditory system, it is important to consider common risk factors associated with congenital or perinatal hearing loss and otitis media and to follow up with additional questions if risk factors exist.

Risk Factors for Congenital or Perinatal Hearing Loss*
Neonatal Risk Factors (Birth to 1 Month)
- Family history of congenital sensorineural hearing loss (SNHL)
- In utero infections associated with SNHL (herpes, syphilis, rubella, cytomegalovirus, or toxoplasmosis)
- Low Apgar scores at birth (0 to 3 at 5 minutes; 0 to 6 at 10 minutes)
- Birth weight less than 1500 g
- Respiratory distress at birth, or need for mechanical ventilation for more than 10 days
- Presence of ear or other craniofacial malformations
- Hyperbilirubinemia requiring blood transfusion
- Bacterial meningitis infection
- Administration of ototoxic medications for more than 5 days (or used in combination with loop diuretics)

Infant Risk Factors (1 to 24 Months)
- Any of the neonatal risk factors listed above
- Recurrent otitis media for at least 3 months
- Infections associated with SNHL (meningitis, mumps, measles)
- Head trauma involving fracture of the temporal bone

Risk Factors for Otitis Media
- Exposure to tobacco smoke (M)
- Day care attendance (M)
- Bottle-fed infant (as opposed to breast-fed infant) (M)
- Anatomy: short, straight eustachian tube
- Age: peak incidence 6 to 12 months
- Gender: males greater than females
- Ethnicity: greatest incidence among Native Americans
- Socioeconomic status: inverse relationship

*Joint Committee on Infant Hearing: Year 2000 position statement: principles and guidelines for early hearing detection and intervention, *Pediatrics* 106:798-817, 2000.
M = modifiable risk factor.

The pediatric health history is adapted to the age and developmental status of the child. The basic format of the history is similar to that of the adult, with additional age-specific data in the areas of perinatal history, growth and development, and behavioral status. In addition, it is important to observe the interaction between parent and child throughout the history and examination. As in the adult, a complete history is obtained during well-child visits. A more limited, focused history is performed when the child presents with an illness.

Much of the pediatric history is obtained from the parent (or other adult) accompanying the child, but it is important to also include the child as much as appropriate for the child's age (Fig. 20-1). After the parent's concerns are explored, additional health history questions can be asked directly to school-age children and adolescents using language and concepts appropriate to their age. It is particularly important to give adolescents an opportunity to talk with the health care provider without the parent present. In many states, adolescents have a legal right to confidential care for specific problems including sexually transmitted infections, contraception and pregnancy, as well as mental health issues and substance abuse. For these reasons, the adolescent should be given an opportunity to discuss these issues privately. The American Medical Association's Guidelines for Adolescent Preventive Services (GAPS) program has published health history questionnaires that can be completed by younger and middle to older adolescents as well as forms for parents. These forms provide a valuable first step in data collection for these age groups (see Fig. 20-4 on p. 503).

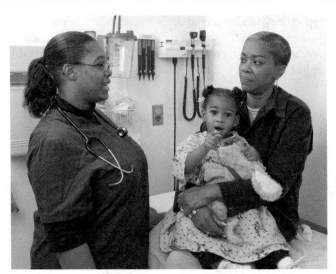

Fig. 20-1 Most data are obtained from the adult accompanying the child.

COMPONENTS OF THE PEDIATRIC HEALTH HISTORY

Biographic Data

In addition to the information included in the adult history (name, gender, age, date of birth, race, and culture), biographic data also include the name of the person giving the history (the informant) and that person's relationship to the child.

Reason for Seeking Health Care

Record the reason for the visit in the words of the parent or the older child/adolescent. Many pediatric visits are for well child care. If this is the case, record the reason for the visit, for example, "6 month well child care." If the child is seen for acute or chronic illnesses, the reason for the visit is often a symptom—for example "cough and runny nose × 10 days." The reason for seeking care should be brief, no more than a sentence or two.

History of Present Illness/Present Health Status

The same information is recorded for the infant and child as for the adult. If illness is present, record a complete symptom analysis (see Box 3-3 in Chapter 3). If the child is being seen for a well visit, an overall statement about the child's current health is included.

Past Health History

For newborns, infants, and toddlers, the past health history includes the mother's health status during the course of the pregnancy as well as information about the birth and neonatal period. Collectively, these data are referred to as the perinatal history and are presented in Box 20-2. The perinatal history may also be important for older children with congenital problems or other problems that may be related to pregnancy or birth complications (for example, fetal alcohol syndrome or cerebral palsy). Also included in the past health history is a developmental history, which details the age of achievement for major developmental milestones. Specific questions asked depend on the age and developmental level of the child. Chapter 19 presents further information regarding developmental assessment and milestones.

Other components of the past health history are similar to the adult history and include a summary of childhood illnesses, chronic illnesses, hospitalizations and surgeries, accidents or injuries, medications, and allergies, as well as the dates of the last medical, vision, and dental care. Particularly important in pediatrics is the immunization history, which should be reviewed at every well child visit and at each visit for acute illness. The immunization schedule is presented in Table 19-6 in Chapter 19.

BOX 20-2 THE PERINATAL HISTORY

Prenatal care (where care occurred, gestation at first prenatal visit, total number of visits)

Maternal complications associated with pregnancy (bleeding problems, hypertension, edema, proteinuria, unusual weight gain, infections, gestational diabetes, preterm labor)
- Use of tobacco, alcohol, medications, and street drugs during pregnancy; include type, dose, duration, and month of gestation when taken
- Emotional state of mother during pregnancy; anxiety or depression, acceptance of pregnancy, mental health issues

Labor and Delivery Process
- Place of birth (hospital, birth center, home)
- Labor: spontaneous or induced, duration, medications, complications (infection, fever, prolonged labor, fetal distress)
- Delivery: vaginal or cesarean section, reason for cesarean section, anesthesia, fetal presentation (vertex, breech), special equipment or procedure required (e.g., forceps, vacuum extraction)

Newborn Course
- Gestational age and growth pattern (SGA, AGA, LGA)
- Apgar score and type of resuscitation required
- Neonatal complications: respiratory problems / oxygen requirements, infections, feeding problems, hyperbilirubinemia, abnormal physical exam, congenital anomalies, etc.

Duration of hospital stay; follow up needed after discharge

Lab results: bilirubin, newborn screening, any other lab tests ordered during duration of baby's stay in hospital and whether the infant was discharged with mother

Immunizations given (Hepatitis B)

Family History

The family history includes the medical history of three generations, including the child and any siblings, the parents, and both sets of grandparents. The ages and health status of all family members are recorded, with particular attention to congenital problems, infant and child deaths, and hereditary illnesses. As in the adult, a family history of chronic illness (including diabetes, cardiovascular disease, malignancy, or mental health disorders) is noted. Smoking among family members, as well as problems with alcohol or substance abuse, are particularly important to note.

Personal and Psychosocial History

The personal and psychosocial history includes an overview of the child's current level of function as well as data about social and family relationships, behaviors and health habits, and mental health. With young children these data are collected primarily from the parent. As children reach adolescence, sensitive parts of the history should be obtained without the parent present. This provides the adolescent with the opportunity to give a confidential history and discuss issues privately. A useful format for collecting the personal and psychosocial history of the adolescent is the HEEADSSS format presented in Table 20-2.

General Status / Child Profile

Ask the parent to describe the child's personality and temperament. Engage older children in a conversation about how they think their life is going, things they like about themselves, and things they are good or not so good at doing. Ask about personal habits and behavior patterns such as nail biting, thumb sucking, rituals ("security blanket" or toy), and unusual behaviors (head banging, rocking, overt masturbation, walking on toes). Also ask for a description of the child's typical day.

Diet and Nutrition

When taking a diet history, inquire about typical daily diet, intolerances or allergies, supplements, family meal time routines, snacks, and any concerns of the parent or child about diet or weight. For newborns and infants, determine the type (breast or formula) and amount/frequency of feeding, intro-

---

TABLE 20-2   *Adolescent Psychosocial History*

History—HEEADSSS

TOPIC	QUESTION
Home	Who lives with you? Where do you live?, What are relationships like at home? To whom are you closest at home? To whom can you talk with at home? Is there anyone new at home? Has someone left recently? Have you moved recently? Have you ever lived away from home? (Why?)
Education and Employment	What are your favorite / least favorite subjects at school? How are your grades? Any recent changes? Any dramatic changes in the past? Have you changed schools in the past few years? Are you working? Where? How much? What are your future education / employment plans/goals?
Eating	What do you like and not like about your body? Have there been any recent changes in your weight? Have you dieted in the last year? How? How often? Have you done anything else to manage your weight? How much exercise do you get in an average day? Week? What do you think would be a healthy diet? How does that compare to your current eating patterns?
Activities	What do you do and your friends do for fun? What do you and your family do for fun? Do you participate in sports or other activities? Do you regularly attend a church group, club, or other organized activity?
Drugs	Do any of your friends use tobacco? Alcohol? Other drugs? Does anyone in your family use tobacco? Alcohol? Other drugs? Do you use tobacco? Alcohol? Other drugs? Is there any history of alcohol or drug problems in your family?
Sexuality	Have you ever been in a romantic relationship? Tell me about the people you've dated OR tell me about your sex life. Have any of your relationships ever been sexual relationships? Are your sexual activities enjoyable? What does the term "safer sex" mean to you?
Suicide and Depression	Do you feel sad or down more than usual? Do you find yourself crying more than usual? Are you bored all the time? Are you having trouble getting to sleep? Have you thought a lot about hurting yourself or someone else?
Safety (savagery)	Have you ever been seriously injured? (How?) How about anyone else you know? Do you always wear a seatbelt in the car? Have you ever ridden with a driver who was drunk or high? When? How often? Do you use safety equipment for sports and or other physical activities? Is there any violence in your home? Does the violence ever get physical? Is there a lot of violence in your school or your neighborhood? Among your friends? Have you ever been physically or sexually abused? Have you ever been raped, on a date or at any other time?

Adapted from Goldenring and Rosen (2004).

duction of solid foods (cereal, fruits, vegetables, meats, eggs) and other liquids (water, juice, cow's milk). Note excess intake of milk or juice, which may impact appetite and decrease the intake of more nutritious foods.

The diet history of children should include a description of the typical diet, including any diet restrictions that may place them at risk for nutritional deficiencies. Ask about habits that increase the risk for dental caries (bottles in bed, constant sipping of milk or juice from bottles or sippy cups, soda consumption, sweet and sticky foods). Assess where most meals are eaten (at home, school, or in restaurants) and identify children who frequently consume "fast food" and "junk food," Obesity is a significant problem in childhood and is associated with the later development of chronic diseases such as Type 2 diabetes, hypertension, and cardiovascular disease.

Adolescents should be asked specifically about their perception of their current weight and behaviors associated with eating disorders, including food restrictions, extreme diet/exercise routines, binging or purging, and the use of laxatives. Calcium and iron intake should also be evaluated because poor calcium intake in adolescence has been linked to osteoporosis later in life. Menstruating teens are at risk for anemia, especially if their iron intake is deficient.

Sleep

The pediatric sleep history includes where and with whom the child sleeps, total amount of sleep including naps, bedtime rituals, difficulty falling or staying asleep, and nightmares or night terrors. Parents should be asked about the sleep position of newborns and infants as well as the sleep environment (Box 20-3).

Sexuality

Ask about pubertal changes, which occur earlier in girls than in boys. Teenage girls should be asked about menstruation, including their last menstrual period and the frequency and duration of menses. Teens should be asked privately about sexual activity. It is important that questions about sexuality be approached with great sensitivity and that the nurse not make assumptions about sexual orientation. The sexually active adolescent should be evaluated for risk of pregnancy and/or sexually transmitted infections. It is also important to determine that sexual activity is consensual and that no coercion or force is involved. See Chapter 18 for a complete discussion of the menstrual and sexual history.

BOX 20-3 CLINICAL NOTE

Sudden infant death syndrome prevention strategies include sleeping in the supine position ("Back to Sleep") on a firm surface. Also recommended is the use of a pacifier at bedtime, avoidance of pillows or other soft objects in the crib, and having infants sleep in their own bed in the parents' room (AAP 2005).

Development

To assess the current developmental stage, it is helpful to ask parents about new skills since the last well child visit as well as the specific milestones that should be occurring. For example, ask the parent of a 5-year-old if the child is able to dress self, jump rope, identify colors, and follow rules when playing games, all of which are expected developmental achievements in a 5-year-old. Asking about school performance is another key component of developmental assessment. Include current grade level, any special educational needs, school problems, and truancy. Adolescents should be asked about future school and career plans.

Health Promotion Habits

To assess health habits, ask about diet, smoking, exercise, hobbies, and other activities including amounts of television and computer time. Also evaluate the use of safety measures including car seats, sun screen, and bicycle helmets / sports equipment. Teenage males should be asked about testicular self-examination.

Social and Family Relationships

A comprehensive pediatric history includes assessment of social relationships, including family and friends, as well as a description of the home environment. Information to gather about this topic includes:

Family composition: individuals who live in the home and their relationship to the child, the primary caregiver(s) in the family, recent changes in family composition, family members or other important persons who interact frequently with the child but live outside the home (noncustodial parents, grandparents, other extended family, nannies, or daycare providers).

Family life: family activities; impact of culture on family; parenting style and skills; discipline methods and their effectiveness; family rules; child care arrangements; parent and family support system; family conflict or chaos; family violence.

Family Socioeconomic Status: parents' occupation and employment, sources of income including government assistance (Medicaid, food stamps, The Special Supplemental Nutrition Program for Women, Infants, and Children [WIC]); insurance coverage; history of homelessness or unstable living arrangements; ability of parents to meet child's basic physical needs (food, shelter, clothing, medical care, supervision).

Home Environment: characteristics of the home including facilities (heat, running water, cooking facilities, adequate space, sleeping arrangements) and home safety (child proofing; storage of firearms, medications, and chemicals; animals in the home; pool safety); characteristics of the community (available resources, crime, pollution, overcrowding, safety hazards).

Friends: child's relationships with friends, classmates, and siblings; ages of friends; ability to make friends easily; activities shared with friends; history of bullying or being bullied; fighting; violence among peers. Adolescents should be asked specifically about alcohol and drug use, dating and sexual activity, gang activity and violence in their school, and peer group.

Mental Health

Many factors that can impact mental health will have been previously noted in either the past medical history (maternal substance abuse in pregnancy, perinatal hypoxia, neurologic illness or injury) or the social history (developmental delays, family problems, body image disturbances, witnessed violence). The mental health history should explore the impact of these problems on the child, identify past psychiatric history, explore current stresses in the child's life, and identify signs and symptoms of mental health issues. Questions should include frequent sense of boredom, suicidal thoughts or attempts, symptoms of depression, anxiety, and risk taking behaviors (drug or alcohol use, fighting, risky sexual behaviors, school failure or truancy, etc). Determine the child's usual ability to cope with stress and any recent changes in coping, mood, or behavior. It is also helpful to ask children to identify who they can talk to about problems in their lives. Children who have poor coping skills, many stressors, and no trusted adult in their lives, as well as those who engage in multiple risk-taking behaviors, are at particular risk. Note that the health care provider's duty to maintain confidentiality ends when a child or adolescent reveals that they are a danger to themselves or others.

The Pediatric Symptom Checklist (PSC) can be used to identify parental concerns about behavioral and emotional issues in children ages 4 to 18. A second version of the form (The PSC Youth Report) is available for self-reporting of symptoms by older children and adolescents (see Fig. 20-5 on p. 504). GAPS Questionnaires (described previously) are also useful components of an adolescent mental health history. Other assessment tools are used in selected cases. For example, the CRAFFT tool (Box 20-4) can be used to screen for alcohol abuse in teens.

BOX 20-4 **CRAFFT SCREENING TOOL**

Answering yes to two or more questions is highly predictive of an alcohol or drug-related disorder.

Have you ever ridden in a **CAR** driven by someone (including yourself) who was high or had been using alcohol or drugs?

Do you ever use alcohol or drugs to **RELAX**, feel better about yourself, or fit in?

Do you ever use alcohol/drugs while you are by yourself, **ALONE**?

Do you ever **FORGET** things you did while using alcohol or drugs?

Do your family or **FRIENDS** ever tell you that you should cut down on your drinking or drug use?

Have you gotten into **TROUBLE** while you were using alcohol or drugs?

From Knight, JR, Shrier LA, Bravender TD, et al: A new brief screen for adolescent substance abuse, *Arch Pediatr Adolesc Med* 153:591-596, 1999.

Review of Systems

The review of systems for the infant and child is similar to that of an adult. The goal is to elicit symptoms and problems that may not have been identified earlier in the history. Critical components of the review of systems in pediatrics include:

General Symptoms

- *Constitutional symptoms:* fever, chills, night sweats, fatigue, tiring with feeding (infants), change in energy level or activity tolerance
- *Growth:* recent weight gain or loss, concerns about height, weight, or head size
- *Pain:* ask the parents of infants and toddlers if they think their baby is in pain and what signs of pain they see; older children can be asked about pain using age-appropriate pain scales (Figure 20-2 and 20-3).

Integumentary System

- *Skin:* jaundice (newborn); rashes, birthmarks, or lesions; easy bruising; petechiae; itching; dry skin; acne (adolescents); piercings and tattoos (adolescents)
- *Hair:* infestations (such as lice), hair loss, seborrhea (infants)
- *Nails:* nail changes; nail biting; ingrown or painful nails

Head and Neck

- *Head:* concerns about head size or shape (newborns, infants); headaches; recent trauma
- *Eyes:* visual concerns including not fixing on objects or following with eyes (newborns, infants), reading difficulty, sitting too close to television or computer screen, bumping into things); redness, drainage, or crusting; itching or pain; abnormal eye movement or alignment
- *Ears:* hearing concerns including not responding to sound (newborns, infants), unusual vocalizations (infants), loud speech or loud TV, child's complaint of decreased hearing, ear pain, discharge
- *Nose:* congestion, drainage, frequent nosebleeds (epistaxis), snoring
- *Mouth/Throat:* teeth (tooth pain, tooth loss, caries); mouth pain or lesions; unusual coatings of tongue or mouth; throat pain; difficulty swallowing; voice changes
- *Neck:* lymph node enlargement, swelling or masses in neck, stiff neck, unusual head/neck position

Breasts

- Breast engorgement (newborns of both sexes); breast changes (school age and adolescents); pain

Cardiovascular

- Cyanosis or pallor; edema; known murmur or cardiovascular disease; syncope

Respiratory System

- Cough; wheezing or noisy breathing; shortness of breath; increased respiratory rate or effort; use of "inhalers"

Text continued on p. 506

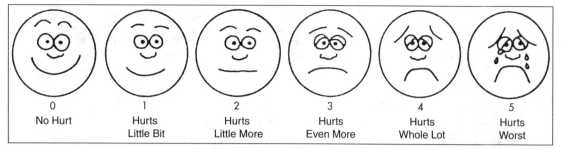

Fig. 20-2 **Wong-Baker FACES Pain Rating Scale.** Recommended for children 3 years of age and older. Ask the child to choose the face that best describes how he or she if feeling. *(From Hockenberry MJ, Wilson D, Winkelstein ML:* Wong's essentials of pediatric nursing, *ed 7, St. Louis, 2005. Used by permission. Copyright, Mosby.)*

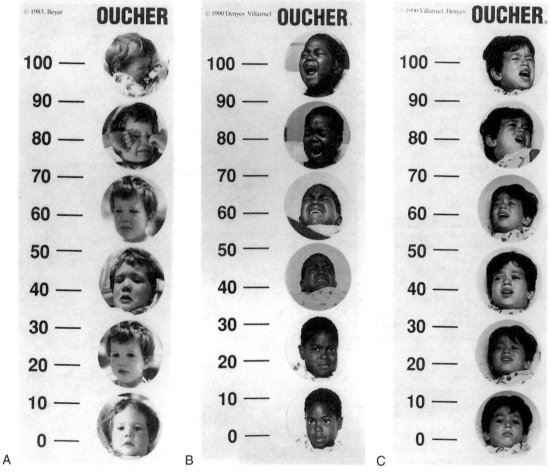

Fig. 20-3 **Oucher Pain Scales. A,** Caucasian, **B,** African American, **C,** Hispanic. *(A, Developed and copyrighted by Judith E. Beyer, 1983. B and C, Courtesy Denyes, Villaruel.)*

| Guidelines for Adolescent Preventive Services |
| Middle-Older Adolescent Questionnaire |

Confidential (Your answers will not be given out.)   Chart # _____

Name _____ Date _____
        Last   First   Middle Initial

Date of Birth _____ Grade in School _____ Year in college _____ Sex: Male Female Age _____

Address _____ City _____ Zip _____

Phone number where you can be reached _____ Pager/beeper number _____

What languages are spoken where you live? _____ Race _____

Medical History

1. Why did you come to the clinic/office today? _____

2. Do you have any health problems? ☐ Yes ☐ No Problem(s) _____

3. Did you have any health problems in the past 12 months? ☐ Yes ☐ No Problem(s) _____

4. Are you taking any medicine now? ☐ Yes ☐ No Name of medicine _____

For Girls

5. Date when last period started _____ Are your periods regular (monthly)? .... ☐ No ☐ Yes
                                    Month   Date

6. Have you had a miscarriage, an abortion, or live birth in the past 12 months? .... ☐ Yes ☐ No

Specific Health Issues

7. Please check whether you have questions or are worried about any of the following:

☐ Height/weight
☐ Blood pressure
☐ Diet/food/appetite
☐ Future plans/job
☐ Skin (rash, acne)
☐ Headaches/migraines
☐ Dizziness/fainting
☐ Eyes/vision
☐ Ears/hearing/ear aches
☐ Nose
☐ Lots of colds

☐ Mouth/teeth/breath
☐ Neck/back
☐ Chest pain/trouble breathing
☐ Coughing/wheezing
☐ Breasts
☐ Heart
☐ Stomach ache
☐ Nausea/vomiting
☐ Diarrhea/constipation
☐ Muscle or joint pain in arms/legs

☐ Frequent or painful urination
☐ Discharge from penis or vagina
☐ Wetting the bed
☐ Sexual organs/genitals
☐ Menstruation/periods
☐ Wet dreams
☐ Physical or sexual abuse
☐ Masturbation
☐ HIV/AIDS

☐ Trouble sleeping
☐ Feeling tired a lot
☐ Cancer
☐ Dying
☐ Sad or crying a lot
☐ Stress
☐ Anger/temper
☐ Violence/personal safety
☐ Other (explain)

_____
_____

Health Profile

These questions will help us get to know you better. Choose the answer that best describes what you feel or do. Your answers will be seen only by your health care provider and his/her assistant.

Eating/Weight

8. Are you satisfied with your eating habits? .... ☐ No ☐ Yes

9. Do you ever eat in secret? .... ☐ Yes ☐ No

10. Do you spend a lot of time thinking about ways to be thin? .... ☐ Yes ☐ No

11. In the past year, have you tried to lose weight or control your weight by vomiting, taking diet pills or laxatives, or starving yourself? .... ☐ Yes ☐ No

12. Do you exercise or participate in sport activities that make you sweat and breathe hard for 20 minutes or more at a time at least three or more times during the week? .... ☐ No ☐ Yes

School

13. Are your grades this year worse than last year? .... ☐ Yes ☐ No ☐ Not in school

14. Have you either been told you have a learning problem or do you think you have a learning problem? .... ☐ Yes ☐ No

15. Have you been suspended from school this year? .... ☐ Yes ☐ No ☐ Not in school

Friends & Family

16. Do you have at least one friend who you really like and feel you can talk to? .... ☐ No ☐ Yes

17. Do you think that your parent(s) or guardian(s) *usually* listen to you and take your feelings seriously? ...... ☐ No ☐ Yes

18. *Have you ever thought seriously about running away from home?* .... ☐ Yes ☐ **No** ☐ Not sure

Turn page

Fig. 20-4   Guidelines for Adolescent Preventive Services. *(American Medical Association, 1997).*

Weapons/Violence/Safety

19. Do you or anyone you live with have a gun, rifle, or other firearm? .... ☐ Yes ☐ No ☐ Not sure
20. In the past year, have you carried a gun, knife, club, or other weapon for protection? .... ☐ Yes ☐ No
21. Have you been in a physical fight during the *past 3 months*? .... ☐ Yes ☐ No
22. Have you ever been in trouble with the law? .... ☐ Yes ☐ No
23. Are you worried about violence or your safety? .... ☐ Yes ☐ No ☐ Not sure
24. Do you usually wear a helmet when you rollerblade, skateboard, ride a bicycle , motorcycle, minibike, or ride in an all-terrain vehicle (ATV)? .... ☐ No ☐ Yes
25. Do you usually wear a seat belt when you ride in or drive a car, truck, or van? .... ☐ No ☐ Yes

Tobacco

26. Do you ever smoke cigarettes/cigars, use snuff or chew tobacco? .... ☐ Yes ☐ No
26. Do any of your close friends ever smoke cigarettes/cigars, use snuff or chew tobacco? .... ☐ Yes ☐ No
28. Does anyone you live with smoke cigarettes/cigars, use snuff or chew tobacco? .... ☐ Yes ☐ No

Alcohol

29. In the past month, did you get drunk or very high on beer, wine, or other alcohol? .... ☐ Yes ☐ No
30. In the past month, did any of your close friends get drunk or very high on beer, wine, or other alcohol? .... ☐ Yes ☐ No
31. Have you ever been criticized or gotten into trouble because of drinking? .... ☐ Yes ☐ No ☐ Not sure
32. In the past year have you used alcohol and then driven a car/truck/van/motorcycle? .... ☐ Yes ☐ No ☐ Does not apply
33. In the past year, have you been in a car or other motor vehicle when the driver has been drinking alcohol or using drugs? .... ☐ Yes ☐ No
34. Does anyone in your family drink or take drugs so much that it worries you? .... ☐ Yes ☐ No

Drugs

35. Do you ever use marijuana or other drugs, or sniff inhalants? .... ☐ Yes ☐ No ☐ Not sure
36. Do any of your close friends ever use marijuana or other drugs, or sniff inhalants? .... ☐ Yes ☐ No ☐ Not sure
37. Do you ever use non-prescription drugs to get to sleep, stay awake, calm down, or get high? (These drugs can be bought at a store without a doctor's prescription.) .... ☐ Yes ☐ No
38. Have you ever used steroid pills or shots without a doctor telling you to? .... ☐ Yes ☐ No ☐ Not sure

Development

39. Do you have any concerns or questions about the size or shape of your body, or your physical appearance? .... ☐ Yes ☐ No ☐ Not sure
40. Do you think you may be gay, lesbian, or bisexual? .... ☐ Yes ☐ No ☐ Not sure
41. Have you ever had sexual intercourse? (How old were you the first time?_____) .... ☐ Yes ☐ No ☐ Not sure
42. Are you using a method to prevent pregnancy? (Which:_____) .... ☐ No ☐ Yes ☐ Not active
43. Do you and your partner(s) *always* use condoms when you have sex? .... ☐ No ☐ Yes ☐ Not active
44. Have any of your close friends ever had sexual intercourse? .... ☐ Yes ☐ No ☐ Not sure
45. Have you ever been told by a doctor or nurse that you had a sexually transmitted infection or disease? ...... ☐ Yes ☐ No ☐ Not sure
46. Have you ever been pregnant or gotten someone pregnant? .... ☐ Yes ☐ No ☐ Not sure
47. Would you like to receive information or supplies to prevent pregnancy or sexually transmitted infections? ... ☐ Yes ☐ No ☐ Not sure
48. Would you like to know how to avoid getting HIV/AIDS? .... ☐ Yes ☐ No ☐ Not sure
49. Have you pierced your body (not including ears) or gotten a tattoo? .... ☐ Yes ☐ No ☐ Thinking about it

Emotions

50. Have you had fun during the past two weeks? .... ☐ No ☐ Yes
51. During the past few weeks, have you *often* felt sad or down or as though you have nothing to look forward to? .... ☐ Yes ☐ No
52. Have you ever *seriously* thought about killing yourself, made a plan or actually tried to kill yourself? .... ☐ Yes ☐ No
53. Have you ever been physically, sexually, or emotionally abused? .... ☐ Yes ☐ No ☐ Not sure
54. When you get angry, do you do violent things? .... ☐ Yes ☐ No
55. Would you like to get counseling about something you have on your mind? .... ☐ Yes ☐ No ☐ Not sure

Special Circumstances

56. In the past year, have you been around someone with tuberculosis (TB)? .... ☐ Yes ☐ No ☐ Not sure
57. In the past year, have you stayed overnight in a homeless shelter, jail, or detention center? .... ☐ Yes ☐ No
58. Have you ever lived in foster care or a group home? .... ☐ Yes ☐ No

Self

59. What four words best describe you? _____
60. If you could change one thing about your life or yourself, what would it be? _____

_____

61. What do you want to talk about today? _____

Fig. 20-4, cont'd   Guidelines for Adolescent Preventive Services. (*American Medical Association, 1997.*)

Pediatric Symptom Checklist (PSC)

Emotional and physical health go together in children. Because parents are often the first to notice a problem with their child's behavior, emotions or learning, you may help your child get the best care possible by answering these questions. Please indicate which statement best describes your child.

Please mark under the heading that best describes your child:

		NEVER	SOMETIMES	OFTEN
1. Complains of aches and pains	1	_____	_____	_____
2. Spends more time alone	2	_____	_____	_____
3. Tires easily, has little energy	3	_____	_____	_____
4. Fidgety, unable to sit still	4	_____	_____	_____
5. Has trouble with teacher	5	_____	_____	_____
6. Less interested in school	6	_____	_____	_____
7. Acts as if driven by a motor	7	_____	_____	_____
8. Daydreams too much	8	_____	_____	_____
9. Distracted easily	9	_____	_____	_____
10. Is afraid of new situations	10	_____	_____	_____
11. Feels sad, unhappy	11	_____	_____	_____
12. Is irritable, angry	12	_____	_____	_____
13. Feels hopeless	13	_____	_____	_____
14. Has trouble concentrating	14	_____	_____	_____
15. Less interested in friends	15	_____	_____	_____
16. Fights with other children	16	_____	_____	_____
17. Absent from school	17	_____	_____	_____
18. School grades dropping	18	_____	_____	_____
19. Is down on him or herself	19	_____	_____	_____
20. Visits the doctor with doctor finding nothing wrong	20	_____	_____	_____
21. Has trouble sleeping	21	_____	_____	_____
22. Worries a lot	22	_____	_____	_____
23. Wants to be with you more than before	23	_____	_____	_____
24. Feels he or she is bad	24	_____	_____	_____
25. Takes unnecessary risks	25	_____	_____	_____
26. Gets hurt frequently	26	_____	_____	_____
27. Seems to be having less fun	27	_____	_____	_____
28. Acts younger than children his or her age	28	_____	_____	_____
29. Does not listen to rules	29	_____	_____	_____
30. Does not show feelings	30	_____	_____	_____
31. Does not understand other people's feelings	31	_____	_____	_____
32. Teases others	32	_____	_____	_____
33. Blames others for his or her troubles	33	_____	_____	_____
34. Takes things that do not belong to him or her	34	_____	_____	_____
35. Refuses to share	35	_____	_____	_____

Total score _____

Does your child have any emotional or behavioral problems for which she/he needs help? ( ) N ( ) Y
Are there any services that you would like your child to receive for these problems? ( ) N ( ) Y

If yes, what
services?_____

Fig. 20-5 Pediatric Symptom Checklist and Pediatric Symptom Checklist Youth Report. *(Jellinek, 1994.)*

Pediatric Symptom Checklist - Youth Report (Y-PSC)

Please mark under the heading that best fits you:

	Never	Sometimes	Often
1. Complain of aches or pains............................	—	—	—
2. Spend more time alone.................................	—	—	—
3. Tire easily, little energy............................	—	—	—
4. Fidgety, unable to sit still..........................	—	—	—
5. Have trouble with teacher....................	—	—	—
6. Less interested in school...............	—	—	—
7. Act as if driven by motor..........................	—	—	—
8. Daydream too much.....................................	—	—	—
9. Distract easily......................................	—	—	—
10. Are afraid of new situations.........................	—	—	—
11. Feel sad, unhappy.....................................	—	—	—
12. Are irritable, angry..................................	—	—	—
13. Feel hopeless...	—	—	—
14. Have trouble concentrating............................	—	—	—
15. Less interested in friends...........................	—	—	—
16. Fight with other children............................	—	—	—
17. Absent from school.	—	—	—
18. School grades dropping.	—	—	—
19. Down on yourself.....................................	—	—	—
20. Visit doctor with doctor finding nothing wrong........	—	—	—
21. Have trouble sleeping................................	—	—	—
22. Worry a lot..	—	—	—
23. Want to be with parent more than before...............	—	—	—
24. Feel that you are bad................................	—	—	—
25. Take unnecessary risks...............................	—	—	—
26. Get hurt frequently..................................	—	—	—
27. Seem to be having less fun...........................	—	—	—
28. Act younger than children your age...................	—	—	—
29. Do not listen to rules...............................	—	—	—
30. Do not show feelings.................................	—	—	—
31. Do not understand other people's feelings.............	—	—	—
32. Tease others...	—	—	—
33. Blame others for your troubles.......................	—	—	—
34. Take things that do not belong to you.................	—	—	—
35. Refuse to share......................................	—	—	—

Fig. 20-5, cont'd Pediatric Symptom Checklist and Pediatric Symptom Checklist Youth Report. *(Jellinek, 1994.)*

Urinary System

- Number of wet diapers per day (newborns, infants); toilet training progress; bedwetting or daytime accidents in a previously toilet-trained child; signs of urinary tract infection (dysuria, urgency, frequency, foul odor); hematuria

Gastrointestinal System

- Usual pattern of bowel movements; changes in bowel function including constipation and diarrhea; abdominal pain; nausea; vomiting; change in appetite

Reproductive System

- Boys: healing of circumcision; rash or irritation; penile discharge; pain; itching; development of secondary sexual characteristics; testicular masses; trauma
- Girls: menstrual concerns (dysmenorrhea, irregular menses, heavy bleeding, amenorrhea); rash or irritation; discharge (*Note:* the basic menstrual and sexual history is collected as part of the HEEADSSS psychosocial history that was previously discussed.)
- Ask adolescents about sexual abuse; younger children are also asked if sexual abuse is suspected. Questions need to be at an appropriate developmental level (Box 20-5)

Musculoskeletal System

- Symmetric movement (newborns/infants); pain in joints or muscles; deformity or asymmetry; range of motion limita-

| BOX 20-5 | **TALKING WITH CHILDREN WHO REVEAL ABUSE** |

- Provide a private time and place to talk.
- Do not promise not to tell; tell the child that you are required to report the abuse.
- Do not express shock or criticize the family.
- Use the child's vocabulary to discuss the body part.
- Avoid using any leading statements that can distort the child's story.
- Reassure the child that he or she has done the right thing by telling.
- Tell the child that the touching or abuse is not his or her fault; he or she is not bad or to blame.
- Determine the child's immediate need for safety.
- Let the child know when you report the situation.

From Wong DL et al: *Whaley & Wong's nursing care of infants and children,* ed 6, St Louis, 1999, Mosby.

tions; muscle or joint trauma; curvature of the spine; concerns about legs or feet (bowlegged, intoeing, limp)

Neurologic System

- Unusual cry; irritability; speech problems (stuttering, articulation, language delay); fainting or dizziness; seizures; difficulty with coordination or gait

EXAMINATION

OVERVIEW: THE ART OF THE PEDIATRIC PHYSICAL EXAM

Because the process and findings associated with infant and child examinations vary by age group, the presentation of the examination is organized by body system. For each component of the body system, a separate discussion of examination issues and techniques is provided for each of the following groups: newborn/infant, toddler/child, and adolescents (with the exception of vital signs and baseline measurements, which are presented across groups).

Newborns and Infants

The nurse should completely undress the infant for examination, keeping the diaper in place until the buttocks and genitalia are examined. Care must be taken to ensure that the infant remains warm during the examination period. Keep the room warm and cover areas not being examined to prevent excessive chilling. If the infant becomes chilled, the skin, hands, and feet may take on transient mottling (blotching or marbling) appearance.

Unlike the physical exam in adults, which for the most part proceeds in a head to toe sequence, the physical exam of an infant requires that the nurse conduct the least invasive portions of the exam before proceeding on to the more invasive components. The nurse should observe the infant for any signs of distress and then proceed to auscultating heart and lungs, saving the ear and oral exam (more invasive procedures) for last. If the infant starts to cry, take time to comfort him or her as the examination of an infant who is crying can be very difficult.

In general the nurse should conduct the physical exam of young infants ($\leq$ 6 months) on an exam table. For the older infant ($\geq$ 6 months) and toddler, the nurse may find that having the caregiver hold the baby or toddler decreases fear and distress, thus making it easier for the nurse to conduct the examination.

Toddlers and Children

If the young child is cooperative and does not appear to be fearful, the nurse can proceed with the physical exam in the same sequence as the adult exam. Showing the equipment to

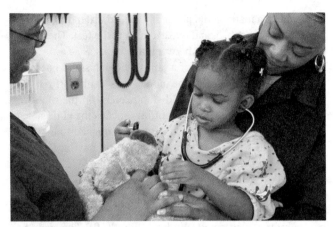

Fig. 20-6 Allow the child to touch examination equipment to reduce fear.

the child, explaining the procedure to the child, and allowing the child to use the equipment (such as a stethoscope) on a doll or teddy bear will help enlist the child's cooperation (Fig. 20-6). Having the child blow bubbles or "blow out" the light of the otoscope or penlight before and during the exam may also help elicit the child's cooperation. This is particularly helpful when trying to auscultate lung sounds.

Adolescent

Although the sequence of examination for the adolescent is the same as for the adult, the nurse needs to be aware that as children enter their teen years it is preferable to conduct the physical exam without the parent present. This ensures privacy and encourages teens to begin assuming responsibility for their health care.

VITAL SIGNS AND BASELINE MEASUREMENTS

Vital signs are measured with every visit.

Temperature

Procedure: The recommended sites for temperature measurement in newborns, infants, and children up to age 5 are the axillary or tympanic sites. Oral measurement using an electronic thermometer is permissible with older children, but the nurse must be sure the probe is correctly held in the mouth (thermometer under the tongue with the mouth closed). To take a tympanic measurement in a child less than 3 years of age, pull down on the earlobe to straighten the ear canal. For children older than 3, pull up on the ear to straighten out the canal. Although research has shown that tympanic measurements in children may be unreliable (Riddell and Eppich, 2001), it is possible that unreliable measurements are attained because the sensor beam is directed at the sides of the ear canal rather than at the tympanic membrane.

Rectal temperatures should be taken as a last resort because children tend to fear intrusive procedures and because of the risk for rectal perforation. A convenient position for taking a rectal temperature is with the child in a side-lying position with knees flexed toward the abdomen. This position is maintained with one of the nurse's hands while the lubricated thermometer is held in the rectum a maximum of 1 inch (2.5 cm).

Findings: The temperature of the infant should be similar to that of the adult (98.6° F or 37.0° C). Temperature variations may be found in newborns, however, because they have less effective heat-control mechanisms. Elevated temperatures among infants and children are often related to viral or bacterial infections, dehydration, and environmental exposure to heat. Low body temperature is most commonly associated with environmental exposure.

Heart and Respiratory Rates

Procedure: Heart and respiratory rates are assessed for the same qualities as in the adult. This assessment should take place when the infant is quiet. If the infant is quiet at the beginning of the assessment, the nurse listens to the apical pulse for a full minute and counts the respirations before proceeding to other parts of the assessment.

Respiratory rates are counted using the same procedure as for adults; infants however, usually breathe diaphragmatically, which requires observation of abdominal movement. Respirations are counted for a full minute because an infant's respiratory rate may be irregular as a normal variation.

Findings: Expected heart, respiratory rate, and blood pressure for infants and children are listed in Table 5-1 in Chapter 5. Elevations in heart rate are most commonly seen with crying, fever, respiratory distress, and dehydration. Elevations in respiratory rate may be associated with crying, fever, or respiratory distress.

Blood Pressure

For an accurate blood pressure reading, the appropriate cuff size must be used (see Chapter 5). Measurements may be taken in the arm or leg of infants and younger children. Blood pressure standards for children ages 1 through 17 are based on gender, age, and height. Blood pressure tables that include both systolic and diastolic blood pressures according to blood pressure percentiles are available on the National Heart Lung and Blood Institute website (*www.nhlbi.nih.gov/guidelines/hypertension/*). Although not common, hypertension can develop in childhood. Hypertension in children is defined as average systolic blood pressure and/or diastolic blood pressure that is ≥ 95th percentile for gender, age, and height on three or more occasions. Because hypertension can develop in adolescence, blood pressure measurement should be included with every visit (Williams, 2002). As with adults, adolescents with blood pressure levels between 120/80 and 130/90 should be considered prehypertensive (National High Blood Pressure Education Program, 2004) (Box 20-6).

Height and Weight

Routine height and weight measurements are taken on all visits until the end of the growth spurt between ages 18 and 20. The height (recumbent length) is recorded in inches or centimeters; the weight is measured in pounds and ounces, or kilograms. Height and weight are plotted on a growth chart and allow the nurse to track the child's growth in comparison with the population standard. Growth charts for infants through adolescence are available on the Centers for Disease Control and Prevention website (*www.cdc.gov*). An example of weight and length plotted on a growth chart is shown at the end of this chapter.

Height

Procedure: Recumbent length of newborns and infants is measured from the top of the head to the heel with the infant in a supine position (Fig. 20-7). The length is recorded in inches or centimeters.

Devices such as measuring mats and boards can be used to measure recumbent length. An infant measuring mat consists of a soft rubber graduated mat attached to a plastic footboard. The infant lies on the mat with the head against the headboard. The infant's knees are held together and pressed gently against the mat with one hand, while the footboard is moved against the heels. A measuring board has a rigid headboard and a movable footboard. It is placed on a table, and the infant lies on the board so that the head touches the headboard. The footboard is then moved until it touches the bottom of the infant's feet.

When height-measuring devices are not available, the nurse places the infant in a supine position on a piece of paper. Using a pen, make a mark on the paper at the head, extend the infant's body as just described, and make a mark at the feet. The recumbent length is the distance between the marks.

To measure the height of a child who can stand but is too short for the adult scale, the nurse uses a platform with a movable headboard. The child stands erect on the platform, and the headboard is lowered until it touches the child's head (Fig. 20-8). A tape measure also can be attached to a wall so that the child's height can be measured by having the child stand against the wall.

Weight

Procedure: The platform scale is used for weighing newborns, infants, and small children (Fig. 20-9). The scale has curved sides to prevent the infant from rolling off. A paper is placed on the scale, and the unclothed newborn is laid on the paper. The newborn is weighed by balancing the scale. The weight is recorded to the nearest 0.5 oz or 14 g.

Findings: Healthy newborns weigh between 5 lb 8 oz and 8 lb 13 oz (2500 and 4000 g). Newborns commonly lose 10% of their birth weight in the first week but regain it in 10 to 14 days. In general, they double their birth weight by 4 to 6 months of age and triple their birth weight by 12 months of age.

Head and Chest Circumference

Head circumference should be measured at every well-baby visit until age 2. Chest circumference is not routinely measured unless an abnormal head or chest size is suspected. Head and chest circumferences are plotted on a growth charts as previously described for height and weight.

Head Circumference

Procedure: To measure head circumference, a measuring tape is wrapped snugly around the infant's head at the largest circumference, usually just above the eyebrows, the pinna of the ears, and the occipital prominence at the back of the skull (Fig. 20-10). The tape measure is read to the nearest 1/8 inch (0.5 cm). Head circumference is measured at least twice to check for accuracy; if the measurements differ, measure a third time.

Findings: Expected head circumference for term newborns averages from 13 to 14 inches (33 to 36 cm) and should be about 1 inch (2 to 3 cm) larger than chest circumference. By 2 years of age the child's head circumference is two thirds its adult size and the chest circumference should exceed the head circumference (Table 20-3 and Box 20-7). A head circumference that is rapidly increasing suggests increased intracranial pressure. A head circumference below the fifth percentile suggests microcephaly.

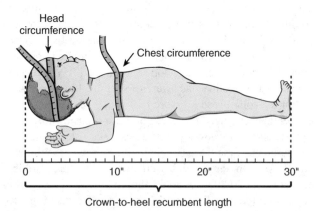

Fig. 20-7   Measurement of head and chest circumference and recumbent length. *(Redrawn from Hockenberry et al, 2003).*

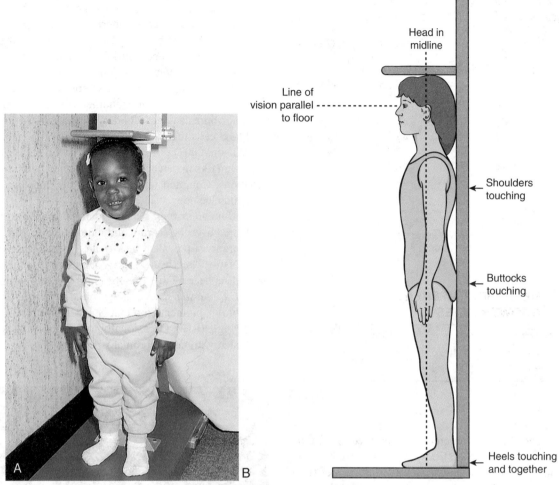

Fig. 20-8 **A,** Measure the height of a child using a platform with movable headboard. **B,** Side view showing correct posture for accurate measurement. **(A,** *From Seidel et al, 2006).*

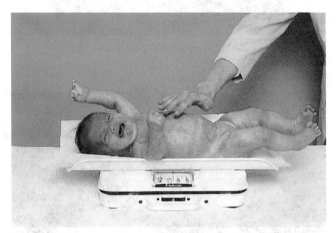

Fig. 20-9 Weighing an infant on an infant scale. *(From Hockenberry et al, 2007).*

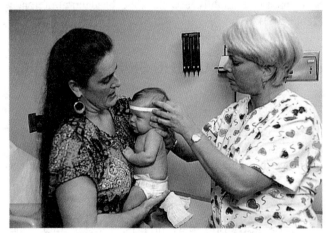

Fig. 20-10 Measuring head circumference in an infant.

TABLE 20-3 *Average Chest and Head Circumference of U.S. Children*

AGE	CHEST CIRCUMFERENCE (cm)	HEAD CIRCUMFERENCE (cm) MALES	HEAD CIRCUMFERENCE (cm) FEMALES
Birth	35	35.3	34.7
3 mo	40	40.9	40.0
6 mo	44	43.9	42.8
12 mo	47	47.3	45.8
18 mo	48	48.7	47.1
2 yr	50	49.7	48.1
3 yr	52	50.4	49.3

Data from Lowrey GH: *Growth and development of children,* ed 8, Chicago, 1986, Mosby; and Waring WW, Jeansonne LO: *Practical manual of pediatrics,* ed 2, St Louis, 1982, Mosby.

BOX 20-7 HEAD CIRCUMFERENCE GROWTH RATES

Full-term newborn to 3 months: 2.0 cm/month
3 to 6 months: 1.0 cm/month
6 months to 1 year: 0.5 cm/month

Chest Circumference

Procedure: The chest circumference is measured at the nipples, pulling the tape measure firmly without causing an indentation in the skin. The measurement is noted between inspiration and expiration and recorded to the nearest ⅛ inch (0.5 cm) (see Fig. 20-7). As noted above, chest circumference is not routinely measured unless abnormal head or chest size is suspected.

Findings: At birth, the infant's chest circumference may be equal to or slightly less than the head circumference (Table 20-3).

EXAMINATION OF THE SKIN, HAIR, NAILS

Newborns and Infants

No special procedures or techniques are necessary when examining the skin, hair, and nails other than keeping the young infant warm during the exam. For this reason, only findings are presented below.

Skin

Normal and Abnormal Findings. The skin color in the neonate depends partially on the amount of fat present. Preterm infants generally appear redder because they have less subcutaneous fat than do full-term infants. In addition, the neonate may appear to have a red skin tone for a short period because of vasomotor instability. This color tends to fade within the first few days. Also, immediately following birth the neonate's lips, nail beds, and feet may be dusky or appear cyanotic. Once the newborn is adequately warmed, the dusky color should fade, and a well-oxygenated pink tone should reappear. Dark-skinned newborns should also have a dark pink tone, which is most evident on the palms of the hands and the soles of the feet. Physiologic jaundice may be present in the newborn following the third or fourth day of life. The skin, mucous membranes, and sclera will appear to have a yellow tone. This normal phenomenon occurs in almost half of all newborns and is secondary to the increased number of red blood cells that hemolyze following birth (Hockenberry and Wilson, 2007).

Birthmarks in newborns may be pigmentation or vascular variations. Common birthmarks that are considered normal variations include:

- *Mongolian spot:* An irregularly shaped, darkened flat area over the sacrum and buttocks (Fig. 20-11). They are most prevalent in African American, Hispanic, Native American, and Asian children and generally disappear by the time the child is 1 or 2 years of age.
- *Café-au-lait spot:* A large round or oval patch of light brown pigmentation that is generally present at birth (Fig. 20-12). Occasionally these spots may be associated with neurofibromatosis.

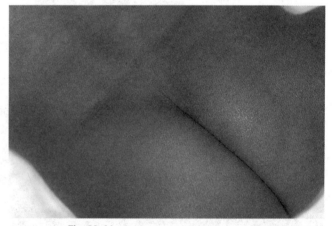

Fig. 20-11 Mongolian spot. *(From Lemmi, 2000.)*

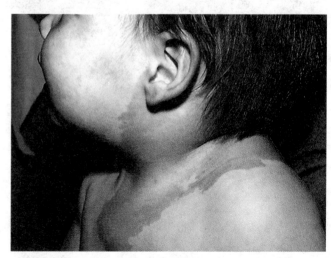

Fig. 20-12 Café-au-lait spot. *(From Weston, Lane, and Morelli, 2002.)*

- *Stork bite (telangiectasis or flat capillary hemangioma):* This common vascular birthmark appears as small red or pink spot that is often seen on the back of the neck (Fig. 20-13). Stork bites usually disappear by 5 years of age.

Some birthmarks are considered deviations from normal and include the following:

- *Port-wine stains (nevus flammeus):* Large, flat, bluish purple capillary areas (Fig. 20-14, *A*). They are most

frequently found on the face along distribution of the fifth cranial nerve. Port-wine stains do not disappear spontaneously.

- *Strawberry hemangioma:* Slightly raised, reddened areas with a sharp demarcation line (Fig. 20-14, *B*). They may be 2 to 3 cm in diameter and usually disappear by 5 years of age.
- *Cavernous hemangioma:* A reddish blue round mass of blood vessels (Fig. 20-15). They may continue to grow until the child reaches 10 to 15 months of age. Frequent reassessment should be conducted.

Common primary skin lesions among newborns that are normal variations include the following:

- *Milia:* Small, whitish papules that may be found on the cheeks, nose, chin, and forehead of newborns (Fig. 20-16). These are benign and generally disappear by the third week of life.
- *Erythema toxicum:* A common rash among newborns (Fig. 20-17). It is a self-limited, benign rash of unknown etiology consisting of erythematous macules, papules, and pustules. The rash may appear anywhere on the body except the palms of the hands and the soles of the feet. Although it may be present at birth, it usually appears by the third or fourth day of life.

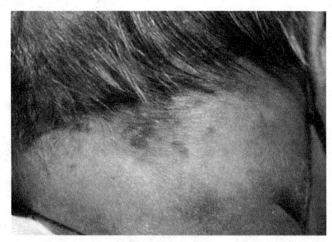

Fig. 20-13 Stork bite. *(From Weston, Lane, and Morelli, 1996.)*

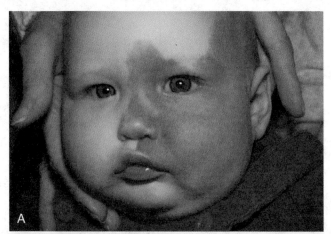

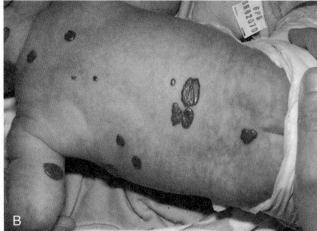

Fig. 20-14 **A,** Port-wine stain. **B,** Strawberry hemangioma. *(From Zitelli and Davis, 2007.)*

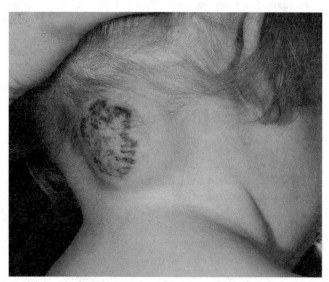

Fig. 20-15 Cavernous hemangioma. *(From Habif, 2004.)*

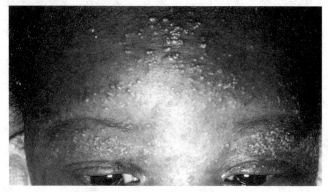

Fig. 20-16 Milia on the forehead of a newborn. *(From Cohen, 1993.)*

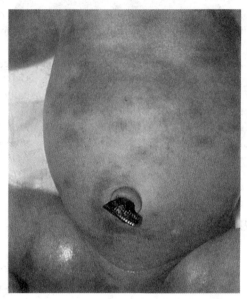

Fig. 20-17 Erythema toxicum on the trunk of an infant. *(From Cohen, 1993.)*

Hair and Nails

Normal and Abnormal Findings. Scalp hair on the newborn may be present or absent. If present, it is generally fine and soft. Seborrheic dermatitis (cradle cap) is a scaly crust that commonly appears on the scalp (Fig. 20-18). The newborn's skin may be covered with fine, soft, immature hair called *lanugo hair* (Fig. 20-19). This may be found anywhere on the body but is most common on the scalp, ears, shoulders, and back. The nails of the newborn should be examined for presence and texture. Postterm infants may have long fingernails at birth.

Toddlers and Children

No special procedures or techniques are necessary when examining the skin, hair, and nails other than keeping the young child warm during the exam.

Skin

Normal and Abnormal Findings. When assessing skin turgor, the skin should move easily when lifted and

should return to place immediately when released. A child who is seriously dehydrated (more than 3% to 5% of body weight) has skin that appears "tented" after the abdominal skin is pinched.

The most common abnormal lesions found in the young child are associated with communicable diseases and bacterial infections such as herpes varicella (chickenpox), rubella, rubeola, roseola, tinea corporis (ringworm), impetigo, pediculosis corporis (body lice), and scabies. Evidence of bruising that may be inconsistent with the child's developmental level or in an unusual area is cause for concern. As the child becomes mobile, bruising is common on the lower legs and perhaps even the face. Bruising in unusual areas (such as upper arms, back, buttocks, and abdomen) or multiple bruises found at different stages of healing should be further investigated to rule out abuse (Giardino and Giardino, 2003).

Hair and Nails

Normal and Abnormal Findings. The young child should have very little body or facial hair. Common problems associated with the scalp and hair of the young child include alopecia, which may be secondary to hair pulling, twisting, or head rubbing; and lice, nits, and scabies. Nail biting is an abnormal behavior and finding. Evidence of cyanosis of the nail bed or nail clubbing requires careful evaluation. These may indicate a cardiac or respiratory disease, or systemic disease such as cystic fibrosis.

Adolescents

Although the examination of the skin, hair, and nails is thought to be a straightforward examination, maturational changes and body hair development often make the adolescent more sensitive than children or adults. Provide adequate

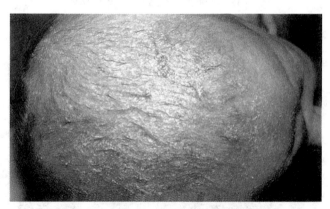

Fig. 20-18 Seborrheic dermatitis (cradle cap). *(From Cohen, 1993.)*

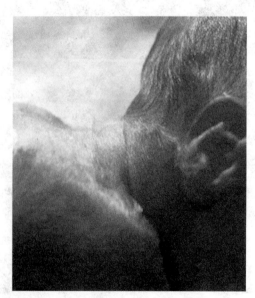

Fig. 20-19 Newborn silky body hair (lanugo). *(From Zitelli and Davis, 2007.)*

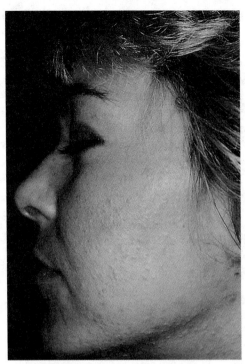

Fig. 20-20 **Comedonal acne.** Note closed comedones. *(From Goldstein and Goldstein, 1997. Courtesy Department of Dermatology, Medical College of Georgia.)*

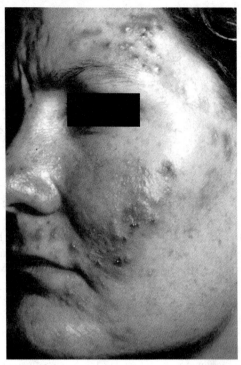

Fig. 20-21 Severe acne. *(From Goldstein and Goldstein, 1997. Courtesy Marshall Guill, MD.)*

privacy and be sensitive to the client's concerns during the examination.

Skin

Normal and Abnormal Findings. As the child becomes an adolescent, the skin undergoes significant maturational development. The skin texture takes on more adult characteristics. In addition, the skin has increased perspiration, oiliness, and acne secondary to an increase in sebaceous gland activity.

The most common abnormal finding and concern for the adolescent is acne. Acne may appear in children as young as 7 to 8 years of age but peaks in adolescence at approximately 16 years of age. Although most acne appears on the face, it may also be prevalent on the chest, back, and shoulders. Acne may appear as blackheads (open comedones) or whiteheads (closed comedones) (Fig. 20-20) (Plewig and Kligman, 2002). Inflamed lesions of acne can be mild or severe. These lesions are painful and are concerning to the client because of the appearance (Fig. 20-21).

Hair and Nails

Normal and Abnormal Findings. The presence and characteristics of facial hair in boys and body hair in both boys and girls change significantly, and by the end of adolescence there is an adult hair distribution pattern (see Chapter 18). The examination findings are the same as those for the adult. Persistent nail biting may be a habit, indicating an abnormal or coping mechanism for dealing with stress. The nurse should take the time to evaluate why nail biting persists.

EXAMINATION OF THE HEAD, EYES, EARS, NOSE, THROAT

Newborns and Infants

Head

Procedure and Techniques. Inspect and palpate the infant's head. Palpate the anterior and posterior fontanels for fullness while the infant is in an upright position and calm. (If the infant is lying down or crying, a false fullness may be felt.)

Normal and Abnormal Findings. The neonate's head may be asymmetric due to *molding,* in which the cranial bones override each other. Molding is secondary to the head passing through the birth canal and generally lasts less than a week. Another common finding in newborns is a cephalhematoma. This is a subperiosteal hematoma under the scalp that occurs secondary to birth trauma. The area, which appears as a soft, well-defined swelling over the cranial bone, generally is reabsorbed within the first month of life. The hematoma does not cross suture lines. Marked asymmetry of the head is usually abnormal and may indicate craniosynostosis, a premature ossification of one or more of the cranial sutures. This rare condition occurs in 1 in 2500 live births; most cases involve male infants (McGee and Burkett, 2000).

The fontanels should have a slight depression, should feel soft, and may have a slight pulsation. A deeply depressed fontanel may indicate dehydration while a bulging fontanel may indicate increased intracranial pressure. The anterior fontanel in infants less than 6 months of age should not exceed 4 to 5 cm. It should get progressively smaller as the child gets older and should be completely closed by the time the infant reaches 24 months of age. The infant's posterior fontanel may or may not be palpable at birth. If it is palpable, it should measure no more than 1 cm, and it should close by 2 months of age. By 4 months, most infants demonstrate head control by holding the head erect and midline when in an upright position. The infant should be able to turn his or her head from side to side by 2 weeks of age.

Eyes

Procedure and Techniques. Newborns frequently have edema of the eyelids, either from the trauma of birth or in response to eyedrops or ointments such as prophylactic instillation of silver nitrate. The edema may delay the examination for a few days. To begin the assessment, hold or rock the infant into an upright position to elicit eye opening. An alternative strategy is to hold the infant supine with the head gently lowered.

Observe if the eyes are small or of different sizes. Inspect the eyelids for edema, epicanthal folds, and position. Note the alignment and slant of the palpebral fissures. Draw an imaginary line through the corners of the eyes (from the medial canthi to the outer canthi). Observe the space between the eyes for wide-spaced eyes. Inspect the sclera for color. Test visual acuity grossly by blinking a penlight on and off several times. Also test for pupillary reaction at this time. Using the opthalmoscope, attempt to visualize the red reflex in each eye.

Normal and Abnormal Findings. Normal findings of the eye examination of an infant reveal eyes that are usually closed; often no eyebrows are present. The eyes are symmetric, and eyelashes may be long. Eyelids may have edema. The outer canthus of the eye aligns with the pinna of the ear (Fig. 20-22). Infant sclera may have a blue tinge caused by thinness; otherwise sclera are white. Tiny black dots (pigmentation) or a slight yellow cast may appear near the limbus of dark-skinned infants. Palpebral conjunctivae are pink and intact without discharge. There are no tears until about 2 to 3 months of age.

The infant should indicate some visual recognition of light from a penlight and follow it momentarily. The blink reflex also is present in normal newborns and infants. Pupils should constrict in response to bright light and are round, about 2 to 4 mm in diameter, and equal in size. A bilateral red reflex should be noted, which is a bright, round, red-orange glow seen through the pupil. It may be pale in dark-skinned newborns. Presence of the red reflex rules out most serious defects of the cornea, aqueous chamber, lens, and vitreous chamber (Hockenberry and Wilson, 2007).

Specific age-related responses may be observed that indicate the infant's attention to visual stimuli.

- Birth to 2 weeks: Eyes do not reopen after exposure to bright light; there is increasing alertness to objects; the infant is capable of fixating on objects.
- Age 1 month: The infant can fixate on and follow a bright toy or light.
- Age 3 to 4 months: The infant can fixate on, follow, and reach for a toy, because binocular vision is normally achieved at this age.
- Age 6 to 12 months: The infant can fixate on and follow a toy in all directions.

Corneal light reflex should be symmetric. Transient strabismus is common during the first few months of life due to lack of binocular vision. If it continues beyond 6 months of age, however, a referral to an ophthalmologist is needed because early recognition and treatment can restore binocular vision. Asian and Native American infants often have *pseudostrabismus,* the false appearance of strabismus due to the flattened nasal bridge or epicanthal fold. Pseudostrabismus disappears at about 12 months of age.

Abnormal findings may include a pronounced lateral upward slant of the eyes with an inner epicanthal fold, which may indicate Down syndrome; asymmetry of eyes; wide-set eyes (hypertelorism); or eyes that are close together (hypotelorism). Note any discolorations of the sclera, such as dark blue sclera, or any dilated blood vessels. Hyperbilirubinemia may cause jaundiced (yellow) sclera in newborns. Asymmetric corneal light reflex followed by malalignment of cover-uncover test (described in Chapter 11) indicates abnormality of eye muscles.

Excessive tearing before the third month or no tearing by the second month is a deviation from normal. A purulent discharge from the eyes shortly after birth is abnormal. It may indicate ophthalmia neonatorum and should be reported. Redness, lesions, nodules, discharge, or crusting of the conjunctiva is abnormal. Birth trauma may cause conjunctivitis or conjunctival hemorrhage as well as eyelid capillary hemangiomas.

If the pupillary response is not present after 3 weeks, the infant may be blind. A dilated, fixed, or constricted pupil may indicate anoxia or brain damage. A white pupil may occur in retinoblastoma, a relatively rare congenital malignant tumor arising from the retina. A white pupil in conjunction with a cloudy cornea or anterior chamber may indicate congenital cataracts. Absence of the red reflex may indicate the presence of retinal hemorrhage or congenital cataracts (Hockenberry and Wilson, 2007).

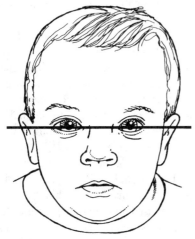

Fig. 20-22 Alignment of the outer canthus with the pinna of the ear is a normal finding.

Ears

Procedures and Techniques. Examine the infant's external ears as previously described for the adult. To examine the auditory canal and tympanic membrane (TM), the infant must be securely immobilized. Because the nurse must have both hands free to hold the ear and maneuver the otoscope, another individual must act as a "holder." The infant can be placed in either a prone or supine position. Instruct the holder to secure the infant's arms down at the sides with one hand and turn and hold the infant's head to one side with the other hand (Fig. 20-23). To optimize visualization of the ear canal and TM, you must alter the method of holding the auricle of the ear. Grasp the lower portion of the pinna and apply gentle traction down and slightly backward (as opposed to pulling the pinna up and back for the adult). This maneuver straightens the canal of the ear.

Two common hearing screening tools used in many newborn nurseries are the Auditory Brainstem Response (ABR) test and the Otoacoustic Emissions (OAE) test. The ABR and OAE tests do not actually test hearing, but rather assess the structural integrity of the auditory pathway. For this reason, hearing cannot be definitively considered normal until the child is old enough to perform an audiogram (Cunningham and Cox, 2003). In settings where special tools for screening are unavailable, a simple hearing screening can be performed and should also be included with an infant examination. This is easily done by eliciting a loud noise (e.g., clapping hands or ringing bell) and observing for a response from the infant such as sudden body movement, startle response, or crying.

Normal and Abnormal Findings. The ears should appear the same bilaterally. The pinna of the ear should align directly with the outer canthus of the eye and be angled no more than 10 degrees from a vertical position. Low-set ears or ears with angulation greater than 10 degrees may indicate a congenital problem such as Down syndrome. An unusually small or absent auricle is referred to as *microtia*, a congenital anomaly of the external ear (Fig. 20-24). Microtia is classified from less severe (grade I) to the absence of an ear—termed *anotia* (grade IV).

The TM of the infant may be difficult to visualize because it is more horizontal than in older children and adults. The TM may appear slightly reddened secondary to crying. Also, because the TM does not become conical for several months, the light reflex may appear diffuse. By age 6 months, the

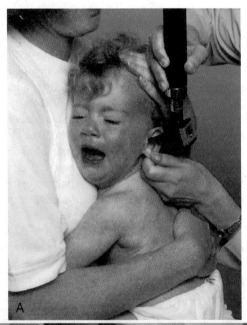

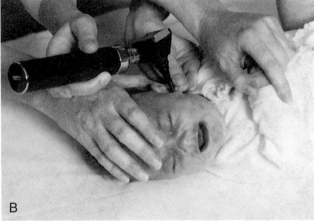

Fig. 20-23 Immobilization of young child or infant during otoscopic examination. Note that lower portion of pinna of ear is pulled down and slightly backward. **A,** Prone position. **B,** Supine position. *(From Hockenberry et al, 2007.)*

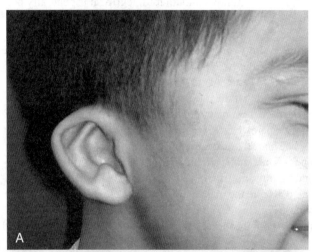

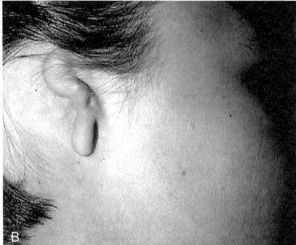

Fig. 20-24 **Microtia. A,** Grade I. **B,** Grade III. *(From Bluestone et al, 2003.)*

infant's TM takes on an adult type of appearance and is easier to visualize and examine.

Hearing behaviors should be readily observed. By age 4 to 6 months the infant should turn the head toward the source of the sound, should respond to the parent's voice, and should respond to music toys. By 6 to 10 months the child should respond to his or her name and follow sounds.

Nose and Mouth

Procedures and Techniques. The examination of the nose and mouth is straightforward; the problem arises when the infant is uncooperative or unable to hold still. The infant must be carefully and securely restrained by a parent or other adult who acts as a "holder" to ensure the infant's safety and to permit the full viewing of the examination area. The re-straining is usually done with the infant in a supine position, with the arms extended securely above the infant's head (Fig. 20-25). The holder will then be able to secure both the infant's arms and head. A second holder or the examiner may need to immobilize the infant's lower extremities.

The infant's nose is small and difficult to examine. Do not attempt to insert a speculum into the nares. Inspect the inside of the nose by tilting the infant's head back and shining a light into the nares. If an infant has nasal congestion, suction the nares with a bulb syringe or small-lumen catheter.

Inspect the infant's mouth for integrity. It is generally possible to examine the mouth while the infant is crying. Palpate the buccal mucosa and gums using a gloved hand and a light source. While your finger is in the infant's mouth, check the strength of the infant's suck.

Normal and Abnormal Findings. Normally you expect to find that the base of the nose is appropriate to the size of the face. You may find milia across the infant's nose. The infant's nares have only minimal movement with breathing.

The buccal mucosa should appear pink, moist, and smooth. The infant's gums should appear smooth and full. Other normal findings may include the presence of small, white epithelial cells on the palate or gums. These are called Bohn's nodules or Epstein's pearls (Fig. 20-26). The infant's tongue should be appropriate to the size of the mouth and fit well into the floor of the mouth. The infant should have a strong suck with the tongue pushing upward against your finger.

Abnormal findings include nasal flaring, which may be seen if the infant has respiratory distress (Hockenberry and Wilson, 2007). Because infants are obligatory nose breathers, any obstruction of the nares secondary to a congenital abnormality such as choanal atresia (occlusion between pharynx and nose), foreign body, or nasal secretions causes the infant to be irritable or distressed.

If whitish patches are seen along the mucosa, scrape the area with a tongue blade to differentiate between a lesion and milk deposits. Milk deposit can be easily scraped off; candidiasis lesions also scrape off, but leave a red area that may bleed. Occasionally, a natal loose tooth may be found. These teeth should be removed to prevent possible aspiration.

Neck

To examine the neck, start with the infant in the supine position and pull the infant's arms to lift the shoulders off the examining table. Permit the infant's head to lag back and inspect the neck for a midline trachea, abnormal skin folds, and generalized neck enlargement. Return the infant to the supine position and palpate the neck for tone, presence of masses, and enlarged lymph nodes. Because the infant's neck is short and thick, examination of the thyroid is extremely difficult.

Normally the newborn's cervical and inguinal lymph nodes are not palpable. Significant head lag after 6 months of age is an abnormal finding requiring further evaluation (Hockenberry and Wilson, 2007). If the infant's neck is proportionately short or has webbing (loose, fanlike skin folds), the infant should be evaluated for congenital abnormalities such as Down syndrome or Turner syndrome. If an enlargement of the infant's anterior neck is palpated, the infant should be referred to a physician for further evaluation.

Toddlers and Children

Head

Examination and findings of the head are similar to those of the adult.

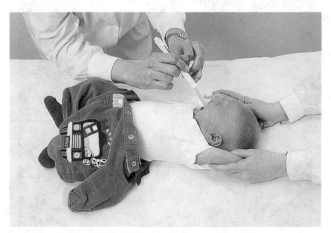

Fig. 20-25   Positioning of infant for examination of nose and mouth.

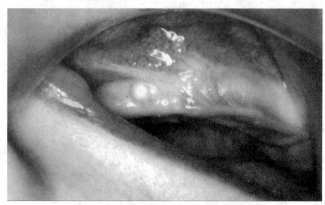

Fig. 20-26   Epstein's pearls (gingival cysts) in an infant. *(From Scully and Welbury, 1994.)*

Eyes

Procedures and Techniques. Most of the examination of children's eyes is the same as that for adults. Vision can be assessed when performing developmental tests such as the Denver II (e.g., noting the child's ability to stack blocks or identify animals). The assessment of vision and eyes should be appropriate for the developmental stage and age of the child.

Use the Allen Picture Cards to screen for visual acuity in children 2½ to 3 years of age. Show the large cards with pictures to the child up close to be sure that the child can identify them. Then present each picture at a distance of 20 feet from the child. Use Snellen's "E" chart for children 3 to 6 years of age (see Chapter 11). Have children point their fingers in the direction of the "arms" of the E. By 7 to 8 years of age, begin to use the standard Snellen's chart, as described for adults. Test each eye separately with and without glasses as appropriate. Be sure to screen children two separate times before referring them. Test for color vision once between ages 4 and 8. The red and green lines on Snellen's chart can be used as a gross screening tool for color blindness to be followed with Ishihara's test as needed. Ask the child to identify each pattern seen in the cards.

Perform the corneal light reflex or Hirschberg at a distance of about 12 inches from the child's eyes. The cover/uncover test should also be performed by having the toddler or child seated on the parent's lap. Have the child fixate on the light of the otoscope. If the child is uncooperative it is often helpful to have the child fixate on a toy. Use the opposite hand to cover the eye and observe the uncovered eye for fixation on the object. Screen for nystagmus by inspecting the movement of the eyes to the six cardinal fields of gaze. It may be necessary to stabilize the child's chin with your hand to prevent the entire head from moving.

Prepare children for the ophthalmoscope examination by showing them the light, explaining how it shines in the eye, and explaining why the room must be darkened. As with the infant, it is important to elicit a bilateral red reflex using the ophthalmoscope.

Normal and Abnormal Findings. Visual acuity of 20/20 (line 7 on the chart) is achieved during toddler years, although 20/40 (line 5) is considered acceptable (Hockenberry and Wilson, 2007). Normally the child will be able to name three of the seven cards within three to five trials during the Allen Picture Cards test. A child with normal color vision will see the number or pattern embedded in Ishihara's test whereas a color-blind child will be unable to see the pattern. A symmetric corneal light reflex is an expected finding (Fig. 20-27). Early recognition and treatment of strabismus can restore binocular vision while diagnosis of strabismus after age 6 has a poor prognosis, often leading to blindness. Children who are found to have strabismus need to be referred to an ophthalmologist.

Ears

Procedures and Techniques. The biggest challenge to examining the auditory canal and tympanic membrane of the young child is immobilization. Immobilize the child in either the supine or prone position as discussed previously

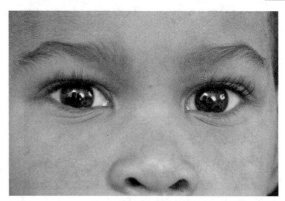

Fig. 20-27   Corneal light reflex.

with the infant (see Fig. 20-23). Inadequate immobilization can result in pain to the child and also may cause injury to the ear canal. If the child is fearful, screaming, or uncooperative, the nurse should place his or her hand against the head of the child to protect the ear canal from sudden movement or jolt. Because the young child may perceive the otoscope examination as traumatic, it may be deferred until the last procedure of the examination. If the child becomes upset during the examination, be sure to quickly return the child to the parent for comforting.

As the child becomes older, the nurse should take the time to elicit the child's cooperation during the examination. If the nurse has any question regarding the child's ability to hold perfectly still during the otoscope examination, the parent or adult who is with the child should assist in immobilizing the child to ensure the child's safety.

The procedure for examination proceeds as previously discussed for the infant. If the child is less than 3 years of age, the pinna should be pulled down during the examination as described for the infant. If the child is older, the pinna should be pulled up and backward as for the adult. Hearing screening may be indicated for children, particularly if risk factors were identified during infancy. As the child gets older, audiometery testing is considered most useful (Cunningham and Cox, 2003).

Normal and Abnormal Findings. The findings of the examination of the ears do not differ significantly for older children than those of the adult. The nurse should be aware that young children are at risk for insertion of foreign bodies into their ears; however, any child with a suspect history should be examined.

Small polyethylene tubes in the TM of a child who has recently had a myringotomy (Fig. 20-28) may be observed. These are surgically placed through the TM to relieve middle ear pressure and to permit drainage of fluid or material collected behind the TM. They are most commonly put in the ears of young children because of recurrent ear infections. Usually the tubes spontaneously work their way out of the TM within 6 to 12 months after insertion.

Hearing evaluation of the young child may be necessary if the parent or nurse perceives that the child has some type of lag related to the child's developmental milestones. Behavioral manifestations that may indicate hearing impairment

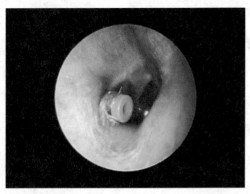

Fig. 20-28 Tympanotomy tube protruding from the right tympanic membrane. *(From Bingham, Hawke, and Kwok, 1992.)*

include delay in verbal skills; speech that is monotone, garbled, or difficult to understand; inattentiveness during conversation; facial expressions that appear strained or puzzled; withdrawal and lack of interaction with others; asking "What?" a lot or asking for statements to be repeated; or having frequent earaches.

Nose and Mouth

Procedures and Techniques. A toddler or young child will probably tolerate the mouth and nose examination better while sitting on the parent's lap. Have the child sit on the adult's lap with his or her back to the parent. The parent may then immobilize the child's legs by placing them between the adult's legs. The parent then has both hands free. One hand should be used to reach around the child's body to restrain the child's arms and chest. The other hand may be used to assist the nurse by immobilizing the child's head (Fig. 20-29). Once the child becomes too large for the parent's lap, the examination is best performed with the child in a supine position on the examination table.

The young child's nose should be assessed in the same manner as the infant's. Use your thumb on the tip of the nose to improve visualization inside the nares. Palpation of the

sinuses can be done after age 7 or 8. When examining the teeth, note the eruption sequence and timing, condition, positioning, and hygiene of the teeth and note the presence of debris around the teeth or gum line.

Normal and Abnormal Findings. The presence of a transverse crease at the bridge of the nose is called an "allergic salute," which occurs when a child has a frequent runny nose or allergies and wipes the nose with an upward sweep of the palm of the hand. A foul odor and unilateral discharge from a nostril may be caused by a foreign body.

Dryness, flaking, or cracking corners of the mouth, if present, may indicate excess licking of the lips, vitamin deficiency, or infection such as impetigo. The buccal mucosa should be pink, moist, and without lesions. Lesions such as Koplik's spots (as seen in measles) or candidiasis (thrush) may be observed (Fig. 20-30).

The child's tonsils are larger than an adult's but should not interfere with swallowing or breathing. Tooth eruption depends on the age of the child. The child's tonsils should be dark pink and without vertical reddened lines, general erythema, edema, or exudate. An excessively dry mouth may indicate dehydration or fever. Excessive salivation may indicate gingivostomatitis or multiple dental caries. Drooling after 12 months of age may indicate a neurologic disorder. Flattened edges on the teeth may indicate teeth grinding (bruxism). Darkened, brown, or black teeth may indicate decay or oral iron therapy. Mottled or pitted teeth may result from tetracycline therapy during tooth development. A strawberry-colored tongue may indicate scarlet fever. If the mouth has a fetid or musty smell, further investigation should be made regarding hygiene practices, local or systemic infections, or sinusitis.

Neck

Procedures and Techniques. The thyroid of the child may be assessed using the same techniques as for the adult, but the challenge is to encourage the child to sit still and swallow as described so that an adequate evaluation may be done. If the child is not able to cooperate, the thyroid examination may be deferred.

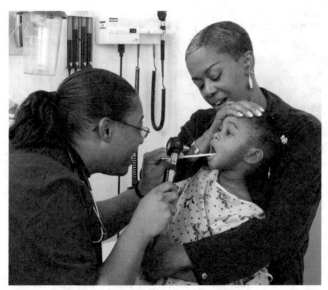

Fig. 20-29 Technique for immobilizing a young child's head for examination.

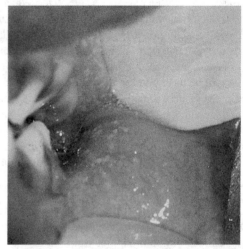

Fig. 20-30 Koplik spots. *(From Hockenberry et al, 2003.)*

Normal and Abnormal Findings. Normally, lymph nodes up to 3 mm may be palpable in children and may reach 1 cm in the cervical areas, but they are discrete, mobile, and nontender. The term *shotty* may be used to describe small, firm, and mobile nodes occurring as a normal variation in children. It is not unusual to find enlarged postauricular and occipital nodes in children less than 2 years of age. Likewise, cervical and submandibular nodal enlargements are more frequent in older children. Thus the age of the client should be considered in your decision to further evaluate lymph node enlargement. Abnormal findings are tender, fixed nodes greater than 1 cm. Enlarged, tender nodes may occur after immunizations or upper respiratory infection (Hockenberry et al, 2003).

Adolescents

The procedures, techniques, and examination findings for the adolescent are the same as for the adult.

EXAMINATION OF THE RESPIRATORY SYSTEM

Newborns and Infants

Procedures and Techniques. Assessing the respiratory status of a newborn or infant usually follows the same sequence as for an adult. Conduct the examination while the infant is calm, if possible, because examination of a crying infant is difficult.

Inspect the infant's chest to observe respiratory effort. Auscultation of the infant's breath sounds is performed in the same manner as for the older child and adult; however, the nurse should use a pediatric stethoscope with a small diaphragm (Fig. 20-31). An adult-sized stethoscope diaphragm head covers at least half of the infant's chest and is inappropriate for an accurate assessment of the infant's respiratory status. Percussion is not routinely performed during infant assessment.

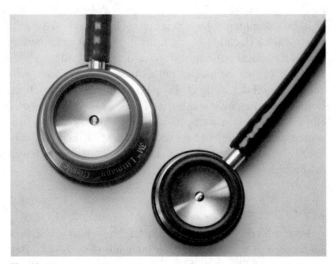

Fig. 20-31 The pediatric stethoscope has a smaller head compared to the adult stethoscope.

Normal and Abnormal Findings. Inspection of the infant's thoracic cage should show a smooth, rounded, and symmetric appearance. Harrison's groove, a normal anatomic deviation, is a horizontal groove in the rib cage at the level of the diaphragm. It extends from the sternum to the midaxillary line. Unlike the adult, the infant has a round thorax with an equal AP and lateral diameter. The average chest circumference ranges from 12 to 14 inches (30 to 36 cm). This measurement should be approximately 1 inch (2 to 3 cm) smaller than the child's head circumference.

Infants are obligate nose breathers until about age 3 months. Should their nasal passages become occluded, they may have difficulty breathing. Sneezing is a common finding for an infant and is therapeutic because it helps to clear the nose. Coughing, however, is considered abnormal and indicates a problem.

The respiratory pattern in the newborn may be irregular, having a Cheyne-Stokes type of pattern. Premature newborns may have periods of apnea for as long as 10 to 15 seconds. Stimulation by the adult caregiver can generally produce a quick breath. The respiratory rate in the newborn and infant ranges from 30 to 60 times per minute. It is important to note if the infant is ill and has a rapid respiratory rate for a prolonged period of time; if so, the infant will tire and may subsequently become hypoxic.

The infant has a thin chest wall, which makes breath sounds difficult to localize with auscultation. They are commonly transmitted from one auscultatory area to another. Because of this, the predominant breath sound heard in the peripheral lung fields is bronchovesicular. The thin chest wall also makes the newborn's xiphoid process more prominent than that of an older child or adult.

Several respiratory findings indicate that an infant is in respiratory distress. These include stridor, grunting, sternal or supraclavicular retractions, and nasal flaring. Any one of these findings warrants immediate medical attention. Stridor is a high-pitched, piercing sound that is primarily heard in a distressed infant during inspiration. It occurs secondary to upper airway obstruction. The obstruction may cause the infant's inspiratory cycle to be three or four times longer than expiration. Respiratory grunting is a mechanism by which the infant tries to force trapped air out of the lungs while still trying to maintain adequate air in the lungs. Sternal and supraclavicular retractions and nasal flaring are indications of respiratory distress. Clinically this may be observed as "see-saw" type of breathing with alternating movements of the chest and abdomen. If any of these are observed, the infant is working very hard to try to maintain adequate breathing and should be referred to a primary care provider.

Toddlers and Children

Procedures and Techniques. The techniques for examining the lungs and respiratory system of the child are the same as those for the adult. By age 2 or 3 years, the child is usually cooperative during the respiratory examination (Fig. 20-32). Even before that age, if the nurse takes the time to develop a relationship with the child, cooperation can usually be obtained.

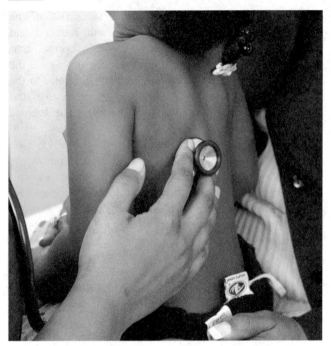

Fig. 20-32 Auscultation of lungs on a young child.

If performing chest palpation, the nurse should adjust the number of fingers used to palpate the chest wall to be appropriate for the size of the chest. For example, if the child is small you may use only two or three fingers. On the other hand, if the child is large, you may use three fingers or all four. Percussion is infrequently performed until the child is at least 10 years of age.

Normal and Abnormal Findings. By age 5 or 6, the rounded thorax of the child approximates the 1:2 ratio of AP to lateral diameter of the adult. If the child's chest proportion remains rounded, it may be an outward indication of a significant problem such as asthma or cystic fibrosis. By age 6 or 7, the child's breathing pattern should change from primarily nasal and abdominal to thoracic in girls and abdominal in boys. The child's respiratory rate should gradually slow as the child becomes older (see Table 5-1 in Chapter 5).

Auscultation findings for the child range between the findings of the infant and the findings of the adult. Depending on the size of the child and the musculature of the chest, slight variations may be found. Findings for a small or young child with undeveloped chest musculature may include more bronchovesicular breath sounds in the peripheral lung areas, whereas if the child is larger and has started to develop more, the breath sounds will be equivalent to those of the adult (vesicular in the peripheral lung fields). Palpation findings for the child are the same as those for the adult. If percussion is performed, the nurse should note that young children normally have a hyperresonance tone.

Adolescents

The procedures, techniques, and examination findings for the adolescent are the same as for the adult. The nurse should be sensitive to the possible modesty of the female adolescent and provide a drape for the breasts when the anterior chest is not being assessed.

EXAMINATION OF THE CARDIOVASCULAR SYSTEM

Newborns and Infants

Procedures and Techniques. The apical pulse of the newborn normally is felt in the fourth or fifth intercostal space (ICS) just medial to the midclavicular line. Examine the heart within the first 24 hours of birth and again at 2 to 3 days to assess changes from fetal to systemic and pulmonic circulation. Auscultation of the heart must be done when the infant is quiet. The stethoscope used must have a small diaphragm and bell to detect specific cardiac sounds of the newborn or infant. If the infant is having dyspnea, estimate the size and position of the heart. Palpate the femoral and brachial pulses and assess capillary refill.

Normal and Abnormal Findings. Normally the heart rate of infants is faster when they are awake and slower when they are asleep. Sinus dysrhythmia is an expected finding when the heart rate increases during inspiration and decreases during expiration. Splitting of heart sounds is common in infants until about 48 hours after birth because of the transition from fetal circulation to systemic and pulmonic circulation. Innocent murmurs, grade I or II, accompanied by no other signs or symptoms frequently disappear within 2 to 3 days. Capillary refill in infants is very rapid—less than 1 second. Acrocyanosis (cyanosis of hands and feet) without central cyanosis is of little concern and usually disappears within hours to days of birth.

Abnormal findings include changes in the skin and cardiovascular system. Central cyanosis may indicate congenital heart defects. Note if cyanosis increases with crying or sucking. Severe cyanosis that appears shortly after birth may indicate transposition of the great vessels, tetralogy of Fallot, a severe septal defect, or severe pulmonic stenosis. Cyanosis that appears after the first month of life suggests pulmonic stenosis, tetralogy of Fallot, or large septal defects.

Murmurs that persist after 3 days or radiate must be referred for further evaluation. A pneumothorax shifts the apical impulse away from the area of the chest where the pneumothorax is located. The infant's heart may be shifted to the right by a diaphragmatic hernia commonly found on the left. Dextrocardia (location of the heart in the right hemithorax) causes the apical pulse to shift toward the right side.

Weak or thin peripheral pulses may be associated with decreased cardiac output or peripheral vasoconstriction. Bounding pulses may indicate a patent ductus arteriosus creating a left-to-right shunt. Coarctation of the heart is suspected when the femoral pulses are absent or there is a difference in pulse amplitude between upper and lower extremities.

Toddlers and Children

Procedures and Techniques. The child's chest is auscultated in the same areas as the adult (Fig. 20-33). Because it may take a considerably longer time to be sure of the sounds, explanations should be given in advance to the caregiver to avoid unneeded concern. All of the techniques used

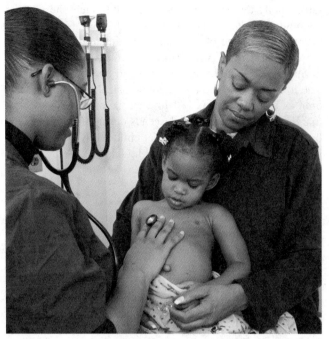

Fig. 20-33   Auscultation on a young child.

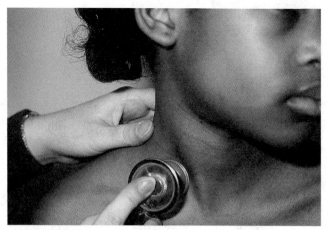

Fig. 20-34   Auscultation for venous hum. *(From Seidel et al, 2003.)*

require that the child wear only underwear and sit on the table or the caregiver's lap. Cooperative children may recline at a 45-degree angle. If this is not possible, the child may lie supine to allow you to hear more cardiovascular sounds.

If an irregular rhythm is noted, have the child hold his or her breath so that only heart sounds are heard. Auscultate with the bell of the stethoscope over the right supraclavicular space at the medial end of the clavicle along the anterior border of the sternocleidomastoid muscle for a venous hum (Fig. 20-34). It is a vibration heard over the jugular vein caused by turbulent blood flow and has a continuous, low-pitched sound that is louder during diastole. A venous hum may be stopped by gentle pressure between the trachea and the sternocleidomastoid muscle at the level of the thyroid cartilage. Note differences between pulses, particularly the radial and femoral.

Normal and Abnormal Findings.   A child's pulse may normally increase on inspiration and decrease on expiration. Sinus dysrhythmia may be an expected finding during childhood. Changes in heart rates in children are listed in Table 5-1 in Chapter 5. An expected finding in children is a venous hum in the jugular vein.

It is important to record the abnormal findings observed during the child's activities. Squatting may be a compensatory position for a child with a heart defect. Cyanosis or pallor may indicate poor perfusion due to congenital heart defects. Note if there is more cyanosis with crying and if there is facial or ankle edema. Note signs of poor feeding (e.g., low weight) and reports of caregiver that the child stops eating to get his or her breath, which may indicate a heart problem. Labored respirations could indicate a cardiovascular problem. Weak or absent femoral pulses may indicate coarctation of the aorta.

Adolescents

The procedures, techniques, and examination findings for the cardiovascular assessment are the same as for the adult.

EXAMINATION OF THE ABDOMEN AND GASTROINTESTINAL SYSTEM

Newborns and Infants

Procedures and Techniques.   The abdominal examination is straightforward, with the infant lying supine on an examining table. Follow the same procedures for examining the abdomen as for adults.

Normal and Abnormal Findings.   Inspecting the abdomen of a healthy infant finds a symmetric, soft, and round abdomen with a slight protrusion, and no masses are present. There is synchronous abdominal and chest movement with breathing. Diastasis swelling and a gap between the rectus muscles may be noted during crying. Visible pulsations in the epigastric areas are common. Note any distention, masses, and concave, sunken, or flat appearance. A scaphoid, turnip-shaped abdomen suggests diaphragmatic hernia.

Inspect the umbilicus in the newborn. Immediately after the umbilical cord is cut, two arteries and one vein should be noted. After the cord is clamped, it will change from white to black as it dries; it should be dry in 5 days and fall off spontaneously in 7 to 14 days. Abnormal findings include discharge, odor, or redness around the umbilicus; a protrusion or nodular appearance of the umbilicus; thick Wharton's jelly; and a thin or green cord.

Auscultate the abdomen for the presence of bowel sounds; an absence of bowl sounds may indicate a bowel obstruction. The abdomen of a newborn should be soft and nondistended upon palpation. The edge of the infant's liver should be 1 to 2 cm below the right rib cage (costal margin). The spleen is generally not palpable, although the tip may be felt in the left upper quadrant (far left costal margin). Both kidneys are noted with deep palpation. An enlarged liver 3 cm or more below the margin, palpable spleen, masses near the kidneys, and enlarged kidneys are considered abnormal findings.

Toddlers and Children

Procedures and Techniques. Children may resist abdominal palpation because they are ticklish. Assessment of children is generally the same as that of adults, with the exception of the areas noted in the normal and abnormal findings. Percussion of the liver span and splenic dullness in children are considered advanced skills.

Normal and Abnormal Findings. Toddlers normally exhibit a rounded (potbelly) abdomen both while standing and while lying down. School-age children may show this roundedness until about 13 years of age when standing; when lying, the abdomen should be scaphoid; generalized distension is an abnormal finding. Inspect and palpate for any umbilical hernia. This type of hernia is common in African American children until 7 years of age and in white children under 2 years of age (Hockenberry and Wilson, 2007) (Fig. 20-35). Note any hernia still present after these ages.

Note movement of the abdomen on respiration. Until about age 7, children are abdominal breathers; after age 7, boys exhibit chiefly abdominal movement whereas girls exhibit chiefly thoracic movement. Check the tenseness of the abdominal muscles. The condition of diastasis recti abdominis (two rectus muscles fail to approximate one another) is common in African American children but should disappear during the preschool years (Hockenberry and Wilson, 2007). The lower edge of the liver may be palpable in young children as a superficial mass 1 to 2 cm below the right costal margin. Normally the liver descends during inspiration. The liver may not be palpable in older children. Abdominal pain is always considered an abnormal finding.

Adolescents

The procedures, techniques, and examination findings for the gastrointestinal assessment are the same as for the adult.

EXAMINATION OF THE MUSCULOSKELETAL SYSTEM

Newborns and Infants

Procedures and Techniques. Examine the infant undressed and lying supine. Palpate clavicles for stability. Extend both arms and legs to compare muscle tone and length. Inspect the back and spine for alignment, tufts of hair, or bulges.

Assess hip location by performing the Barlow-Ortolani maneuver; this maneuver can be performed up until 2 months of age. With the infant supine, flex the knees, holding your thumbs on the inner midthighs and your fingers outside on the hips touching the greater trochanters. Adduct the legs until thumbs touch (Fig. 20-36, A). Then abduct, moving the knees apart and down to touch the table with their lateral aspects (Fig. 20-36, B). Allis' sign is another assessment of hip location. With the infant supine, flex the knees with the feet flat on the table, and align the femurs. Observe the height of the knees (Fig. 20-37).

Assess the feet for position. Scratch the outside and inside borders of the foot or immobilize the heel with one hand and gently push the forefoot to neutral position with the other hand.

Normal and Abnormal Findings. Normal findings include stable and smooth clavicles, without crepitus. Limited shoulder range of motion and deformity can be palpated if the clavicle is fractured. Erb's palsy (paralysis of shoulder and upper arm muscles) may be noted. Asymmetry of extremities, limited movement, syndactyly (fused digits), and polydactyly (extra digits) are abnormal findings. Arms and legs should have strong muscle tone and have equal length bilaterally.

The feet should be flexible and not fixed. Note the relationship of the forefoot to the hindfoot. The hindfoot aligns with the lower leg and the forefoot turns inward slightly. Metatarsus varus (toeing in or pigeon-toed) or talipes equinovarus (clubfoot) may be noted.

The Barlow-Ortolani maneuver should feel smooth and produce no clicking. Any click that occurs when you per-

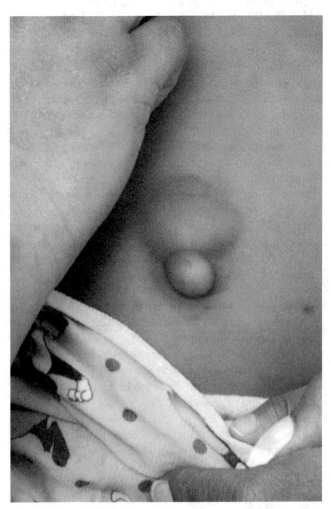

Fig. 20-35   Umbilical hernia on a toddler.

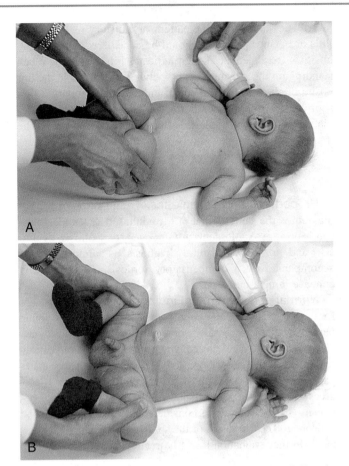

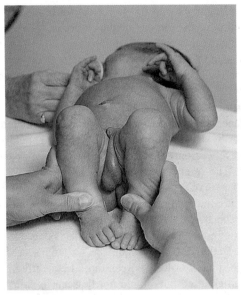

Fig. 20-37 Positive Allis' sign shows that the left leg is shorter than the right leg, indicating left hip dysplasia. *(From Seidel et al, 2006.)*

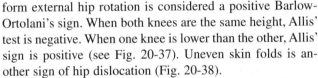

Fig. 20-36 Barlow-Ortolani maneuver to detect hip dislocation. **A,** Phase I, adduction. **B,** Phase II, abduction. This is a negative finding because no dislocation is found.

form external hip rotation is considered a positive Barlow-Ortolani's sign. When both knees are the same height, Allis' test is negative. When one knee is lower than the other, Allis' sign is positive (see Fig. 20-37). Uneven skin folds is another sign of hip dislocation (Fig. 20-38).

The spine should be flexible with convex dorsal and sacral curves, no masses, and easy movement in and out of fetal position. Note asymmetric back curve, masses (hair tufts, dimples), and abnormal posturing perhaps indicating malformation of vertebrae or the spinal column.

Toddlers and Children

Procedures and Techniques. When evaluating children, compare data with tables of normal age and sequence of motor development. (Chapter 19 discusses expected motor development for children.) Measure the child and compare values to tables of percentiles for growth to assess bone growth. Observe the gait for steadiness. Inspect the spine for alignment. Inspect the knees for symmetric alignment.

ETHNIC & CULTURAL VARIATIONS

Navajo Indians and Canadian Eskimos are among the cultures with the highest incidence of hip dislocation. In these cultures newborns are tightly wrapped in blankets or strapped to cradle boards. Hip dislocation is virtually unknown in cultures where infants are carried on their mother's backs or hips in the widely abducted straddle position such as in the Far East and Africa (Hockenberry et al, 2003).

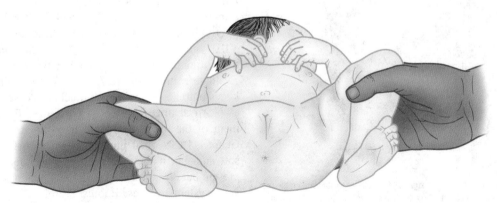

Fig. 20-38 Sign of hip dislocation: the three skin folds on the left upper leg and limited abduction indicate left hip dysplasia. *(Seidel et al, 2006.)*

Trendelenburg's sign (or gait) tests for hip dysplasia and the function of the gluteus medius muscle, which normally acts to abduct and rotate the thigh (Fig. 20-39). Assist the client to stand. You stand behind the client to observe the tilt of the pelvis as the client stands on one foot and then the other.

Normal and Abnormal Findings. Toddlers have a wide stance and a wide-waddle gait pattern, which tends to disappear by age 24 to 36 months. The gait should become progressively stronger, steadier, and smoother as the child matures. The spine should be straight. By 12 to 18 months the lumbar curve develops as the child learns to walk; lumbar lordosis is common in toddlers; after 18 months, the cervical spine is concave, the thoracic spine is convex (although less than that of adults), and the lumbar spine is concave (similar to that of adults). There should be no bulges or dimpling along the spine. Lordosis is seen more frequently in African American children but should not be seen in children over 6 years of age. The knees should be in a direct straight line between the hip, the ankle, and the great toe. Valgus rotation (medial malleolus greater than 1 inch [2.5 cm] apart with knees touching) is normal in children 2 to 3.5 years of age and may be present up to age 12 years. Varus rotation (medial malleolus touching, with knees greater than 1 inch [2.5 cm] apart) requires further evaluation for tibial torsion; it may be normal until 18 to 24 months of age. The expected finding of Trendelenburg's sign is that the opposite thigh and hip elevate because the pelvic muscles to the greater trochanter are sufficient to elevate the hip not bearing weight (see Fig. 20-39). For example, when the client stands on the left leg, the right thigh and hip should tilt upward.

Any deviation from the pattern or a history of increasing falls or balance problems should be considered abnormal. A positive Trendelenburg's sign indicates hip dysplasia. When standing on the affected leg, no pelvic tilt is noted in the opposite thigh and hip. The client with a Trendelenburg's sign shortens the step on the unaffected leg and has a lateral deviation of the entire trunk and affected side. This is one of the more common gait deviations.

Adolescents

Procedures and Techniques. Examination of the adolescent is the same as that of the adult. Observe the adolescent's posture. Adolescents are screened for scoliosis, kyphosis, and lordosis. Postural kyphosis is almost always accompanied by a compensatory lordosis, an abnormally concave lumbar curvature.

Normal and Abnormal Findings. The normal findings for the adolescent are the same as those for the adult. A young person with low self-esteem or feelings of rejection may assume a slumped, careless, and apathetic posture. Poor posture, regardless of the cause (e.g., low self-esteem or heavy backpack), contributes to kyphosis. A curvature less than 10 degrees is considered a normal variation, and a curvature between 10 and 20 degrees is considered mild (Hockenberry and Wilson, 2007). Curvature of the spine greater than 10 degrees needs further evaluation for early treatment.

EXAMINATION OF THE NEUROLOGIC SYSTEM

Newborns and Infants

Procedures and Techniques. Observe spontaneous motor activity for symmetry. Palpate the infant's fontanels for presence and contour. Measure the infant's head circumference using a soft tape measure and compare it with previous measurements if available. Observe the infant's response to touch and pressure. Determine the presence of the Moro's, tonic neck, rooting, sucking, palmar grasp, Babinski's, clonus, and plantar reflexes as applicable. Initial reflexes that should be evident in the newborn are shown in Table 20-4. Cranial nerves are assessed by observing eye movements and blinking (CNs III, IV, and VI), sucking (CN V), wrinkling of the forehead (CN VII), turning the head toward a sound (CN VIII), and swallowing (CN IX). With the infant supine, pull to a sitting position holding the wrists; observe head control. Evaluate resting posture for muscle tone. Flex the infant's knees onto the abdomen and quickly release them.

Normal and Abnormal Findings. Expected development of the infant by month is outlined in Table 19-3, in Chapter 19. Normal findings begin with fontanels that are soft and flat, if they are present. The infantile reflexes are present but disappear during the first year as the infant's nervous system matures. Babinski's reflex is an exception; it disappears by 18 months. Some head flexion (head lag) is normally present. Three-month-old infants raise the head and

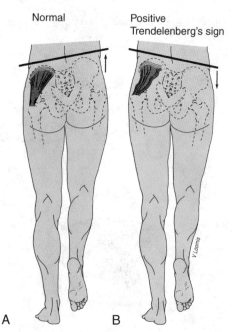

Fig. 20-39 **Trendelenburg's test or sign. A,** Normally when standing on the left foot, the right pelvis rises. **B,** Lack of pelvic tilt when standing on the affected leg indicates hip dysplasia, a positive Trendelenburg's test. *(From Greenberger and Hinthorn, 1993.)*

TABLE 20-4 *Infantile Reflexes*

REFLEX	TECHNIQUE FOR EVALUATION	APPEARANCE AGE	DISAPPEARANCE AGE	NORMAL RESPONSE
REFLEXES TO EVALUATE POSITION AND MOVEMENT				
Moro's	Startle infant by making loud noise, jarring examination surface, or slightly raising infant off examination surface and letting him fall quickly back onto examining table	Birth	1 to 4 months	Infant abducts and extends arms and legs; index finger and thumb assume C position; then infant pulls both arms and legs up against trunk as if trying to protect self
Palmar grasp 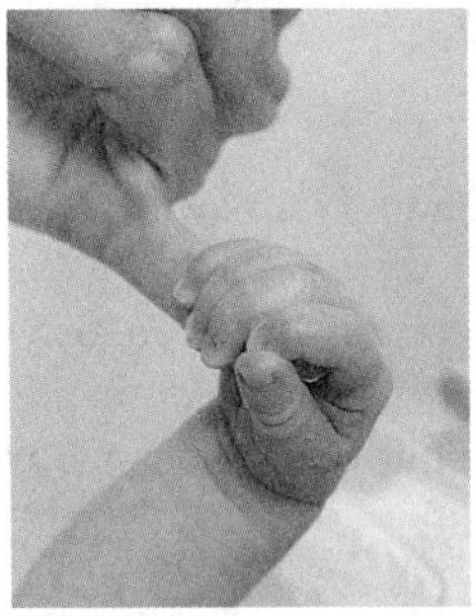	Touch object against ulnar side of infant's hand; then place finger in palm of hand	Birth	3 to 4 months	Infant will grasp finger; grasp should be tight, and nurse may be able to pull infant into sitting position by infant's grasp
Tonic neck 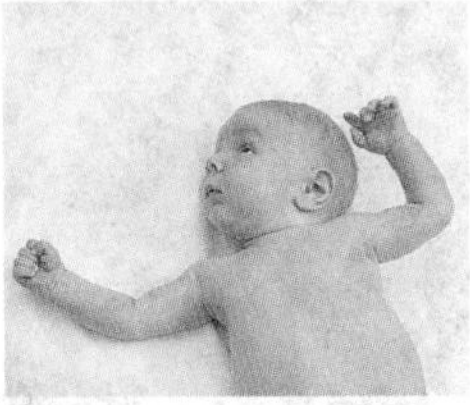	Infant supine; rotate head to side so that chin is over shoulder	Birth to 6 weeks	4 to 6 months	Arm and leg on side to which head turns extend; opposite arm and leg flex; infant assumes fencing position (some normal infants may never show this reflex)
Plantar grasp 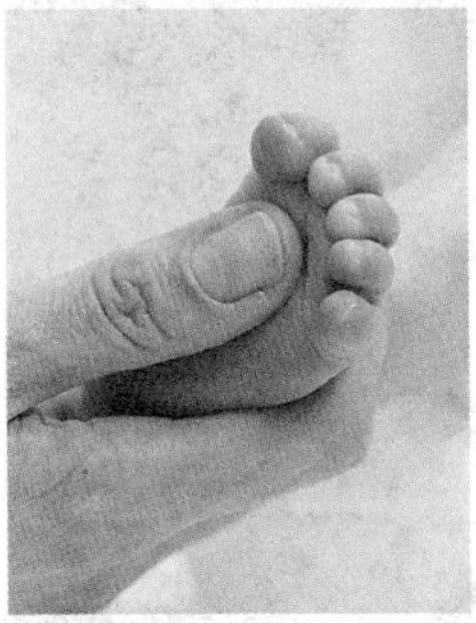	Touch object to sole of infant's foot	Birth	8 to 10 months	Toes will flex tightly downward in attempt to grasp
Babinski's	Stroke lateral surface of infant's sole, using inverted J-curve from sole to great toe (see Fig. 25-26, *F*)	Birth	18 months	Infant response: positive response showing fanning of toes
Step in place 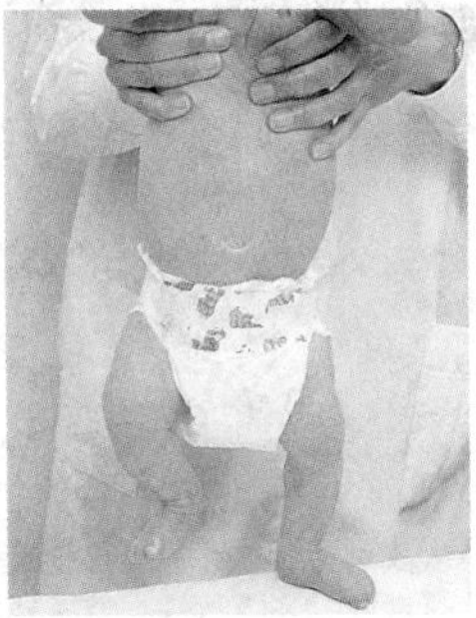	Infant in upright position, feet flat on surface	Birth	3 months	Will pace forward using alternating steps

Continued

TABLE 20-4 *Infantile Reflexes—cont'd*

REFLEX	TECHNIQUE FOR EVALUATION	APPEARANCE AGE	DISAPPEARANCE AGE	NORMAL RESPONSE
Clonus	Dorsiflex foot; pinch sole of foot just under toes	Birth	4 months	May get clonus movement of foot (not always present)
FEEDING REFLEXES				
Rooting response (awake)	Brush infant's cheek near corner of mouth	Birth	3 to 4 months	Infant will turn head in direction of stimulus and will open mouth slightly
Sucking	Touch infant's lips	Birth	10 to 12 months	Sucking motion follows with lips and tongue

arch the back; this reflex persists until 18 months of age. Spontaneous movement should be smooth and symmetric. The infant's knees should unfold gradually after being flexed to the chest.

Abnormal findings may include fontanels that feel full and distended. This finding, together with head circumference greater than expected and lethargy, irritability, shrill cry, weakness, and "sunset eyes," may indicate hydrocephalus (see Fig. 20-58 later in this chapter). Motor activity abnormalities indicating brain damage include hypotonia, as evidenced by poor head control and limp extremities, hypertonia, stiff legs, jittery arm movements, and hands tightly flexed. An arched back (opisthotonos) with a stiff neck and extension of extremities may indicate meningitis. Any asymmetric posture is also abnormal. Note any spasticity, which may be an early sign of cerebral palsy. If present, the legs quickly extend and adduct, possibly even in a scissoring pattern.

Toddlers and Children

Procedures and Techniques. Follow the same sequence of evaluation as for adults when dealing with children. Observe the child carefully during spontaneous activity, because the child may not be able to cooperate with requests as an adult would. Making the examination a game helps in data collection. Observe the child for achievement of expected developmental milestones for fine and gross motor, social-adaptive, and language skills described in Chapter 19, Table 19-3. Evaluate the child's general behavior while he or she is at play, interacting with parents, and cooperating with parents and with the nurse.

In testing cranial nerves, sense of smell usually is not tested; if it is, use a scent familiar to the child, such as an orange or peanut butter. In testing visual fields and gaze (CNs II, III, IV, and VI), gently immobilize the head so that the child cannot follow objects with the whole head but only with the eyes. When testing CN VII, approach it like a game, asking the child to make "funny faces" as the nurse models them (Fig. 20-40).

Use the Denver II or other appropriate tools to assess fine motor coordination in children under 6 years of age. For children older than 6 years, use the finger-to-nose test, with the nurse's finger held 1 to 2 inches (2.5 to 5 cm) away from the child's nose.

Sensory function is not normally tested before age 5. Carefully explain what is being done when children are tested, and use descriptions that the child can understand,

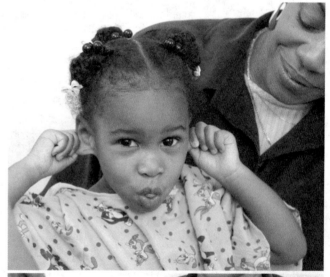

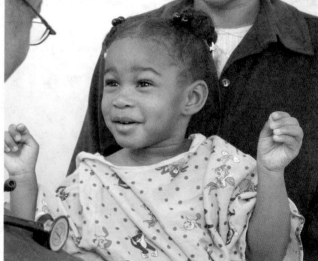

Fig. 20-40 Ask the child to make a "funny face" to assess Cranial Nerve VII.

such as "this will feel like a tickle or a mosquito bite." Use simple numbers (such as 0, 7, 5, 3, or 1) for graphesthesia testing and X and O for younger children.

The screening for neurologic "soft" signs in school-age children is used to describe vague and minimal dysfunction signs, such as clumsiness, language disturbances, motor overload, mirroring movement of extremities, or perceptual development difficulties (Table 20-5).

Typically deep tendon reflexes (DTR) are not tested in young children unless they present with neurological symptoms (i.e. muscle weakness, dizziness). However, if it is warranted perform the DTR in the same manner as in the adult examination.

Normal and Abnormal Findings. Normal findings should generally be the same as those for adults. Soft neurologic signs may be considered normal in the young child, but as the child matures, the signs should disappear.

Abnormal findings are the same as those for the adult. Spasticity, paralysis, seizures with mental retardation, or impaired vision, speech, or hearing may indicate cerebral palsy. The identification of soft signs indicates failure of the child to perform age-specific activities (see Table 20-5), and the child should be referred to a health care professional for further evaluation. Inattention, motor restlessness, and easy distractibility may indicate Attention Deficit Hyperactivity Disorder.

Adolescents

The procedures, techniques, and examination findings for the adolescent is the same as the adult.

EXAMINATION OF THE BREASTS

Newborns and Infants

Procedures and Techniques. The examination of the newborn's and the child's breasts generally requires only inspection. The infant or child should be undressed to the waist.

Normal and Abnormal Findings. Neonates of both genders may have full, slightly enlarged breasts secondary to the mother's estrogen level before the infant was born (Fig. 20-41). Maternal hormones are also responsible for the production of a small amount of watery or milky nipple discharge (referred to as "witch's milk") during the first month of life in approximately 5% of neonates (Pena and Rosenfeld, 2001). The nipples are normally located slightly lateral to the midclavicular line between the fourth and fifth ribs; the nipple should be flat and surrounded by a slightly darker pigmented areola.

Older Children and Adolescents

Procedures and Techniques. School-age and adolescent females may be sensitive about having their breasts exposed. The nurse should take time to reassure the client that although her privacy is important, it is necessary to adequately expose the chest for a complete breast examination. The breast examination should proceed in the same manner as with the adult female. Note the developmental stage of the client.

Normal and Abnormal Findings. Tanner (1962) describes breast development in five stages (Fig. 20-42). As the girl reaches prepubertal age, sometimes as young as age 8, her breasts will show prepubertal budding. Precocious development of breasts in girls before age 8 should be investigated further. The full development of the breast takes an average of 3 years (with a range 1.5 to 6 years). Menarche begins when the breasts reach stages 3 or 4, usually just after the peak of the adolescent growth spurt, which is about age 12 (Fig. 20-43). Because Tanner developed the stages from studies conducted on British white females, the nurse is cautioned about generalizing the stages to other cultural groups. For example, Harlan (1980) found that African American girls developed secondary sex characteristics earlier than white girls of the same age. The right and left breasts may develop at different rates. It is important to reassure the client that this is common and, in time, the development may equalize. The breast tissue in the adolescent female should feel firm and elastic throughout both breasts. By age 14, most females have developed breasts that resemble those of the adult female.

Male adolescents, especially obese males, may have transient unilateral or bilateral subareolar masses (Fig. 20-44). These firm and sometimes tender masses may be of great concern. Reassure the young adolescent that these are generally transient and should disappear within a year or so. Gynecomastia, on the other hand, is an unexpected enlargement of one or both breasts in the male. It may be caused by hormonal or systemic disorders; however, it is most commonly a result of adipose tissue associated with obesity or the body change transition that occurs during early puberty (Hockenberry and Wilson, 2007).

EXAMINATION OF THE REPRODUCTIVE SYSTEM AND PERINEUM

Newborns and Infants

Female Exam

Procedures and Techniques. During infancy, the examination is limited to an evaluation of the external genitalia to determine if the structures are intact. The infant is placed on the examination table in frog-leg position (hips flexed with the soles of the feet together and up to the buttocks). Using gloved hands, place both thumbs on either side of the labia majora and gently push the tissue laterally while pushing the perineum down. This should permit visualization of the perineal area, the urethra, the clitoris, the hymen, and possibly the vaginal opening.

Normal and Abnormal Findings. Secondary to maternal hormones, the newborn's genitalia may appear somewhat engorged, with edematous labia majora and prominent and protruding labia minora. The clitoris also looks relatively enlarged, and the hymen may appear thick; the vaginal open-

TABLE 20-5   *Screening Assessment of Neurologic "Soft" Signs*

INSTRUCTIONAL TECHNIQUE	IMPORTANT OBSERVATIONS	VARIABLES AND CONSIDERATIONS
• Evaluation of fine motor coordination: observe child during:		
a. Undressing, unbuttoning	Note child's general coordination	
b. Tying shoe		
c. Rapidly touching alternate fingers with thumb	Note if similar movement on other side	For items c to e and h and i, movement of other side noted as associated motor movements, adventitious overflow movements, or synkinesis
d. Rattling imaginary doorknob	Note if similar movement on other side	
e. Unscrewing imaginary light bulb	Note if similar movement on other side	
f. Grasping pencil and writing	Note excessive pressure on pen point; fingers placed directly over point, or placed greater than 1 inch (2.5 cm) up shaft	May indicate difficulty with fine-motor coordination
g. Moving tongue rapidly		
h. Demonstrating hand grip	Note if similar movement on opposite side	
i. Inverting feet	Note if similar movement on opposite side	
j. Repeating several times "pa, ta, ka" or "kitty, kitty, kitty"	Accurate reproduction of these sounds indicates auditory coordination	
• Evaluation of special sensory skills		
a. Dual simultaneous sensory tests (face-hand testing): first demonstrate technique, then instruct child to close eyes; nurse performs simultaneously:		
(1) Touch both cheeks	Failure to perceive hand stimulus when face simultaneously touched referred to as *rostral dominance*	About 80% of normal children able to perform this test by age 8 years without rostral dominance
(2) Touch both hands		
(3) Touch right cheek and right hand		
(4) Touch left cheek and right hand		
(5) Touch left cheek and left hand		
(6) Touch right cheek and left hand		
b. Finger localization test (finger agnosia test): touch two spots on one finger or two fingers simultaneously; child has eyes closed; ask, "How many fingers am I touching, one or two?"	Evaluate number of correct responses with four trials for each hand Six out of eight possible correct responses passes	About 50% of all children pass test by age 6 years About 90% of all children pass test by age 9 years This test reflects child's orientation in space, concept of body image, sensation of touch, and position sense
• Evaluation of child's laterality and orientation in space		
a. Imitation of gestures: instruct child to use same hand as nurse and to imitate the following movements ("Do as I do"):	Note difficulty with fine finger movements, manipulation, or reproduction of correct gesture Note any marked right-left confusion regarding nurse's right and left hands	This test helps to evaluate child's finger discrimination and awareness of body image, right, left, front, back, and up and down orientation Especially important after age 8 years if there continues to be marked right-left confusion
(1) Extend little finger		
(2) Extend little and index fingers		
(3) Extend index and middle fingers		
(4) Touch two thumbs and two index fingers together simultaneously		
(5) Form two interlocking rings—thumb and index finger of one hand, with thumb and index finger of other hand		
(6) Point index finger of one hand down toward cupped finger of opposite hand held below		

Data from McMillan J, Nieburg P, Oski F: *The whole pediatrician catalog,* Philadelphia, 1977, WB Saunders.

TABLE 20-5 *Screening Assessment of Neurologic "Soft" Signs—cont'd*

INSTRUCTIONAL TECHNIQUE	IMPORTANT OBSERVATIONS	VARIABLES AND CONSIDERATIONS

b. Following directions: ask child to:
  (1) Show me your left hand
  (2) Show me your right eye
  (3) Show me your left elbow
  (4) Touch your left knee with your left hand
  (5) Touch your right ear with your left hand
  (6) Touch your left elbow with your right hand
  (7) Touch your right cheek with your right hand
  (8) Note any difficulty with following sequence of directions
  (9) Point to my left ear
  (10) Point to my right eye
  (11) Point to my right hand
  (12) Point to my left knee
	Note any incorrect response
	Note any difficulty with following sequence of directions
		Items 1 through 7 mastered by approximately age 6 years
		
		Items 8 through 11 mastered by age 8 years

ing may be difficult to see. A mucoid, white vaginal discharge may be observed during the early period following birth but should disappear by 1 month. Vaginal discharges noted after the infant is 1 month old may occur secondary to diaper or powder irritation.

Male Exam

Procedures and Techniques. For examination of the genitalia, the infant should be undressed so that the genitalia are completely exposed. The genitalia should remain covered until you are ready to begin, and the cover should be replaced

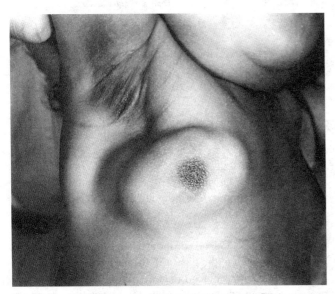

Fig. 20-41 **Marked enlargement of breast bud in neonate.** This is an exaggerated response to maternal hormones. *(From Gallager et al, 1978.)*

immediately after you have completed the examination, in case of unexpected urination. Inspect the urinary meatus; however, do not attempt to retract the foreskin more than necessary to see the meatus. Force may tear the prepuce from the glans, which in turn could cause binding adhesions to form between the prepuce and the glans.

Palpate the scrotum to determine presence of the testes (Fig. 20-45). If a mass other than a testicle or spermatic cord is palpated in the scrotum, transillumination is indicated to determine the presence of fluid (hydrocele) or mass (possible hernia) in the testicle.

Normal and Abnormal Findings. If the infant is uncircumcised, the foreskin (prepuce) should cover the glans. The foreskin will have little mobility. As the infant becomes older, the foreskin has more mobility. The foreskin should retract enough to permit unobstructed urinary stream and general cleaning. The urinary meatus should be at the tip of the penis. If possible, observe the infant's urine stream. It should be full and strong. A weak stream with dribbling is an abnormal finding and may indicate stenosis of the urethral meatus.

The full-term infant has a pendulous scrotum with deep rugae; the size of the scrotum usually appears large when compared with the penis. The scrotum appears pink in white infants and dark brown in dark-skinned infants. A testis should be palpable in each scrotum. If one or both testicles are not palpable, gently place a finger over the upper inguinal ring and gently push downward toward the scrotum. If the testicle can be pushed into the scrotum, it is considered descended even though it retracts into the inguinal canal. A hydrocele is a common finding in infants. A hydrocele transilluminates and usually becomes bigger as the child cries or becomes stressed. A mass (such as a hernia) will not transilluminate.

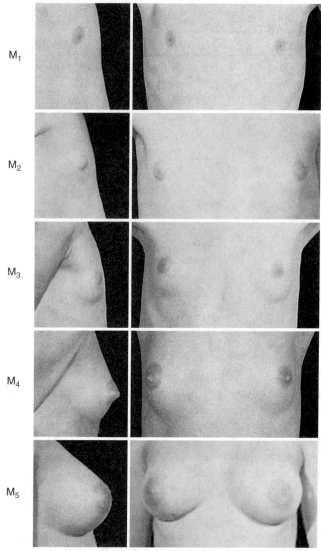

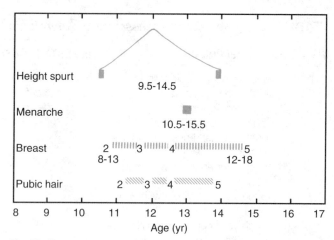

Fig. 20-43 **Summary of maturational development of girls.** See Fig. 20-42 for explanation of numbers 2 through 5 in breast development. Number ranges in graph (e.g., 9.5-14.5) indicate average or common range of age for development of characteristic. *(From Marshall and Tanner, 1969.)*

Fig. 20-42 **Tanner's five stages of breast development in females.** M_1—Only the nipple is raised above the level of the breast, as in the child. M_2—Budding stage: bud-shaped elevation of the areola. On palpation, a fairly hard disk- or cherry-shaped "button" can be felt. The areola is increased in diameter and the surrounding area is slightly elevated. M_3—Further elevation of the mammary gland. Diameter of areola increases further. Shape of mammary tissue is now visibly feminine. M_4—Increasing fat deposits. The areola forms a secondary elevation above that of the breast. This secondary mound apparently occurs in roughly half of all young females and in some cases persists in adulthood. M_5—Adult stage. The areola (usually) subsides to the level of the breast and is strongly pigmented. *(From Van Wieringen et al, 1971. Reprinted by permission of Kluwer Academic Publishers.)*

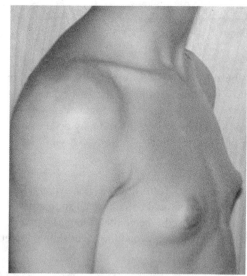

Fig. 20-44 Prepubertal gynecomastia. *(Courtesy Wellington Hung, MD, Children's National Medical Center, Washington, DC. From Seidel et al, 2006.)*

Toddlers and Children

Female Exam

Procedures and Techniques. The extent of the genitalia examination in children depends on their age and the presence of problems, but typically the examination is limited to inspection of the external genitalia to determine if the structures are intact and without obvious abnormalities. An inspection of a young girl's external genitalia should be included with each routine examination. If this examination is performed consistently, the child experiences less anxiety and embarrassment in later years when internal examination

becomes necessary. Internal examination is not routinely performed because the internal female genitalia are underdeveloped in the prepubertal girl.

The nurse must take the time to gain the cooperation and understanding of the child; how this is done depends largely on the age of the child and previous experiences. By the time a child is 4 to 6 years of age, time is spent reassuring the child that the procedure involves looking at her genitalia and touching her on the outside only. Approach the child in a matter-of-fact manner informing her about the procedure and what to expect. It may be difficult to get the child to understand the difference between a permissible genitalia examination by a nurse and inappropriate touching by others; it is important to include the parent in this discussion.

When nurses examine younger children, parents often are present and can participate by helping to position the child. In all cases, ensure privacy for the child. The child should

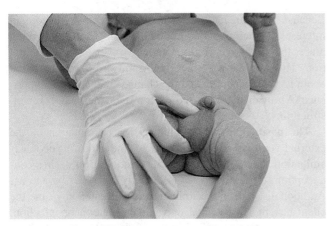

Fig. 20-45 Palpation of the scrotum in an infant.

participate in the decision about whether or not the parent is present in the room during the examination. Some girls may want a parent present, while the preteen child may not. Confer with the child before the examination and, if appropriate, ask the parent to wait outside.

Position the child on her back and place her legs in a frog-leg position (hips flexed with the soles of the feet together and up to her buttocks), with the head slightly elevated so she can observe the nurse. The older girl may have difficulty obtaining adequate relaxation of the knees with the feet together, and thus it may be necessary for her to assume the lithotomy position with feet in stirrups. The techniques of the external genitalia examination are the same as for the infant. Using gloved hands, gently spread the labia so that the genitalia may be inspected.

There are, however, occasional situations that warrant a more complete examination. The decision to do this is usually based on external examination findings or the history. For example, if the child has a history of urinary tract infections, vaginal discharge or irritation, or complaints of itching, rash, or pain, a more complete examination is necessary. A complete examination is also necessary if there is any indication of sexual abuse or mishandling of the child. (In this case, such an examination is performed by a sexual assault nurse examiner.) If internal inspection of the vagina and cervix is necessary, a pediatric Pederson speculum may be used for an older girl. For young girls, a nasal speculum with an attached light source is a useful instrument if the speculum is too large. A rectal examination is necessary if there is any suspected history of fondling, abuse, or the possibility of a foreign body in the rectum. Internal inspection is considered an advanced skill and should only be attempted by those nurses who have received adequate training for this type of exam.

Normal and Abnormal Findings. Until approximately age 7, the labia majora are flat, the labia minora are thin, and the clitoris is relatively small. Usually the hymen membrane has a visible opening, although there are a number of normal variations in the appearance of the hymen. In older girls, the labia majora and minora appear thicker, and evidence of pubic hair may be seen by the time the child reaches pubescence—usually between ages 8 and 11 (Table 20-6). There should be no vaginal discharge, vaginal odor, or evidence of bruising.

TABLE 20-6 *Tanner's Sex Maturity Development (Female)*

STAGE		PUBIC HAIR DEVELOPMENT
Stage 1	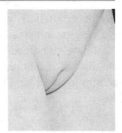	No growth of pubic hair
Stage 2	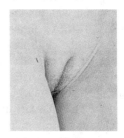	Initial, scarcely long, straight, downy, and slightly pigmented hair, especially along the labia
Stage 3	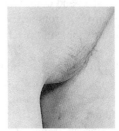	The hair is darker, coarser, and curly, and spread sparsely over the entire pubis in the typical female triangle
Stage 4	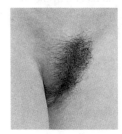	Pubic hair is denser, curled, and in an adult distribution, but less abundant and restricted to the pubic area
Stage 5	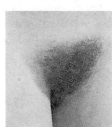	The pubic hair is adult in quantity, type, and pattern, with lateral spreading to the inner aspect of the thighs
Stage 6	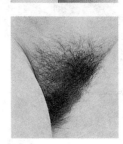	Further extension laterally, upward, or over the upper thighs (this stage may not occur in all women)

Photographs from Van Wierengen et al, 1971. Reprinted by permission of Kluwer Academic Publishers.

Male Exam

Procedures and Techniques. The techniques for examining the male child's genitalia are the same as those for the infant. The major difference in the examination is the approach. In many cultures, children are taught at a very early age that the genitalia should not be exposed or touched. In the presence of the child's parent, reassure him that you must examine his genitalia just as you have examined all of his other body areas. It is important that the parent reassure the child that you need to examine him to make sure that he is healthy. Whenever possible, reassure the child that he is growing up normally.

The examination is easiest to perform if the child is sitting in either a slightly reclining position with his knees flexed and heels near the buttock (Fig. 20-46) or sitting with his knees spread and ankles crossed. If the child has not been circumcised, do not force the foreskin to be retracted. Retract the foreskin only to the point of tightness. Then evaluate whether it is retracted far enough to permit adequate urination and cleaning. Determine if the child has any discharge, crusting, or lesions around or under the foreskin. In addition, examine the scrotum for shape, size, and color and to determine the presence of testicles in the scrotum. Evidence of pubic hair may be seen by the time the child reaches pubescence (Table 20-7).

Normal and Abnormal Findings. The findings for children are the same as those for the infant. By age 6, the foreskin should be easily retracted. If the scrotum has well-formed rugae, it indicates that the testes have descended into the scrotum. If the scrotum remains small, flat, and underdeveloped, it is considered an abnormal finding and may indicate cryptorchidism (undescended testes).

Adolescents

Female Exam

Procedures and Techniques. If a parent is present, the adolescent should be given a choice to be examined alone, and she should be assured of privacy and confidentiality. Assess her menstrual history and sexual maturity development using Tanner's stages (see Table 20-6). Reassure the client that the changes her body is undergoing are normal.

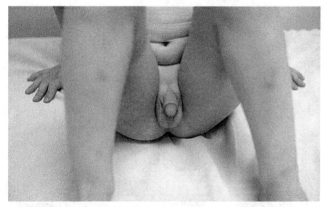

Fig. 20-46   Position of young child for examination of genitalia. *(From Seidel et al, 2006.)*

Because many preadolescents and adolescents are becoming interested in their own bodies and the changes that are taking place, they may want to take an active part in the examination. This may be a perfect opportunity to teach the client about her own anatomy and the changes that she will experience. A mirror may be used during the examination for instruction.

The positioning and techniques for examination of the external genitalia are the same as for the adult. A pelvic examination should be performed if the adolescent desires contraception, if the adolescent is sexually active, or by age 21. Additionally, a pelvic examination is warranted any time the client has signs of genital or vaginal irritation or infection. This will include periodic Pap tests when intercourse begins.

The procedures to be followed are the same as for an adult woman, but additional time must be taken to explain the procedure, show the equipment, and tell the client exactly what she may expect. The size and type of vaginal speculum used is based on the size of the client and the sexual history. The speculum most commonly used to reduce discomfort is a pediatric speculum with blades that are 1.0 to 1.5 cm wide.

Normal and Abnormal Findings. All findings for the genitalia examination of the adolescent are the same as the findings previously described for the adult.

Male Exam

Procedures and Techniques. Genitalia assessment of the adolescent male is important to ensure that the maturational development is progressing according to Tanner's stages (Fig. 20-47). This is also the time when teen modesty is at its peak. The nurse must take time to develop a relationship with the client and reassure him in a matter-of-fact manner that the examination of the genitalia is an essential part of a complete examination. It is also important to ensure privacy and adequate draping when the genitalia are not being examined. It is usually best to defer the examination of the genitalia to the last procedure of the examination. The process of examination is essentially the same as previously discussed for the adult.

Normal and Abnormal Findings. Expected findings for the young adolescent male depend on the maturational stage of the client. Review Table 20-7 for the expected and normal findings of the maturing male. Findings for the older adolescent are essentially the same as previously discussed for the adult.

PERIANAL EXAMINATION

Newborns and Infants

Procedures and Techniques. The external perianal examination is routinely performed with comprehensive assessment; an internal anal examination, however, is not routinely performed. The infant is generally placed on his or her back with the feet held in the nurse's hand and the infant's knees flexed upward toward the abdomen (Fig. 20-48). In the newborn, inspect the perineum and anal re-

TABLE 20-7 *Tanner's Sex Maturity Development (Male)*

STAGES	PUBIC HAIR	PENIS	SCROTUM
Stage 1 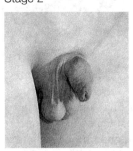	No pubic hair.	Appears like smaller child's penis	Testes begins to enlarge. but scrotum remains small and undeveloped.
Stage 2 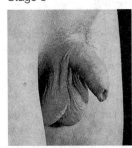	Pubic hair starting to develop. Appears as straight, long, and downy texture.	Little enlargement.	Both testes and scrotum enlarge. The scrotum begins to acquire darker skin tone and change in texture.
Stage 3	Increasing hair growth over entire pubic region. Hair is darker, curly, and beginning to become coarse.	Penis begins to enlarge. Enlargement is more in length than general size.	Growth and skin texture continue to develop.
Stage 4 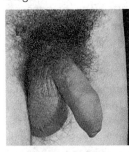	Hair is thick and coarse over entire pubic area.	Penis grows in both length and diameter. The glans also develops.	The scrotum is like the adult, with darker tone, and the testes are almost adult size.
Stage 5 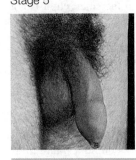	Mature pubic hair distribution, including on upper medial thighs.	Adult appearance of penis.	Full development and adult-appearing testes.

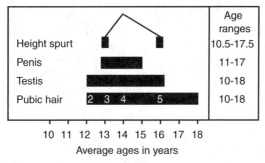

	Age ranges
Height spurt	10.5-17.5
Penis	11-17
Testis	10-18
Pubic hair	2 3 4 5	10-18

10 11 12 13 14 15 16 17 18
Average ages in years

Fig. 20-47 Development of male genitalia and pubic hair. (2, 3, 4, 5 refer to Tanner's stages. See Table 20-7.) *(From Tanner, 1962.)*

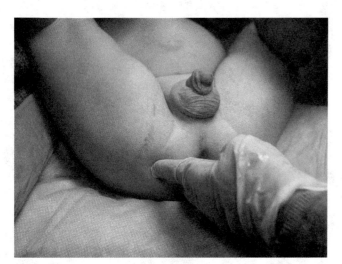

Fig. 20-48 Position for rectal examination of the infant. *(From Seidel et al, 2006.)*

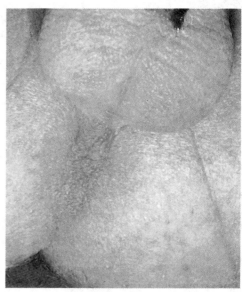

Fig. 20-49 Imperforate anus. *(From Diagnostic picture tests in clinical medicine, 1984. By permission of Mosby International.)*

gion for presence of anus, lesions, and inflammation. Confirm anal contraction by lightly stroking the anal opening with a cotton-tipped applicator. Observe the lower back and buttocks for appearance and surface characteristics. If stool is present when the diaper is removed, note the characteristics, color, odor, and consistency.

Normal and Abnormal Findings. The perineal and perianal skin should be free of lesions or inflammation, although diaper rash is a common finding with infants. A patent anus is the expected finding; imperforate anus is an abnormal finding that is assessed at birth (Fig. 20-49). Stroking the anus with the cotton-tipped applicator should produce an "anal wink" or contraction. Lack of anal contraction may indicate a lower spinal cord deformity. The lower back and buttocks should be free of lesions. Normal variations include mongolian spots and birthmarks. A tuft of hair or dimpling in the pilonidal (sacrococcygeal) area may indicate a lower spinal deformity or sinus tract. Buttocks should be firm and rounded.

Toddlers and Children

Procedures and Techniques. External perianal examination is routinely performed during a comprehensive assessment. For the external examination, be sure to respect the child's modesty and apprehension; take the time to explain what is going to happen and what the child can

expect. Children should be positioned so that the perianal area is adequately exposed and so that the child is comfortable. The child should be positioned either in a knee-chest position or on the left side with the hips and knees flexed toward the abdomen (the same positioning as for the adult).

Internal rectal examination is not performed in children unless there are specific symptoms such as severe abdominal pain, constipation, or injury. If an internal rectal examination is warranted, the nurse should use the little finger to perform the examination. Even when this is done, there may occasionally be slight rectal bleeding. The parent should be told about this possibility before the examination. The procedure for the internal examination is the same as that for the adult.

Normal and Abnormal Findings. The findings for external examination are the same for the child as for the adult. Variations are based on developmental maturity. Redness or irritation may be an indication of a bacterial or fungal infection or pinworms. Assess for signs of physical or sexual abuse such as bruising, anal tearing, rapid anal wink, anal dilation, or extreme or inappropriate apprehension from the child. If there is suspicion of child abuse or assault, report the findings to the appropriate local health authorities. The findings for the internal examination are the same as for the adult with the exception that the prostate in the small child is not palpable.

Adolescents

Rectal exams are not routinely performed unless warranted by symptoms (i.e. rectal bleeding). Females may have a rectal exam performed as part of a pelvic exam. The prostate exam is not routinely performed in adolescent males. If performed, the procedures, techniques, and findings for the adolescent are the same as for those in the adult.

COMMON PROBLEMS & CONDITIONS

SKIN CONDITIONS

Atopic Dermatitis

Atopic dermatitis is a chronic superficial inflammation of the skin with an unknown cause. It is commonly associated with hay fever and asthma and it is thought to be familial. It is most commonly seen in infancy and childhood. **Clinical Findings:** During infancy and early childhood, red, weeping, crusted lesions appear on the face, scalp, extremities, and diaper area. In older children lesion characteristics include erythema, scaling, and lichenification. The lesions are usually localized to the hands, feet, arms, and legs (particularly at the antecubital fossa and popliteal space) and are associated with intense pruritus. (Fig. 20-50).

Diaper Dermatitis

One of the most common causes of irritant contact dermatitis, diaper dermatitis is an inflammatory reaction to urine, feces, moisture, or friction. It is most common among infants between 4 to 12 months of age. **Clinical Findings:** This dermatitis is characterized by a primary irritant rash involving skin areas in contact with the diaper. The rash is composed of red plaques that may be raised and confluent in severe cases (Fig. 20-51).

Impetigo

This is a common and highly contagious bacterial infection caused by staphylococcal or streptococcal pathogens. It is most prevalent in children, especially among individuals living in crowded conditions with poor sanitation. It occurs most commonly in mid-to-late summer, with the highest incidence in hot, humid climates. **Clinical Findings:** This infection appears as an erythematous macule that becomes a vesicle or bulla and finally a honey-colored crust after the vesicles or bullae rupture (Fig. 20-52).

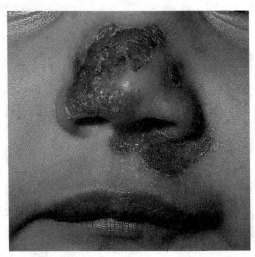

Fig. 20-51 Severe diaper rash. *(From Habif, Campbell, Chapman et al, 2005.)*

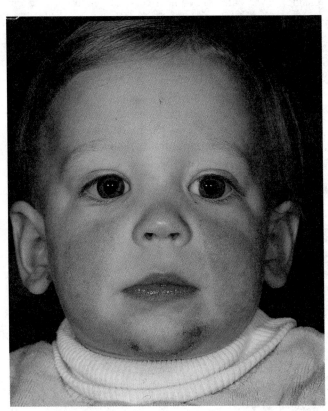

Fig. 20-50 Atopic dermatitis. *(From Habif, 2004.)*

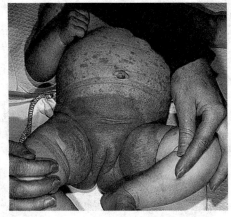

Fig. 20-52 Impetigo. *(From Weston and Lane, 1996.)*

Herpes Varicella (Chickenpox)

This is a highly communicable viral infection spread by droplets that most commonly occurs during childhood. **Clinical Findings:** The lesions first appear on the trunk and then spread to the extremities and the face. Initially the lesions are macules; they progress to papules, then vesicles, and finally the old vesicles become crusts. The lesions erupt in crops over a period of several days. For this reason, lesions in various stages are seen concurrently (Fig. 20-53).

EAR CONDITIONS

Acute Otitis Media

Acute otitis media (AOM) is an infection of the middle ear with the presence of middle ear effusion that can be viral or bacterial in origin. It is one of the most common of all childhood infections (Rovers et al, 2007). **Clinical Findings:** The major symptom associated with AOM is ear pain (otalgia).

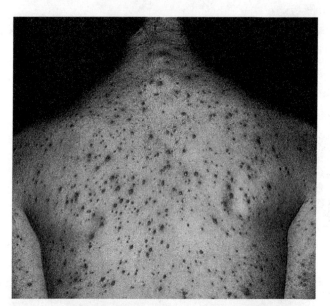

Fig. 20-53   Chickenpox (Varicella). *(From Habif, Campbell, and Chapman, 2005.)*

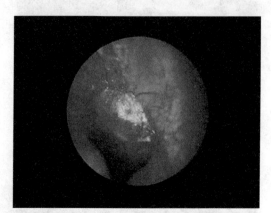

Fig. 20-54   Acute otitis media of the left ear with redness and edema of the pars flaccid. *(From Bingham, Hawke, and Kwok, 1992.)*

Infants, unable to verbally communicate pain, demonstrate irritability, fussiness, crying, lethargy, and pulling at the affected ear. Associated manifestations include fever, vomiting, and decreased hearing. On inspection in the early stages, the TM appears inflamed—it is red and may be bulging and immobile (Fig. 20-54). Later stages may reveal discoloration (white or yellow drainage) and opacification to the TM. Purulent drainage from the ear canal with a sudden relief of pain suggests perforation.

EYE CONDITIONS

Conjunctivitis

An inflammation of the palpebral or bulbar conjunctiva is termed *conjunctivitis*. It is caused by local infection of bacteria or virus, as well as by an allergic reaction, systemic infection, or chemical irritation. **Clinical Findings:** The eye appears red, with thick, sticky discharge on the eyelids, in the morning.

MOUTH

Tonsillitis

Tonsillitis is one of the most common oropharyngeal infections among children. It can be viral or bacterial in origin; common bacterial pathogens include beta-hemolytic and other streptococci. **Clinical Findings:** The classic presentation of tonsillitis includes sore throat, pain with swallowing (odynophagia), fever, chills, and tender cervical lymph nodes. Some children may also complain of ear pain (Johnson and Aijaz, 2003). On inspection, the tonsils appear enlarged and red and may be covered with white or yellow exudates (Fig. 20-55).

Cleft Lip and Cleft Palate

Cleft lip and cleft palate are incomplete fusion of the maxillary process or the secondary palate during fetal development. These conditions are the most common congenital craniofacial defects and fourth most common congenital de-

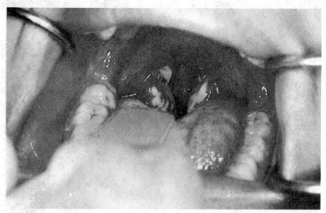

Fig. 20-55   Tonsillitis and pharyngitis. *(Courtesy Dr. Edward L Applebaum, Head, Department of Otolaryngology. University of Illinois Medical Center.)*

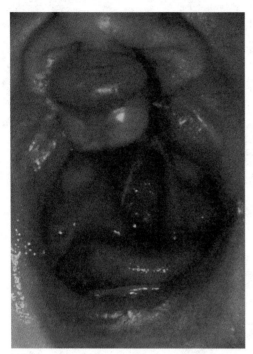

Fig. 20-56 Bilateral cleft lip and complete cleft palate. *(From Zitelli and Davis, 2007.)*

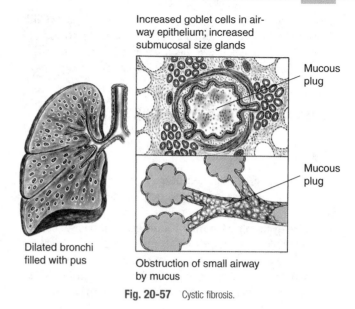

Increased goblet cells in airway epithelium; increased submucosal size glands

Mucous plug

Mucous plug

Dilated bronchi filled with pus

Obstruction of small airway by mucus

Fig. 20-57 Cystic fibrosis.

fects seen in the United States. **Clinical Findings:** Usually diagnosed before or at birth, the defects are characterized by a defect in the upper lip or a complete separation extending to the floor of the nostril. This can be unilateral or bilateral (Fig. 20-56).

RESPIRATORY CONDITIONS

Cystic Fibrosis

This is an autosomal recessive genetic disorder of the exocrine glands. It is a multisystem disease affecting most body systems but especially the lungs, pancreas, and sweat glands. It causes respiratory system dysfunction because of abnormally thick mucus production, which leads to a chronic, diffuse obstructive pulmonary disease (Fig. 20-57). Symptoms most commonly appear by age 4, although a milder form of disease may delay diagnosis until late childhood or early adolescence. **Clinical Findings:** The classic symptom of cystic fibrosis is the production of thick, sticky mucus. Stools of children with cystic fibrosis are often frothy, foul smelling, and greasy (steatorrhea). Respiratory signs and symptoms include a chronic moist productive cough with frequent respiratory infections. As the disease progresses, children will develop a barrel chest and finger clubbing.

Childhood Asthma

This chronic inflammatory disorder is characterized by airway obstruction and inflammation caused by multiple factors including environmental exposures, viral illnesses, allergens,

and genetic predisposition. Although it can occur at anytime during childhood, most children develop symptoms by age 5. **Clinical Findings:** Signs include increased respiratory rate with prolonged expiration, audible wheeze, shortness of breath, tachycardia, anxious appearance, possible use of accessory muscles, and cough.

Croup Syndromes

The term *croup* is used to describe a wide range of upper airway illnesses that result from edema of the epiglottis and larynx that often extends into the trachea and bronchi. The three most common conditions—laryngotracheobronchitis (LTB), epiglottitis, and bacterial tracheitis—affect the greatest number of children across all age groups (although it is most common in young children). **Clinical Findings:** The classic findings include inspiratory stridor, a barking-like cough, and hoarseness. In severe cases, the child may display respiratory distress including rapid, labored breathing with retractions and lethargy. Associated findings may include fever, runny nose.

CARDIOVASCULAR CONDITIONS

Congenital Heart Defects

There are a number of congenital heart defects; the most common involve an abnormal connection between the left and right side of the heart (septal defects) or between the great arteries (patent ductus arteriosus). Large defects are typically diagnosed before or shortly after birth while smaller defects may be undiagnosed until the preschool years. **Clinical Findings:** Among infants and children, poor feeding and poor weight gain are often seen; elevations in heart and respiratory rates may be observed with feeding. A murmur is often auscultated and splitting heart sounds may be noted. Children fatigue easily and often assume a squatting position to relieve cyanotic spells. Signs associated with congestive heart failure may be observed with larger defects.

MUSCULOSKELETAL CONDITIONS

Muscular Dystrophies

This is a group of inherited diseases characterized by progressive muscle wasting due to degeneration of muscle fibers. The most common form in childhood is Duchenne muscular dystrophy. **Clinical Findings:** In infancy, sucking and swallowing difficulties may be observed. In early childhood weakness involving the lower extremities becomes evident with frequent tripping or toe walking. The muscle weakness progresses to muscle wasting; eventually the child loses the ability to walk.

Spina Bifida

Spina bifida is a type of neural tube birth defect characterized by a protrusion of the spinal cord through a vertebral defect. These defects occur within the first month of gestation. **Clinical Findings:** At birth a saclike protrusion is noted on the infant's back along the spine. These defects can occur anywhere from the upper thoracic to the sacral spine. A wide range of sensory impairment is also noted such as motor impairment and sensory impairment of the lower extremities and possibly sensory loss involving the anus and genitalia.

NEUROLOGIC CONDITIONS

Hydrocephalus

Hydrocephalus is abnormal accumulation of cerebrospinal fluid (CSF). In infants, hydrocephalus is usually a result of an obstruction of the drainage of CSF in the head. **Clinical Findings:** In infants, a gradual increase in intracranial pressure occurs leading to an actual enlargement of the head (Fig. 20-58). As the head enlarges, the facial features appear small in proportion to the cranium, the fontanels may bulge, and the scalp veins dilate.

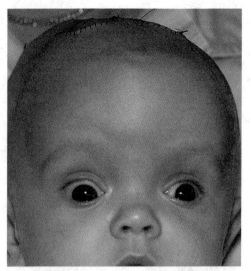

Fig. 20-58   Infantile hydrocephalus. *(From Zitelli and Davis, 2007.)*

Cerebral Palsy

This is a group of motor function disorders caused by permanent, nonprogressive brain injuries that occur during fetal development or near the time of birth. Classifications of cerebral palsy are spastic, accounting for 50% of cases; dyskinetic (athetoid), accounting for 20% of cases; ataxic, accounting for 10% of cases; and mixed, accounting for 20% of cases. **Clinical Findings:** Deficits may include spasticity, seizures, mental retardation, muscle contractions, delayed motor development, and impaired vision, speech, and hearing.

Attention Deficit Hyperactivity Disorder

Attention deficit hyperactivity disorder (ADHD) is a condition that begins in childhood characterized by inattentiveness, impulsivity, and hyperactivity that are developmentally inappropriate. ADHD is diagnosed three times more often in boys than girls. **Clinical Findings:** The manifestations may be numerous or few, mild or severe, and vary with the developmental level of the child. An important clinical manifestation is distractibility. The child seems to have selective attention and often does not seem to listen or follow through.

CLINICAL APPLICATION & CLINICAL REASONING

See Appendix E for answers to exercises in this section.

REVIEW QUESTIONS

1 Which of the following findings on a 2-month-old baby is considered abnormal and requires further follow-up?
1 The anterior fontanel is not palpable.
2 The thyroid gland cannot be palpated.
3 The head circumference is slightly greater than the chest circumference.
4 Head lag is observed when the shoulders are lifted off the examination table.

2 A nurse is palpating the lymph nodes of an 18-month-old toddler and finds enlarged postauricular and occipital nodes. What is the significance of this finding?
1 This is a normal finding at this age.
2 The toddler may have an ear infection.
3 The toddler may have an inflammation of the scalp.
4 The toddler needs to be referred to a pediatrician.

3 While examining the ear of an infant with an otoscope, the nurse pulls down on the ear for which of the following reasons?
1 Increases the depth the otoscope can be inserted.
2 Stabilizes the ear to avoid injury if the infant moves her head suddenly.
3 Enhances visualization of the tympanic membrane by straightening the ear canal.
4 Facilitates drainage of cerumen from the ear canal, allowing better visualization of inner ear structures.

4 What are expected findings of the newborn's vision that the nurse teaches to the parents?
1 There will be small tears noted when their newborn cries.
2 Peripheral sight does not develop until age 3 or 4 months.
3 The newborn can only distinguish the colors of blue and green.
4 The newborn is nearsighted and cannot see items unless they are close.

5 When examining a 16-year-old male client, the nurse notes multiple pustules and comedones on the face. The nurse recognizes this is due to increased activity of the:
1 Epidermal cells.
2 Eccrine glands.
3 Apocrine glands.
4 Sebaceous glands.

6 Which are expected findings of a newborn's pulmonary assessment?
1 Thoracic breathing.
2 A 1:2 ratio of AP to lateral diameter.
3 Flaring of the nares noted on inspiration.
4 Bronchovesicular breath sounds in the peripheral lung fields.

7 Which of the following is an abnormal finding of a preschooler during a cardiovascular system examination?
1 Heart rate of 106 beats per minute.
2 Failure to gain weight because of fatigue while eating.
3 Continuous low-pitched vibration heard over the jugular vein.
4 Pulse increasing on inspiration and decreasing on expiration.

8 Which would be an abnormal finding for a 7-year-old African American boy?
1 Potbelly.
2 Umbilical hernia.
3 Abdominal breathing.
4 Tenseness of abdominal muscles.

9 When examining the genitalia of a 3-year-old boy, which of the following positions is ideal?
1 Prone position.
2 Supine position.
3 Lithotomy position.
4 Sitting position with knees spread and ankles crossed.

10 On assessment of the neurologic status of a 4-month-old infant, the nurse notes which of the following as an abnormal finding?
1 The infant abducts and extends arms and legs when startled.
2 When the infant's sole is touched, the toes flex tightly in an attempt to grasp.
3 The infant steps in place when held upright with feet on a flat surface.
4 When stroking the infant's foot from sole to great toes, there is fanning of the toes.

SAMPLE DOCUMENTATION

Review the data obtained during an interview and examination by the nurse below.

Denzel Morgan is a 9-month-old boy brought to the clinic by his mother for a well-baby exam. He has no current or chronic medical conditions, takes no medications, and has no allergies. He is up to date on his immunizations. His mother states that he has been well, and loves to sit in a high chair and feed himself. She describes his activity as "normal" and he is crawling all over the house. Vital signs: tympanic temperature, 98.2° F (36.8° C); heart rate, 122; respiratory rate, 30. He weighs 10.8 kg (23.5 lb), his length is 29 inches and his head circumference is 18". He is a healthy-appearing, playful male child actively exploring the examining room.

Below, note how the nurse recorded these same selected data in a documentation format and on the Growth Chart (at end of this chapter).

9-month-old M brought by mother for 9-month well child care.

SELECTED SUBJECTIVE DATA

Medical Hx: none. Medications: none. Allergies: NKDA. Immunizations: up to date. No recent illness. Mother reports child crawling and feeding self.

INITIAL OBJECTIVE DATA

Vitals: T 98.2° F (36.8° C) tympanic; HR 122; RR 30; Wt 10.8 kg (23.5 lb); head circumference 18"; length, 29".

General observations: Healthy-appearing child actively exploring examining room.

CASE STUDY

M. G. is an 8-year-old girl being treated for seizures.

Interview Data

M. G.'s mother states that M. G. was at home watching television when she started "shaking and jerking all over." The seizure occurred several hours ago, but lasted longer than 20 minutes. The mother is concerned because her daughter has never had a seizure last this long before. M. G. denies recent headaches or problems with balance; she takes primidone 125 mg twice a day.

Examination Data

Vital Signs: Blood pressure, 110/68 mm Hg; pulse, 84 beats/min; respiratory rate, 18; temperature, 98.6° F (37° C).

Cognition: She is a cooperative, alert child with flat affect. She communicates slowly but appropriately.

Neurologic: M. G. has voluntary, symmetric, coordinated movement of all extremities with full range of motion; muscle strength is 5 bilaterally. Deep tendon reflexes are 2+ bilaterally. Sensation is present in arms and legs to vibration, cotton, and pinprick bilaterally.

Clinical Reasoning

1. What data deviate from normal findings, suggesting a need for further investigation?
2. What additional information should the nurse ask or assess for?
3. Based on the data, what risk factors for injury does Madison have?
4. What nursing diagnoses and collaborative problems should be considered for this situation?

INTERACTIVE ACTIVITIES

Open the interactive student CD-ROM, click on Chapter 20, and choose from the following activities on the menu bar:

- **Multiple Choice Challenge.** Click on the best answer for each question. You will be given immediate feedback, rationale for incorrect answers, and a total score. Good luck!

- **Risk Factors.** Review this client's history and identify risk factors. Complete your assessment by deciding which risk factors are modifiable or nonmodifiable. You only get one shot, so choose carefully!

- **Printable Lab Guide.** Locate the Lab Guide for Chapter 20, and print and use it (as many times as needed) to help you apply your assessment skills. These guides may also be filled in electronically and then saved and e-mailed to your instructor!

- **Quick Challenge.** Use this critical thinking exercise to assess your skills through case study-style questions, then compare with expert answers!

Birth to 36 months: Boys
Length-for-age and Weight-for-age percentiles

NAME Morgan, Denzel

RECORD # 236582

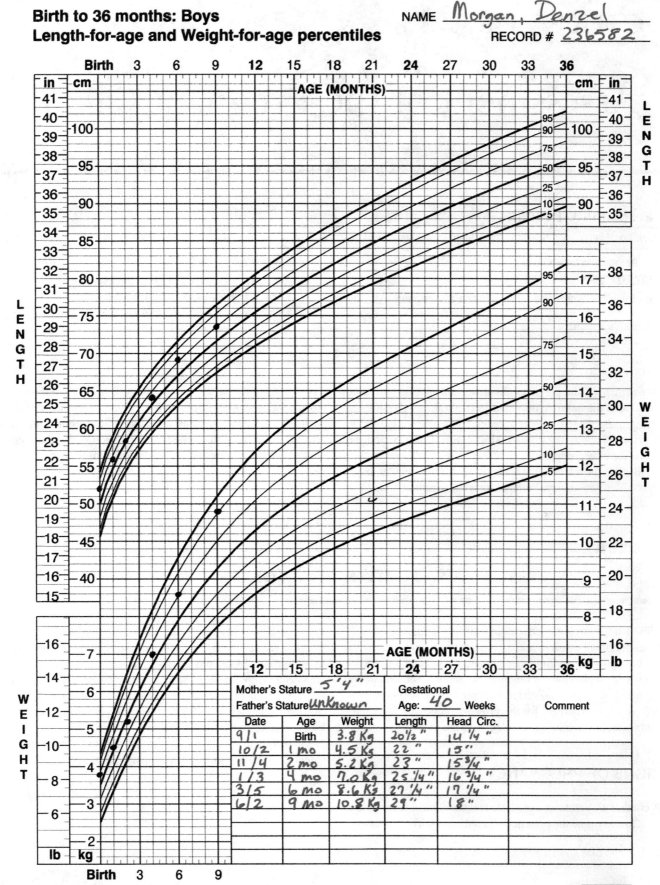

Mother's Stature	5'4"		Gestational		Comment
Father's Stature	Unknown		Age: 40 Weeks		
Date	Age	Weight	Length	Head Circ.	
9/1	Birth	3.8 Kg	20½"	14¼"	
10/2	1 mo	4.5 Kg	22"	15"	
11/4	2 mo	5.2 Kg	23"	15¾"	
1/3	4 mo	7.0 Kg	25¼"	16¾"	
3/5	6 mo	8.6 Kg	27¼"	17¼"	
6/2	9 mo	10.8 Kg	29"	18"	

Published May 30, 2000 (modified 4/20/01).
SOURCE: Developed by the National Center for Health Statistics in collaboration with
the National Center for Chronic Disease Prevention and Health Promotion (2000).
http://www.cdc.gov/growthcharts

SAFER · HEALTHIER · PEOPLE™

CHAPTER 21

Assessment of the Pregnant Client

Assessment of the pregnant client warrants special attention because of the multiple hormonal, structural, and physiologic changes associated with pregnancy. This chapter builds on previous chapters regarding taking a health history and the sequence of examination.

Ideally, the pregnant woman is seen on a regular basis throughout pregnancy. Prenatal visits are recommended every 4 weeks up to 28 weeks; every 2 weeks from 28 to 36 weeks; and weekly after 36 weeks. The initial prenatal visit includes a comprehensive history and examination; follow-up visits are more limited in scope, monitoring the progress of the pregnancy and assessing for complications.

ANATOMY & PHYSIOLOGY

Maternal physiologic adaptations during pregnancy result from hormonal changes and mechanical pressures caused by the enlarging uterus and other tissues. These changes protect the woman's physiologic functioning, allow adaptation to the metabolic demands associated with pregnancy, and provide a protective environment for the growing fetus. Box 21-1 presents selected changes associated with pregnancy.

SIGNS OF PREGNANCY

A combination of laboratory tests and the clinical findings are used to determine the presence of a pregnancy. The laboratory test most commonly used detects an antigen antibody reaction between human chorionic gonadotropin (hCG) hormone and an antiserum. Many physiologic changes are recognized as signs and symptoms of pregnancy. Some of these findings are categorized as: (1) presumptive symptoms—symptoms experienced by the woman; (2) probable signs—changes observed by the nurse; and (3) positive signs—findings that prove the presence of a fetus. Table 21-1 lists the signs of pregnancy by category and when they may become evident.

BOX 21-1 SELECTED ANATOMIC AND PHYSIOLOGIC CHANGES ASSOCIATED WITH PREGNANCY

Integumentary System
- Increased estrogen increases vascularity to the skin, causing itchiness and causing hands and feet to take on reddened appearance.
- Increased secretion of melanotropin causes pigmentation changes to the skin, including chloasma (mask of pregnancy), linea nigra (dark-pigmented line on abdomen), and increased pigmentation to nipples, areolae, axillae, and vulva.
- Increasing size of breasts and abdomen contribute to striae gravidarum (stretch marks) over abdomen and breasts.
- Increased hair or nail growth is reported by some individuals.

Respiratory System
- Uterine enlargement pushes up on diaphragm, causing periodic shortness of breath.
- Respiratory rate may increase slightly, tidal volume increases; breathing becomes more thoracic than abdominal; thoracic cage widens.

Cardiovascular System
- Blood volume increases by 1500 ml to meet the need of an enlarged uterus and fetal tissue, causing increased cardiac workload (increased heart rate).
- Uterine enlargement pushes up on the heart, causing the heart to shift upward and forward.
- Enlarged uterus increases pelvic pressure, causing decreased venous return that results in varicosities and edema in lower extremities.

Gastrointestinal System
- Rise in human chorionic gonadotropin early in pregnancy causes nausea and vomiting (morning sickness).
- Uterine enlargement results in displacement of intestines and decreased peristalsis, causing heartburn and constipation, respectively.
- Increased pelvic pressure and vascularity cause hemorrhoids.
- Increased estrogen increases vascularity and tissue proliferation of gums resulting in swollen and bleeding gums.

Urinary System
- Increased pressure of growing uterus on bladder in early pregnancy and fetal head exerting pressure on bladder in late pregnancy result in nocturia and urinary frequency.

Musculoskeletal System
- Increased size of uterus and growing fetus results in the center of gravity moving forward, causing lordosis (increased spinal curvature) and back discomfort; waddling gait and balance problems may occur.
- Abdominal wall muscles stretch and lose tone, which may lead to separation of abdominal muscles (diastasis recti) in the third trimester.

Reproductive System
- Uterus enlarges and fundus becomes palpable because of growing fetus.
- Vagina, vulva, and cervix take on bluish color caused by increased vascularity.

Breasts
- Breasts become full and tender early in pregnancy.
- Breasts enlarge as pregnancy progresses.
- Nipples and areolae are more prominent and deeply pigmented.
- Increased mammary vascularization causes veins to become engorged; visible under skin surface.

TABLE 21-1 Signs of Pregnancy

CATEGORY	SIGN	TIME OF OCCURRENCE (WEEKS OF GESTATION)
Presumptive signs	Breast fullness/tenderness	3-4
	Amenorrhea	4
	Nausea, vomiting	4-12
	Urinary frequency	6-12
	Quickening (fetal movement)	16-20
Probable signs	Chadwick's sign (violet-blue color to cervix)	6-8
	Goodell's sign (softening of cervix)	5
	Hegar's sign (softening of lower uterine segment)	6-12
	Positive pregnancy test (hCG)	
	Serum	4-12
	Urine	6-12
	Ballottement	16-28
Positive signs	Visualization of fetus by ultrasound	5-6
	Auscultation of fetal heart tones:	
	Doppler	8-17
	Fetoscope	17-19
	Palpation of fetal movements	19-22
	Observable fetal movements	Late pregnancy

HEALTH HISTORY

RISK FACTORS   *High-Risk Pregnancy*

As you conduct a health history during a prenatal visit, it is important to consider common risk factors associated with high-risk pregnancy and to follow up with additional questions if risk factors exist.

Maternal Characteristics
- Under 16 or over 35 years of age
- Marital status: single (or lack of supporting relationship) (M)
- Short stature (less than 5 feet [150 cm] tall)
- Weight less than 100 lb (4.5 kg) or over 200 lb (91 kg) (M)
- Socioeconomic: poverty, low education level (M)
- Lives at a high altitude (M)

Maternal Habits
- Alcohol consumption (M)
- Illicit drug use (M)
- Failure to obtain early prenatal care (M)
- Smoking (M)
- High-risk sexual behaviors (M)
- Poor diet (M)

Obstetric History
- Previous birth to infant weighing less than 2500 g
- Previous birth to infant weighing more than 4000 g
- Previous pregnancy ending in perinatal death
- More than two previous spontaneous abortions
- Birth to infant with congenital or perinatal disease
- Birth to infant with isoimmunization or ABO incompatibility

Current Medical Problems
- Chronic illnesses, including diabetes mellitus, thyroid disorder, heart disease, hypertension, pulmonary disease, renal failure, anemia, sickle cell disease
- Sexually transmitted disease
- Infectious disease (such as rubella or cytomegalovirus)

Problems with Current Pregnancy
- Bleeding
- Pregnancy-induced hypertension
- Eclampsia or preeclampsia
- Fetal position breech or transverse at term
- Polyhydramnios
- Multiple fetus (twins, triplets, etc.)
- Postmaturity (gestation >40 weeks)
- Premature rupture of membranes
- Weight gain that is inadequate or excessive

M = modifiable risk factor.

COMPONENTS OF PRENATAL HEALTH HISTORY

A comprehensive history should be obtained at the first prenatal visit to establish baseline data; it can then be updated as needed during subsequent visits. The history is similar to that of the adult (see Chapter 3), but with a special emphasis on collecting data that could affect pregnancy outcomes. The physical and psychologic health of the mother and the presence of chronic diseases could affect her health and that of the fetus.

Reason for Seeking Care

The pregnant woman may be seeing her health care provider for routine prenatal care or for a specific problem that may or may not directly relate to the pregnancy. Prenatal visits are needed to monitor the health of the mother and the growth of the fetus, as well as to educate the mother and family about the care of mother and neonate during the delivery process and neonatal period.

Present Health Status

Data collected are the same as was discussed in Chapter 3. Data specific to the pregnant woman include her present general physical and psychologic well-being and motherhood-coping abilities. Also, it is essential to determine what medications the client uses. Many pregnant women assume the use of over-the-counter medications is safe and are not aware of the potentially harmful effects to the fetus (Tillett et al, 2003).

Past Health History

Data collected in this section are the same as was discussed in Chapter 3. It is important to note any chronic illness (such as diabetes mellitus, thyroid or cardiovascular conditions, renal disease, and depression) as well as other current risks the pregnant client may have (see the Risk Factors box).

Family History

In addition to the family history described in Chapter 3, a pregnant woman's family history should specifically address the childbearing history of her mother and sister(s), including multiple births, chromosome abnormalities such as Down syndrome, genetic disorders, congenital disorders, and

---

BOX 21-2 ESTIMATED DATE OF BIRTH (EDB)

Nagele's Rule
Determine the first day of the last menstrual period (LMP), subtract 3 months, and then add 7 days.

Example:

First day of LMP	= November 1
− 3 months	= August 1
+ 7 days	= August 8 EDB*

*Most women give birth during the period extending from 7 days before to 7 days after the EDB.

---

chronic illnesses such as diabetes mellitus or renal disease and cancer.

Gynecologic and Obstetric History

General information regarding the reproductive system, such as problems with menstruation, infections, painful intercourse, and sexual patterns, should be included (see Chapter 18).

The history includes information regarding the current and past pregnancies. Determine the exact date of the last menstrual period (LMP) to estimate expected delivery date (Box 21-2).

An obstetric history includes gravidity (G) (number of pregnancies, including current pregnancy); the number of full-term births (T); the number of preterm births (P); the number of abortions (A) (both spontaneous "miscarriages" and "therapeutic" pregnancy interruptions); and the number of living children (L). The acronym GTPAL may be of help in remembering this system of documentation (Table 21-2).

The obstetric history also includes specific data regarding each pregnancy. Document the following information:

- The course of each pregnancy (including the duration of gestation, date of delivery, and significant problems or complications)
- The process of labor (including manner in which labor was started [i.e., spontaneous or induced], length of labor, and complications associated with labor)
- The delivery (presentation of the infant, the method of delivery [i.e., vaginal or cesarean section], and pain management strategies used for delivery, if any)
- Condition of the infant at birth (including weight)
- Postpartum course (including any maternal or infant problems)

Personal and Psychosocial History

Attitude Toward the Pregnancy

Inquire how the woman and her partner feel about the pregnancy. Was it planned? What kind of expectations does she have regarding being pregnant, the process of labor, child-

---

TABLE 21-2 *Determining Gravidity and Parity Using a Five-Digit (GTPAL) System*

CONDITION	G GRAVIDA	T TERM BIRTH	P PRETERM BIRTH	A ABORTIONS	L LIVING CHILDREN
Woman pregnant for the first time	1	0	0	0	0
Woman who has carried her first pregnancy to term, and the infant survives	1	1	0	0	1
Woman who is currently pregnant for the second time; has one child from the first pregnancy born full term	2	1	0	0	1
Woman who has been pregnant twice; has one child who was born preterm and had one miscarriage	2	0	1	1	1
Woman who has been pregnant once and delivered full-term twins	1	1	0	0	2

Modified from Lowdermilk and Perry, 2007.

FOCUS ON PAIN *Childbirth*

Most women have some concerns about pain during the childbirth process. Green (1993) reported that 23% of women were "not at all worried" about such pain, 67% were a "bit worried," and 12% were "very worried." The discomfort and pain associated with childbirth are unique not only to each woman, but also as a pain experience in itself. Compared with other known painful events or experiences, the potential for achieving satisfactory pain relief is high because of the uniqueness of this pain experience (Reeder et al, 1997). Unique points include the following:

- The woman knows the pain will happen.
- The woman knows approximately when (within a week or so) the pain will happen.
- The woman knows there will be a predictable pattern to the pain.
- The woman knows there is a time limit to the pain experience (hours as opposed to days or weeks) and that it will end.
- The woman knows there is a tangible end product associated with the birth (i.e., the birth of her child).

birth, and parenthood? Explore if the client has any fear (such as fear of pain) regarding the pregnancy and delivery process (Box 21-3). Adjustments to parenthood such as role changes within the family should also be explored. Emotional stability data are collected, which includes the incidence of excessive crying, social withdrawal, or decisions related to infant care.

Nutritional History

A woman's nutritional status during pregnancy affects maternal and fetal health. An understanding of the woman's normal dietary practices is essential for nutritional assessment. Cultural diversity should be taken into account when evaluating dietary practices. Clients should be interviewed regarding food allergies or intolerance. Development of an individualized meal pattern may be necessary to ensure nutrient needs are met if the client must avoid particular foods or food groups. Lactose intolerance is a commonly reported problem.

Dietary assessment should also include questions regarding ingestion of nonnutritive substances known as pica. Clay, starch, baking soda, and dirt are some of the reported crav-

ETHNIC & CULTURAL VARIATIONS

Cultural diversity should be taken into account with dietary assessment. An understanding of how different foods are viewed is important. Specific foods may be considered healthful or harmful during pregnancy and lactation by some cultures. For instance, in some cultures, eating hot foods is believed to provide warmth for the fetus and enable the baby to be born into a warm, loving environment. Additionally, many cultural groups believe that certain cravings for foods should be met while pregnant to avoid harm to the baby (Purnell and Paulanka, 2003).

ings during pregnancy. To assess potentially harmful effects of eating nonnutritive substances, determine what is being ingested, the quantity, and the frequency.

Personal Habits

Some behaviors may contribute to a high risk pregnancy. The nurse identifies high-risk behaviors and targets these areas for teaching. Some of the specific habits to discuss are tobacco use, alcohol use, and drug use.

Tobacco use should be assessed. Smoking during pregnancy is associated with premature and low–birth-weight (LBW) infants. However, women who stop smoking by the sixteenth week of pregnancy minimize the increased risk of having an LBW infant (Maloni, 2001). Furthermore, smoking increases the need for vitamin C, a nutrient that has increased intake requirements during pregnancy. For these reasons, smoking is an important modifiable risk factor targeted by nursing interventions (Newburn-Cook et al, 2002). Researchers reported smoking cessation efforts among pregnant women is less successful among older women, those reporting Medicaid coverage, and those who had a partner/husband who also smoked (Ma, Goins, Pbert, & Ockene, 2005).

All pregnant women should be questioned about alcohol intake. Alcohol is a teratogen. No safe level of alcohol ingestion has been identified for the pregnant woman (Eustace et al, 2003). Advise the woman to avoid drinking alcoholic beverages entirely while pregnant. Fetal alcohol syndrome (birth defects in an infant born to a mother who consumed excessive amounts of alcohol during pregnancy) is a major public health problem.

The use of street drugs should also be explored with pregnant women. Many drugs are known teratogens (such as cocaine); others have significant long-term effects on the infant after birth. Stimulants may affect the client's appetite and therefore lead to decreased nutrient intake. Barbiturates and opiates may impair the client's desire and ability to obtain food; in fact, in some cases the client's resources may be used to obtain drugs instead of food. Clients who admit to drug use should be counseled and possibly be referred to a drug treatment program.

Environment

Pregnant women should be questioned about safety issues, including activities at work and in the home, routine safety practices such as use of seat belts while in a car, and the presence of physical abuse and violence in the home.

Review of Systems

The health history also includes questions related to body systems. Following is an outline of common symptoms organized by body systems. Conduct a symptom analysis (onset, location, duration, characteristics, aggravating and alleviating factors, related symptoms, and treatment measures) to further assess the symptom (see Box 3-3 in Chapter 3).

Fetal assessments

- Report of fetal movements; frequency, time of day

Integumentary system
- Skin marks, lines, varicosities
- Pruritus

Nose and mouth
- Nose bleeding or stuffiness
- Gum bleeding or swelling

Ears
- Changes in hearing
- Sense of fullness in ears

Eyes
- Excessive dryness
- Visual changes

Respiratory system
- Shortness of breath

Cardiovascular system
- Palpitations
- Edema of extremities
- Orthostatic hypotension (dizziness when standing up)

Breasts
- Enlargement, engorgement, tenderness
- Nipple discharge

Gastrointestinal system
- Nausea, vomiting (morning sickness), loss of appetite, food aversions
- Heartburn (gastric reflex), epigastric pain (second and third trimesters)
- Constipation (second and third trimesters)
- Hemorrhoids (second and third trimesters)

Genitourinary system
- Urinary pain, frequency, and urgency
- Vaginal discharge or bleeding

Musculoskeletal system
- Backache
- Leg cramps

Neurologic system
- Headaches

HEALTH PROMOTION   *Maternal-Infant Health*

Prenatal care can contribute to reductions in maternal and perinatal illness, disability, and death by identifying and minimizing potential risks and helping women to address behavioral factors, such as smoking and alcohol use, that contribute to poor outcomes. Major maternal complications of pregnancy include hemorrhage, ectopic pregnancy, pregnancy-induced hypertension, embolism, and infection. The maternal mortality rate among African American women consistently has been three to four times that of white women. Prematurity and low birth weight (LBW) are among the leading causes of neonatal death. LBW is also associated with long-term disabilities.

Goals and Objectives—*Healthy People 2010*

The *Healthy People 2010* goal related to maternal-fetal health is to improve the health and well-being of women, infants, children, and families.

Recommendations to Reduce Risk (Primary Prevention)
American College of Obstetricians and Gynecologists (ACOG)
- Counsel pregnant women about eating healthy diet; encourage all women planning or capable of pregnancy to take daily multivitamins with folic acid to reduce risk of neural tube defects.
- Encourage healthy body weight during pregnancy.
- Encourage regular exercise while pregnant.
- Counsel clients regarding need to abstain from smoking, drug use, and alcohol use while pregnant. Remind clients that over-the-counter medications are potentially harmful and to consult with health care provider.
- Counsel clients to avoid exposure to chemicals while pregnant.

Screening Recommendations (Secondary Prevention)
U.S. Preventive Services Task Force
- *Ultrasound:* It is unknown if routine ultrasound examination of the fetus in the second trimester is beneficial in low-risk pregnant women. Routine third-trimester ultrasound examination is not recommended.
- *Preeclampsia:* Recommends screening for preeclampsia with blood pressure measurement in all pregnant women at first prenatal visit and throughout pregnancy.
- *Rh incompatibility:* Recommends Rh typing and antibody screening for all pregnant women at first prenatal visit. Repeat screening is recommended at 24 to 28 weeks of gestation for unsensitized Rh-negative women.
- *Down syndrome:* Recommends offering amniocentesis or chorionic villus sampling for chromosome studies for pregnant women age 35 or older and those at high risk for having a Down syndrome infant.
- *Neural tube defects:* Recommends offering screening for neural tube defects by maternal serum alphafetoprotein measurement at 16 to 18 weeks of gestation.
- *Gestational diabetes:* Research has been inconclusive regarding routine screening for gestational diabetes.
- *Bacterial vaginosis (BV):* Recommends against routinely screening average-risk asymptomatic pregnant women for BV; it is unknown if screening high-risk asymptomatic pregnant women is beneficial.
- *Fetal monitoring:* Fetal monitoring in low-risk women is not recommended. It is unknown if routine electronic fetal monitoring for high-risk women in labor results in a difference in long-term outcomes.
- *Home uterine activity monitoring (HUAM):* HUAM is not recommended in normal-risk pregnancies; it is unknown if HUAM has long-term benefits in high-risk pregnancies.

Data from American College of Obstetricians and Gynecologists website (available at *www.acog.org*); US Department of Health and Human Services: *Healthy People 2010: understanding and improving health,* ed 2, Washington, DC, 2000, US Government Printing Office (available at *www.healthypeople.gov*); US Preventive Services Task Force: *Guide to clinical preventive services,* ed 2, 1996 (available at *www.ahrq.gov*).

EXAMINATION

PROCEDURES AND TECHNIQUES WITH NORMAL FINDINGS

Positioning of the pregnant client for examination purposes is the same as discussed in previous chapters, with one exception: Be sure not to position the pregnant woman flat on her back for an extended length of time.

VITAL SIGNS AND BASELINE MEASUREMENTS

MEASURE temperature, blood pressure, pulse, and respiration.

Vital signs are measured with every visit.
Pulse: The heart rate increases as much as 10 to 15 beats per minute.
Respiration: Respiratory rate may increase slightly, especially during the third trimester; the client may also experience shortness of breath.
Blood pressure: Document blood pressure trends throughout pregnancy. Blood pressure should remain fairly consistent during pregnancy. It may decrease slightly in the second trimester and then return to the usual level during the third trimester. Because position affects blood pressure readings, it is essential to use a consistent method and position of blood pressure measurement throughout pregnancy.

MEASURE height and weight.

Height should be measured on the first visit. Weight should be measured with every visit. Prepregnancy weight may give the clinician insight into the woman's nutritional status. On the initial visit, complete a weight-for-height assessment to determine if the weight is within or outside ideal weight range. Calculate a body mass index to determine an appropriate weight gain goal for pregnancy.

Evaluate the rate of weight change at each prenatal visit in addition to assessment of overall weight change. Expected patterns of weight gain are presented in Box 21-4. Generally, a total weight gain of 25 to 35 lb (11.4 to 16 kg) is associated with positive pregnancy outcome for women with normal prepregnancy weight. Underweight women should gain more weight, whereas overweight women should gain somewhat less weight.

BOX 21-4	EXPECTED WEIGHT GAIN DURING PREGNANCY	
First trimester	3-5 lb (1.6-2.3 kg)	
Second trimester	12-15 lb (5.5-6.8 kg)	⎤ Additional pounds
Third trimester	12-15 lb (5.5-6.8 kg)	⎦

ABNORMAL FINDINGS

Excessive shortness of breath and dyspnea are of concern and may indicate pulmonary complications such as embolus. Preexisting hypertension in pregnancy significantly increases risk of preterm delivery and infant mortality. Pregnancy-induced hypertension (PIH) is a serious disorder that requires prompt and close medical management. It is characterized by systolic blood pressure of at least 140 mm Hg, or a rise of 30 mm Hg or more above the usual level in two readings 6 hours apart, or diastolic blood pressure of 90 mm Hg or more, or a rise of 15 mm Hg above baseline in two readings done 6 hours apart.

A prepregnancy BMI over 29 increases the risk of both inadequate and excessive weight gain during pregnancy (Wells, Schwalberg, Noonan, and Gabor, 2006). A rapid increase in weight could indicate multiple gestation, preeclampsia, or diabetes associated with pregnancy (gestational diabetes). If a woman gains more than 2 lb (0.9 kg) in any 1 week or more than 6 lb (2.7 kg) in 1 month, preeclampsia should be suspected (Cunningham et al, 2005). Preeclampsia is described further later in the chapter. During the first trimester, a weight loss of up to 5 lb (2.3 kg) may be caused by nausea and vomiting. Poor weight gain or weight loss may be associated with a small for gestational age (SGA) infant or more serious complications such as placental dysfunction or fetal death in utero. LBW infants have more health problems than normal-weight infants and represent the largest group of infants who die during the first year of life (Maloni, 2001).

| **PROCEDURES AND TECHNIQUES WITH NORMAL FINDINGS** | **ABNORMAL FINDINGS** |

EXAMINATION OF THE EXTREMITIES

INSPECT the hands and nails for color and surface characteristics, movement, and sensation.

Pinkish red blotches or diffuse mottling of the hands due to an increase in estrogen is termed *palmar erythema* and is considered a normal finding. The client's nails may become thin and brittle. Women who take prenatal vitamins may report fast-growing, strong nails. Movement and sensation of fingers and hands should remain the same.

Some pregnant clients may periodically report numbness of the fingers, caused by a brachial plexus traction syndrome (caused by drooping shoulders associated with increased breast size and weight). A carpal tunnel syndrome caused by compression of the median nerve in the wrist and the hand may lead to symptoms of numbness, tingling, burning, and impaired finger movement. This most typically affects the thumb and the second and third fingers.

INSPECT and PALPATE the lower extremities for edema, surface characteristics, redness, and tenderness.

Edema in the lower extremities is seen almost universally during the later stages of pregnancy. Typically, women notice edema late in the day or after long periods of standing. Palpation of the legs helps to determine the extent of the edema. Vascular spiders or varicosities may appear on the lower legs and thighs and are considered normal findings. The legs should be free from redness and tenderness.

Although some edema is considered normal, excessive edema (particularly if noted in the hands and face in addition to the lower extremities) is considered pathologic and may be an indication of PIH. Edema not associated with preeclampsia or normal lower-extremity swelling should be evaluated for adequate protein intake. Redness in the legs, particularly if accompanied by tenderness, may be an indication of thrombophlebitis.

EXAMINATION OF THE HEAD

INSPECT the head and face for skin characteristics, pigmentation, and edema.

Blotchy, brownish pigmentation of the face—chloasma, or the mask of pregnancy—is a normal finding. There should be no facial edema. Fine, lanugo-type hair may be observed on the face and is a normal finding.

Facial edema is considered an abnormal finding and should be reported.

INSPECT the eyes and TEST vision for acuity.

The eye examination should proceed as discussed in Chapter 11. Findings generally remain the same; however, the eyelids of some women may darken from melanin pigment. Visual acuity should be tested with the first visit to establish a baseline. Visual checks should be repeated if the client verbalizes a change in vision during the pregnancy. Contact lenses may be uncomfortable to wear because of increased dryness. Both eyesight and the corrective prescription may change.

PIH may cause blurred vision. Chromatopsia may be noted, characterized by unusual color perception, seeing spots, or blindness in the lateral visual field. This requires immediate follow-up. Retinal arteriole constriction, disc edema, and retinal detachment (which is an emergency) are concerns; these may be caused by PIH. Pale conjunctivae may indicate anemia.

PROCEDURES AND TECHNIQUES WITH NORMAL FINDINGS	ABNORMAL FINDINGS

INSPECT the ears, nose, and mouth.

The examination of the ears, nose, and mouth should proceed as discussed in Chapter 11. Findings generally are the same as previously discussed for the adult. However, the nurse may note an increase in vascularization of the external ear, the auditory canal, and the tympanic membrane. The nose and mouth of the pregnant woman also are associated with an increase in vascularization, causing redness in the nose, pharynx, and gums; the gums become edematous, spongy, and may bleed easily. A hypertrophied gum lesion, known as an epulis, is a raised nodule that may be seen toward the end of the third trimester.

> Some women develop a pregnancy-induced tumor in the mouth. Any growth in the mouth is an abnormal finding.

INSPECT and PALPATE the neck.

The examination of the neck and thyroid should proceed as discussed in Chapter 11. Findings generally are the same as previously discussed. There may be transient thyroid enlargement that makes the thyroid more easily palpable, but this will disappear following delivery.

> Excessive or asymmetric enlargement of the thyroid gland or nodules on the thyroid gland are abnormal findings.

EXAMINATION OF THE ANTERIOR AND POSTERIOR CHEST

INSPECT, AUSCULTATE, PERCUSS, and PALPATE the anterior and posterior chest.

The examination of the anterior and posterior chest proceeds as discussed in Chapters 12 and 13. If the client is near term or has difficulty breathing when lying down, perform chest examination when the client is in a sitting position.

The breathing pattern changes from abdominal to costal or lateral; likewise, the breathing pattern may be shallow with an increased respiratory rate. A wide thoracic cage and increased costal angle may be noted. Diaphragmatic excursion may decrease secondary to the growing fetus.

The heart shifts laterally in response to the positions of the uterus and diaphragm (Fig. 21-1). The point of maximum impulse also shifts upward and rotates slightly to the left. Murmurs, splitting of S_1 and S_2, and the presence of S_3 may be heard after the twentieth week of gestation.

> Abnormal findings as discussed in Chapters 12 and 13 also apply to the pregnant client. Dyspnea, orthopnea, fatigue, and palpitations may be attributed to the pregnancy but should be evaluated for other causes. Preexisting cardiac conditions may have pronounced symptoms because of the increased blood volume. Note any signs of heart failure. Note low blood pressure or tachycardia occurring during this period.

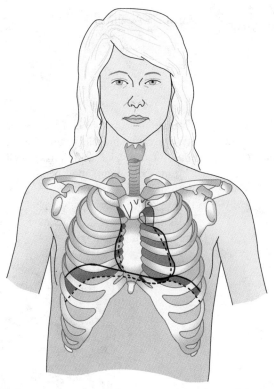

Fig. 21-1   Changes in position of heart, lungs, and thoracic cage during pregnancy. *Broken line,* nonpregnant; *solid line,* changes during pregnancy. *(From Lowdermilk and Perry, 2007.)*

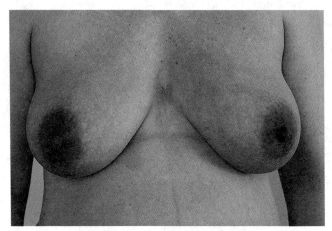

Fig. 21-2   Enlarged breasts in pregnancy with venous network and darkened areolae and nipples. *(From Seidel et al, 2007.)*

PROCEDURES AND TECHNIQUES WITH NORMAL FINDINGS	ABNORMAL FINDINGS

EXAMINATION OF THE BREAST

INSPECT and PALPATE the breast for surface and tissue characteristics.

Examine the breasts as described in Chapter 17. During the first trimester the breasts become fuller and have transient tenderness. As the pregnancy advances, the breasts increase in size and striae may develop. A subcutaneous venous pattern may be seen as a network of blue tracings across the breasts (Fig. 21-2). Palpation of the breasts reveals fullness and coarse nodularity. Following delivery, breast engorgement peaks at about the third to fifth day. Engorged breasts may be very uncomfortable and painful. This is more pronounced in women who are not breastfeeding.

Note any asymmetry or appearance of attachment (fixation), bulging, or retraction of either breast. Abnormal findings during the breast palpation include masses or isolated areas of tenderness or pain.

INSPECT and PALPATE the nipples for surface characteristics and nipple shape.

During the first trimester the nipples may become somewhat flattened or inverted. The areolae become darker and Montgomery's tubercles may appear. The nipples should be assessed in preparation for breast-feeding. Press on the nipple just behind the areola to express any discharge and note whether the nipple protracts or inverts. Following the first trimester, colostrum may be expressed from the breast (a yellowish discharge).

Thickening of the nipple tissue, a mass, and loss of elasticity are signs consistent with malignancy. Nipple discharge is considered an abnormal finding (except for expression of colostrum as described).

PROCEDURES AND TECHNIQUES WITH NORMAL FINDINGS

EXAMINATION OF THE MUSCULOSKELETAL SYSTEM

INSPECT and PALPATE the spine, extremities, and joints.

Examination of the musculoskeletal system proceeds as described in Chapter 15. Changes that are expected during pregnancy include progressive lordosis, anterior cervical flexion, kyphosis, and slumped shoulders (Fig. 21-3). A characteristic "waddling" gait develops at the end of pregnancy.

Exaggerated posture or excessive activity can cause muscle strain. Preexisting musculoskeletal conditions (such as chronic back pain) may become worse both during the pregnancy and after delivery. Muscle cramps, numbness, and weakness of the extremities are considered abnormal findings.

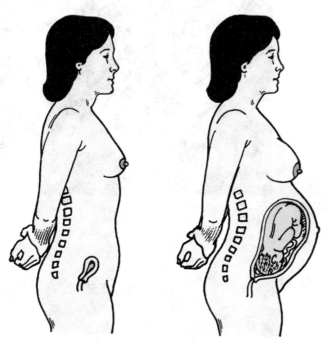

Fig. 21-3 Lordosis during pregnancy. *(From Lowdermilk and Perry, 2007.)*

EXAMINATION OF THE NEUROLOGIC SYSTEM

EXAMINE the client for neurologic changes.

Examine the client as described in Chapter 16. Although the examination proceeds as for other adults, pregnancy alters balance. Assessment of reflexes may also provide valuable data if the nurse suspects eclampsia.

Seizures or increased frequency of seizures associated with pregnancy are abnormal. Other abnormal findings are signs of myasthenia gravis, carpal tunnel syndrome (burning, pain, tingling in hand, wrist, or elbow), or hand numbness as a result of brachial plexus traction. These conditions return to prepregnant state after delivery. Hyperreflexia is an abnormal finding that may indicate eclampsia.

| PROCEDURES AND TECHNIQUES WITH NORMAL FINDINGS | ABNORMAL FINDINGS |

EXAMINATION OF THE ABDOMEN

INSPECT the abdomen for surface characteristics and fetal movement.

Common changes to the skin on the abdomen are linea nigra (Fig. 21-4), striae gravidarum, and venous patterns. After the twenty-eighth week, fetal movements may be observed.

Absence of fetal movement could indicate fetal demise.

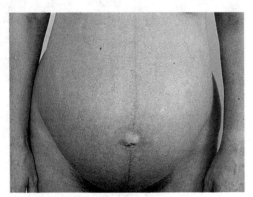

Fig. 21-4   Linea nigra on abdomen. *(From Seidel et al, 2006.)*

PALPATE the abdomen for fetal movement and uterine contraction.

The mother should report fetal movements (also known as quickening) by approximately 20 weeks of gestation. Fetal movement and uterine contraction can be evaluated by placing the hands directly on the abdomen.

MEASURE the fundus for height.

Measure fundal height from the top of the symphysis pubis to the top of the fundus (Fig. 21-5). From the twentieth to thirty-sixth week of gestation, the expected pattern of uterine growth is an increase in fundal height of about 1 cm per week (Fig. 21-6). Uterine size should roughly correlate with gestational age. Any discrepancy greater than 2 cm between fundal height and the estimate of gestational age (based on last menstrual period) should be evaluated further. It is important to note that measurement of fundal height is an estimate and may vary among examiners by 1 to 2 cm.

A uterus that is larger than expected may be due to inaccurate dating of the pregnancy, more than one fetus, gestational diabetes, or polyhydramnios (excessive fluid in the uterus). A uterus that is smaller than expected for gestational age may be due to inaccurate dating of the pregnancy or growth retardation of the fetus.

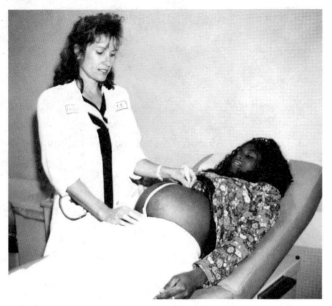

Fig. 21-5   Measuring fundal height. *(Courtesy Marjorie Pyle, RNC, Lifecircle.)*

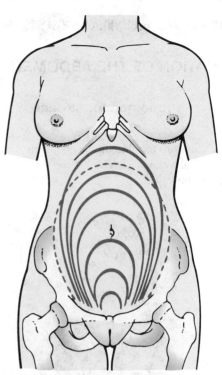

Fig. 21-6   Changes in fundal height during pregnancy. Weeks 1 through 12, the uterus is within the pelvis. Weeks 36 through 40, fundal height drops as the fetus begins to engage in the pelvis (lightening). *(From Seidel et al, 2006.)*

PROCEDURES AND TECHNIQUES WITH NORMAL FINDINGS

AUSCULTATE the abdomen for fetal heart sounds.

Auscultation of fetal heart tones is performed by use of a Doppler ultrasonic stethoscope after 10 to 12 weeks of gestation or with a fetoscope after 17 to 19 weeks (Fig. 21-7). The fetal heart rate is usually heard over the lower abdomen for fetuses that are in a head-down position. The expected fetal heart rate ranges between 120 and 160 beats/min. (The Doppler and fetoscope are discussed in Chapter 4.)

ABNORMAL FINDINGS

Increases and decreases in fetal heart rate can be caused by multiple factors stressing the fetus. A fetal heart rate over 160 beats/min or below 120 beats/min requires further investigation. Absence of fetal heart tones is always abnormal and usually indicates fetal demise.

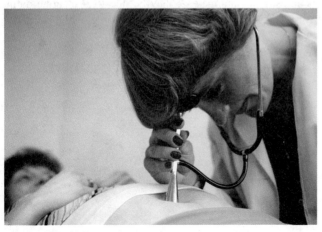

Fig. 21-7   Auscultating fetal heart tones with a fetoscope.

PROCEDURES AND TECHNIQUES WITH NORMAL FINDINGS

ABNORMAL FINDINGS

★ **PALPATE fetal position for fetal lie and presentation, position, and attitude.**

The outline of the fetus can be determined after 26 to 28 weeks through a technique known as Leopold's maneuvers (Fig. 21-8). The client should be lying supine, with head slightly elevated and knees flexed slightly. The fetal lie, presentation, position, and attitude can be determined through these maneuvers. See Table 21-3 for description of these terms.

Fundal palpation: This is done to determine what part of the fetus is at the fundus. Typically, the feet or buttocks are at the fundus. The buttocks feel firm, but not hard, and slightly irregular. If the head is at the fundus, you will palpate a firm, movable part (Fig. 21-8, *A*).

Lateral palpation: Palpate the sides of the uterus to identify the spine of the fetus. It is smooth and convex, compared with the irregular feel on the other side of the fetus—the hands, elbows, knees, and feet (Fig. 21-8, *B*).

Symphysis pubis palpation: This is done to assess which part of the fetus is in or just above the pelvic inlet and helps to determine if the presenting part is engaged. Gently grasp the presenting anatomic part over the symphysis pubis using your dominant hand. If the head is the presenting part, it will feel very smooth, round, and firm. If it is movable from side to side and you are able to

Inability to palpate the fetal position could be associated with polyhydramnios. A fetus with breech presentation or a transverse lie before delivery is of concern because of higher risks during the labor and delivery process.

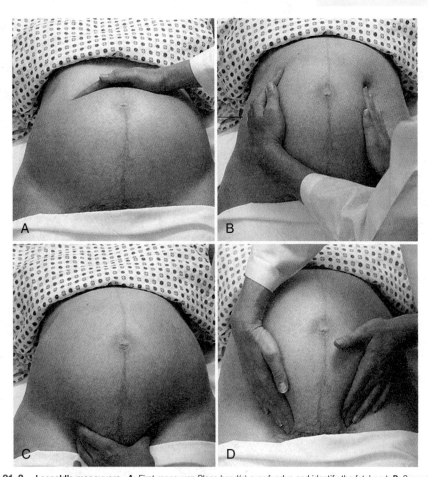

Fig. 21-8   Leopold's maneuvers. A, First maneuver. Place hand(s) over fundus and identify the fetal part. **B,** Second maneuver. Use the palmar surface of one hand to locate the back of the fetus. Use the other hand to feel the irregularities such as hands and feet. **C,** Third maneuver. Use thumb and third finger to grasp presenting part over the symphysis pubis. **D,** Fourth maneuver. Use both hands to outline the fetal head. With a head presenting deep in the pelvis, only a small portion may be felt. *(From Seidel et al, 2003.)*

★ = advanced practice

TABLE 21-3   *Fetal Assessment Terms*

TERM	Illustration

Fetal Lie

The lie is the relationship of the long axis of the fetus to the long axis of the uterus. **A,** Longitudinal lie. **B,** Oblique lie. **C,** Transverse lie.

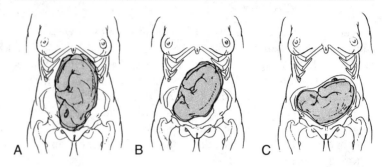

A   B   C

Presentation

The presentation is determined by the fetal lie and by the body part of the fetus that enters the pelvic passage first. The presentation may be vertex, brow, face, shoulder, or breech. **A,** Vertex. **B,** Brow. **C,** Face. **D,** Shoulder. **E,** Breech.

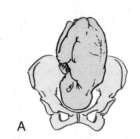 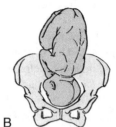 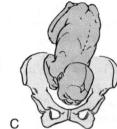

A   B   C

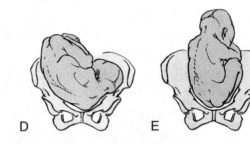

D   E

Position

Position refers to the relationship of the landmark on the presenting fetal part to the front, sides, or back of the maternal pelvis. The landmark on the fetal presenting part is related to four imaginary quadrants of the pelvis: left anterior, right anterior, left posterior, and right posterior. These quadrants indicate whether the presenting part is directed toward the front, back, left, or right of the pelvic passage. **A,** Left occiput anterior. **B,** Left occiput transverse. **C,** Left occiput posterior.

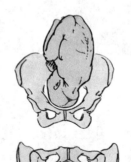 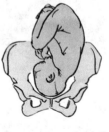 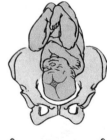

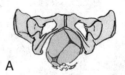 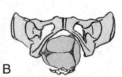 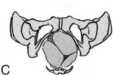

A   B   C

Attitude

The attitude is the relationship of the fetal head and limbs to the body. **A,** Fully flexed. **B,** Poorly flexed. **C,** Extended.

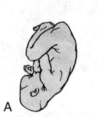 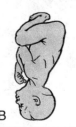 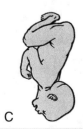

A   B   C

PROCEDURES AND TECHNIQUES WITH NORMAL FINDINGS	**ABNORMAL FINDINGS**

palpate all the way around it, the head is not engaged in the pelvis. If engaged, the head is not movable and is below the level of the symphysis, preventing palpation all the way around the head. The presenting part could also be the buttocks. The buttocks feel softer and irregular (Fig. 21-8, *C*).

Deep pelvic palpation: If the head is the presenting part, palpation allows you to determine the position and attitude (Fig. 21-8, *D*). Use both hands to identify the outline of the fetal head. Depending on the fetal position, the cephalic prominence can be either the forehead or the occiput.

EXAMINATION OF THE GENITALIA

INSPECT the external and internal genitalia for general appearance and discharge.

Follow the guidelines described in Chapter 18. By the second month of pregnancy, the cervix, vagina, and vulva take on a bluish color (Chadwick's sign), and there will be increased vaginal secretions.

Note presence of infection of genitalia, including lesions or vaginal discharge with a foul odor. Leakage of watery fluid may be associated with preterm labor. During early pregnancy, slight bleeding may occur for unknown reasons and be of no consequence, or it could indicate an impending abortion. During late pregnancy, bleeding could be caused by abruptio placentae or placenta previa (discussed later in this chapter). Bleeding should never be considered a normal finding in pregnancy and should always be investigated thoroughly.

★ **PALPATE the cervix to determine length (effacement) and dilation.**

This procedure is done near the expected date of delivery and once labor begins. The cervix should not efface until about the thirty-sixth week. The cervical os should remain closed until near delivery. During the last 4 weeks the cervix shortens (known as effacement) as the fetal head descends. The cervical os softens and is pulled upward, becoming incorporated into the isthmus of the uterus. As the cervix shortens, it also begins to dilate. Cervical dilation is measured in centimeters from 0 cm, when completely closed, to 10 cm, when it is completely open. The effacement and dilation of the cervix is estimated by palpation of the cervix (Fig. 21-9).

Effacement and dilation of the cervix before the thirty-sixth week may result in premature delivery. Failure of the cervical os to efface and dilate impedes the progression of labor. If the cervix has inadequate effacement and dilation at the onset of delivery, trauma to the cervix often results.

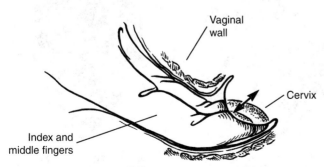

Fig. 21-9 Measurement of cervical length (effacement) and dilation. *(From Barkauskus et al, 2002.)*

★ = advanced practice

| PROCEDURES AND TECHNIQUES WITH NORMAL FINDINGS | ABNORMAL FINDINGS |

EXAMINATION OF THE RECTUM AND ANUS

INSPECT and PALPATE the anus and rectum.

The perianal and rectal examination should be carried out in the pregnant woman as described in Chapter 18. The rectum and anus are commonly examined while the client is in the lithotomy position with her legs up in stirrups. Early during pregnancy, the client should have minimal difficulty attaining and maintaining the position for the examination. Later in pregnancy, however, positioning for the rectal examination could be uncomfortable.

The presence of hemorrhoids, a common variation, is usually considered normal with pregnancy. The client may not have hemorrhoids during the early phase of pregnancy, but toward the last trimester the hemorrhoids may appear secondary to pressure on the pelvic floor or possible constipation with straining when having a bowel movement. The hemorrhoids may be either internal in the lower segment of the rectum or prolapsed as external hemorrhoids.

Presence of lesions or rectal bleeding is considered an abnormal finding.

COMMON PROBLEMS & CONDITIONS

ABRUPTIO PLACENTAE

The premature separation of the implanted placenta before the birth of the fetus is referred to as abruptio placentae (Fig. 21-10). This usually occurs during the third trimester, but it could occur as early as 20 weeks. The most important risk factor for abruptio placentae is maternal hypertension (Benedetti, 2002). Because it is the most common cause of intrapartum fetal death, abruptio placentae is considered an obstetric emergency. **Clinical Findings:** Bleeding, abdominal pain, and uterine contractions are the three classic features of this complication. The blood is usually described as dark red, and the pain can range from mild to excruciating.

PLACENTA PREVIA

A placenta attachment in the lower uterine segment near or over the cervical os, (as opposed to a more typical attachment higher in the uterus), is referred to as placenta previa. (Fig. 21-11). This condition is often associated with premature rupture of membranes, preterm birth, anemia, infections, and postpartum hemorrhage (Crane et al, 2000). **Clinical Findings:** The classic finding is painless vaginal bleeding most commonly during the third trimester, but bleeding can occur anytime after 24 weeks. In a small percentage of women, the bleeding is accompanied by mild uterine contractions. On palpation, the uterus is typically soft and nontender.

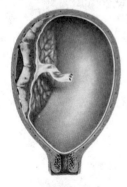

Partial separation
(concealed hemorrhage)

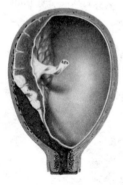

Partial separation
(apparent hemorrhage)

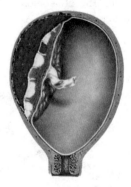

Complete separation
(concealed hemorrhage)

Fig. 21-10 Abruptio placentae. Premature separation of normally implanted placenta. *(From Lowdermilk and Perry, 2007.)*

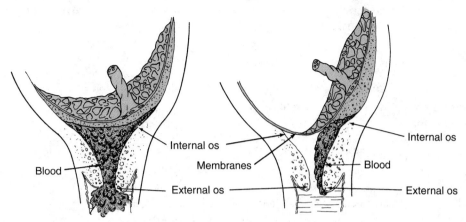

Fig. 21-11 Types of placenta previa after onset of labor. **A,** Complete, or total. **B,** Incomplete, or partial. *(From Lowdermilk and Perry, 2007.)*

HYDRAMNIOS (POLYHYDRAMNIOS)

An excessive quantity of amniotic fluid is referred to as hydramnios. This is common in pregnancies with more than one fetus. In single-fetus pregnancies, it is associated with fetal malformation of the central nervous system and gastrointestinal tract. Hydramnios may result in perinatal death from premature labor and fetal abnormalities. **Clinical Findings:** Excessive uterine size, tense uterine wall, difficulty palpating fetal parts, and difficulty hearing fetal heart tones are common findings associated with this condition. The woman may also experience dyspnea, edema, and discomfort caused by pressure on the surrounding organs.

PREGNANCY-INDUCED HYPERTENSION (PIH)

PIH involves a group of hypertensive conditions during pregnancy in a previously normotensive client. *Preeclampsia* refers to a condition of PIH with proteinuria and edema. *Eclampsia* is the occurrence of seizures precipitated by PIH in a preeclamptic client. **Clinical Findings:** Hypertension in pregnancy is defined as follows: Systolic blood pressure is 140 mm Hg or higher; *or* there is an increase of more than 30 mm Hg of systolic blood pressure from baseline in the first half of pregnancy; *or* diastolic blood pressure is more than 90 mm Hg; *or* there is an increase of more than 15 mm Hg of diastolic blood pressure from baseline (Sibai, 2007).

PREMATURE RUPTURE OF MEMBRANES

A spontaneous rupture of uterine membranes before the onset of labor is referred to as premature rupture of membranes (PROM). It can occur at any time during the pregnancy, but this is usually seen with term pregnancy. This situation is associated with a high risk of perinatal and maternal morbidity and mortality. The cause of PROM is not known, although infection and hydramnios are thought to be associated factors. **Clinical Findings:** PROM manifests as passage of amniotic fluid from the vagina before labor.

CLINICAL APPLICATION & CLINICAL REASONING

See Appendix E for answers to exercises in this section.

REVIEW QUESTIONS

1 The nurse specifically assesses for which of the following data on every prenatal visit?
   1 Blood pressure.
   2 Diastasis recti.
   3 Personal habits (smoking, alcohol consumption).
   4 Visual acuity.

2 Which of the following, identified during an initial prenatal visit, is consistent with a high-risk pregnancy?
   1 Client is 18 years old.
   2 Client height is 5 feet 4 inches.
   3 Birth weight of infant with last pregnancy was 2800 g.
   4 Client smokes one-half pack of cigarettes a day.

3 A client with a missed menstrual period and nausea has which of the following signs of pregnancy?
1 Questionable.
2 Presumptive.
3 Probable.
4 Positive.

4 The nurse measures from the symphysis pubis to the top of the fundus in order to:
1 Measure fetal development.
2 Determine fetal lie and position.
3 Calculate the attitude of the fetus.
4 Estimate gestational age.

5 Which of the following is considered an abnormal finding associated with late pregnancy?
1 Watery vaginal discharge.
2 Hemorrhoids.
3 Lordosis.
4 Abdominal striae.

SAMPLE DOCUMENTATION

Review the following data obtained during an interview and examination by the nurse below:

Jenny Garner is a 23-year-old African-American woman who comes to the women's health clinic for a prenatal visit. She states that her last menstrual period was 10 weeks ago, on March 4. She performed a home pregnancy test 2 weeks ago and it was positive. Jenny is married, has a healthy 3-year-old son, and is a stay-at-home mother. She states that this planned pregnancy is the second time she has been pregnant; she has never had an abortion or a miscarriage. Her last pregnancy was without complications; her baby was full-term and had an uncomplicated vaginal delivery. Jenny reports having a great deal of nausea and loss of appetite since becoming pregnant. She states that she has had a 2 lb weight loss in the last 2 weeks. Measured height is 5 feet 4 inches, measured weight is 154 lb. Jenny currently smokes one-half pack of cigarettes a day and states that she knows this is bad for her pregnancy; she states that she wants to quit smoking while she is pregnant to improve the health of her baby. She admits to occasional alcohol intake but reports that during pregnancy she avoids alcohol completely. She denies illicit drug use. Jenny states that she has never had any medical problems and takes no medications except for a multivitamin tablet every day—she started this the day she found out she was pregnant. She states that she has never had an allergic reaction to any medication. Her temperature is 98.3° F (36.8° C); her pulse rate is 82 beats/min, her respiratory rate is 18/min, and her blood pressure is 114/76 mm Hg. Her skin is warm, dry, with no lesions. Her hair is clean and full. She has elastic skin turgor. She has pink, moist gums with no lesions. There are positive bowel sounds on auscultation, and her abdomen is soft and nontender. Her uterus is not palpable. Her vaginal examination is unremarkable except for a bluish hue to her cervix and vulva and slight enlargement of the cervix. She does not have any swelling of her legs or feet.

Below, note how the nurse recorded these same data in a documentation format.

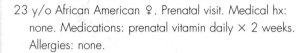

23 y/o African American ♀. Prenatal visit. Medical hx: none. Medications: prenatal vitamin daily × 2 weeks. Allergies: none.

SUBJECTIVE DATA
J. G. reports she is pregnant; LMP March 4 (10 weeks ago); + home pregnancy test 2 weeks ago. Planned pregnancy; G2, T0, P0, A0, L1; last pregnancy uncomplicated with vaginal delivery. Married with healthy 3 y/o son; does not work. Reports nausea and ↓ appetite; reports 2 lb wt loss in last 2 weeks. J. G. smokes one-half pack cigarettes/day; indicates desire to quit smoking. Reports no ETOH use during pregnancy; denies illicit drug use.

OBJECTIVE DATA
General survey: Vital signs: T 98.3° F (36.8° C); BP 114/76; HR 82; RR 18. Ht 5 feet 4 inches; wt 154 lb; BMI 25.5.
Skin: Warm, dry, no lesions; hair clean, full head of hair, elastic turgor.
Mouth: No lesions; mucous membranes pink, moist.
Abdomen: soft, nontender, + bowel sounds; uterus not palpable.
Pelvic examination: Within normal limits; + Chadwick's; + Goodell's.
Lower extremities: No edema.

CASE STUDY

Kristin is a 17-year-old pregnant client (G_1, T_0, P_0, A_0, L_0) who is in her thirtieth week of pregnancy. She comes to the clinic for a routine prenatal visit. The following data are collected by the nurse.

Interview Data

Kristin tells the nurse, "I have been feeling pretty good the last few weeks, but I have noticed I'm getting so puffy in my feet, hands, and face. I feel like I'm full of water." When asked about other symptoms or problems, Kristin responds, "I have a backache sometimes." Kristin indicates that she feels the baby move "all the time now." She conveys to the nurse that she is excited about the baby but is very worried about how bad the labor pain will be. "My friend Shawna told me the pain is so bad that I will want to be knocked out when it is time to have the baby."

Examination Data

- *Vital signs:* Blood pressure, 154/96 mm Hg (prepregnancy blood pressure reading, 114/70 mm Hg—within normal limits up until this visit); pulse, 92 beats/min; respiration rate, 18; temperature, 98.3° F (36.8° C).
- *Weight:* 152 lb (prepregnancy weight, 116 lb). She has had an increase of 10 lb in last month.
- *Fundal height:* 31 cm.
- *Urine dipstick:* 3+ protein.

Clinical Reasoning

1. What data deviate from normal findings, suggesting a need for further investigation?
2. What additional information should the nurse ask or assess for?
3. Based on the data, what risk factors for high-risk pregnancy does this client have?
4. What nursing diagnoses and collaborative problems should be considered for this situation?

INTERACTIVE ACTIVITIES

Open the interactive student CD-ROM, click on Chapter 21, and choose from the following activities on the menu bar:

- **Multiple Choice Challenge.** Click on the best answer for each question. You will be given immediate feedback, rationale for each incorrect answer, and a total score. Good luck!

- **Marvelous Matches.** Drag each word or phrase to the appropriate place on the screen. Test your ability to match the clinical finding to the clue.

- **Risk Factors.** Review this client's history and identify risk factors. Complete your assessment by deciding which risk factors are modifiable and which are nonmodifiable. You only get one shot, so choose carefully!

- **Printable Lab Guide.** Locate the Lab Guide for Chapter 21, and print and use it (as many times as needed) to help you apply your assessment skills. These guides may also be filled in electronically and then saved and e-mailed to your instructor!

- **Quick Challenge.** Use this critical thinking exercise to assess your skills through case study-style questions, then compare with expert answers!

CHAPTER 22

Assessment of the Older Adult

Aging is a normal developmental process that begins at conception. There is no specific age at which one becomes old: everyone ages at a different rate. Biologic, social, and functional ages are more important than chronological age. A suggested classification based on age is shown below (Lueckenotte, 2000):

Young-old	65-74 years
Middle-old	75-84 years
Older-old	85 years and older

Approximately 13% of the U.S. population is age 65 years and older, the fastest growing age group in terms of percentage are those age 100 and older. By 2050 there may be 1.1 million people age 100 and older in the United States. Some sources suggest that as much as 75% of life expectancy can be explained by lifestyle and 25% by genetics (Holmes and Dickson, 2007). Terms related to aging are described below:

- *Life expectancy*: the number of years one can be expected to live based on year of birth or current age. In 1900 it was 47 years, while in 1950 it increased to 68 years. In 2005 the life expectancy for women was 80.1 years and for men it was 74.8 years, with an average of 77.5 years. By 2040, life expectancy is predicted to be 91.5 years for women and 86 years for men.
- *Life span*: the number of years that human beings are probably capable of living (estimated to be about 110-120).
- *Ageism* is a negative, prejudiced view of aging based on lack of correct facts.

Being physically, mentally, and socially active into the 100s is considered normal. High blood pressure, pain, urinary incontinence, and severe memory loss are not a part of normal aging. While aging is not a disease, the incidence of chronic health problems increases with advanced age. Therefore, it is essential to know the difference between normal aging and disease and not assume that clinical manifestations of disease are caused by age alone. Healthy lifestyle behaviors such as nutrition, regular exercise, and sleep are very important and it is never too late to improve them.

ANATOMY & PHYSIOLOGY

As adults grow older, they experience gradual changes in every body system. Thus, it is necessary to recognize the expected anatomic and physiologic changes of older adults and to understand how they may alter the functioning of clients in these age groups. Box 22-1 presents expected changes associated with older adults.

| BOX 22-1 | SELECTED ANATOMIC AND PHYSIOLOGIC CHANGES ASSOCIATED WITH OLDER ADULTS |

Mental health

- Emotional experiences of sadness, grief, response to loss, and temporary "blue" moods are normal responses in older adults. However, persistent depression that interferes significantly with ability to function is not an expected response (*www.nimh.nih.gov/publicat/elderlydepsuicide*).

Sleep

- The typical 80-year-old adult may take 18 to 20 minutes to fall asleep and sleep about six hours; about 80% of that time is spent sleeping, with a few minutes in deep REM sleep and about one hour dreaming.
- Older adults have more difficulty falling asleep, spend less time sleeping deeply, and report a greater number of early-morning awakenings (Cole & Richards, 2007).
- Frequency of nocturnal awakenings increases with age and may be caused by dyspnea, pain, coughing, noise, or the need to void.

Integument System

- Decreased sebaceous and sweat gland activity causes dry skin and less perspiration.
- The dermis loses elasticity, collagen, and mass, causing folding and wrinkling appearance (Lueckenotte, 2000).
- Subcutaneous fat distribution shifts from the face and extremities to the abdomen and hips. Decrease in subcutaneous and cutaneous tissue causes deepening in the hollows of the thoracic, axillary, and supraclavicular regions. These changes result in sharp, angular appearance of joints and bony prominences.
- Decreased melanin production tends to produce gray hair, and reduced hormonal functioning causes thinning of scalp, axillary, and pubic hair.
- The nails become thicker, brittle, hard, and yellowish; they also develop ridges and are prone to splitting into layers.

Head, Eyes, Ears, Nose, and Throat

- Tearing is diminished resulting in "dry eyes," which causes irritation and discomfort.
- Corneal sensitivity often is diminished so that older adults may be unaware of infection or injury. Corneal reflexes are often diminished or absent.
- As the lens becomes more rigid, usually by age 45, and the ciliary muscle of the iris weakens, the near point of accommodation changes. This loss of lens elasticity is termed *presbyopia*.
- Color perception is altered, with difficulty seeing blue, violet, and green (Lueckenotte, 2000).
- A decrease in active sebaceous glands causes the cerumen to become very dry; it may completely obstruct the external auditory canal, resulting in diminished hearing.
- Both conductive and sensorineural hearing losses occur with aging. *Conductive hearing loss* occurs when the tympanic membrane becomes more translucent and sclerotic. An excess deposit of bone cells along the ossicle chain can cause fixation of the stapes in the oval window, resulting in hearing loss. *Sensorineural hearing loss* develops as the hair cells in the organ of Corti begin to degenerate, usually after age 50. Hearing loss first occurs with high-frequency sounds and than progresses to lower-frequency tones.
- A decreased sense of smell is caused by a decrease in the number of sensory cells in the nasal lining.
- Gingival tissue is less elastic and more vulnerable to injury. Because of gingival recession, the root surfaces of the teeth are exposed to caries formation. Tooth enamel becomes harder and more brittle. As teeth lose their translucency, they darken and become worn from use.
- The tongue becomes more fissured. Older adults may have altered motor function of the tongue, leading to problems with swallowing. Taste perception may diminish due to gradual atrophy of the tongue and a decrease in the number of papillae and taste buds.
- Muscle weakness may result in chewing and swallowing difficulties.
- The size of the thyroid decreases due to atrophy.
- The client may have increased concave cervical curvature, causing forward and downward positioning of the head.
- Lymph nodes may decrease in both size and number with advanced age.

Respiratory System

- Kyphoscoliosis, a common finding associated with aging, causes the thorax to shorten and the AP diameter to increase.
- The chest wall may become stiffer, possibly because of calcification at rib articulation points resulting in decreased chest wall compliance.
- Diminished strength of the respiratory muscles results in reduced maximal inspiratory and expiratory force.

Continued

- As the alveoli become less elastic and more fibrous, dyspnea on exertion becomes more frequent.
- There are fewer cilia and the mucociliary clearance is less effective. Also, mucous membranes become drier and less able to clear retained mucus (Lueckenotte, 2000).

Cardiovascular System

- The heart size tends to decrease. Response to stress or increased oxygen demand is less efficient, and the return to baseline heart rate takes longer.
- Cardiac function is also affected by fibrosis and sclerosis of the SA node and mitral and aortic valves.

Gastrointestinal System

Many of the changes in the function of digestion and absorption of nutrients result from alterations in the cardiovascular and neurologic systems rather than the GI system.

- Motility of the entire GI system is slowed because of central and peripheral nervous system changes, causing a decrease in transit time through the intestines. Along with the decreased motility in the esophagus, there is a decrease in the lower esophageal pressure, resulting in increased likelihood of regurgitation.
- In the large intestine, weakened muscle and decreased peristalsis contribute to constipation. Bacterial flora in the intestines become less biologically active, contributing to food intolerance and impaired digestion.
- With increasing age, the rectal wall's afferent neurons degenerate, interfering with the ability to detect changes in rectal pressure and creating a decrease in internal sphincter tone in response to rectal distention. Some older adults experience reduced external sphincter control and may experience occasional fecal incontinence.
- The liver decreases in size after age 50, reducing its storage capacity and ability to synthesize proteins (Brozenee, 2000).
- The bladder decreases in size, shape, and muscle tone, which can cause more frequent urination and increase likelihood of stress incontinence.
- In men, the prostate gland atrophies with loss of function. A benign enlargement of the prostate associated with aging frequently occurs.

Musculoskeletal System

- A decrease in bone mass increases the risk for stress fractures. Intervertebral disks lose water, causing a narrowing of the disk space that results in a loss of height.

Height may decrease as much as six inches or more from ages 25 to 80. The lordotic or convex curve of the back flattens, and both flexion and extension of the back decrease. Increased flexion of the back changes the posture to a more flexed position, which in turn changes the center of gravity.

- Tendons and muscles decrease in elasticity and tone, with the muscles losing both mass and strength. This alteration in muscle tone and strength means the person may experience loss of agility.

Neurologic System

- Functional changes in sensory and motor function, memory, cognition, and proprioception occur at different rates. Short-term memory (e.g., of names and recent events) may decline with age, but long-term memory is usually maintained.

Reproductive System

Female Genitourinary System

- After menopause, the labia and clitoris become smaller and paler. The epithelial layers become thinner and flatter, losing their subcutaneous fat as a result of decreased estrogen.
- The vaginal introitus may diminish in size, with a shortening and narrowing of the vagina, and a thinning and drying of the vaginal mucosa. In some women the ligaments and connective tissue of the pelvis may lose their muscle tone and elasticity.
- The uterus and ovaries decrease in size; the ovarian follicles gradually disappear.

Male Genitourinary System

- Hyperplasia is the major change in the prostate associated with aging. If the prostate enlargement is excessive, a decrease or obstruction of urinary flow occurs.

Breast

- Before menopause, a moderate decrease in glandular breast tissue occurs. After menopause, the glandular tissue in the breast continues to atrophy and is replaced by fat and connective tissue.
- Changes to the breast tissue and the relaxation of the suspensory ligaments result in a tendency for the breast to hang more loosely from the chest wall, giving it a flattened appearance.

HEALTH HISTORY

RISK FACTORS *Older Adult*

As you conduct a health history related to the musculoskeletal system, it is important to consider common risk factors associated with this system and follow up with additional questions should risk factors exist.

Falls

The combination of visual deficits, loss of muscle strength, and slowed reaction time contributes to the increased risk of falls for older adults.

- Gender: Males have a higher risk
- Mental status: confusion, disorientation, depression
- Poor muscle strength and balance, dizziness, vertigo
- Altered elimination
- Adverse effect of medications
- Life style: alcohol consumption (M)

Malnutrition in Older Adults

- Institutionalized (nursing homes or hospitalization)
- Poverty
- Social isolation
- Chronic illnesses
- Alcoholism (M)
- Illness affecting mental capacities (depression, dementia)
- Decreased functional abilities—affecting food purchasing and preparation
- Anorexia
- Feeding problems—including chewing and swallowing problems
- Taking multiple medications

M = modifiable risk factor.

A complete assessment is essential for older adults as a part of preventive care as well as management of health-related problems. The health history for older adults is similar to that presented in Chapter 3. However, clinical manifestations may be vague and/or different from those that usually occur in younger adults. The most common and important differences in older people that may be noted on assessment are presented in this chapter.

When obtaining a health history from an older adult, seek information directly from the client first, if possible, rather than from relatives who may accompany the client. During the interview sit, if possible, so that eye contact is more direct and friendly. The client can also see the movements of the mouth, which helps if there is a hearing problem. Observe for hearing or vision deficits that will affect data collection.

GENERAL HEALTH HISTORY

Present Health Status

Data collected are the same as described in Chapter 3.

Past Health History

Data collected in this section are the same as described in Chapter 3. Note any chronic illnesses such as diabetes mellitus, osteoarthritis, cardiovascular, and neurologic conditions. The time span included in the history is, of course, longer, and the client's memory may affect accuracy. Review all medications the client is taking. Older adults often take many medications prescribed by more than one health care provider. Specifically ask about allergies and adverse effects with the medications and if the client has problems getting access to the drugs (because of financial or transportation restraints). Also ask about immunizations the client has had such as influenza and pneumococcal vaccines.

Family History

Although the family history provides data about illnesses and the causes of death of relatives, the value of this information for an older adult is questionable. A genogram is not routinely used to document the family history for an older adult.

Personal and Psychosocial History

Many of the aspects of personal and psychosocial history are the same as those previously described for the younger adult. However, there is a shift in focus in this section that reflects changes in roles and perceptions during the retirement years.

Personal Status

Ask the client for a general statement of feelings about self. Explore the following subjects: work/retirement concerns, reduced/fixed income, moving/selling home, living alone, and role changes.

Family and Social Relationships

Current living arrangements (family members, living alone); satisfaction with living arrangements; sufficient and satisfactory access to family and friends; presence of pet in home; participation in family activities and in family decisions; presence of conflict with family members; problems in relationship with spouse because of retirement.

Functional Ability

The functional ability or (functional assessment) focuses on a person's ability to perform self-care activities or basic activities of daily living (BADLs) and instrumental activities of daily living (IADLs) (Ebersole and Hess, 2001). BADLs include skills such as dressing, toileting, bathing, eating, and ambulating. The IADLs consist of skills that enable the client to function independently and include preparing meals, shopping, safe use of medications, management of finances, and ability to travel within the community. Ask the client (or other family member) to describe the client's ability (independent, partially independent, or dependent) to perform these activities. Box 22-2 provides detailed information regarding functional assessment.

BOX 22-2 **ACTIVITIES OF DAILY LIVING ASSESSMENT**

A. Self-care
1. Dressing, undressing, clothing
   a. Keeping clothes in good repair (mending)
   b. Accessing clothes
   c. Getting into and out of underwear (bra, girdle, underpants, pantyhose, stockings, garter belt)
   d. Putting on and removing pants
   e. Getting arms in sleeves
   f. Managing zippers, buttons, snaps (especially in back), ties
   g. Putting on socks, shoes, tying laces
   h. Applying prostheses (e.g., glasses, hearing aids)
2. Grooming and hygiene
   a. Washing, drying, brushing hair
   b. Brushing teeth
   c. Cleaning and putting in dentures
   d. Shaving
   e. Caring for nails (feet and hands)
   f. Applying makeup
   g. Preparing bathwater and testing temperature
   h. Getting into and out of tub, shower
   i. Reaching and cleaning all body parts
3. Elimination
   a. Position altered for urination or sitting on toilet
   b. Ability to wipe self
   c. Lowering onto and rising from toilet

B. Mobility
1. Difficulty climbing or descending stairs (Is bedroom or bathroom on upper level? How many stairs or flights to apartment or house?)
2. Sitting up and rising from bed
3. Lowering to or rising from chair
4. Walking (short and long distances); describe necessity for walking
5. Opening doors
6. Reaching items in cupboards
7. Necessity for lifting (and any difficulty)

C. Communication
1. Dialing telephone
2. Reading numbers
3. Hearing over telephone
4. Answering door
5. Immediate access to neighbors, help

D. Eating
1. Access to market
2. Preparing food (opening cans and packages, using stove, reaching dishes, pots, utensils)
3. Handling knife, fork, spoon (cutting meat)
4. Getting food to mouth
5. Chewing, swallowing

E. Housekeeping, laundry, house upkeep
1. Making bed
2. Sweeping, mopping floors
3. Dusting
4. Washing dishes
5. Cleaning tub, bathroom
6. Picking up clutter (to client's satisfaction)
7. Taking out trash, garbage
8. Use of basement (stairs, cleaning)
9. Laundry facilities (in home or near residence, washtub, clothesline)
10. Yard care (garden, bushes, grass)
11. Other home-maintenance concerns (e.g., access to fuse box, storm windows, furnace filters, painting)

F. Medications
1. Large number of prescriptions (may be many)
2. Ability to remember
3. Ability to see labels or directions
4. Medications kept in one area

G. Access to community
1. Bus line
2. Walking
3. Driving (self or service from others)
4. Church, dry cleaning, drugstore, bank, health care facility, dentist, other community agencies

H. Other
1. Caring for spouse, relative, or companion
2. Financial management (able to write checks, make payments, cash checks)
3. Care of pet(s)

Sleep

Ask the client about the quality of sleep and any problems he or she may be experiencing. Sleep depth and efficiency decline with age. As a person ages, the proportion of time spent in deep sleep (stages 3 and 4, the most restorative sleep) decreases while the time spent in light sleep (stage 1) increases. Also the proportion of time spent in rapid eye movement (REM) sleep decreases slightly. Sleep is less efficient as evidenced by the need to spend more time in bed to achieve the same amount of restorative sleep as when they were younger (Cole and Richards, 2007). Sleep complaints of older adults are frequently secondary to chronic health problems and they often are interrelated: health problems interrupt sleep and sleep disruptions contribute to health problems. Pain, sleep apnea, shortness of breath, and restless leg syndrome frequently interfere with sleep of older adults (Cole and Richards, 2007). Also, inquire about daytime napping; an increase in the number or length of naps during the day may indicate a sleep problem during the night or may contribute to a sleep problem during the night.

Mental Health

Include a general statement about the client's ability to cope with stress (you may also want to obtain input from spouse, adult child, or close friend); recent changes or stresses in the client's life (e.g., moving, retirement, illness of self or family member, financial stress, death of friend or family member); feelings or symptoms of depression (e.g., insomnia, crying, fearfulness, marked irritability or anger); changes in personality, behavior, or mood; and use of medications or other techniques during times of anxiety, stress, or depression. The Yesavage Geriatric Depression Scale, Short Form, has been validated for use with this age group (Fig. 22-1).

Environment

Data on environmental safety and comfort should be gathered with a specific focus on problems unique to older adults.

- Hazards in the home: inadequate heating or cooling; stairs to climb (stairs without handrails, steep stairs); fear of falling; gait or balance problems; slippery or irregular surfaces in home (including throw rugs); inadequate space for maneuvering walker or wheelchair; inadequate lighting in dark hallway/stairs
- Hazards in the neighborhood: noise, water, and air pollution; safety, heavy traffic on surrounding streets; overcrowding; isolation from neighbors

Review of Systems

The review of systems is the same as that for the adult; below are specific components commonly associated with older adults.

Head, Eyes, Ears, Nose, and Throat

- Vision: Use of corrective devices (glasses, contacts); date of last examination. Ask about recent changes in or problems with near, distant, and peripheral vision as

---

Yesavage Geriatric Depression Scale, Short Form

Read the following 15 questions. Circle the response (*yes* or *no*) at the end of the question if it applies to you; that is, if it describes how you are feeling. If the answer given at the end of the question does NOT apply to you, then do not write anything for that question.

1. Are you basically satisfied with your life? (no)
2. Have you dropped many of your activities and interests? (yes)
3. Do you feel that your life is empty? (yes)
4. Do you often get bored? (yes)
5. Are you in good spirits most of the time? (no)
6. Are you afraid that something bad is going to happen to you? (yes)
7. Do you feel happy most of the time? (no)
8. Do you often feel helpless? (yes)
9. Do you prefer to stay home at night, rather than go out and do new things? (yes)
10. Do you feel that you have more problems with memory than most? (yes)
11. Do you think it is wonderful to be alive now? (no)
12. Do you feel pretty worthless the way you are now? (yes)
13. Do you feel full of energy? (no)
14. Do you feel that your situation is hopeless? (yes)
15. Do you think that most persons are better off than you are? (yes)

Score 1 point for each response that matches the yes or no answer after the question.

Fig. 22-1 Yesavage Geriatric Depression Scale, Short Form. *(From Yesavage JA, Brink TL: Development and validation of a geriatric depression screening scale: a preliminary report, J Psychosom Res 17:37-49, 1983. Copyright 1983 Elsevier Science. Reprinted from Journal of Psychosomatic Research with permission from Elsevier Science.)*

---

well as problems with night vision or the ability to recognize colors. These are common visual changes among older adults and may contribute to falls or motor vehicle accidents.

- Dry or burning eyes. Dry or irritated eyes are a frequent symptom experienced by older adults because of the decrease in quantity of tears.
- Hearing: Ask about problems with hearing; use of hearing aids; date of last eye examination. Asking older clients (or family members) about hearing problems is an effective hearing screening method during periodic health assessments (Gates et al, 2003).
The Hearing Handicap Inventory for the Elderly—Screening (HHIE-S) (Box 22-3) is a self-administered instrument effective in identifying clients with hearing impairment (Yueh et al, 2003). Scores between 0 and 8 indicate a 13% probability of a hearing impair-

HEARING HANDICAP INVENTORY FOR THE ELDERLY—SCREENING VERSION (HHIE-S)

1. Does a hearing problem cause you to feel embarrassed when meeting new people?
2. Does a hearing problem cause you to feel frustrated when talking to members of your family?
3. Do you have difficulty hearing when someone speaks in a whisper?
4. Do you feel handicapped by a hearing problem?
5. Does a hearing problem cause you difficulty when visiting friends, relatives, or neighbors?
6. Does a hearing problem cause you to attend religious services less often than you would like?
7. Does a hearing problem cause you to have arguments with family members?
8. Does a hearing problem cause you difficulty when listening to the TV or radio?
9. Do you feel that any difficulty with your hearing limits hampers your personal or social life?
10. Does a hearing problem cause you difficulty when in a restaurant with relatives or friends?

Scores are yes, 4 points; sometimes, 2 points; or no, 0 points to each question about a particular handicap. Scores range from 0 (no handicap) to 40 (maximum handicap).
From Yueh et al: *JAMA* 289(15): 1979, 2003.

ment, scores of 10 to 24 indicate a 50% probability of a hearing impairment, and scores between 26 and 40 indicate an 84% probability of a hearing impairment (Lichstenstein et al, 1988).

- Dry nose and mouth. An adverse effect of many medications is a dry mouth, which may be relieved with fluids.
- Mouth: Use of prosthetic devices (dentures) and date of last dental exam. Ask specifically if the client is experiencing difficulty chewing and swallowing. These problems may be caused by a number of things (such as ill-fitting dentures, dental pain, neuromuscular conditions, and esophageal motility) and can lead to inadequate nutritional intake or aspiration.

Respiratory System

- Fatigue, shortness of breath, cough.

Cardiovascular System

- Dizziness, blackouts, fainting, palpitations: Atherosclerosis may interfere with blood flow to the brain, causing confusion, dizziness, or fainting.
- Chest pain, fatigue, shortness of breath with exertion or at night, edema in the legs or feet: These symptoms may be associated with coronary artery disease or heart failure; risk of heart disease increases with age.
- Pain, discoloration, coldness, chronic wounds in legs or feet: These symptoms may indicate poor peripheral circulation or heart disease and are more common among older adults.

Gastrointestinal System

- Abdominal pain: Older adults often have nonspecific signs and symptoms of abdominal pain. Frequent manifestations of abdominal disorders may be low-grade fever, tachycardia, and vague abdominal discomfort. Degenerative vascular disease of local arteries may contribute to the development of gastric pain in older adults. These clients frequently do not complain of epigastric pain until hemorrhage or perforation occurs from gastrointestinal bleeding or intestinal obstruction (Eddy and Hricko, 2001).
- Constipation: Constipation is a common problem of older adults that may not be voluntarily reported to the health care provider. Ask about frequency of bowel movements and consistency of stool.

Urinary System

- Urine leakage and incontinence: Relaxation of the pelvic floor muscles and decreased sphincter tone may lead to urinary incontinence or a feeling of urgency. Clients may be reluctant to initiate a discussion about incontinence. Urinary incontinence is reported by 15% to 30% of older adults living at home and almost 50% for those in nursing homes.
- Difficulty starting urinary stream: Enlargement of the prostate—a common condition among older men—may cause hesitancy, weak urinary stream, and incomplete bladder emptying.

Musculoskeletal System

- Changes in muscle strength, joint pain: Independence in activities of daily living may be interrupted by muscle weakness or joint pain.
- Mobility, gait, balance, use of assistive devices (walker, cane, wheel chair): The degree, ease, and confidence related to mobility and assistive devices provide information about how clients maintain independence or suggest ways that these devices could be used. Mobility aids can prevent falls and improve independence.
- Recent falls and fall prevention, use of assistive devices in home (such as grab bars): Discussing fall prevention with older adults is important. Fall risk is categorized according to intrinsic (illness- or disease-related) or extrinsic (environmental) factors. Inquire about potential hazards in the environment such as steps, throw rugs, inadequate light, and curbs.
- A risk of fall assessment tool is shown in Box 22-4.

Reproductive System

- Women: Vaginal itching or dryness: Physiologic changes may cause a decrease in vaginal fluids.
- Women: Vaginal bleeding: Postmenopausal bleeding may result from numerous causes, from friable vaginal tissue to cancer of the uterus. If the client has postmenopausal bleeding, she should be referred to a health care provider for further evaluation.
- Sexual activity: As the client becomes older, it is important to assess if the client is sexually active, and if so, the

BOX 22-4 RISK OF FALLS ASSESSMENT TOOL

Fall Assessment Scoring System

I. Age
65–79 years   1
≥80   2

II. Mental Status
A. Oriented at all times or comatose   0
    Confusion at all times   2
    Intermittent confusion   4
B. Agitated/uncooperative/anxious—moderate   2
    Agitated/uncooperative/anxious—severe   4

III. Elimination
Independent and continent   0
Catheter and/or ostomy   1
Elimination with assistance   3
Ambulatory withg urge incontinence or episodes   5
   of incontinence

IV. History of Falling Within 6 Months
No history   0
Has fallen one or two times   2
Multiple history of falling   5

A score of 10 or more indicates a high risk for falling. If the patient does not meet a score of 10, but in the nurse's judgment is at risk to fall, initiate the high-risk fall protocol.

V. Sensory Impairment
Sensory impairment   1
   (blind, deaf, cataracts, not using corrective device)

VI. Activity
Ambulation/transfer without assistance   0
Ambulation/transfer with assist of one   2
   or assistive device
Ambulation/transfer with assist of two   1

VII. Medications
❑ Narcotics   ❑ Tranquilizers   ❑ Sleeping aids
❑ Diuretics   ❑ Chemotherapy   ❑ Antiseizure/
                                          antiepileptic

For the above medications, check how many the patient is taking currently at home or that the patient will be taking in the hospital.

No medications   0
1 medication   1
2 or more medications   2
Add one more point if there has been a change in these medications or dosages in the past 5 days.

SCORE   [   ]

From MacAvoy S, Skinner T, Hines M: Clinical methods: fall risk assessment tool, *Appl Nurs Res* 9(4):213, 218, 1996. In Phipps WJ, Sands JK, Marek JF: *Medical-surgical nursing: concepts and clinical practice,* ed 6, St Louis, 1999, Mosby.

level of satisfaction. Sexual activity is normal at any adult age. If the client has physical difficulties that interfere, it is important to assess what these are, how much they interfere, and what the client or partner has done to resolve the difficulty. Intercourse may be painful for women due to vaginal dryness secondary to hormonal changes. Older adults may welcome the opportunity to discuss sexual issues; this can be a time of education and encouragement. Some drugs depress sexual function (for example, antihypertensives, sedatives, tranquilizers, and alcohol).

EXAMINATION

OVERVIEW: THE OLDER ADULT PHYSICAL EXAMINATION

An examination of an older adult proceeds as described for the younger adult. The nurse assesses the client's level of comfort in different positions needed for the examination. The examination description that follows highlights common and abnormal findings of the older adult.

VITAL SIGNS AND BASELINE MEASUREMENTS

Vital signs are measured with every visit.

Temperature

The procedures for assessing vital signs are the same as the younger adult. The expected temperature is usually lower for older adults (97.2° F, 36.2° C), because of decreased metabolism and less physical activity. Older adults are especially prone to hypothermia. If the client's normal oral temperature is 94° F, a temperature of 98° F may indicate a fever.

Heart and Respiratory Rates

Heart and respiratory rates are assessed for the same qualities as in the younger adult. In the absence of heart disease pulse rates do not differ from those of younger adults. Note the pulse rate, rhythm, amplitude, and contour of the radial pulse. In the absence of lung disorders respiratory rates do not differ from those of other adults, although breathing may be more shallow.

Blood Pressure

For an accurate blood pressure reading, the appropriate cuff size must be used (see Chapter 5).

In the absence of heart disease expected blood pressure values are the same as for younger adults. While blood pressure elevations frequently occur in older adults, they are not considered a normal variation. Isolated systolic hypertension (>140 mm Hg) is frequently seen in older adults due to atherosclerotic changes (Tabloski, 2007).

Pain

Pain assessment is the same as described for the younger adult.

Some older adults may perceive pain as an expected aspect of aging that they must endure. They may manifest pain as fatigue, lethargy, or anorexia. Pain assessment in older adults, including those who were cognitively impaired, is significantly improved by using a descriptive scale (see Fig. 6-5, *A*), a visual analog scale (see Fig. 6-5, *C*), or pain faces (see Fig. 20-4) (Kamel et al, 2003).

Height and Weight

Height, weight, and BMI are measured in the same manner as described previously for the younger adult. If the scale does not have a handle close by to hold onto, stand close to the scale, because some older people may have a problem standing on a small surface off the floor.

Normal and Abnormal Findings
Height: Decreased bone formation reduces height in most older adults, which may cause shortening of the vertebrae

and thinning of the vertebral disks. Decreases in height may occur more often in women because of osteoporosis. *Weight:* For those in their eighties and beyond, body weight may decrease because of muscle wasting or chronic diseases. The total body water declines, which contributes to weight loss. Subcutaneous fat distribution shifts from the face and extremities to the abdomen and hips. Refer to Chapter 9 to calculate BMI.

EXAMINATION OF THE SKIN, HAIR, NAILS

Procedure and Techniques

Procedures and techniques for assessing skin, hair, and nails of an older adult are the same as those described in Chapter 10. Because many physiologic skin changes occur with aging, the nurse must take special care when examining the skin, hair, and nails of the older adult. Inspect the sun-exposed areas such as the nose, lips, and ears for color and lesions.

Normal and Abnormal Findings
Skin
As skin thins, it takes on a parchment-like appearance, especially over bony prominences, the dorsal surfaces of the hands and feet, the forearms, and the lower legs (Fig. 22-2). The skin hangs loosely on the frame, secondary to a loss of adipose tissue and loss of elasticity. Dry skin may indicate dehydration or malnutrition. Tenting of the skin may indicate moderate to severe dehydration. Skin tears may occur due to thin, fragile texture. The skin may be cool due to impaired circulation. Edema may indicate fluid retention from cardiovascular or renal disease. Normal variations in the skin of the older adult include findings such as the following:
- *Solar lentigo (liver spots):* Irregularly shaped, flat, deeply pigmented macules that may appear on body surface areas having repeated exposure to the sun (Fig. 22-3).

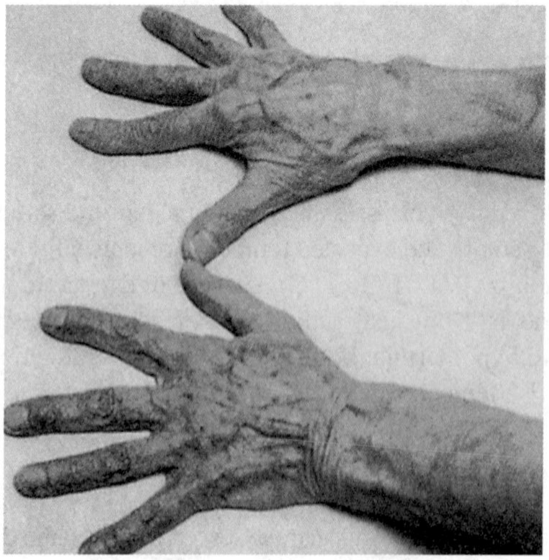

Fig. 22-2 **Hands of older adult.** Note prominent veins and thin appearance of the skin. *(From Seidel et al, 2006.)*

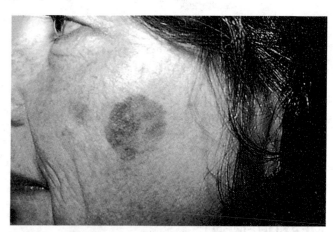

Fig. 22-3 **Solar lentigo (liver spots).** Brown macules that appear in chronically sun-exposed areas. *(From Goldstein and Goldstein, 1997. Courtesy Department of Dermatology, University of North Carolina at Chapel Hill.)*

- *Seborrheic keratoses:* Pigmented, raised, warty-appearing lesions that may appear on the face or trunk (Fig. 22-4). Differentiate these benign lesions from similar-appearing actinic keratoses, which are premalignant lesions.
- *Acrochordon (skin tag):* Small, soft tag of skin that generally appears on the neck and upper chest (Fig. 22-5). These tags may or may not be pigmented.
- *Sebaceous hyperplasia:* Yellowish, flattened papules that have a central depression (Fig. 22-6).

Abnormal findings of the skin are the same as those discussed for adults. Refer to Chapter 10 for descriptions of squamous cell and basal cell cancers and malignant melanoma.

Hair

The hair becomes thin, gray, and coarse in texture. Symmetric balding may occur in men; a decrease in the amount of body, pubic, and axillary hair occurs in both men and women. Men

have an increase in the amount and coarseness of nasal and eyebrow hair, and women may develop coarse facial hair.

Nails

Nails may become thick and brittle, especially the toe nails.

EXAMINATION OF THE HEAD, EYES, EARS, NOSE, AND THROAT

Procedures and techniques for assessing the head, eyes, ears, nose, and throat of the older adult are the same as those described in Chapter 11.

Neck

Procedure and Technique

Assess range of motion of the neck with one movement at a time, rather than a full rotation of the neck, to avoid causing dizziness on movement. Note any pain, crepitus, dizziness, or limited movement.

Normal and Abnormal Findings

A stiff neck in the older adult may indicate cervical arthritis.

Eyes and Vision

Procedures and techniques for assessing an older adult are the same as those described in Chapter 11.

Normal and Abnormal Findings

Eyebrows may be thin along the outer edge and the remaining brow hair may appear coarse. Pseudoptosis, or relaxed upper eyelid, may be seen, with the lid resting on the lashes. Orbital fat may have decreased, so that the eyes appear sunken, or may herniate, causing bulging on the lower lid or inner third of the upper lid. The lacrimal apparatus may func-

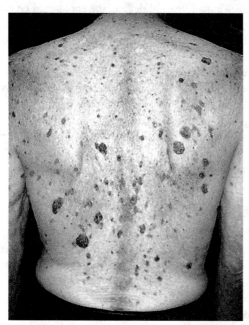

Fig. 22-4 Multiple seborrheic keratosis lesions on the trunk. *(From Goldstein and Goldstein, 1997. Courtesy Department of Dermatology, Medical College of Georgia.)*

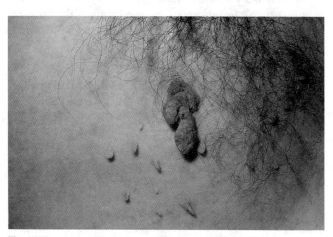

Fig. 22-5 Multiple skin tags. *(From Goldstein and Goldstein, 1997. Courtesy Department of Dermatology, University of North Carolina at Chapel Hill.)*

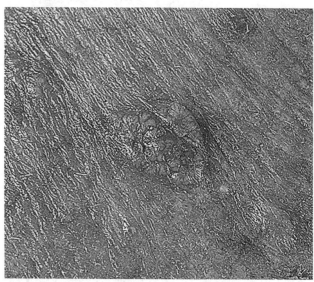

Fig. 22-6 Sebaceous hyperplasia. *(From Habif, Campbell, Chapman et al, 2006.)*

tion poorly, giving the eye a lack of luster. Brown spots may appear near the limbus as a normal variation. Bulbar conjunctiva may appear dry, clear, and light pink without discharge or lesions. The cornea is transparent, clear, often yellow; arcus senilis (a gray-white circle around the limbus) is common but not associated with any pathologic condition (Fig. 22-7). Abnormal findings include ectropion, in which the lower lid drops away from the globe (Fig.22-8), or entropion, in which the lower lid turns inward (Fig. 22-9).

Central and peripheral vision may decrease after age 70. Acuity of 20/20 or 20/30 with corrective lenses is common. Accommodation takes longer. Color perception of blue, violet, and green may be impaired. Presbyopia is decreased near vision that usually occurs after age 40 and is treated with corrective lenses. Gradual loss of central vision may be caused by macular degeneration due to changes in the retina. The difficulty or inability to visualize the internal structures of the eye may denote cataracts.

During an ophthalmic examination, the retinal structures usually appear dull, with pale blood vessels. The arterioles display a narrower light reflex and are straighter. More defective crossings of arteries and veins are also seen. Benign degenerative hyaline deposits may be noted on the retinal surface (drusen); these do not interfere with vision.

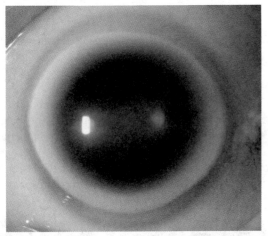

Fig. 22-7   Arcus senilis (a gray-white circle around the limbus). *(From Paley and Krachmer, 1997.)*

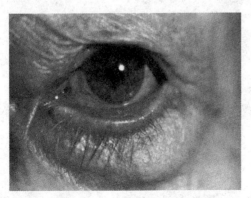

Fig. 22-8   Ectropion. *(Courtesy Dr. Ira Abrahamsom, Jr, Cincinnati, Ohio. From Stein, Slatt, and Stein, 1988.)*

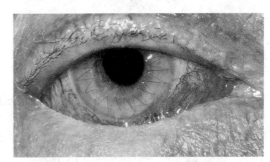

Fig. 22-9   Entropion. *(From Paley and Krachmer, 1997.)*

Ears and Hearing

Procedures and techniques for assessing an older adult are the same as those described in Chapter 11.

Normal and Abnormal Findings

Box 22-5 presents hearing loss statistics for older adults. If the client wears a hearing device, the ear should be carefully assessed for any skin irritation or sores that may be secondary to the molded device. There may be the presence of or an increase in wiry hair in the opening of the auditory canal; and the tympanic membrane may appear whiter, opaque, and thickened. If the client wears a hearing device, there is an increased likelihood of cerumen impaction. Presbycusis is hearing loss associated with aging. Ability to hear high-frequency sounds diminishes first, making high-pitched sounds such as "s" and "th" difficult to hear and tell apart. The speech of others seems mumbled or slurred.

Mouth

Procedures and techniques for assessing an older adult are the same as those described in Chapter 11. Clients with dentures should have an examination both with the dental appliance in and out.

Normal and Abnormal Findings

The surface of the lips may be marked with deep wrinkling and fissures at the corners of the mouth (perlèche) associated with overclosure of the mouth or vitamin deficiency. The older client is at higher risk for squamous cell carcinoma of the lip, especially if the client has been a longtime pipe smoker. Aging

---

BOX 22-5   **HEARING LOSS STATISTICS IN MIDDLE-AGE ADULTS, OLDER ADULTS, AND OLD-OLD ADULTS**

Middle-age adults (51 to 65 years of age)—25% of population in this age group have early changes in hearing loss that may go unnoticed.

Older adults (65 to 85 years of age)—33% of population in this age group have documented hearing loss.

Old-old adults (85 years and older)—50% of population in this age group have documented hearing loss.

Data from US Preventive Services Task Force: *Guide to clinical preventive services,* ed 2, Baltimore, 1996, Williams & Wilkins.

causes the gum line to recede secondary to bone degeneration, causing the teeth to appear longer. The gums may become more friable and bleed with slight pressure. The teeth may become darkened or stained. Many older adults may become edentulous or have caps or bridges. Dental occlusion surfaces may be markedly worn down. Malocclusion of the teeth may be common secondary to the migration of teeth after tooth extraction. A red, edematous tongue with erosions in the corners of the mouth may indicate iron deficiency anemia.

EXAMINATION OF THE RESPIRATORY SYSTEM

Procedures and techniques for assessing an older adult are the same as those described in Chapter 12.

Normal and Abnormal Findings

The thorax and scapulae should be symmetric. The anteroposterior diameter of the chest should be approximately one half the lateral diameter. There may be decreased elasticity and ability to clear the air passages in older adults. Breath sounds are the same as for younger adults. Kyphoscoliosis, a skeletal deformity affecting the spinal curvature, is common and may alter the chest wall configuration and make adequate lung expansion more difficult. It may also increase the AP diameter. This in turn may result in decreased tidal volume, causing shallow breathing.

EXAMINATION OF THE CARDIOVASCULAR SYSTEM

Procedures and techniques for assessing an older adult are the same as those described in Chapter 13.

Normal and Abnormal Findings

Occasional ectopic beats are common and may or may not be significant. The S_4 heart sound is common in older adults and may be associated with decreased left ventricular compliance. Carotid bruits may be heard, indicating arteriosclerosis. Cool feet and weak pedal pulses may be noted due to peripheral arterial disease.

EXAMINATION OF THE ABDOMEN AND GASTROINTESTINAL SYSTEM

Procedures and techniques for assessing an older adult are the same as those described in Chapter 14.

Normal and Abnormal Findings

Older adults may have increased fat deposits over the abdominal area even with decreased subcutaneous fat over the extremities. The abdomen may feel soft due to decreased abdominal muscle tone, making palpation of organs easier (Brozenee, 2000). Bowel sounds may be hypoactive.

EXAMINATION OF THE MUSCULOSKELETAL SYSTEM

Procedures and techniques for assessing an older adult are generally the same as those described in Chapter 15. Assess balance and gait when indicated.

Normal and Abnormal Findings

Muscle mass is decreased compared to findings in younger adults. Muscles that are not equal bilaterally may indicate muscle atrophy. Common findings include osteoarthritis changes in joints, which may result in decreased range of motion in affected joints. Many joints may not have the expected degree of movement or range of motion seen in younger adults.

Assess range of motion of the neck with one movement at a time, rather than a full rotation of the neck, to avoid causing dizziness on movement. A stiff neck in the older adult may indicate cervical arthritis. Note any pain, crepitus, dizziness, or limited movement. The Tinetti Balance and Gait Assessment Tool is in Box 22-6.

EXAMINATION OF THE NEUROLOGIC SYSTEM

Procedures and techniques for assessing an older adult are the same as those described in Chapter 16. Mental status is assessed while taking the client's history. Cranial nerves are assessed earlier, during the examination of the head, eyes, ears, nose, and throat.

Normal and Abnormal Findings

For indications of the client's ability to perform activities of daily living, note his or her personal hygiene, appearance, and dress. Be aware that some older adults have slowed responses, move more slowly, or show a decline in function (for example, the sense of taste). Other expected changes with aging may include deviation of gait from midline; difficulty with rapidly alternating movements; and some loss of reflexes and sensations (for example, the knee-jerk or ankle-jerk reflexes and light touch and pain sensations). Often a normal flexor response is indistinct, and the plantar reflex may be missing or difficult to interpret. Superficial abdominal reflexes may be missing (Cacchione, 2000).

EXAMINATION OF THE BREASTS

Procedures and techniques for assessing an older adult are the same as those described in Chapter 17. Postmenopausal

BOX 22-6 FUNCTIONAL ASSESSMENT: TINETTI BALANCE AND GAIT ASSESSMENT TOOL

Balance Tests

Eight positions and position changes are evaluated.
Instructions: The client is seated in a hard, armless chair. The following maneuvers are tested.

1. Sitting balance	Leans or slides in chair	= 0
	Steady, safe	= 1 _____
2. Arises (ask client to rise without using arms)	Unable without help	= 0
	Able, uses arms to help	= 1
	Able without using arms	= 2 _____
3. Attempts to arise	Unable without help	= 0
	Able, requires more than one attempt	= 1
	Able to arise, one attempt	= 2 _____
4. Immediate standing balance (first 5 seconds)	Unsteady (swaggers, moves feet, trunk sways)	= 0
	Steady but uses walker or other support	= 1
	Steady without walker or other support	= 2 _____
5. Standing balance (once stance balances)	Unsteady	= 0
	Steady but wide stance (medial heels more than 4 inches apart) or uses cane or other support	= 1
	Narrow stance without support	= 2 _____
6. Nudged (subject at maximum position with feet as close together as possible, nurse pushes lightly on subject's sternum with palm of hand 3 times)	Begins to fall	= 0
	Staggers, grabs, catches self	= 1
	Steady	= 2 _____
7. Eyes closed (at maximum position, as in 6)	Unsteady	= 0
	Steady	= 1 _____
8. Turning 360 degrees	Discontinuous steps	= 0
	Continuous steps	= 1
	Unsteady (grabs, staggers)	= 0
	Steady	= 1 _____
9. Sitting down	Unsafe (misjudges distance, falls into chair)	= 0
	Uses arm or not a smooth motion	= 1
	Safe, smooth motion	= 2 _____

Balance Score: _____ of 16

Gait Tests

Eight components of gait are observed.
Initial instructions: The client stands with nurse, walks down hallway or across room for at least 10 feet, first at "usual" pace, then back at "rapid but safe" pace (using usual walking aids).

10. Initiation of gait (immediately after being told "go")	Any hesitancy or multiple attempts to start	= 0
	No hesitancy	= 1 _____
11. Step length and height	Right swing foot does not pass left foot with stance	= 0
	Passes left stance foot	= 1
	Right foot does not clear floor completely with step	= 0
	Right foot completely clears floor	= 1
	Left swing foot does not pass right stance foot with step	= 0
	Passes right stance foot	= 1
	Left foot does not clear floor completely with step	= 0
	Left foot completely clears floor	= 1 _____
12. Step symmetry	Right and left step length not equal (estimate)	= 0
	Right and left step length appear equal	= 1 _____
13. Step continuity	Stopping or discontinuity between steps	= 0
	Steps appear continuous	= 1 _____
14. Path (estimated in relation to floor tiles, 12 inches square; observe excursion of one of the subject's feet over about 10 feet of the course)	Marked deviation	= 0
	Mild/moderate deviation or uses walking aid	= 1
	Straight without walking aid	= 2 _____

BOX 22-6 FUNCTIONAL ASSESSMENT: TINETTI BALANCE AND GAIT ASSESSMENT TOOL—cont'd

Gait Tests—cont'd

15. Trunk

Marked sway or uses walking aid = 0

No sway, but flexion of knees or back, or spreads arms out while walking = 1

No sway, no flexion, no use of arms, and no use of walking aid = 2 _____

16. Walking stance

Heels apart = 0

Heels almost touching while walking = 1 _____

Gait Score: _____ of 12

Balance and Gait Score: _____ of 28

From Tinetti, 1986.

women, as well as older men, should continue to have regular breast examinations.

Normal and Abnormal Findings

The breasts in postmenopausal women may appear flattened and elongated or pendulous secondary to a relaxation of the suspensory ligaments. Palpation findings that may be normal variations in the older adult include a granular feeling of the glandular tissue of the breast. If the woman had cystic disease earlier in life, her breasts are now more likely to feel smoother and less cystic. The inframammary ridge thickness may now be more prominent, and the nipples may be smaller and flatter.

EXAMINATION OF THE REPRODUCTIVE SYSTEM AND PERINEUM

Procedures and techniques for assessing an older adult are the same as described in Chapter 18.

Female Exam

Procedure and Techniques

Often there is a temptation to defer the routine pelvic examination of the older woman because it may be difficult for her to be positioned in stirrups, she is postmenopausal, or she is no longer sexually active. None of these is a sufficient reason to defer the examination. Instead, older women may have different problems, such as urinary incontinence, pelvic relaxation, vaginal irritation, dryness, or rectal problems that warrant evaluation. When examining an older adult is that she may need assistance to help hold her legs if she is unable to tolerate positioning in the stirrups. In addition, she may need more assistance in assuming a modified lithotomy position and may not be able to stay in the position as long as a younger woman. If the cli-

ent is no longer sexually active, a smaller speculum with narrower blades may be necessary to prevent discomfort from the introital constriction. Also, because of the decrease in the amount of natural lubrication in the vagina, it becomes necessary to lubricate the speculum and the fingers of the examining hand adequately to avoid causing discomfort during the examination.

Normal and Abnormal Findings

The labia and clitoris of the older woman are small and pale. The skin may appear dry and have a shiny appearance. The pubic hair may be sparse, patchy, or absent.

The nurse may find that the client's vagina is narrower and shorter and that there is an absence of rugation of the vaginal wall. Likewise, the cervix may appear smaller and paler, and the fornices may be smaller or absent. The uterus should be small, smooth, firm, freely movable, and nontender. Any uterine enlargement; nodular, irregular, hardened, or indurated areas; areas that are tender on palpation; fixed, nonmobile areas in the pelvis; or masses should be further evaluated.

Because ovaries atrophy with age, these are not usually palpable in aging women. The rectovaginal septum should be thin, smooth, and pliable. The anal sphincter tone may be somewhat diminished, and because of pelvic musculature relaxation, the client may have prolapse of the vaginal walls or uterus.

Male Exam

Procedures and techniques for assessing an older adult are the same as described in Chapter 18.

Normal and Abnormal Findings

Externally, pubic hair becomes finer and less abundant, sometimes leading to pubic alopecia. The scrotal sac of the client may appear elongated or pendulous. The client may have injury or excoriation of the scrotal sac surface secondary to sitting on the scrotum. The testes may feel slightly smaller and softer than in the younger client.

Perianal Examination

Procedure and Techniques

The client may need assistance getting into an adequate position for the examination. If the client is lying on his or her back on the examination table, the client may need assistance turning to a left lateral lying position. Procedures and techniques for assessing an older adult are the same as described in Chapter 18.

Normal and Abnormal Findings

The examination findings for the older adult are the same as those for the adult. Prostate hyperplasia is a common abnormal finding. The prostate may feel smooth and rubbery; the median sulcus may or may not be palpable. The nurse may also note a relaxation of the client's perianal muscles and decreased sphincter control when the older adult bears down.

COMMON PROBLEMS & CONDITIONS

Below is a list of common problems and conditions of older adults. Most of these have been discussed in previous chapters and the chapter number is included beside the category. Those not previously discussed (in *italics* below) are described and include macular degeneration, anemia, constipation, and urinary incontinence.

Integumentary—See Chapter 10
 Skin Cancer
Vision—See Chapter 11
 Cataracts
 Macular degeneration
 Glaucoma
 Diabetic retinopathy
Hearing—See Chapter 11
 Conductive hearing loss
 Sensorineural hearing loss
Respiratory—See Chapter 12
 Asthma
 Chronic Obstructive Pulmonary Disease
 Pneumonia
Cardiovascular—See Chapter 13
 Hypertension
 Angina
 Myocardial infarction
 Valvular heart disease
 Heart failure
 Peripheral arterial disease
 Anemia
Gastrointestinal—See Chapter 14
 Gastrointestinal reflux disease
 Constipation
Genitourinary—See Chapters 14 and 18
 Urinary tract infections—Chapter 14
 Urinary incontinence
 Benign prostatic hyperplasia—Chapter 18
Musculoskeletal—See Chapter 15
 Osteoporosis
 Fractures
 Osteoarthritis
 Gout

Neurologic—See Chapter 16
 Alzheimer disease
 Cerebrovascular accident (stroke)
 Parkinson's disease

MACULAR DEGENERATION

The macula is an oval yellow spot in the center of the retina that helps provide central vision. As the maculae degenerate, central visual impairment occurs. Risk factors are over 50 years of age, Caucasian, smoking, hypertension, and cardiovascular disease.
Clinical Findings: Loss of central vision, decline in visual acuity, a dark spot in the center of vision, and straight lines appear crooked or wavy (Fig. 22-10) (Tabloski, 2007).

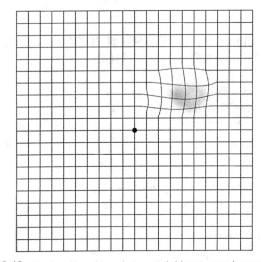

Fig. 22-10 Amsler grid used to evaluate central vision as occurs in macular degeneration; here showing visual changes caused by fluid leakage under the retina. *(Courtesy of Brent A. Bauer, MFA, The Wilmer Institute, The John Hopkins University and Hospital, Baltimore, MD. From Seidel et al, 2006.)*

ANEMIA

A reduction in the total number of circulating erythrocytes (red blood cells) or a decrease in the quantity or quality of hemoglobin describes anemia. Causes of anemia that affect older adults are due to lack of nutrients needed to produce erythrocytes or to a slow blood loss from a bleeding ulcer or colon cancer those results in the loss of erythrocytes. Nutrients needed to produce erythrocytes include iron, vitamin B_{12}, and folate. Older adults may lack these nutrients because they cannot afford to purchase them, are not mobile enough to go to the store, do not have the energy to prepare the food containing these nutrients, or are unable to chew or swallow food. **Clinical Findings:** Manifestations that may occur regardless of the type of anemia are tachycardia; tachypnea; dyspnea; fatigue; cool, pale skin; lightheadedness; and tinnitus. Iron deficiency also causes glossitis; erosions in the corners of the mouth; thin, brittle nails; conjunctiva pallor; and (in older adults) confusion. Folate deficiency produces irritability, memory loss, depression, and sleep deprivation. Vitamin B_{12} deficiency causes neurologic manifestations including paresthesia of the hands and feet, altered vibratory perception, and ataxia.

URINARY INCONTINENCE

This common urinary disorder occurs when the client is unable to control urination associated with relaxation of the bladder and/or urinary sphincter. Risk factors include multiple pregnancies, abdominal wall weakness, obesity, urinary tract infections, cerebrovascular accident, or multiple sclerosis. **Clinical Findings:** The client may report feeling an immediate urge to void (urge incontinence); leaking of urine when laughing, coughing, or sneezing (stress incontinence); a continuous leakage of urine; or a leakage of urine during sleep (nocturnal enuresis). Consequences of incontinence are skin breakdown, risk for falls, social isolation, and feelings of embarrassment.

CLINICAL APPLICATION & CLINICAL REASONING

See Appendix E for answers to exercises in this section.

REVIEW QUESTIONS

1 When obtaining a health history from a 72-year-old male client with a red lesion at the base of his tongue, the nurse specifically asks the client about:
   1 Alcohol and tobacco use.
   2 The date of his last dental examination.
   3 How well his dentures fit.
   4 A history of pyorrhea.
2 On inspection of the eye of an 82-year-old woman, the nurse notes which finding as normal?
   1 Opaque coloring of the lens.
   2 Clear cornea with a gray-white ring around the limbus.
   3 Dilated pupils when looking at an item in her hand.
   4 Impaired perception of the colors yellow and red.
3 The nurse notes which finding as abnormal during a thoracic assessment of an older adult?
   1 A skeletal deformity affecting curvature of the spine.
   2 Shortness of breath on exertion.
   3 An increase in anterior-posterior diameter.
   4 Bronchovesicular breath sounds in the peripheral lung fields.
4 The nurse notes which finding as normal during a cardiovascular assessment of an older adult?
   1 A drop in blood pressure when moving from lying to standing.
   2 A loud aortic ejection murmur that radiates to the neck.
   3 A radial pulse of 56 beats per minute.
   4 A low-pitched blowing sound heard over a carotid artery.

5 Which would be an abnormal finding during an abdominal examination of an older adult?
   1 Report of incontinence when sneezing or coughing.
   2 Loss of abdominal muscle tone.
   3 Bowel sounds every 15 seconds in all quadrants.
   4 Silver-white striae and a very faint vascular network.
6 Which finding is an expected age-related change for a woman 80 years old?
   1 Kyphosis.
   2 Back pain.
   3 Loss of height.
   4 Crepitation on movement.

SAMPLE DOCUMENTATION

Review the data obtained during an interview and examination by the nurse.

A 70-year-old Native American male reports that his physician diagnosed him with anemia. Since his diet was healthy and he had not noticed any bleeding, he had colonoscopy to determine if the cause of the anemia could be from a slow bleed in the colon. The colonoscopy revealed a villous adenoma. This client is being admitted for surgery to remove the adenoma found on colonoscopy. This client takes lisinopril for hypertension, metformin for type 2 diabetes mellitus, Crestor for hyperlipidemia, an aspirin daily as an antiplatelet, and a multivitamin. This client is oriented to person, place, and time. His short- and long-term memories are intact. All but the first cranial nerve were observed and are intact. This client does not report any pain or fatigue.

When asked about skin wounds, lesions, rashes or itching, he said he did not have any of these. He wears glasses. He did report hesitancy when starting stream, and has not had any pain with urination, blood in urine, urinary frequency, testicle pain, or scrotal swelling. His abdomen is obese. On palpation the abdomen is soft and tender with no masses felt. Bowel sounds were heard in all quadrants. His liver and spleen are not enlarged. He has no hernias. He has no back pain, joint pain, or swelling. He has no muscle cramps, weakness, or stiffness. He never has ear aches, decreased hearing, nose bleeds, sore throat, bleeding gums, hoarseness, difficulty swallowing. He cannot remember ever feeling too cold or too hot for no apparent reason. While he is thirsty and hungry sometimes from the diabetes, this does not happen very often.

Skin is intact; color tone even and consistent with race. The skin is elastic. His head is a normal shape. His conjunctiva are pale. He does have an opaque ring that surrounds the peripherally of the cornea. Both of his pupils are equal, round, and react to light and accommodation. He is able to follow the nurse's finger with his eyes in all directions. His vision is 20/20 bilaterally with glasses. Proliferative diabetic retinopathy is noted on opththalmoscopic exam. He does become short of breath during activity such as walking up stairs. At the end of the day he notices his feet are swollen. He has not had any chest pain, palpitations, easy bruising, or leg pain when walking. He does become short of breath during activity, but does not wake up during the night out of breath. He has not coughed up any blood or had wheezing. He has not been dizzy or had any weakness or numbness. He has no allergies to food or drugs. He has been constipated lately, but has not had nausea, diarrhea, bloating, blood in stool, or a change in bowel habits. He reports no depressed mood, anxiety, or memory loss. No thrills or palpable murmurs were palpated. The point of maximum impulse is at the 5th intercostal space in the midclavicular line. The first and second heart sounds are heard in all locations with no murmurs or rub heard. The carotid and radial pulses are 2+ and symmetric, but the pedal pulses are 1+ and symmetric.

His temperature is 98.8° F (37.1° C); his pulse rate is 96 beats/min, regular; his blood pressure is 130/78 mm Hg; his respiratory rate 12 breaths/min; height, 6'1"; weight, 224 lbs. Appears older than stated age. He is able to hear conversation. The inside of his mouth is moist, pink, and pale. There is no redness noted in the mouth. His teeth are discolored, but are straight. His tongue is symmetric and moves evenly. The uvula is in the middle of the posterior pharynx, which is pink. The trachea is midline. The thyroid gland cannot be palpated. There is no retraction or use of accessory muscles when he breaths. The anterior-posterior diameter is increased. His breath sounds are clear bilaterally in all lobes. His gait is balanced. He can perform active range of motion and his muscle strength is 5/5. In 2006 he had his left hip replaced (total hip arthroplasty [THA]) after a fall.

To the right, note how the nurse recorded these same data in a documentation format.

A 77 y/o Native American ♂ admitted for a hemicolectomy to remove a villous adenoma found on colonoscopy performed to determine cause of iron deficiency anemia.
PMH: HTN, diabetes mellitus type 2. Hospitalizations: L (left) THA 2006 after a fall. Allergies: None. Medications: lisinopril, metformin, Crestor, multivitamin, aspirin.

SUBJECTIVE DATA

Client reports his physician said he had anemia and scheduled a colonoscopy that found colon cancer. Denies fatigue or pain. *Skin:* Denies wounds, lesions, rash or itching; *HEENT:* Wears glasses. Denies ear aches, decreased hearing, nose bleeds, sore throat, bleeding gums, hoarseness, difficulty swallowing, cold or heat intolerance, thirst or hunger all of the time. *CV:* C/O DOE, swelling in feet at the end of the day. Denies chest pain, palpitations, easy bruising, or leg pain when walking. *Resp:* Denies shortness of breath at night, hemoptysis, and wheezing. *GI:* C/O constipation. Denies nausea, diarrhea, bloating, blood in stool, change in bowel habits. *GU:* C/O hesitancy when starting stream. Denies pain with urination, blood in urine, urinary frequency, testicle pain, or scrotal swelling. *MS:* Denies back pain, joint pain, joint swelling, muscle cramps, muscle weakness, or stiffness. *Neuro:* Denies weakness, numbness, or dizziness. *Psychiatric:* Denies depressed mood, anxiety, or memory loss.

OBJECTIVE DATA

General survey: Vital Signs: T 98.8° F (37.1° C); P 96 beats/min, regular; BP 130/78; RR 12 breaths/min; Ht. 6'1"; Wt 224 lbs. Appears older than stated age.

Skin: Intact; color tone even, consistent with race, elastic turgor.

HEENT: Normocephalic; conjunctiva pale, PERRLA, arcus senilis present, EOM intact, vision 20/20 bilaterally with glasses, proliferative diabetic retinopathy noted; hearing intact; oral mucous membranes moist and pale, without redness, teeth discolored and aligned, tongue symmetric, pink, moist, movable, uvula midline, posterior pharynx pink; trachea midline, thyroid nonpalpable.

Resp: No retractions or accessory muscle use, expected fremitus, increased AP diameter, breath sounds clear in all lobes.

Heart and Peripheral vascular: no thrill or palpable murmurs, PMI is 5ICS, MCL, S_1 and S_2 present without murmurs or rubs; carotid and radial pulses 2+ and symmetric, pedal pulses 1+ and symmetric.

Abdomen: obese; soft, tender, no masses; BS in all quadrants, no enlargement of liver or spleen, no hernias.

Musculoskeletal: balanced gait, full active ROM, muscle strength 5/5 bilaterally.

Neurologic: O×3, short- and long-term memories present, cranial nerves II to XII grossly intact.

CASE STUDY

Sara Reinarz is an 80-year-old Caucasian woman who recently developed confusion and urinary incontinence. She lives with her daughter, Megan, who reported her mother has fallen several times at home. She is admitted to the hospital for assessment for possible fractures and confusion.

Interview Data

The daughter reports her mother has fallen several times going to the bathroom. This is the first time Sara reported pain from after the fall. Megan is concerned about her mother's confusion. Two weeks ago Sara was independent and caring for herself at home. Megan recalled that last year her mother became confused and was diagnosed with a urinary tract infection at the same time. As soon as the urinary tract infection was treated, her mother's confusion stopped. Sara has no allergies to food or medications. She takes calcium with vitamin D for osteoporosis, aspirin for an antiplatelet, and thyroid hormone for hypothyroidism. She does not smoke or drink alcohol.

Examination Data

Vital signs: Blood pressure, 141/86 mm Hg; pulse, 88 beats/min; respiration rate, 22; temperature, 98.3° F (36.8° C). *Weight:* 152 lb. The client is confused and oriented to person. She appears anxious. She has a bruise on her right hip and thigh. There is full range of motion of the right leg, but movement is painful. Muscle strength 4/5. Pedal pulses are 1+ and symmetric.

Clinical Reasoning

1. What data deviate from normal findings, suggesting a need for further investigation?
2. What additional data should the nurse ask or assess for?
3. Based on the data, what risk factors for falls does Sara have?
4. What nursing diagnoses and collaborative problems should be considered for this situation?

INTERACTIVE ACTIVITIES

Open the interactive student CD-ROM, click on Chapter 22, and choose from the following activities on the menu bar:

- **Multiple Choice Challenge.** Click on the best answer for each question. You will be given immediate feedback, rationale for incorrect answers, and a total score. Good luck!

- **Risk Factors.** Review this patient's history and identify risk factors. Complete your assessment by deciding which risks are modifiable and which are nonmodifiable. You only get one shot, so choose carefully!

- **Quick Challenge.** Use this critical thinking exercise to assess your skills through case study-style questions, then compare with expert answers!

- **Printable Lab Guide.** Locate the Lab Guide for Chapter 22, and print and use it (as many times as needed) to help you apply your assessment skills. These guides may also be filled in electronically and then saved and e-mailed to your instructor!

CHAPTER 23

Conducting a Head-to-Toe Assessment

ELECTRONIC RESOURCES

Additional information related to the content in Chapter 23 can be found

in the companion website at

evolve

evolve: http://evolve.elsevier.com/Wilson/assessment/

or on the interactive student CD-ROM

 Activities for Chapter 23 include the following:
- Marvelous Matches • Printable Lab Guide
- Quick Challenge

Now that you have studied and practiced assessing each body system separately, it is time to put everything together. Although you began with knowledge and techniques specific for each system, the client comes to you as a whole person. You must organize your techniques to assess the entire person, literally from "head to toe." Therefore, when you begin with the head, you should examine the facial characteristics—skin, hair, eyes, ears, mouth, throat, and range of motion of the neck—in a systematic, organized manner incorporating neurologic, integumentary, musculoskeletal, visual, and auditory systems within the head, neck, nose, and mouth regions. Then you must move on to the next region of the body and repeat the same. After all body regions are examined, you document your findings by body system.

Each nurse's approach to a head-to-toe assessment is unique. No two nurses do things in exactly the same manner, nor are any two clients exactly the same. As a student, you determine what assessment sequence works best for you. Use a systematic method so that you do not omit any data. When performing a focused assessment, you refer only to those regions needed based on the client's chief complaint and additional data learned from the history.

PERFORMING A HEALTH ASSESSMENT

The assessment should begin with the general survey when you first meet the client. During this initial meeting, observe the client enter the room, noting gait, posture, and ease of movement. Shake hands with the client, noting eye contact

and firmness of the hand grip. Introduce yourself to the client and begin data collection by asking the client the reason for seeking care. Note the language spoken, as well as gross hearing and speech capability. In addition, observe characteristics such as obvious vision difficulties or blindness; difficulty standing, sitting, or rising; obvious musculoskeletal difficulties; general affect; appearance of interest and involvement; dress and posture; general mental alertness, orientation, and integration of thought processes; obvious shortness of breath or posture that would facilitate breathing; and obesity, emaciation, or malnourishment.

After the initial observations, obtain the history, assess vital signs, assess vision, and prepare the client for the examination. Instruct the client to first empty the bladder (collect specimen if necessary based on client history) and then to remove clothing, put on a gown if needed, and sit on the examination table. You are now ready to conduct an assessment that accommodates the client's needs.

Use the following sequence only as a guide. It was developed to demonstrate how examination of one body system is integrated with other body systems to permit a comprehensive regional assessment. Note in the following example that all relevant body systems in one region are assessed. For example, when the nurse is examining the client's anterior chest, he or she must consider the other body systems in that region that must be assessed simultaneously and incorporate them into an integrated assessment. Body systems that would be assessed during the anterior chest examination include skin; respiratory, lymphatic, cardiovascular, musculoskeletal systems; and breasts. Techniques for a routine examination are listed.

BOX 23-1	EQUIPMENT FOR HEALTH EXAMINATION IN SUGGESTED ORDER OF USE

Writing surface for examiner
Scale with height measurement
Thermometer
Watch with second hand
Vision charts—Snellen's or Jaeger card
Sphygmomanometer
Stethoscope with bell and diaphragm
Client gown
Drape sheet
Examination table (with stirrups for female clients)
Otoscope with pneumatic bulb
Tuning fork
Ophthalmoscope ★
Nasal speculum
Tongue blade
Penlight
Gauze pads
Nonsterile examination gloves
Ruler and tape measure
Marking pen
Goniometer
Aromatic items
Cotton balls
Sharp and dull testing items
Objects for stereognosis such as a key or comb ★
Percussion hammer
Lubricant
Vagina speculum (for female clients) ★
Pap smear materials (for female clients) ★
Gooseneck light

When additional techniques are indicated for special circumstances or advanced practice, those are identified as well.

Exactly how the assessment proceeds depends on the purpose of the assessment, the needs of the client, the nurse's ability, and the policies of the facility where the examination is conducted. Equipment for a health assessment is listed in Box 23-1.

Most important are the following points:
- Be organized.
- Develop a routine. This helps with consistency.
- Before you begin the actual assessment, have a clear picture in your mind of what you plan to do and in what order.
- Practice, practice, practice so that you learn to become systematic and inclusive.
- Imagine yourself as the client, and consider how you would want a nurse to be prepared if he or she were to assess you.

GUIDELINES FOR ADULT HEAD-TO-TOE EXAMINATION

Procedures

Assessment Data Collected in the General Survey During the History

Level of consciousness and mental status 🔑
Mood or affect
Personal hygiene
Skin color 🔑
Posture/position 🔑
Mobility 🔑
Ability to hear and speak 🔑

Assess Vital Signs and Other Baseline Measurements

Temperature, radial pulse, respirations, and blood pressure
    If indicated, take blood pressure in both arms
Height, weight, and body mass index
Visual acuity

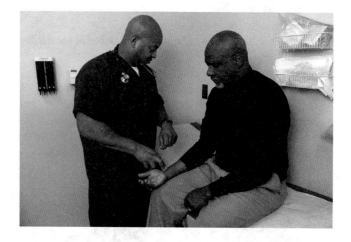

Examine Hands

When taking pulse and blood pressure, inspect skin surface characteristics, temperature, and moisture of hands
Inspect hands for symmetry
Inspect and palpate nails for shape, contour, consistency, color, thickness, and cleanliness
Test capillary refill 🔑
Observe for clubbing of the fingers

Examine Head and Face

Inspect skull for contour and hair for color and distribution
    If indicated, palpate hair for texture
    If indicated, palpate scalp for tenderness and intactness
Palpate temporal pulses for amplitude 🔑
Inspect for facial features and symmetry 🔑
Inspect bony structures of face for size, symmetry, and intactness 🔑
    If indicated, ask client to clench teeth

If indicated, ask client to clench eyes tightly, wrinkle forehead, smile, stick out tongue, and puff out cheeks noting symmetry

If indicated, evaluate sensitivity of forehead, cheeks, and chin to light touch

🔑 Inspect skin for color and lesions

If indicated, palpate skin surfaces for texture, tenderness, and lesions

If indicated, palpate facial bones for size, intactness and tenderness

If indicated, palpate sinus regions for tenderness and transilluminate sinuses

Examine Eyes

Assess near vision and peripheral vision

Inspect eyebrows for hair distribution, underlying skin, and symmetry

Inspect eyelids and eyelashes for symmetry, position, closure, blinking, and color

🔑 Inspect conjunctiva and sclera for color and clarity; inspect cornea for transparency

If indicated, inspect anterior chamber for transparency and chamber depth

🔑 Inspect symmetry of eye movements

If indicated, test extraocular eye movements in six cardinal fields of gaze

🔑 Inspect iris for shape and color

🔑 Assess pupillary response, consensual reaction, corneal light reflex, and accommodation

If indicated, perform cover-uncover test

★ Ophthalmic examination: inspect red reflex, disc cup margins, vessels, retinal surface, macula

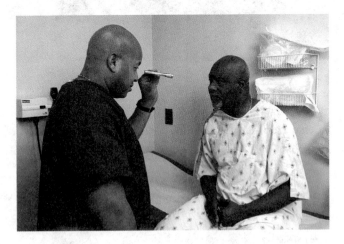

Examine Ears

Inspect external ear for alignment, position, size, shape, symmetry, intactness, and skin color

Inspect external auditory canal for discharge or lesions

Inspect skin over superficial lymph nodes for edema, erythema, and red streaks

Palpate lymph nodes of the head for size and tenderness

Palpate external ear and mastoid areas for tenderness, edema, or nodules

If indicated, perform whisper test to evaluate gross hearing

If indicated, perform Rinne and Weber's tests for conduction and sensorineural hearing losses

Otoscopic examination: inspect characteristics of external ★
canal, cerumen, eardrum (landmarks)

Examine Nose, Mouth, and Oropharynx

Inspect nasal structure and septum for symmetry

Inspect nose for patency, turbinates, and discharge

If indicated, evaluate sense of smell

Inspect lips, buccal mucosa, and gums for color, symmetry, 🔑
moisture, and texture

Inspect teeth for number, color, position, alignment, hygiene, and condition 🔑

Inspect floor of mouth and hard and soft palates for color 🔑
and surface characteristics

Inspect oropharynx for odor, anterior and posterior pillars, uvula, tonsils, and posterior pharynx

If indicated, grade tonsils

Inspect tongue for symmetry, movement, color, and surface 🔑
characteristics

If indicated, palpate tongue and gums for tenderness and lesions

If indicated, evaluate gag reflex

If indicated, test temporomandibular joint for movement

Examine Neck

Observe symmetry of neck, trachea, and thyroid

If indicated, palpate trachea for alignment and thyroid for size

Inspect neck for range of motion 🔑

If indicated, test range of motion of head and neck; shrug shoulders against resistance

Palpate carotid pulses, one at a time, for amplitude 🔑

If indicated, auscultate carotid for bruits

Palpate lymph nodes of the neck for size and tenderness

Observe for jugular veins for distention

Examine Upper Extremities

Inspect client's arms for skin characteristics, symmetry, and 🔑
deformities

Palpate arms, elbows, and wrists for temperature, tenderness, and deformities 🔑

Palpate brachial or radial pulse for presence and amplitude 🔑

If indicated, palpate epitrochlear lymph nodes for size and tenderness

If indicated, test range of motion, muscle strength, and sensation

If indicated, test deep tendon reflexes

If indicated, perform Phalen's sign or Tinel's sign for ★
carpal tunnel syndrome

If indicated, test for rotator cuff damage ★

🔑 = core examination skill   ★ = advanced practice

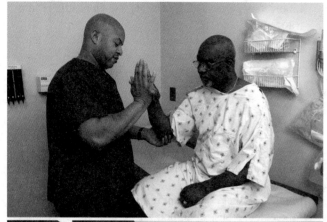

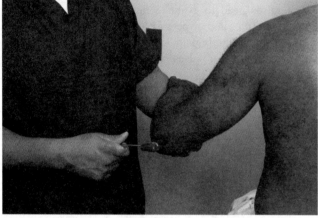

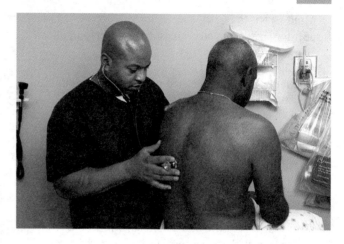

Assess Anterior Chest

Move to front of client; client should lower gown to waist

Inspect skin for color, intactness, lesions, and scars

Observe respiratory movement for symmetry, client's ease
    with respirations, and posture

Observe precordium for pulsations or heaving

Palpate left chest wall to locate point of maximum impulse
    (PMI)

    If indicated, palpate chest wall for fremitus, as with pos-
        terior chest

    If indicated, palpate anterior chest wall for thoracic
        expansion

    If indicated, percuss anterior chest for resonance   ★

Auscultate anterior chest for breath sounds

Auscultate heart for rate, rhythm, intensity, frequency, tim-
    ing, and splitting of S_1 or S_2 or presence of S_3, S_4, or
    murmurs

Assess Posterior Chest

*Nurse moves behind client; client seated; gown to waist for
men; gown opened in the back for women*

Observe posterior and lateral chest for symmetry of shoul-
    ders, muscular development, scapular placement, spine
    alignment, and posture

Inspect skin for color, intactness, lesions, and scars

Palpate vertebrae for alignment and tenderness

Observe respiratory movement for symmetry, depth, and
    rhythm of respirations

    If indicated, palpate posterior chest and thoracic muscles
        for tenderness, bulges, and symmetry

    If indicated, palpate posterior chest wall for thoracic
        expansion

    If indicated, palpate posterior chest wall for fremitus

    If indicated, palpate vertebral column for alignment and
        tenderness

★   If indicated, percuss posterior and lateral chest for
      resonance

★   If indicated, percuss and measure thorax for diaphrag-
      matic excursion

    If indicated, percuss with fist along costovertebral angle
        for tenderness

Auscultate posterior and lateral chest walls for breath
    sounds

    If adventitious sounds heard, assess for bronchophony,
        egophony, and whispered pectoriloquy

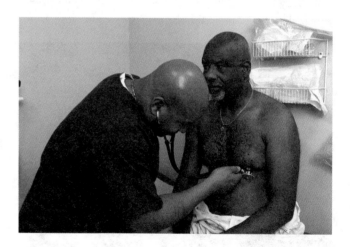

Female Breasts

Inspect for size, symmetry, contour, surface characteristics,
    and breast or nipple deviation

Observe for symmetry of breast tissue during movement:
    arms over head, behind head, behind back; hand pushed
    together tightly, client leaning forward

= core examination skill   ★ = advanced practice

Male Breasts

Inspect for size, symmetry, breast enlargement, nipple discharge, or lesions

All Clients

Palpate lymph nodes associated with lymphatic drainage of breasts and axillae

Assess Anterior Chest in Recumbent Position

Elevate head of bed 45 degrees to inspect for jugular vein pulsations

    If indicated, measure jugular venous pressure for height seen above sternal angle

Palpate anterior chest wall for thrills, heaves, and pulsations

    If indicated, measure blood pressure with client lying to compare with earlier reading

Female Breasts

Provide chest drape for females; expose abdomen from pubis to epigastric region

Inspect for symmetry, contour, venous pattern, skin color, areolar area (note size, shape, and surface characteristics), and nipples (note direction, size, shape, color, surface characteristics, and discharge)

Palpate breasts; note firmness, tissue qualities, lumps, areas of thickness, or tenderness; areolar and nipple areas

Assess Abdomen

Observe skin characteristics from pubis to midchest region for scars, lesions, vascularity, bulges, and navel

Inspect abdominal contour

Observe for movement of abdomen, peristalsis, and pulsations

Auscultate abdomen (all quadrants) for bowel sounds, bruits, and venous hums

Lightly palpate all quadrants for tenderness, guarding, and masses

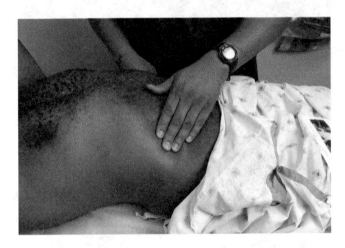

    If indicated, deeply palpate all quadrants for tenderness, guarding, and masses

    ★ If indicated, deeply palpate midline epigastric area for aortic pulsation

If indicated, percuss all quadrants and epigastric region for tone

If indicated, percuss upper and lower liver borders and estimation of liver span   ★

If indicated, percuss left midaxillary line for splenic dullness   ★

If indicated, deeply palpate right costal margin for liver border   ★

If indicated, deeply palpate left costal margin for splenic border   ★

If indicated, deeply palpate abdomen for right and left kidneys   ★

If indicated, test abdominal reflexes   ★

If indicated, assess abdomen for fluid   ★

Client raises head to evaluate flexion and strength of abdominal muscles and inspect for umbilical hernia

    If indicated, lightly palpate inguinal region for lymph nodes, femoral pulses, and bulges that may be associated with hernia

Assess Lower Extremities

Client remains lying; abdomen and chest should be draped

Inspect legs, ankles, and feet for skin characteristics, vascular sufficiency, hair distribution, and deformities

Palpate lower legs and feet for temperature, pulses, tenderness, and deformities

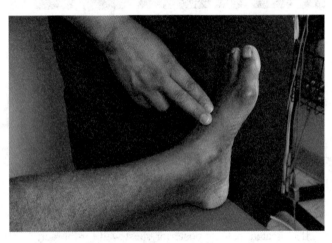

If indicated, test range of motion, motor strength, and sensation of hips, legs, knees, ankles, and feet

If indicated, test for deep tendon reflexes   ★

If indicated, palpate hips for stability and tenderness   ★

If indicated, assess for knee effusion with the bulge test or ballottement   ★

If indicated, assess for knee stability with the drawer test, McMurray's test, or Apley test   ★

If indicated, assess for hip flexion contracture with the Thomas test   ★

If indicated, assess for nerve root compression with straight leg raises   ★

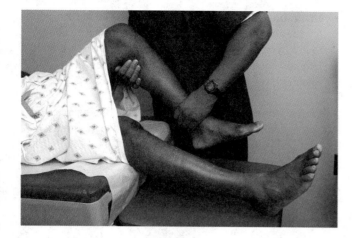

Assess Remaining Neurologic System

🔑 Observe client moving from lying to sitting position; note use of muscles, ease of movement, and coordination

🔑 Assess client's gait: observe and palpate client's spine and posterior thorax for alignment as client stands and bends forward to touch toes

If indicated, evaluate hyperextension, lateral bending, and rotation of upper trunk

★ If indicated, test sensory function by using light and deep (dull and sharp) sensation

If indicated, bilaterally test and compare vibratory sensation

★ If indicated, test proprioception by moving the toe up and down

★ If indicated, test two-point discrimination

★ If indicated, test stereognosis and graphesthesia

If indicated, test fine motor functioning and coordination of upper extremities by instructing client to perform at least two of the following:
- Alternating pronation and supination of forearm
- Touching nose with alternating index fingers
- Rapidly alternating finger movements to thumb
- Rapidly moving index finger between nose and examiner's finger

If indicated, test fine motor functioning and coordination of lower extremities by instructing client to run heel down tibia of opposite leg

★ If indicated, evaluate Babinski's sign and ankle clonus tests

★ If indicated, test for meningeal signs with Kernig's and Brudzinski's signs

If indicated, assess cerebellar and motor functions by using at least two of the following:
- Romberg's test (eyes closed)
- Walking straight heel-to-toe formation
- Standing on one foot and then other (eyes closed)
- Hopping in place on one foot and then other
- Knee bends

Assess Genitalia, Pelvic Region, and Rectum

Males

Client is lying and adequately draped

Inspect pubic hair for distribution and general characteristics 🔑

Inspect and palpate penis color, tenderness, discharge, and 🔑 general characteristics

Inspect scrotum for texture and general characteristics

Inspect sacrococcygeal and perianal areas and anus for sur- 🔑 face characteristics

Position client lying on left side with right hip and knee flexed

Palpate anal canal and rectum for surface characteristics with lubricated gloved finger

Note characteristics of stool when gloved finger removed

If indicated, palpate anterior rectal surface for prostate ★ gland size, contour, consistency, mobility, and tenderness

With client standing, inspect inguinal canal for bulges

Palpate testes, epididymides, and vas deferens for location, consistency, tenderness, and nodules

If indicated, transilluminate scrotum for fluid and masses ★

If indicated, palpate inguinal canal for hernias ★

Females

Client should be lying in lithotomy position; examiner should don gloves

Inspect the pubic hair for distribution 🔑

Inspect and palpate the labia majora, labia minora, clitoris, 🔑 urethral meatus, vaginal introitus, perineum, and anus for surface characteristics

If indicated, palpate the Skene's and Bartholin's glands for surface characteristics

If indicated, inspect and palpate muscle tone for vaginal wall tone, rectal muscle, and urinary incontinence

If indicated, insert vaginal speculum and inspect surface ★ characteristics of vagina and cervix

If indicated, collect Papanicolaou (Pap) smear and cul- ★ ture specimen

If indicated, perform bimanual palpation to assess for ★ size and characteristics of vagina, cervix, uterus, and adnexa

If indicated, perform vaginal-rectal examination to assess ★ rectovaginal septum and pouch, surface characteristics, and broad ligament tenderness

If indicated, perform rectal examination to assess anal sphincter tone and surface characteristics; note characteristics of stool when lubricated gloved finger removed

Client resumes seated position; client should have gown on and be draped across lap

---

🔑 = core examination skill   ★ = advanced practice

⊙ INTERACTIVE ACTIVITIES

Open the CD-ROM, click on Chapter 23, and choose from the following activities on the menu bar:

- **Marvelous Matches.** Drag each word or phrase to the appropriate place on the screen. Test your ability to match the body system being examined with the assessment area.

- **Printable Lab Guide.** Locate the Lab Guide for Chapter 23, and print and use it (as many times as needed) to help you apply your assessment skills. These guides may also be filled in electronically and then saved and e-mailed to your instructor!

- **Quick Challenge.** Use this critical thinking exercise to assess your skills through case study-style questions, then compare with expert answers!

Documenting the Health Assessment

ELECTRONIC RESOURCES

Additional information related to the content in Chapter 24 can be found

in the companion website at

evolve

evolve: http://evolve.elsevier.com/Wilson/assessment/

or on the interactive student CD-ROM

Activities for Chapter 24 include the following:
- Multiple Choice Challenge • Crossword Wizard
- Marvelous Matches • Quick Challenge

At the completion of a health assessment, the nurse documents the data so that other health care providers can use the information. The written record serves as a legal document and permanent record of the client's health status at the time of the nurse-client interaction. The nurse must record data accurately, concisely, legibly, and without bias or opinion.

As mentioned in Chapter 1, a variety of formats to document assessment findings are used in various health care settings. Both paper and electronic records are common. The amount of information documented reflects the depth and scope of the health assessment. The purpose of this chapter is to provide you with an example of documentation of a comprehensive history and examination for a well client. At the end of the documentation, the nurse forms a problem list and identifies nursing diagnoses. The actions that follow data collection reflect analysis, clinical judgment, and clinical reasoning

HEALTH HISTORY

Biographic Data

Name: Maria S. Griego
Gender: Female
Address: 1000 1st Street, Angus, TX 87123
Telephone numbers: (111) 999-9999, home;
    (111) 444-4444, work
Birth date: 10-13-54
Birthplace: Houston, Texas
Race/ethnicity: Hispanic
Religion: Catholic

Marital status: Married, 30 years
Occupation: Counselor in a high school
Contact person: Christopher Griego, spouse
Source of interview data: Client

Reason for Seeking Care

"I need a Pap smear."

History of Present Illness

Not applicable.

Present Health Status

Overall health described as "good." *Chronic illnesses*: None. *Medications:* Takes no prescription drugs; does not use herbal preparations; takes one multivitamin each morning. *Allergies:* Reports allergy to penicillin; "give me hives"; no known food allergies.

Past Health History

Childhood illnesses: Measles, mumps, rubella, chickenpox, streptococcal throat, otitis media. *Surgeries and hospitalizations:* 1962 appendectomy; vaginal deliveries 1976, 1980. *Accidents/injuries*: Denies. *Immunizations:* Childhood immunizations for school, tetanus immunization unknown. *Last examinations*: Physical and Pap smear 2 years ago. Dental: 2 years ago. Vision: 2 years ago. Mammogram: 2 years ago. *Obstetric history:* G2, P2. Both vaginal deliveries without complications.

Family History

MGM deceased age 70, hypertension and heart failure; MGF deceased age 72, colon cancer; PGM deceased age 84, "old age"; PGF deceased age 81, prostate cancer; mother, age 80, hypertension, arthritis, dementia; father, deceased age 62, myocardial infarction. Client has no brothers or sisters. Denies family history of stroke, diabetes, kidney disease, mental disorders, or seizure disorders. Both children are in good health.

Personal and Psychosocial History

Personal Status

Client states that she feels good about herself most of the time. Her cultural affiliation is self-described as middle-class Hispanic female. She has a master's degree in counseling and has been a high school counselor with the same school for 16 years. Overall enjoys her job, but experiences frustration with the social issues of her students. Hobbies include playing piano and gardening.

Family and Social Relationships

Lives with husband and mother in a four-bedroom home in a suburban area; both sons live in the same community and remain close. Neither son is married. The client considers relationship with husband as close; also speaks of two other very close female friends. Mother is elderly and has moderate dementia and occasional falls, requiring increasing supervision. Client expresses concerns about meeting her mother's needs in the future and the ongoing physical demands.

Diet/Nutrition

Describes appetite as excellent; no changes in appetite or weight. Reports balanced food intake. 24-hour recall: *Breakfast:* muffin, 1% milk, fruit juice, coffee; *Lunch:* spaghetti, green beans, salad, tea; *Dinner:* chicken, mashed potatoes, applesauce, roll, tea, chocolate cake for dessert; *Snack:* crackers with peanut butter; *Fluid:* 4 glasses of water, 2 cups coffee, and 1 glass tea daily

Functional Ability

Client's activities include maintaining a home, working full time, and caring for her mother.

Mental Health

Verbalizes frequent episodes of frustration and despair in meeting her mother's needs. Does not feel husband is supportive of situation and has caused some conflict. She counts on her friends to help her "talk through" stress periods. The client and her spouse have had marriage counseling on two different occasions, which she feels was beneficial. Also verbalizes stress at work regarding issues with students and administration. Has not recently been able to find time to exercise, but when she can, she finds this helpful in coping with the stress. Has had no previous psychiatric or mental health counseling.

Personal Habits

Denies drug use; 1 to 2 glasses of wine per week; previously a smoker with a 22 pack-year history; has not smoked for over 10 years.

Health Promotion Activities

Reports walking 1.5 miles two to three times per week to stay fit, but has not been able to maintain this routine recently.

Environment

Client believes that her home and neighborhood environment are safe and without hazards.

Review of Systems

General Symptoms

Client considers herself in "good health," but frequently feels fatigued due to obligations of caring for her mother and working full time.

Integumentary System

Skin: Denies lesions, masses, discolorations, or rashes to skin. *Hair:* Denies texture changes or loss, uses hair color monthly to cover gray; no scalp irritation reported from hair coloring. *Nails:* Denies changes in texture, color, shape. *Health promotion:* Uses sunscreen "occasionally" when outside.

HEENT

Denies headache, vertigo, syncope. *Eyes:* Wears glasses/contacts for nearsighted vision. Denies discharge, pruritus, pain, visual disturbances. *Ears:* Denies pain, discharge, tinnitus. *Nose, nasopharynx, paranasal sinuses:* Denies nasal discharge epistaxis, olfactory deficit, snoring. *Mouth and oropharynx:* Denies sore throat, lesions, gum irritation, chewing or swallowing difficulties, hoarseness, voice changes. *Neck:* Denies tenderness or range-of-motion difficulties. *Health promotion:* Brushes teeth twice daily.

Breasts

No tenderness; denies lumps, masses, or nipple discharge. *Health Promotion:* None.

Cardiovascular System

Denies chest pain, shortness of breath, and palpitations; feet frequently feel cold; denies discoloration or peripheral edema. *Health promotion:* Until recently has walked two to three times a week; has trouble finding time to do this of late.

Respiratory System

Denies breathing difficulties, cough, shortness of breath.

Gastrointestinal System

Denies eating and digestion problems or abdominal pain. Daily bowel movement is formed, brown; does not use stool softener or laxatives; denies hemorrhoids.

Urinary System

Describes urine as yellow and clear; voiding frequency four to five times daily; denies problems with voiding, changes in urinary pattern, or pain.

Musculoskeletal System

Denies muscular weakness, twitching, and pain; gait difficulties; and extremity deformities. States that she has occasional joint stiffness, but has not experienced pain, edema, or crepitus.

Neurologic System

Denies changes in cognitive function, coordination, and sensory deficits.

Reproductive System

LMP 4 years ago. Denies genital lesions or discharge. States that she is sexually active with husband and is satisfied with sexual relationship; denies history of STD. *Health promotion:* Attempts to have regular Pap smear, but admits she does not do this every year—"just can't seem to make the time."

PHYSICAL EXAMINATION

General Survey

Cooperative, oriented, alert woman; sitting with erect posture; maintains eye contact; appropriately groomed and dressed. Vital signs: BP 110/78; P 78; R 14; T 98° F (36.7° C); wt 137 lb (62 kg); ht 5 ft 3 inches.

Skin, Hair, Nails

Smooth, soft, moist, tanned, warm, intact skin with elastic turgor. Hair brown with female distribution, soft texture; nails smooth, rounded, manicured.

Head

Skull symmetric; scalp intact; face and jaw symmetric.

Eyes

Vision 20/20 OU with contact lenses; near vision, able to read magazine at 13 inches with contacts. Peripheral vision present; EOM intact; brows, lids, and lashes symmetric; lacrimal ducts pink and open without discharge. Conjunctiva clear, sclera white, moist, and clear; cornea smooth and transparent, iris transparent and flat, PERRLA. Corneal light reflex symmetric. *Ophthalmic examination:* Red reflex present, disc margins distinct, round, yellow; artery to vein ratio 2:3, retina red uniformly; macula and fovea slightly darker.

Ears

Hearing intact as noted in general conversation; pinna aligned with eyes, ears symmetric, earlobes pierced once.

Cerumen in auditory canal, TM pearly gray, cone of light reflex present.

Nose and Sinuses

Septum midline, nasal passages patent; turbinates pink with no drainage. No pain with sinus palpation.

Mouth and Throat

TMJ moves without difficulty, no halitosis. Lips symmetric, moist, smooth; 32 white, smooth, and aligned teeth. Mucous membranes pink and moist, symmetric pillars, clear saliva. Tongue symmetric, pink, moist, and movable. Hard palate smooth, pale; soft palate smooth, pink and rises, uvula midline; posterior pharynx pink, smooth, tonsils pink with irregular texture.

Neck

Trachea midline; thyroid smooth, soft, size of thumb pad; full ROM of neck; no palpable lymph nodes.

Chest and Lungs

Breathing is quiet and effortless. AP: Lateral diameter is 1:2; muscle and respiratory effort symmetric, equal excursion, resonant percussion tones throughout, lungs clear to auscultation throughout lung fields with no adventitious sounds.

Breasts

Moderate size; R slightly > L; no dimpling present. Granular consistency bilaterally but more pronounced in outer quadrants; nipples without discharge, areolas symmetric; symmetric venous pattern; no palpable axillary lymph nodes.

Heart

Apical pulse palpated at fifth LICS, MCL; no lifts, heaves, or thrills or abnormal pulsations, S_1 and S_2 heard without splitting, no murmurs.

Peripheral Vascular

Distal pulses palpable, smooth contour; pulse amplitude 2+ in all pulses; no jugular distention noted; lower extremities warm and pink with symmetric hair distribution, no edema or tenderness; capillary refill <1 second in all nail beds.

Abdomen

Rounded, striae noted; skin smooth with no lesions; bowel sounds in all quadrants; tympanic percussion tones; abdomen soft, no tenderness, masses, or aortic pulsations noted with light or deep abdominal palpation. Umbilical ring feels round with no irregularities or bulges. Tympany heard over abdomen and spleen, and dullness over suprapubic area. Liver spans 3.0 inches at the midclavicular line, the lower border descends downward 1 inch. Gallbladder not palpable. Abdominal reflexes present. No CVA tenderness, no inguinal lymphadenopathy.

Musculoskeletal

Full ROM in all joints without tenderness; muscle strength 5/5 bilaterally, extremities aligned and symmetric, vertebral column straight; coordinated smooth gait.

Neurologic

Oriented to time, place, person; speech understandable and of sufficient volume; cranial nerves I to XII grossly intact; negative Romberg's sign; peripheral sensation intact, deep tendon reflexes 2+ bilaterally.

Gynecologic

Pubic hair in female distribution; labia smooth and soft; urethral meatus midline; perineum smooth and without lesions; Skene's and Bartholin's glands nontender; vaginal tone firm; cervix pink, midline, parous os, pliable, smooth; no discharge noted; vaginal wall smooth, homogeneous, moist, and nontender; anteverted uterus, smooth, movable, nontender; ovaries smooth, firm, movable. Rectal wall smooth, nontender, sphincter tone tight, two small hemorrhoids. Specimen for Pap smear collected.

PROBLEM LIST

- Education regarding health promotion
- Concerned about providing care for mother

NURSING DIAGNOSES

- Health-seeking behaviors related to interest in obtaining regular preventive health services (Pap smear, mammogram, exercise)
- Caregiver role strain related to increasing care needs of elderly mother

INTERACTIVE ACTIVITIES

Open the CD-ROM, click on Chapter 24, and choose from the following activities on the menu bar:

- **Multiple Choice Challenge.** Click on the best answer for each question. You will be given immediate feedback, rationale for incorrect answers, and a total score. Good luck!

- **Crossword Wizard.** Complete a crossword puzzle using the clues associated with health assessment concepts. It's a whiz!

- **Marvelous Matches.** Drag each word or phrase to the appropriate place on the screen. Test your ability to correctly match subjective and objective data.

- **Quick Challenge.** Use this critical thinking exercise to assess your skills through case study-style questions, then compare with expert answers!

North American Nursing Diagnosis Association (NANDA) Nursing Diagnoses

Activity intolerance
Risk for **Activity** intolerance
Ineffective **Airway** clearance
Latex **Allergy** response
Risk for latex **Allergy** response
Anxiety
Death **Anxiety**
Risk for **Aspiration**
Risk for impaired parent/child **Attachment**
Autonomic dysreflexia
Risk for **Autonomic** dysreflexia
Risk-prone health **Behavior**
Disturbed **Body** image
Risk for imbalanced **Body** temperature
Bowel incontinence
Effective **Breastfeeding**
Ineffective **Breastfeeding**
Interrupted **Breastfeeding**
Ineffective **Breathing** pattern
Decreased **Cardiac** output
Caregiver role strain
Risk for **Caregiver** role strain
Readiness for enhanced **Comfort**
Impaired verbal **Communication**
Readiness for enhanced **Communication**
Decisional **Conflict**
Parental role **Conflict**
Acute **Confusion**
Chronic **Confusion**
Risk for acute **Confusion**
Constipation
Perceived **Constipation**
Risk for **Constipation**
Contamination
Risk for **Contamination**
Compromised family **Coping**
Defensive **Coping**
Disabled family **Coping**
Ineffective **Coping**

Ineffective community **Coping**
Readiness for enhanced **Coping**
Readiness for enhanced community **Coping**
Readiness for enhanced family **Coping**
Risk for sudden infant **Death** syndrome
Readiness for enhanced **Decision** making
Ineffective **Denial**
Impaired **Dentition**
Risk for delayed **Development**
Diarrhea
Risk for compromised human **Dignity**
Moral **Distress**
Risk for **Disuse** syndrome
Deficient **Diversional** activity
Disturbed **Energy** field
Impaired **Environmental** interpretation syndrome
Adult **Failure** to thrive
Risk for **Falls**
Dysfunctional **Family** processes: alcoholism
Interrupted **Family** processes
Readiness for enhanced **Family** processes
Fatigue
Fear
Readiness for enhanced **Fluid** balance
Deficient **Fluid** volume
Excess **Fluid** volume
Risk for deficient **Fluid** volume
Risk for imbalanced **Fluid** volume
Impaired **Gas** exchange
Risk for unstable blood **Glucose**
Grieving
Complicated **Grieving**
Risk for complicated **Grieving**
Delayed **Growth** and development
Risk for disproportionate **Growth**
Ineffective **Health** maintenance
Health-seeking behaviors (specify)
Impaired **Home** maintenance
Readiness for enhanced **Hope**

NANDA International (2007). *NANDA-I Nursing Diagnoses: Definitions and Classification 2007-2008*. Philadelphia: NANDA-I.

Hopelessness

Hyperthermia

Hypothermia

Disturbed personal **Identity**

Readiness for enhanced **Immunization** status

Functional urinary **Incontinence**

Overflow urinary **Incontinence**

Reflex urinary **Incontinence**

Stress urinary **Incontinence**

Total urinary **Incontinence**

Urge urinary **Incontinence**

Risk for urge urinary **Incontinence**

Disorganized **Infant** behavior

Risk for disorganized **Infant** behavior

Readiness for enhanced organized **Infant** behavior

Ineffective **Infant** feeding pattern

Risk for **Infection**

Risk for **Injury**

Risk for perioperative positioning **Injury**

Insomnia

Decreased **Intracranial** adaptive capacity

Deficient **Knowledge** (specify)

Readiness for enhanced **Knowledge**

Sedentary **Lifestyle**

Risk for impaired **Liver** function

Risk for **Loneliness**

Impaired **Memory**

Impaired bed **Mobility**

Impaired physical **Mobility**

Impaired wheelchair **Mobility**

Nausea

Unilateral **Neglect**

Noncompliance

Imbalanced **Nutrition**: less than body requirements

Imbalanced **Nutrition**: more than body requirements

Readiness for enhanced **Nutrition**

Risk for imbalanced **Nutrition**: more than body requirements

Impaired **Oral** mucous membrane

Acute **Pain**

Chronic **Pain**

Readiness for enhanced **Parenting**

Impaired **Parenting**

Risk for impaired **Parenting**

Risk for **Peripheral** neurovascular dysfunction

Risk for **Poisoning**

Post-trauma syndrome

Risk for **Post-trauma** syndrome

Readiness for enhanced **Power**

Powerlessness

Risk for **Powerlessness**

Ineffective **Protection**

Rape-trauma syndrome

Rape-trauma syndrome: compound reaction

Rape-trauma syndrome: silent reaction

Impaired **Religiosity**

Readiness for enhanced **Religiosity**

Risk for impaired **Religiosity**

Relocation stress syndrome

Risk for **Relocation** stress syndrome

Ineffective **Role** performance

Readiness for enhanced **Self-care**

Bathing/hygiene **Self-care** deficit

Dressing/grooming **Self-care** deficit

Feeding **Self-care** deficit

Toileting **Self-care** deficit

Readiness for enhanced **Self-concept**

Chronic low **Self-esteem**

Situational low **Self-esteem**

Risk for situational low **Self-esteem**

Self-mutilation

Risk for **Self-mutilation**

Disturbed **Sensory** perception (specify: visual, auditory, kinesthetic, gustatory, tactile, olfactory)

Sexual dysfunction

Ineffective **Sexuality** pattern

Impaired **Skin** integrity

Risk for impaired **Skin** integrity

Sleep deprivation

Readiness for enhanced **Sleep**

Impaired **Social** interaction

Social isolation

Chronic **Sorrow**

Spiritual distress

Risk for **Spiritual** distress

Readiness for enhanced **Spiritual** well-being

Stress overload

Risk for **Suffocation**

Risk for **Suicide**

Delayed **Surgical** recovery

Impaired **Swallowing**

Effective **Therapeutic** regimen management

Ineffective **Therapeutic** regimen management

Ineffective community **Therapeutic** regimen management

Ineffective family **Therapeutic** regimen management

Readiness for enhanced **Therapeutic** regimen management

Ineffective **Thermoregulation**

Disturbed **Thought** processes

Impaired **Tissue** integrity

Ineffective **Tissue** perfusion (specify: renal, cerebral, cardiopulmonary, gastrointestinal, peripheral)

Impaired **Transfer** ability

Risk for **Trauma**

Impaired **Urinary** elimination

Readiness for enhanced **Urinary** elimination

Urinary retention

Impaired spontaneous **Ventilation**

Dysfunctional **Ventilatory** weaning response

Risk for other-directed **Violence**

Risk for self-directed **Violence**

Impaired **Walking**

Wandering

Health History Using Functional Health Patterns

1. Health Perception–Health Management
   - How would you describe your health overall?
   - How would you describe your health at this time?
   - What is the reason for this healthcare visit? What are your expectations?
   - If ill, describe your illness. What do you think caused this illness?
   - What treatments, health care practices, or folk remedies have you used to treat your illness?
   - Are you usually able to follow prescribed instructions given by a healthcare professional?
   - Do you anticipate problems caring for yourself or others? If so, describe.
   - Describe what you do to keep healthy and prevent disease in yourself and your family, including exercise, leisure activities, regular dental care, routine professional examinations, self-examinations, nutrition, weight control, and immunizations.
   - What medications (prescribed and over-the-counter) do you take?
   - Do you use tobacco products? Alcohol? If so, how much and how frequently?
   - What safety measures do you take? (Smoke alarms in home? Use of helmets when cycling, skiing, or in-line skating? Weapons in home? Use of seat belt in automobile? Storage of poison in home?)
   - Describe the health of your family (maternal grandparents, mother, paternal grandparents, father, siblings, spouse, children).
   - Are you aware of any risk factors you have for disease?

2. Nutrition-Metabolic
   - Describe what you usually eat. Breakfast? Lunch? Dinner? Snacks?
   - What is your typical fluid intake? (Name the type of fluids and amounts.)
   - Describe your appetite. Do you have any problems that affect your appetite (such as nausea, fullness, indigestion)?
   - Are you on, or have you been on in the past, any specially prescribed diet?
   - Describe your food preferences.
   - Do you take any nutritional supplements (such as vitamins or protein)?
   - Do you have any food restrictions? Any food allergies?
   - Have you experienced any difficulties with eating (such as chewing or swallowing)?
   - How much do you think you weigh?
   - Have you experienced weight changes (loss or gain) in the last 6 to 9 months?
   - Have you noticed problems with your skin (such as dryness, swelling, lesions, or itching)?
   - Do your wounds heal quickly?
   - Do you have any risk factors making you susceptible to skin ulcers (such as decreased circulation, sensory deficits, or decreased mobility)?

3. Elimination
   - How many times a day do you urinate?
   - What color is your urine?
   - Do you experience any problems with urination (such as pain or burning, dribbling, incontinence, retention, or frequency)?
   - Do you use any assistive devices for urinating (such as incontinence pads, intermittent or indwelling catheter, or cystostomy)?
   - Describe your normal bowel elimination pattern, including time and frequency.
   - What does your stool look like (color, consistency)?
   - Are any assistive devices used for bowel elimination (such as laxatives, suppositories, enemas, or colostomy/ ileostomy)?

4. Activity-Exercise
   - Describe your activity level.
   - Do you exercise? If so, describe the type, frequency, intensity, and duration of exercise.
   - What do you do for leisure activities?
   - Do you experience any of the following: shortness of breath, fatigue or weakness, cough, chest pain, palpitations, leg pain, or pain in muscles or joints? If so, describe.

- To what extent do you require assistance for the following daily activities:
  - Feeding
  - Bathing
  - Toileting
  - Bed mobility
  - Dressing
  - Grooming
  - General mobility
  - Cooking
  - Home maintenance
  - Shopping

  Level 0: Full self-care
  Level I: Requires use of equipment or device
  Level II: Requires assistance or supervision from another person
  Level III: Requires assistance from another person (and equipment or device)
  Level IV: Is dependent and does not participate

5. Sleep-Rest
   - How many hours per night do you generally sleep?
   - What time do you usually go to bed? Wake up?
   - Do you generally feel rested after sleep?
   - Do you have any sleep rituals? If so, describe.
   - Do you experience any problems associated with sleeping (such as difficulty falling asleep, difficulty remaining asleep, or early awakening)? If so, describe.

6. Cognitive-Perceptual
   - Are you able to read and write?
   - What languages do you speak?
   - How do you learn best?
   - Do you experience any problems with hearing? Do you use a hearing aid?
   - Do you wear glasses or contact lenses? Do you experience any problems with vision?
   - When was your last visual examination?
   - Do you experience problems with dizziness? If so, describe.
   - Have you noticed any insensitivity to cold, heat, or pain? If so, describe.
   - Do you experience pain? If so, describe.

7. Self-Perception–Self-Concept
   - How would you describe yourself?
   - Have any recent occurrences made you feel differently about yourself? If so, describe.
   - What concerns you most?
   - Do you frequently have feelings of anger? Anxiety? Depression? Fearfulness? If so, describe.

8. Role-Relationship
   - Describe your living arrangements. Do you live alone? If not, with whom do you live?
   - Do you have a significant other? If yes, is this relationship satisfying?
   - What are the different roles within your family? Do others depend on you? If so, explain.
   - Describe how relationships are among your family members (close, marital difficulties, or estrangement).
   - How are family decisions made in your family?
   - How are conflicts resolved?
   - Are finances adequate to meet family needs?
   - Outside the family, do you have close friends, or do you belong to any social groups? If so, describe.

9. Sexuality-Reproductive
   - Are you sexually active? If yes, how many partners do you have?
   - Do you routinely use protection against sexually transmitted infections, pregnancy, or both? If yes, describe.
   - Are you comfortable with your sexual functioning?
   - Are you experiencing any difficulties with sexual activity? If yes, describe.
   - Do you anticipate a change in your sexual activity or relations with illness?
   - Women: date of last menstruation, description of menstrual flow, age of menarche, age of menopause (if applicable), pregnancy history, problems associated with menstruation.

10. Coping–Stress Tolerance
    - Have there been any major changes in your life within the last couple of years? If so, describe.
    - How do you handle it problems that arise in your life? Is this effective most of the time?
    - Is there an individual who is helpful to talk problems over with? Is this person available to you now?
    - Would you describe yourself as tense or relaxed most of the time? If tense, how do you relieve the tension?
    - Do you use medications, drugs, or alcohol to help you relax? If yes, describe.

11. Value-Belief
    - Do you generally get what you want out of life?
    - Do you have any plans or goals for the future?
    - Are there any personal beliefs or values you feel may be compromised?
    - Is religion an important part of your life? If so, describe.

Conversion Tables

TABLE C-1 Length

in	cm	cm	in
1	2.54	1	0.4
2	5.08	2	0.8
4	10.16	3	1.2
6	15.24	4	1.6
8	20.32	5	2
10	25.4	6	2.4
20	50.8	8	3.1
30	76.2	10	3.9
40	101.6	20	7.9
50	127	30	11.8
60	152.4	40	15.7
70	177.8	50	19.7
80	203.2	60	23.6
90	228.6	70	27.6
100	254	80	31.5
150	381	90	35.4
200	508	100	39.4

1 inch = 2.54 cm
1 cm = 0.3937 inch

TABLE C-2 Weight

lb	kg	kg	lb
1	0.5	1	2.2
2	0.9	2	4.4
4	1.8	3	6.6
6	2.7	4	8.8
8	3.6	5	11.0
10	4.5	6	13.2
20	9.1	8	17.6
30	13.6	10	22
40	18.2	20	44
50	22.7	30	66
60	27.3	40	88
70	31.8	50	110
80	36.4	60	132
90	40.9	70	154
100	45.4	80	176
150	66.2	90	198
200	90.8	100	220

1 lb = 0.454 kg
1 kg = 2.204 lb

TABLE C-3 Temperature: Fahrenheit and Celsius Equivalents in the Body Temperature Range

F°	C°	F°	C°	F°	C°	F°	C°	F°	C°
94	34.44	97	36.11	100	37.78	103	39.44	106	41.11
94.2	34.56	97.2	36.22	100.2	37.89	103.2	39.56	106.2	41.22
94.4	34.67	97.4	36.33	100.4	38	103.4	39.67	106.4	41.33
94.6	34.78	97.6	36.44	100.6	38.11	103.6	39.78	106.6	41.44
94.8	34.89	97.8	36.56	100.8	38.22	103.8	39.89	106.8	41.56
95	35	98	36.67	101	38.33	104	40	107	41.67
95.2	35.11	98.2	36.78	101.2	38.44	104.2	40.11	107.2	41.78
95.4	35.22	98.4	36.89	101.4	38.56	104.4	40.22	107.4	41.89
95.6	35.33	98.6	37	101.6	38.67	104.6	40.33	107.6	42
95.8	35.44	98.8	37.11	101.8	38.78	104.8	40.44	107.8	42.11
96	35.56	99	37.22	102	38.89	105	40.56	108	42.22
96.2	35.67	99.2	37.33	102.2	39	105.2	40.67		
96.4	35.78	99.4	37.44	102.4	39.11	105.4	40.78		
96.6	35.89	99.6	37.56	102.6	39.22	105.6	40.89		
96.8	36	99.8	37.67	102.8	39.33	105.8	41		

To convert Centigrade or Celsius degrees to Fahrenheit degrees: Multiply the number of Centigrade degrees by 9/5 and add 32 to the result. To convert Fahrenheit degrees to Centigrade degrees: Subtract 32 from the number of Fahrenheit degrees and multiply the difference by 5/9.

Abbreviations

A & W	alive and well		GE	gastroesophageal
AB	abortion		GI	gastrointestinal
abd	abdomen; abdominal		GU	genitourinary
ac	before meals		GYN	gynecologic
ADL	activities of daily living		HA	headache
AJ	ankle jerk		HCG	human chorionic gonadotropin
AK	above knee		HEENT	head, eyes, ears, nose, and throat
ANS	autonomic nervous system		HOPI	history of present illness
AP	anteroposterior		HPI	history of present illness
bid	twice a day		Hx	history
BK	below knee		ICS	intercostal space
BP	blood pressure		IOP	intraocular pressure
BPH	benign prostatic hyperplasia		IUD	intrauterine device
BS	bowel sounds; breath sounds		IV	intravenous
c̄	with		JVP	jugular venous pressure
CC	chief complaint		KJ	knee jerk
CHD	childhood disease; congenital heart disease; coronary heart disease		KUB	kidneys, ureters, and bladder
			lat	lateral
CHF	congestive heart failure		LCM	left costal margin
CNS	central nervous system		LE	lower extremities
c/o	complains of		LLL	left lower lobe (lung)
COPD	chronic obstructive pulmonary disease		LLQ	left lower quadrant (abdomen)
CV	cardiovascular		LMD	local medical doctor
CVA	costovertebral angle; cerebrovascular accident		LMP	last menstrual period
CVP	central venous pressure		LOC	loss of consciousness; level of consciousness
Cx	cervix		LS	lumbosacral; lumbar spine
D & C	dilation and curettage		LSB	left sternal border
DM	diabetes mellitus		LUL	left upper lobe (lung)
DOB	date of birth		LUQ	left upper quadrant (abdomen)
DOE	dyspnea on exertion		M	murmur
DTRs	deep tendon reflexes		MAL	midaxillary line
DUB	dysfunctional uterine bleeding		MCL	midclavicular line
Dx	diagnosis		MGF	maternal grandfather
ECG, EKG	electrocardiogram; electrocardiograph		MGM	maternal grandmother
EENT	eye, ear, nose, and throat		MSL	midsternal line
ENT	ear, nose, and throat		MVA	motor vehicle accident
EOM	extraocular movement		N & T	nose and throat
FB	foreign body		N & V	nausea and vomiting
FH	family history		NA	no answer; not applicable
FROM	full range of motion		NKA	no known allergies
FTT	failure to thrive		NKDA	no known drug allergies
Fx	fracture		NPO	nothing by mouth
G	gravida		NSR	normal sinus rhythm
GB	gallbladder		OM	otitis media

OTC	over the counter	ROS	review of systems
p̄	after	RRR	regular rate and rhythm
P	para	RSB	right sternal border
pc	after meals	RUL	right upper lobe (lung)
PE	physical examination	RUQ	right upper quadrant (abdomen)
PERRLA	pupils equal, round, react to light, and accommodation	s̄	without
		SCM	sternocleidomastoid
PGF	paternal grandfather	Sx	symptoms
PGM	paternal grandmother	T & A	tonsillectomy and adenoidectomy
PI	present illness	TM	tympanic membrane
PID	pelvic inflammatory disease	TPR	temperature, pulse, and respiration
PMH	past medical history	UE	upper extremities
PMI	point of maximum impulse; point of maximum intensity	URI	upper respiratory infection
		UTI	urinary tract infection
PMS	premenstrual syndrome	WD	well developed
prn	as necessary	WN	well nourished
PVC	premature ventricular contraction	*Symbols:*	
RCM	right costal margin	<	less than
REM	rapid eye movement	>	greater than
RLL	right lower lobe (lung)	×	times; by (size)
RLQ	right lower quadrant (abdomen)	♀	female
RML	right middle lobe (lung)	♂	male
ROM	range of motion	#	pound

Answer Key

Chapter 1

Review Questions

1. 1
2. 2
3. 2
4. 3
5. 1

Case Study 1

1. *Subjective data:* Abdominal pain in right abdomen. Pain feels like a knife and goes to shoulder. Client is nauseated and feels exhausted. Client has not slept for three nights; pain keeps her awake. Client hurts too much to get up and move.
2. *Objective data:* Dark circles under eyes. Vital signs: BP, 132/90 mm Hg; Pulse, 104 beats/min; RR 22 per minute; Temp, 101.8° F (38.8° C). Elevated WBCs. Client lying in fetal position.

Case Study 2

1. *Subjective data:* Complains of pain in right leg. Pain medication helps only a little bit and "butt hurts" because she can't move. *Objective data:* Client has fractured femur. Right leg is in skeletal traction. Taking Percocet orally for pain every 6 hours.
2. *Subjective data:* No bowel movement for 3 days. Stool looked like "hard, dry rabbit turds." Normal bowel elimination daily. *Objective data:* Client is on bedrest in skeletal traction. Fluid intake average = 1000 ml/day. Eating 30% of meals. Abdomen slightly distended. Active bowel sounds. Taking Percocet for pain.

3. *Subjective data:* "My butt hurts because I can't move around." "The food is horrible." *Objective data:* Client is on bedrest in skeletal traction. Fluid intake average = 1000 ml/day. Eating 30% of meals. 2-inch diameter redness over sacrum (skin intact).
4. *Subjective data:* Client complains she is so bored she can't stand it. "I am used to being active, so being stuck in bed is driving me crazy." "TV shows are not worth watching." *Objective data:* Client is on complete bed rest with right leg in skeletal traction. Client is alert, agitated, and restless.

Chapter 2

Review Questions

1. 2
2. 3
3. 1
4. 2

Chapter 3

Review Questions

1. 2
2. 4
3. 3
4. 1
5. 4

Case Study

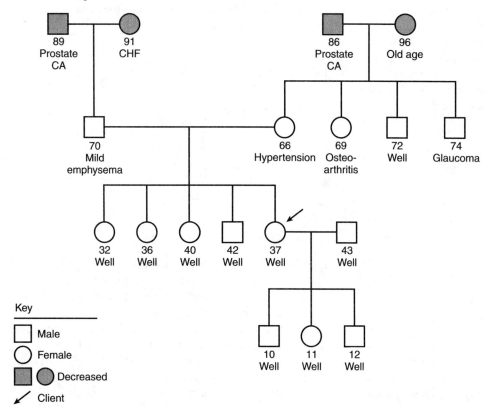

Key
- ☐ Male
- ○ Female
- ⬛ ⬤ Decreased
- ✓ Client

Chapter 4

Review Questions

1. 2
2. 1
3. 4
4. 3
5. 1

Chapter 5

Review Questions

1. 2
2. 3
3. 1
4. 3
5. 4

Chapter 6

Review Questions

1. 1
2. 2
3. 2
4. 1
5. 3

Case Study

Mr. M.'s description of pain indicates some sort of acute problem—this indicates a need to search for the source of the problem.

1. Data that deviate from normal are signs and symptoms consistent with acute pain. The signs are elevated heart and respiratory rates, as well as diaphoresis. The symptoms are his reports of pain at 12 (on a scale of 10) and nausea.

2. Ask if the pain radiates to any other site. Ask if there are any symptoms associated with urination, such as blood in the urine or pain with urination. Ask Mr. M. if he has ever had pain like this before. If so, ask him to describe the pain. Ask Mr. M. if he has noticed anything that reduces the intensity or if he has taken any medications or tried any self-treatment? Ask him what his past experiences with pain have been.

3. Recommendations for health promotion include drinking 3 liters of fluid daily, eating a healthy diet and exercising 30 minutes most days of the week.
4. Acute pain related to inflammatory process as evidenced by temperature, tachycardia, hyperpnea, and reports of client pain of 12 (on a scale of 10). Nausea related to inflammatory process and acute pain as evidenced by client's reports. Collaborative problem: renal calculi.

Chapter 7

Review Questions

1. 2
2. 1
3. 3
4. 2
5. 4

Case Study

1. Unkempt general appearance; crying behavior; excessive sleeping; self-deprecating, slow speech with flat affect.
2. Ask about the onset of symptoms and current stressors. Ask about recent changes in her life, and identify coping mechanisms. Ask about interpersonal relationships with friends and with boyfriend. Consider doing a Holmes stressor scale. Ask her if she takes any medications.
3. Her risk factors for depression are that she is female and in late adolescence. She may have a distorted perception of her parent's reaction to her performance in school and a pessimistic outlook.
4. Risk for ineffective coping. Risk for low self-esteem. Risk for sleep deprivation. Risk for altered nutrition: more than body requirements.

Chapter 8

Review Questions

1. 2
2. 3
3. 1
4. 1
5. 4

Case Study

1. Complains of not sleeping well and not feeling rested; descriptions of ineffective sleep; stress in life; divorce and possible bankruptcy; alcohol intake in evening.
2. How long has this been going on? How often does this occur (how many nights a week)? What medications is he currently taking? Ask questions about coping mechanisms (how does he best handle stress, who does he have in his life to talk to about his problems).

3. Risk factors for insomnia include psychological factors, such as the stress of the divorce and the alcohol consumed prior to sleep.

Chapter 9

Review Questions

1. 1
2. 2
3. 4
4. 3
5. 2

Case Study

1. *Subjective data:* Fatigue. Shortness of breath. Change in diet. Weight loss. Perception of health. *Objective data:* Height for weight. Scaling of skin. Hair findings. Cracks in corner of mouth. Pale conjunctiva.
2. Ask about other symptoms she may be experiencing; ask if her appetite has been affected; ask if weight loss has been intentional; ask what her usual body weight is; ask her if she has a history of weight loss; assess her knowledge regarding vegetarian diet. Calculate the BMI, the DBW, her % of DBW, and the % weight change in 4 months from her UBW.
3. *Risk factors:* Lack of money to buy food.
4. Ineffective health maintenance related to lack of knowledge regarding change in diet. Altered comfort related to cracks in mouth. Activity intolerance related to decrease in energy. Collaborative problem: malnutrition.

Chapter 10

Review Questions

1. 3
2. 4
3. 1
4. 1
5. 2
6. 4
7. 4
8. 3

Case Study

1. Foul-smelling odor; loss of appetite; flat affect; 6 feet 2 inches, 153 pounds; skin breakdown; minimal activity.
2. Ask the client if he is aware of the skin breakdown. Ask about recent weight loss with loss of activity. Assess ulcers to determine stage and presence of infection. Assess other pressure areas for evidence of skin breakdown. Perform a nutritional assessment.

3. The primary risk factor is immobility caused by paraplegia and a lack of sensation in pressure points over bony prominences. A second risk factor is poor nutritional intake.

4. Impaired skin integrity related to reduced mobility and nutritional status. Risk for infection related to nutritional status. Risk for self-care deficit related to weakness. Risk for impaired home maintenance related to weakness and depression. Imbalanced nutrition: less than body requirements related to decreased appetite, depression.

Chapter 11

Review Questions

1. 1
2. 1
3. 4
4. 2
5. 1
6. 4
7. 3
8. 2
9. 3
10. 3
11. 1
12. 4

Case Study

1. Fever; complaints of ear pain; presence of drainage in ear canal; TM perforation; reduction of hearing in left ear; quiet affect; limited talking.

2. Ask what treatment the child has received for the ear pain from the medicine man in the past. Ask if she has ever seen drainage from ear with past problems. Ask if the child has been treated at a hospital or clinic for ear pain in the past. Ask mother if child acts withdrawn or demonstrates disruptive behavior. Hearing assessment using an audiometer is indicated for this child. Assessment of T. N.'s developmental level should also be done.

3. Recurrent otitis media is the only risk factor identified in the data.

4. Impaired verbal communication related to hearing loss in left ear as manifested by lack of interaction. Risk for injury related to decreased hearing acuity. Acute pain related to inflammation of the middle ear. Risk for parental role conflict related to illness of the child. Risk for delayed growth and development related to impaired hearing.

Chapter 12

Review Questions

1. 2
2. 4
3. 3

4. 1
5. 3
6. 1
7. 4
8. 2
9. 1
10. 3

Case Study

1. History of shortness of breath; limitation in activity; interrupted sleep (requires pillows); smoking history; labored breathing with tachypnea; presence of cyanosis; underweight/protruding ribs; increased AP diameter; reduced chest wall movement; diminished tactile fremitus; adventitious breath sounds and diminished breath sounds.

2. Ask about chest pain with shortness of breath. Ask about the presence of a cough. Ask how old the client was when she started smoking. Ask how long she has been smoking as much as she currently is. Assess oxygen saturation, body weight, and rhythm of breathing pattern. Assess for presence of retraction. Percuss chest for tone and diaphragmatic excursion. Count how many words she can say without taking a breath to assess dyspnea.

3. Her smoking is a risk factor for lung cancer.

4. Impaired gas exchange related to alveolar hypoventilation. Ineffective airway clearance related to expiratory airflow obstruction. Activity intolerance related to dyspnea. Sleep deprivation related to dyspnea. Risk for imbalanced nutrition: less than body requirements related to poor appetite and labored breathing. Risk for anxiety related to dyspnea. Risk for self-care deficit related to dyspnea and fatigue. Collaborative problem: hypoxia.

Chapter 13

Review Questions

1. 4
2. 2
3. 3
4. 2
5. 3
6. 2
7. 3
8. 4
9. 1
10. 3

Case Study

1. Complaint of shortness of breath; complaint of fatigue that interferes with routine activities; complaint of sleeping difficulty; labored breathing with elevated respiratory rate, pulse rate, and blood pressure; pitting edema in lower extremities; frothy-looking phlegm.

2. Complete a symptom analysis on the shortness of breath and fatigue. Ask the client if he has symptoms associated with chest pain, cough, or nocturia. Ask the client about cardiovascular history. Perform a precordial assessment, including inspection, percussion, palpation, and auscultation.
3. Risk factors for coronary artery disease: age, gender, and family history.
4. Activity intolerance related to fatigue. Anxiety related to breathlessness. Sleep deprivation related to nocturnal dyspnea. Impaired gas exchange related to dyspnea. Risk for ineffective coping related to altered lifestyle. Risk for self-care deficit related to dyspnea and fatigue.

Chapter 14

Review Questions

1. 4
2. 1
3. 3
4. 1
5. 3
6. 2
7. 3
8. 4
9. 2
10. 3

Case Study

1. Abdominal pain (progressively worse); loss of appetite and nausea; guarded position; hot skin, possibly indicating fever; absence of bowel sounds; pain on palpation and guarding RLQ; positive rebound tenderness in RLQ.
2. Ask if vomiting accompanies her nausea. Ask about her menstrual cycle (LMP) and about the possibility of pregnancy. Ask her about bowel elimination (last bowel movement) and appearance of stool. Check vital signs (of particular interest is temperature). Auscultate for arterial bruits and venous hums. Percuss kidney for CVA tenderness. Perform iliopsoas muscle test and obturator muscle test.
3. Risk factors: smoking is a risk factor for most cancers of the gastrointestinal system.
4. Acute pain related to abdominal inflammation. Anxiety related to uncertainty of diagnosis and pain.

Chapter 15

Review Questions

1. 1
2. 4
3. 2
4. 4

5. 1
6. 4
7. 3
8. 2

Case Study

1. Diagnosis of RA; significant joint pain; limitations in self-care activities; limitations in socialization; difficulty with posture and gait; deformities to joints; tender inflamed joints with palpation; subcutaneous nodules at the ulnar surface of the elbows.
2. Ask the client what medications she is taking for the RA; find out whether she is using any other nonpharmaceutical therapies; ask her whether these things help or make a difference; ask if she has any assistive devices that she uses and if she receives any assistance with self-care activities. Document ROM in various joints. Use of a goniometer would be particularly helpful.
3. Risk factors for osteoporosis: age, gender, race (Asian), family history, and medication (methotrexate).
4. Chronic pain related to joint inflammation. Risk for impaired physical mobility related to joint pain and stiffness. Risk for self-care deficit related to loss of dexterity. Disturbed body image related to statements made by client. Risk for social isolation related to consequences of chronic illness and body image.

Chapter 16

Review Questions

1. 2
2. 3
3. 1
4. 1
5. 4
6. 3
7. 2

Case Study

1. The client has been diagnosed with right CVA; he had a headache preceding incident; the client is unable to talk; he has absence of sensation and trace to no muscle strength on the left arm and leg; he requires assistance for mobility; and the client avoids eye contact and cries.
2. Ask Mr. T if he feels he can swallow normally. Ask him whether he has any pain or discomfort. Ask Mrs. T about medical and family history; ask about medications he may be currently taking. Ask Mrs. T if her husband lost consciousness or had a seizure with this incident. Assess gag reflex. Test reflexes (deep tendon). Assess for drooling.
3. Risk factors: age, gender, race, and history of diabetes mellitus, hypertension, and smoking.

4. Impaired physical mobility related to altered neuromuscular function. Impaired verbal communication related to expressive aphasia. Self-care deficit syndrome (total) related to left hemiplegia. Chronic low self-esteem related to loss of function. Risk for impaired skin integrity related to immobility. Risk for imbalanced nutrition: less than body requirements related to inability to feed self.

Chapter 17

Review Questions

1. 3
2. 4
3. 4
4. 3
5. 2
6. 1

Case Study

1. Client has a history of nontender breast lump, noticeable for about 9 months; mass has increased in size over 9 months; risk factors include early onset of menarche and the fact that the client is childless; palpable lump is present in the left upper outer quadrant; dimpling noted on left breast; left nipple is retracted; bloody discharge is noted from nipple when squeezed.
2. Ask about personal or family history of breast disease. Ask client whether she performs BSE. Ask whether she has ever had a mammogram. Ask about the location of the lump. Ask whether the lump is tender now. Ask whether she has noticed nipple discharge. Ask about changes in the lump size in relation to menstrual cycle. Inspect the areolae. Besides location, the following characteristics must be assessed with a breast mass: size, shape, consistency, tenderness, mobility, and borders. Palpate the axilla. It is especially important to note any lumps or masses in the left axilla.
3. Age, early onset of menarch, and no children make her at risk for breast cancer. Recommend having CBH and/or mammograms more often that (for) women of low risk.
4. Ineffective denial related to delay in seeking health care for known problem. Deficient knowledge related to inaccurate perception of health status. Risk for disturbed body image related to probable breast surgery. Risk for ineffective coping related to perceptions regarding breast surgery.

Chapter 18

Review Questions

1. 2
2. 1
3. 4
4. 2
5. 1
6. 3
7. 4
8. 3
9. 3
10. 1

Case Study

1. The history suggests some type of acute inflammation. It is also suggestive of multiple sex contacts, and primary partner has multiple sex contacts. Mass with inflammation, discharge, and extreme pain on palpation needs further evaluation.
2. Discussion is needed regarding past sexual history and associated medical problems, if any. Identification of protection (or lack of it) is also important to discuss. Obtain a culture of the discharge for evaluation. If client is too uncomfortable for internal examination, this may need to be delayed until the inflammation has resolved.
3. The risk factors are sexual activity and being in a non-monogamous sexual relationship. Based on the data provided, it is unknown if protection from STI is used. It is also unclear how many sexual partners the client has.
4. Acute pain related to verbalization of discomfort in perineal area. Ineffective health maintenance related to sexual activity. Risk for infection transmission related to sexual activity.

Chapter 19

Review Questions

1. 2
2. 3
3. 1
4. 3
5. 4

Case Study

1. *Subjective data:* Client recently lost spouse (5 months ago). Son says his mother has "gone downhill." Son indicates client is no longer keeping her house clean and is not cooking appropriate meals. Son reports significant change in client's personal hygiene habits (loss of interest in getting hair done or getting dressed for the day). Son reports client becomes angry when he talks about other living options; client states, "You think I am helpless and want to lock me away."
2. *Objective data:* 78-year-old woman; sits quietly during conversation. Overall hygiene—client appears clean; hair is matted; clothes do not match and are badly wrinkled. Speech is clear. Overall affect is dull; makes no eye contact with her son or nurse. Age-consistent findings with physical examination; no overt physical problems identified.

3. Mrs. C. is in Erikson's stage of ego integrity versus despair.
4. Mrs. C. may be struggling with the following developmental tasks: dealing with the death of her spouse; adapting to living arrangements; adjusting to relationships with adult children and grandchildren; adjusting to slower physical and intellectual responses; managing leisure time and remaining active; maintaining physical and mental health; finding the meaning of life.
5. Additional assessment needs to be done in the area of skills of daily living versus mental health/depression. Some of the changes noted by the son may be indicative of physical/cognitive decline, or they may be a result of depression and apathy from the loss of a husband.

Chapter 20

Review Questions

1. 1
2. 1
3. 3
4. 4
5. 4
6. 4
7. 2
8. 1
9. 4
10. 4

Case Study

1. Reported seizure, "shaking all over" lasted 20 minutes. History of seizures, but length of seizure was atypical (according to mother).
2. Ask if there was a loss of consciousness. Ask how long ago since last seizure. Ask if there were any warning signs before the seizure. Ask about change in medication dose, or change in adherence; ask about recent changes in health status, changes in appetite, excessive fatigue, etc.
3. Risk for falls; risk for musculoskeletal injury, risk for head injury.
4. Risk for delayed development related to frequent seizures; Risk for falls related to loss of coordination; Risk for injury related to frequent seizures.

Chapter 21

Review Questions

1. 1
2. 4
3. 2
4. 4
5. 1

Case Study

1. *Subjective data:* Symptoms of puffiness to hands and feet. Backache. Fear of excessive labor pain. *Objective data:* Increase in BP. Sudden, excessive increase in weight. 3 + protein in urine.
2. Assess FHT; palpate fetal movement. Assess the extent of the edema, including how far up on the legs and the degree of edema, if pitting. Check her visual acuity. Conduct a neuroassessment, particularly to check reflexes. Ask her about her diet, specifically sodium intake, because this may be contributing to the edema. Get more information about the back discomfort; do a symptom analysis. Determine her knowledge level of labor and delivery process; assess pain experiences.
3. She has PIH, excessive weight gain, and evidence of preeclampsia (proteinuria and edema).
4. Excess fluid volume related to fluid retention. Altered comfort related to edema and changes in spinal position. Anxiety related to perceived threat to comfort secondary to labor and delivery. Collaborative problem: preeclampsia.

Chapter 22

Review Questions

1. 1
2. 2
3. 4
4. 3
5. 1
6. 3

Case Study

1. The client is confused and incontinent. She has a history of urinary tract infection (UTI) that has contributed to her confusion. A urine specimen needs to be obtained to determine if she has another UTI. Treating her incontinence is another priority. Moving her right hip is painful due to the fall and bruise.
2. A fall risk assessment needs to be completed
3. Female, Caucasian, thyroid replacement, postmenopausal, confusion, history of falls, and osteoporosis
4. Risk for falls related to incontinence, confusion, and osteoporosis. Ineffective therapeutic regime management related to lack of knowledge regarding treatment of incontinence and urinary tract infections.

Glossary

A

abduction   Movement of a limb away from the body.

accommodation   The adjustment of the eye to variations in distance.

active listening   Concentrating on what the client is saying and the subtleties of the message being conveyed.

adduction   Movement of a limb toward the body.

adnexa   General term meaning adjacent or related structures. *Example:* The ovaries and fallopian tubes are adnexa of the uterus.

adolescent   Refers to a person between the ages of 12 and 18 years.

adventitious sounds   Breath sounds that are not normal.

adulthood   Stage of life that can be divided into several recognized categories:

Young adult	ages 20 to 35 years
Middle adult	ages 35 to 65 years
Young-old adult	ages 65 to 74 years
Middle-old adult	ages 75 to 84 years
Old-old adult	ages 85 and up

affect   Observable behaviors indicating an individual's feelings or emotions.

alopecia   Absence or loss of hair.

alveolar ridge   Bony prominences of the maxilla and mandible that support the teeth; in edentulous clients, these structures support dentures.

amblyopia   Reduced vision in an eye not correctable by refraction and with no obvious pathologic or structural cause.

amenorrhea   Absence of menstruation.

anesthesia   Partial or complete loss of sensation.

angina pectoris   Paroxysmal chest pain often associated with myocardial ischemia; pain patterns and severity vary among individuals; pain sometimes radiates to the neck, jaw, or left arm; may be accompanied by choking or smothering sensations.

angle of Louis   Visible and palpable angulation between the sternum and manubrium; also referred to as the *manubriosternal junction.*

ankylosis   Fixation of a joint, often in an abnormal position, usually resulting from destruction of articular cartilage, as in rheumatoid arthritis.

annulus   Dense fibrous ring surrounding the tympanic membrane.

anosmia   Absence or impairment of the sense of smell.

anterior   Referring to the front.

anterior triangle (of the neck)   Landmark area for palpating the submaxillary, submental, and anterior cervical lymph nodes; sectioned by the anterior surface of the sternocleidomastoid muscle, the mandible, and an imagined line running from the chin to the sternal notch.

anthropometrics   Measurement of body composition and growth; includes measurement of height, weight, body mass index, head circumference, and skinfold thickness.

anular   Type of lesion that forms a ring around a center of normal skin.

anuria   Complete absence of urine production; may also be used to describe situations in which urine output is less than 100 cc per day.

anxiety   A feeling of uneasiness or discomfort experienced in varying degrees, from mild anxiety to panic; anxiety is a response to no specific source or actual object.

apathy   Lack of emotional expression; indifference to stimuli or surroundings.

aphakia   Absence of the crystalline lens of the eye.

aphasia   A neurological condition in which language function is absent or severely impaired.

aphthous ulcer (canker sore)   Painful ulcer on the mucous membrane of the mouth.

apical   Refers to the top portion (apex) of an organ or part.

apnea   Absence of breathing.

apocrine sweat glands   Secretory dermal structures located in the axillae, nipples, areolae, scalp, face, and genital area; they develop at puberty and respond to emotional stimulation.

arcus senilis   Gray ring composed of lipids deposited in the peripheral cornea; commonly seen in older adults. Also called *arcus cornealis.*

areola   Circular, darkly pigmented area around the nipple of the breast.

arteriosclerosis   General term denoting hardening and thickening of the arterial walls.

ascites   Accumulation of serous fluid in the peritoneal cavity.

assessment   First step in the nursing process involving collection of comprehensive data pertinent to the client's health or situation.

asthma   Paroxysmal dyspnea that is accompanied by wheezing and caused by spasm of the bronchial tubes or by swelling of their mucous membranes.

astigmatism   Visual distortion resulting from an irregular corneal curvature that prevents light rays from being focused clearly on the retina.

ataxia   Inability to coordinate muscular movement.

atelectasis   Shrunken, airless alveoli or collapse of lung tissue.

atherosclerosis   Formation of plaques within arterial walls resulting in thickening of the walls and narrowing of the lumen; end organs supplied by these vessels receive diminished circulation.

atrophy   A wasting or decrease in size or physiologic activity of a part of the body because of disease or other influences.

auricle   The external ear; also called the *pinna.*

auscultatory gap   Phenomenon sometimes noted by a nurse listening for blood pressure sounds; temporary silent interval between systolic and diastolic sounds that may cover a range of 40 mm Hg; commonly occurs with hypertensive clients with a wide pulse pressure.

B

balano   Prefix that denotes the glans penis. *Example: Balanitis* means inflammation of the glans penis.

ballottement   Technique of palpating a floating structure in the abdomen by bouncing it gently and feeling it rebound.

Bartholin's glands   Two mucous-secreting glands located within the posterolateral vaginal vestibule.

bilateral   Relating to or referring to two sides.

Biot breathing   Breathing characterized by several short breaths followed by long, irregular periods of apnea.

bipolar disorder   A mood disorder characterized by episodes of mania, depression, or mixed moods.

blepharitis   Inflammation of the eyelid.

blocking   Interruption in a train of thought, a loss of an idea, or a repression of a feeling or idea from conscious awareness; can be a normal behavior or, in extreme form, indicative of abnormality.

body mass index (BMI)   Method to evaluate height-weight ratio; calculated by dividing the weight (kilograms) by the height (meters).

borborygmi   Abdominal sounds produced by hyperactive intestinal peristalsis that is audible at a distance.

boutonniere deformity   Common deformity of the hands seen in clients with rheumatoid arthritis; involves flexion of the proximal interphalangeal joint and hyperextension of the distal interphalangeal joint.

bradycardia   Abnormally slowed heart rate, usually under 60 beats per minute.

bradykinesia   Abnormal slowness of movement.

bradypnea   Breathing that is abnormally slow.

bronchial breath sounds   High-pitched breath sounds normally heard over the trachea and the area around the manubrium; considered abnormal if heard anywhere over the posterior or lateral chest.

bronchitis   Inflammation of the bronchi.

bronchophony   An abnormality in vocal resonance. When lungs are auscultated, the client says "ninety-nine" or "one, two, three". If there a lung consolidation, the sounds will be clear; without consolidation, the sounds are muffled.

bronchovesicular breath sounds   Refers to breath sounds at a moderate pitch heard in the posterior chest over the outer center of the back on either side of the spine between the scapulae and in the anterior chest around he sternal border.

Brudzinski's sign   Examination technique used to detect meningeal irritation by flexing the neck of a supine client forward.

bruit   Audible murmur (a blowing sound) heard when auscultating over a peripheral vessel or an organ.

buccal   Pertaining to the inside of the cheek, the surface of a tooth, or the gum beside the cheek.

bulbar conjunctiva   Thin, transparent mucous membrane that covers the sclera and adjoins the palpebral conjunctiva, which lines the inner eyelid.

bulla   Elevated, circumscribed, fluid-filled lesion greater than 1 cm in diameter.

bunion   Abnormal prominence on the inner aspect of the first metatarsal head, with bursal formation; results in lateral or valgus displacement of the great toe.

bursa   Fibrous, fluid-filled sac found between certain tendons and the bones beneath them.

bursitis   Inflammation of a bursa.

C

cachexia   Severe malnutrition and wasting of muscles associated with a chronic illness such as cancer.

callus   Hyperkeratotic area caused by pressure or friction; usually not painful.

canthus   Outer or inner angle between the upper and lower eyelids.

carpal tunnel syndrome   Painful disorder of the wrist and hand induced by compression of the median nerve between the inelastic carpal ligament and other structures within the carpal tunnel.

cataract   Opacity of the crystalline lens of the eyes.

cauliflower ear   Thickened, disfigured ear caused by repeated trauma such as blows to the ear.

cellulitis   Diffuse spreading infection of the skin or subcutaneous or connective tissue.

cerumen   Waxy secretion of the glands of the external acoustic meatus; earwax.

chalazion   Small, localized swelling of the eyelid caused by obstruction and dilation of the meibomian gland.

circumduction Circular movement of a limb.

circumscribed Well-defined, limited, and encircled.

clonus Abnormal pattern of neuromuscular functioning characterized by rapidly alternating involuntary contraction and relaxation of skeletal muscles.

clubbing Broadening and thickening of the fingernails or toe nails associated with an increased angle of the nail greater than 160 degrees; associated with chronic hypoxia.

coarctation Stricture or narrowing of the wall of a vessel as the aorta.

cochlea Conical bony structure of the inner ear; perforated by numerous apertures for passage of the cochlear division of the acoustic nerve.

cognitive functioning Appraisal of an individual's perception of his or her intellectual awareness, potential for growth, and recognition by others for his or her mental skills and contributions.

coherency Conversation and behavior that conveys thoughts, feelings, ideas, and perceptions in a logical and relevant manner.

compulsive behavior Repetitive act that usually originates from an obsession; extreme anxiety emerges if the act is not completed.

condyloma acuminatum (wart) Soft, warty, papillomatous projection that appears on the labia and within the vaginal vestibule; viral in origin and sexually transmitted.

condyloma latum Slightly raised, moist, flattened papules that appear on the labia or within the vaginal vestibule; a sign of secondary syphilis; sexually transmitted.

confabulation Fabrication of events or sequential experiences often recounted to cover up memory gaps.

confluent Describes lesions that run together.

consensual reaction The constriction of the iris and pupil of one eye when a light is shone in the opposite eye.

consolidation Increasing density of lung tissue caused by pathologic engorgement.

contusion (bruise) Swelling, discoloration, and pain without a break in the skin.

Cooper ligaments Suspensory ligaments of the breast.

corn Hyperkeratotic, slightly raised, circumscribed lesion caused by pressure over a bony prominence.

costal angle Costal margin angle formed on the anterior chest wall at the base of the xiphoid process, where the ribs separate.

crackles Abnormal respiratory sound heard during auscultation characterized by discontinuous bubbling sounds; heard over distal bronchioles and alveoli that contain serous secretions; formerly called *rales*.

crepitus Dry, crackling sound or sensation heard or felt as a joint is moved through its range of motion.

cricoid cartilage Lowermost cartilage of the larynx.

crust Dried serum, blood, or purulent exudate on the skin surface.

cryptorchism Failure of one or both of the testicles to descend into the scrotum.

cyanosis Bluish-gray discoloration of the skin resulting from the presence of or abnormal amounts of reduced hemoglobin in the blood.

cycloplegia Paralysis of the ciliary muscle resulting in a loss of accommodation and a dilated pupil; usually induced with medication to allow for examination or surgery of the eye.

cystocele Bulging of the anterior vaginal wall caused by protrusion of the urinary bladder through relaxed or weakened musculature.

D

darwinian tubercle Blunt point projecting up from the upper part of the helix of the ear.

database Collection or store of information.

deciduous teeth Twenty teeth that appear normally during infancy: four incisors, two canines, and four molars in the upper and lower jaw.

delirium An acute, reversible organic mental disorder characterized by confusion, disorientation, restlessness, anxiety, and excitement.

delusion Persistent belief or perception that is illogical or improbable.

dementia Broad term that indicates impairment of intellectual functioning, memory, and judgment.

depersonalization Sense of being out of touch with one's environment; loss of a sense of reality and association with personal events.

depression An abnormal mood state in which a person characteristically has a sense of sadness, hopelessness, helplessness, worthlessness, and despair resulting from some personal loss or tragedy.

desquamation Sloughing process of the cornified layer of the epidermis; when accelerated, the process can cause peeling, scaling, and loss of the deeper layers of the skin.

diaphoresis Sweating.

diaphragmatic excursion Extent of movement of the diaphragm with maximum inspiration and expiration.

diarthrotic joint Joint that permits relatively free movement; types of diarthrotic joints include hinge joints, pivot joints, condyloid joints, ball and socket joints, and gliding joints.

diastole Period of time within the cardiac cycle in which ventricles are relaxed and filling with blood.

diffuse Spread out, widely dispersed, copious.

diplopia Double vision.

distal Refers to the area furthest away from a point of reference.

dizziness Sensation of faintness.

dorsal Referring to the back or posterior part of an anatomic structure. *Example:* Dorsal aspect of the hand.

dorsiflexion Upward or backward bending or flexion of a joint.

dysarthria Speech disorder involving difficulty with articulation and pronunciation of specific sounds; results from loss of control over the muscles of speech.

dysesthesia Sensation of something crawling on the skin or of pricks of pins and needles.

dyskinesia Refers to a reduced ability to perform voluntary movements.

dysmenorrhea Abnormal pain associated with the menstrual cycle. Mild, self-limiting premenstrual pain is considered normal. Pain becomes abnormal when it is severe, disabling, or accompanied by other severe symptoms, such as nausea, vomiting, fainting, or intestinal cramping.

dyspareunia Pain associated with sexual intercourse; most often used to describe female conditions including vaginal spasms, lack of lubrication, or genital lesions.

dysphagia Difficulty swallowing.

dysphasia A neurological condition in which language function is absent or severely impaired.

dysphonia Difficulty in controlling laryngeal speech sounds; can be a normal event, such as male vocal changes occurring at puberty.

dyspnea Breathing that is labored or difficult.

dysuria Difficulty, pain, or burning sensation associated with urination.

E

ecchymosis Discoloration of skin or a mucous membrane caused by leakage of blood into the subcutaneous tissue; can also be a bruise.

eccrine sweat glands Secretory dermal structures distributed over the body that secrete water and electrolytes and regulate body temperature; heat, emotional reactions, and physical exercise are the primary stimulants for secretion from these glands.

ectopic An event that occurs away from its usual location, such as a premature ventricular contraction.

ectropion Abnormal outward turning of the margin of the eyelid.

eczematous Superficial inflammation characterized by scaling, thickening, crusting, weeping, and redness.

edema Excessive accumulation of fluid within the interstitial space.

egophony Abnormality in vocal resonance; when lungs are auscultated, the client says "e-e-e," but the nurse hears "a-a-a"; suggests pleural effusion.

embolus Foreign object (composed of air, fat, or clustered cellular elements) that circulates through the blood and usually lodges in a vessel, causing some degree of occlusion.

emesis Vomit.

emphysema Chronic pulmonary disease characterized by permanent enlargement of air spaces due to destruction of alveolar walls.

enophthalmos Abnormal backward placement of the eyeball.

entropion Abnormal inward turning of the margin of the eyelid.

enuresis Any involuntary urination, especially during sleep.

epicondyle Round protuberance above the condyle (at the end of a bone).

epididymitis Inflammation of the epididymis (tightly coiled, comma-shaped structure overlying the posterolateral surface of the testis).

epiphysis End of a long bone that is cartilaginous during early childhood and becomes ossified during late childhood.

epispadias Congenital defect in which the urinary meatus opens on the dorsum of the penis.

epistaxis Bleeding from the nose.

erosion Wearing away or destruction of the mucosal or epidermal surface; often develops into an ulcer.

erythematous Redness (of the skin).

euphoria Sense of elation or well-being; can be a normal feeling or exaggerated to the extent of distorting reality.

eustachian tube Tube lined with mucous membrane that joins the nasopharynx and the tympanic cavity.

eversion Outward turning, as with a foot, or an inside out position, as with an eyelid.

exacerbation Increase in intensity of signs or symptoms.

excoriation Scratch or abrasion on the skin surface.

exophthalmos Abnormal forward placement of the eyeball.

extension Movement that brings a joint into a straight position.

external rotation Turning a limb outward or away from the midline of the body.

extrapyramidal system Motor pathways lying outside the pyramidal tract that help to maintain muscle tone and to control body movements such as walking; includes nerve pathways between the cerebral cortex, the basal ganglia, the brainstem, and the spinal cord.

F

fasciculation Localized, uncoordinated, uncontrollable twitching of a single muscle group innervated by a single motor nerve fiber.

fifth vital sign Assessment of pain, including location, quality, quantity, chronology, and setting.

fissure Linear crack in the skin.

flaccid Referring to muscles that lack tone.

flail chest Unstable, flapping chest wall caused by fractures of the sternum and ribs.

flank Part of the body between the bottom of the ribs and the upper border of the ilium, it overlies the kidneys.

flatulence Presence of excessive amounts of gas in the stomach or intestines.

flexion Movement that brings a joint into a bent position.

fontanel Unossified space or soft spot lying between the cranial bones of an infant.

Fordyce spots Small yellow spots on the buccal membrane that are visible sebaceous glands; a normal phenomenon seen in many adults that is sometimes mistaken for abnormal lesions. Also called *Fordyce granules*.

fornix (plural: fornices) General term designating a fold or an archlike structure. The vaginal fornix is the ringed recess (pocket) that forms around the cervix as it projects into the vaginal vault; although continuous, this fornix is anatomically divided into the anterior, posterior, and lateral fornices.

fourchette Small fold of membrane connecting the labia minora in the posterior part of the vulva.

frenulum (lingual) Band of tissue that attaches the ventral surface of the tongue to the floor of the mouth.

friction rub Sound produced by the rubbing of the pleura around the lung or the pericardium around the heart.

functional assessment Appraisal of an individual's perception of his or her capacity to maneuver within a defined environment.

G

gallop rhythm Audible extra heart sound produced by an abnormal third or fourth heart sound.

gate (referring to pain) An area in the dorsal horn of the spinal cord that controls the stimulation of spinothalamic sensory tracts within the spinal cord.

gate theory of pain When A-delta or C sensory nerve fibers stimulate (open) the "gate," pain impulses enter the spinal cord and ascend in the spinothalamic tract to the thalamus.

gingiva Pertaining to the gum.

glaucoma Eye disease characterized by abnormally increased intraocular pressure caused by obstruction of the outflow of aqueous humor.

glossitis Inflammation of the tongue.

goiter Hypertrophy of the thyroid gland, usually evident as a pronounced increase in its size.

gout Metabolic disease associated with abnormal uric acid metabolism that is a form of acute arthritis; marked by inflammation of the joints.

graphesthesia Ability to recognize symbols, numbers, or letters traced on the skin.

gravida Denotes number of pregnancies. *Example: Multigravida* indicates more than one pregnancy.

guarding Protective withdrawal or positioning of a body part during an injury.

gynecomastia Abnormally large mammary glands in the male.

H

hallucination Sensory perception that does not arise from an external stimulus; can be auditory, visual, tactile, gustatory, or olfactory.

health history Collection of subjective data by interview from a client as a component of health assessment.

heave Palpable, diffuse, sustained lift of the chest wall or a portion of the wall.

helix Margin of the external ear.

hemangioma Benign tumor found predominately in subcutaneous tissue or skin; caused by newly formed blood vessels.

hematuria Presence of blood in the urine.

hemoptysis Coughing up blood or referring to bloody sputum.

hernia Abnormal opening in a muscle wall or cavity that permits protrusion of its contents.

herpetiform Describes a cluster of vesicles resembling herpes lesions.

hirsutism Excessive body hair, usually in a masculine distribution, owing to heredity, hormonal dysfunction, porphyria, or medication.

Homans' sign Calf pain associated with rapid dorsiflexion of the foot, indicative of thrombophlebitis in 10% of clients.

hordeolum (stye) Infection of a sebaceous gland at the margin of the eyelid.

hydramnios Excess formation of amniotic fluid during pregnancy.

hydrocele Nontender, serous fluid mass located within the tunica vaginalis (layered, hollow membrane adjacent to the testis).

hymenal remnants Small, irregular, fleshy projections that are remnants of a ruptured hymen; a normal phenomenon that may or may not be present at the vaginal introitus in varied sizes and shapes.

hyoid U-shaped bone suspended from the styloid process of the temporal bone.

hyperesthesia Abnormally increased sensitivity to sensory stimuli such as touch or pain.

hyperextension Refers to the extension of a body part beyond normal limits of extension.

hyperkinesis Hyperactivity or excessive muscular activity.

hyperkinetic Hyperactive.

hyperopia (farsightedness) Refractive error in which light rays focus behind the retina.

hyperresonance Sound elicited by percussion; very loud intensity and very low pitch with a booming quality; heard over lungs when air is trapped in emphysema.

hypertension Blood pressure above 120 mm Hg systolic or above 80 mm Hg diastolic on two or more readings taken at two or more visits.

hypoesthesia Decreased or dulled sensitivity to stimulation.

hyposmia Decreased sense of smell.

hypospadias Congenital defect in which the urinary meatus opens on the ventral aspect of the penis; opening may be located in the glans, penile shaft, scrotum, or perineum.

hypotension Refers to abnormally low blood pressure.

hypoxemia Abnormal reduction of oxygen content in the arterial blood.

hypoxia Abnormal reduction of oxygen delivery to body tissue.

hypovolemic Pertaining to decreased blood volume; usually refers to a state of shock resulting from massive blood loss and inadequate tissue perfusion.

I

illusion Perceptual distortion of an external stimulus. *Example:* A mirage in a desert.

"inching" Recommended method for moving the stethoscope over the precordium while listening for heart sounds; small, sliding movements (rather than lifting and lowering the stethoscope from side to side) may enable the listener to hear more sounds.

incus One of three ossicles in the middle ear; resembling an anvil, it communicates sound vibrations from the malleus to the stapes.

induration   Hardening of the skin, usually caused by edema or infiltration by a neoplasm.

infancy   First year of life.

infarct   Localized area of tissue necrosis caused by prolonged anoxia.

inferior   Lower surface of an organ; refers to a position that is lower in relation to another.

infection   Redness, heat, edema, and fever secondary to pathogenic microorganisms.

intermittent claudication   Condition characterized by symptoms of pain, aching, cramping, and localized fatigue of the legs that occur while walking but that can be relived by rest (2 to 5 minutes); discomfort occurs most often in the calf but may arise in the foot, thigh, hip, or buttock.

internal rotation   Inward turning of a limb.

introitus   General term denoting an opening or the orifice of a cavity or hollow structure.

inversion   Turning inside out or upside down.

inverted nipple   Nipple that is turned inward.

ischemia   Diminished supply of blood to a body organ or surface; characterized by pallor, coolness, and pain.

isthmus glandulae thyroideae   Narrow portion of the thyroid gland connecting the left and right lobes.

J

jaundice   A yellow discoloration of the skin, mucous membrane, and sclera caused by increased bilirubin in the blood.

K

keloid   Hypertrophic scar tissue; prevalent in nonwhite races.

keratosis   Overgrowth and thickening of the cornified epithelium.

Kernig's sign   Diagnostic sign of meningeal irritation characterized by pain and inability of a supine client to completely extend the leg when the knee and hip are flexed on the abdomen.

kinesthetic sensation   Ability to detect muscle movement and position.

Koplik spots   Lesions that appear in the prodromal stage of measles; they appear as small bluish-white lesions with irregular borders on the buccal mucosa opposite the molar teeth.

Korotkoff sounds   Sounds heard during the taking of blood pressure.

Kussmaul respiration   Rapid deep respiration often associated with ketoacidosis.

kyphosis   Abnormal convexity of the posterior curve of the spine.

L

labile emotions   Unpredictable, rapid shifting of expression of feelings.

labyrinth   Complex structure of the inner ear that communicates directly with the acoustic nerve by transmitting sound vibrations from the middle ear through the fluid-filled network of three semicircular canals that join at a vestibule connected to the cochlea.

lateral   Referring to the side; position away from the middle.

Leopold's maneuvers   Series of palpation techniques used to determine fetal presentation, position, and lie.

lesion   A pathologically or traumatically altered area of tissue.

leukoplakia   Thickened, white, well-circumscribed patch that can appear on any mucous membrane; sometimes precancerous; often a response to chronic irritation, such as pipe smoking.

leukorrhea   White vaginal discharge; can be a normal phenomenon that occurs (or increases) with pregnancy, the use of birth control medication, or as a postmenstrual phase; can also be an abnormal sign indicating malignancy or infection.

lichenification   Thickening of the skin characterized by accentuated skin markings; often the result of chronic scratching.

light reflex   Triangular landmark area on the tympanic membrane that most brightly reflects the nurse's light source.

lordosis   Abnormal anterior concavity of the spine.

lower motor neurons   Nerve cells that originate in the anterior horn cells of the spinal column and travel to innervate the skeletal muscle fibers; injury or disease of this area will result in decreased muscle tone, reflexes, or strength.

lymphadenitis   Inflammation of the lymph nodes.

lymphadenopathy   Enlargement of lymph nodes greater than 1.5 cm.

lymphedema   Swelling caused by obstruction of the lymphatic system and accumulation of interstitial fluid.

lymphoma   General term for the growth of new tissue in the lymphatic area; generally refers to malignant growth.

M

macule   Flat, circumscribed lesion of the skin or mucous membrane that is 1 cm or less in diameter.

malleus   Innermost ossicle of the middle ear; resembling a hammer, it is connected to the tympanic membrane and transmits sound vibrations to the incus.

mastitis   Inflammation of the breast.

mastoid process   Conical projection of the temporal bone extending downward and forward behind the external auditory meatus.

McBurney point   Point of specialized tenderness in acute appendicitis that is situated on a line between the umbilicus and the right anterosuperior iliac spine about 1 or 2 inches above the latter.

medial   Referring to the middle; the median plane of the body.

mediastinum   Space within the thoracic cavity positioned behind the sternum, in front of the vertebral column, and between the lungs.

menarche   Onset of menstruation.

menopause   The period that marks the cessation of menstrual cycles.

menorrhagia   Abnormally heavy or extended menstrual periods.

metrorrhagia   Menstrual bleeding at irregular intervals, sometimes prolonged, but of expected amount.

Mini Mental State Exam (MMSE)   A standardized screening tool used to estimate cognitive function and detect organic brain disease.

midaxillary line   Vertical line extending downward from the midaxillary fold; used in assessment as an anatomic reference point.

midclavicular line   Vertical line extending downward from the middle of the clavicle; used in assessment as an anatomic reference point.

miosis   Condition in which the pupil is constricted, usually drug induced.

modulation   The fourth step in the pain process when the body releases endogenous opioids to inhibit transmission of nociceptive impulses to reduce pain perception.

Montgomery tubercles   Small sebaceous glands located on the areola of the breast.

Murphy's sign   Sign of gallbladder disease consisting of pain when taking a large breath when the nurse's fingers are pressing on the approximate location of the gallbladder.

myalgia   Tenderness or pain in the muscle.

mydriasis   Dilation of the pupil, usually drug induced.

myoclonus   Twitching or clonic spasm of a muscle group.

myopia (nearsightedness)   Refractive error in which light rays focus in front of the retina.

N

nabothian cyst (retention cyst)   Small white or purple firm nodule that commonly appears on the cervix; forms within the mucus-secreting nabothian glands, which are present in large numbers on the uterine cervix.

narcolepsy   Sudden onset of excessive daytime sleepiness that lasts from 10 to 30 minutes.

nares (singular: naris)   Nostrils; anterior openings of the nose.

necrosis   Localized death of tissue.

neonate   Newborn infant during the first 28 days of life.

neurosis   Ineffective or troubled coping mechanism stemming from anxiety or emotional conflict.

nevus   Congenital pigmented area on the skin. *Example:* Mole, birthmark.

nicking   Abnormal condition showing compression of a vein at an arteriovenous crossing; visible through an ophthalmoscope during a retinal examination.

nociceptor   Free nerve endings located at the ends of small, thinly myelinated or unmyelinated nerve fibers initiate an action potential.

nocturia   Excessive urination during the night.

nodule   Solid skin elevation that extends into the dermal layer and that is 1 to 2 cm in diameter.

nystagmus   Involuntary rhythmical movement of the eyes; oscillations may be horizontal, vertical, rotary, or mixed.

O

objective data   Data obtained from examination, measurements, or diagnostic tests; observable by the nurse.

obsession   Persistent thought or idea that preoccupies the mind; not always realistic and may result in compulsive behavior.

obsessive-compulsive disorder   An anxiety disorder that develops when the client tries to resist an obsession or compulsion.

oligomenorrhea   Abnormally light or infrequent menstruation.

oliguria   Inadequate production or secretion of urine (usually less than 400 ml in a 24-hour period).

orchi   Combining form that denotes the testes. *Example: Orchitis* means inflammation of one or both of the testes.

orthopnea   Difficulty breathing in any position other than an upright one.

osteoarthritis   Form of arthritis in which one or many of the joints undergo destruction of cartilage.

otalgia   Pain in the ear.

otitis externa   Infection of the external canal or auricle of the ear.

otitis media   Infection of the inner ear.

P

Paget's disease of the nipple   Condition characterized by an excoriating or scaling lesion of the nipple extending from an intraductal carcinoma of the breast.

palmar   Relating to the palm of the hand.

palpebral conjunctiva   Thin, transparent mucous membrane that lines the inner eyelid and adjoins the bulbar conjunctiva, which covers the sclera.

palpebral fissure   Opening between the upper and lower eyelids.

palpitation   Sensation of pounding, fluttering, or racing of the heart; can be a normal phenomenon or caused by a disorder of the heart.

papilla   General term for a small projection; dorsal surface of the tongue is composed of a variety of forms of papillae that contain openings to the taste buds.

papule   Solid, elevated, circumscribed, superficial lesion 1 cm or less in diameter.

paradoxic pulse   Diminished pulse amplitude on inspiration with increased amplitude on expiration; an exaggeration of a normal response to respiration.

paralysis   Loss of muscle function, loss of sensation, or both.

paranoia   Sense of being persecuted or victimized; suspicion of others.

paraphimosis   Condition characterized by the inability to pull the foreskin forward from a retracted position.

paresis   Motor weakness.

paresthesia   Abnormal sensation such as numbness or tingling.

parity   Denotes the number of viable births.

paronychia   Inflammation of the skinfold that adjoins the nail bed.

paroxysmal nocturnal dyspnea (PND)   Periodic acute attacks of shortness of breath that awaken a person, usually after several hours of sleep in a recumbent position.

pars flaccida   Small portion of the tympanic membrane between the mallear folds.

pars tensa   Larger portion of the tympanic membrane.

patch   Flat, circumscribed lesion of the skin or mucous membrane that is more than 1 cm in diameter.

peau d'orange   Dimpling of the skin that resembles the skin of an orange.

pectoralis major muscle   One of the four muscles of the anterior upper portion of the chest.

pectus carinatum   Abnormal prominence of the sternum.

pectus excavatum   Abnormal depression of the sternum.

perception of pain   The third step in the pain process that occurs when the parietal lobe is stimulated, causing a conscious experience of pain.

periodontitis (pyorrhea)   Inflammation and deterioration of the gums and supporting alveolar bone; occurs in varying degrees of severity; if neglected, this condition will result in loss of teeth.

peristalsis   Alternating contraction and relaxation of the smooth muscles of the intestinal tract to propel contents forward.

perlèche (cheilosis, cheilitis)   Fissures at the corners of the mouth that become inflamed; caused by overclosure of the mouth in an edentulous client, marked loss of the alveolar ridge, or riboflavin deficiency; saliva irritates the area, and moniliasis is a common complication.

petechiae   Tiny, flat, purple or red spots on the surface of the skin resulting from minute hemorrhages within the dermal or submucosal layers.

phimosis   Tightness of the foreskin that results in an inability to retract it.

phobia   Uncontrollable and often unreasonable intense fear of a specific object or event.

photophobia   Ocular discomfort caused by exposure of the eyes to bright light.

physical functioning   Appraisal of an individual's perception of his or her ability to control and manipulate the physical environment, as well as judgment of the ability of his or her inner resources to control and use his or her body effectively.

pilonidal fistula (or sinus)   Abnormal channel containing a tuft of hair that is situated most frequently over or close to the tip of the coccyx; may also occur in other regions of the body.

pinna   Auricle or projected part of the external ear.

plantar flexion   A toe-down motion of the foot at the ankle.

plantar   Referring to the bottom surface of the foot.

plaque   Solid, elevated, circumscribed, superficial lesion more than 1 cm in diameter.

plaque (dental)   Film that accumulates on the surface of the teeth; made up of mucin and colloidal material from saliva; subject to bacterial invasion.

pleximeter   Finger placed on the skin surface to receive the taps from the percussion hammer or plexor; used in percussion.

point of maximum impulse (PMI)   Specific area of the chest where the heartbeat is palpated strongest; usually the apical impulse, located in the fourth or fifth intercostal space along the midclavicular line.

polyuria   Excessive urine excretion.

posterior   Referring to the back.

posterior triangle (of neck)   Landmark area for palpating the posterior cervical chain, the supraclavicular chain, and the occipital lymph chain; sectioned along the anterior border by the sternocleidomastoid muscle, the posterior border by the trapezius muscle, and the bottom by the clavicle.

precipitating factor   Event or entity that hastens the onset of another event.

precordium   Area of the chest that overlies the heart and adjacent great vessels.

predisposing factor (risk factor)   Event or entity that contributes to the cause of another event. *Example:* A family history of obesity increases a client's risk for obesity.

prehypertension   An elevated blood pressure of 120 to 139 mm Hg systolic or 80 to 89 mm Hg diastolic on two or more readings taken at two or more visits.

presbycusis   Impairment of hearing in older adults.

presbyopia   Loss of accommodation (ability to focus on near objects) associated with older adults.

preschool age   Refers to children between ages 3 and 5 years.

problem list   Compilation of findings that appear at the end of a database; may be diagnoses (medical or nursing), clusters of interrelated findings, or isolated findings that the nurse wishes to pursue but cannot label or attach to other findings.

pronate   To turn the forearm so that the palm faces downward or to rotate the leg or foot inward.

proprioception   Awareness of body posture, movement, and changes in equilibrium originating from sensory nerve endings (proprioceptors) within muscles and tendons.

pruritus   Itching.

psychosis   Any major mental disorder characterized by greatly distorted perceptions and severe disorganization of the personality.

psychosocial functioning   Appraisal of an individual's capacity to attain and maintain satisfactory intimate and social relationships with others.

ptosis   Drooping of the upper eyelid; can be unilateral or bilateral.

ptyalism   Excessive salivation.

pudendum   Collective term denoting the external genitalia; for the female it includes the mons pubis, labia majora, labia minora, vaginal vestibule, and vestibular glands; for the male it includes the penis, scrotum, and testes.

pulse deficit   Discrepancy between the ventricular rate auscultated over the heart and the arterial rate palpated over the radial artery.

pulse pressure   Difference between systolic and diastolic pressures, usually within the range of 30 to 40 mm Hg;

tends to increase as systolic pressure rises with arteriosclerosis of the large vessels (specifically the aorta).

pulsus alternans Alternating pulse; abnormal pulse characterized by a regular rhythm in which a strong beat alternates with a weaker one.

purpura Hemorrhage into the tissue, usually circumscribed; lesions may be described as petechiae, ecchymoses, or hematomas, according to size.

pustule Vesicle or bulla that contains pus.

pyramidal tract Bundle of upper motor neurons that coordinate voluntary movements originating in the motor cortex of the brain; nerve fibers travel from the frontal lobe through the brainstem and the spinal cord, where they synapse with anterior horn cells; responsible for the coordinated response of voluntary movements.

pyrosis Burning sensation in the epigastric and sternal region with the raising of acid liquid from the stomach; also called *heartburn*.

pyuria Presence of white cells (pus) in the urine.

R

rebound tenderness Sign of inflammation in the peritoneum in which pain is elicited by a sudden withdrawal of a hand pressing on the abdomen; often found in clients with appendicitis.

rectocele Bulging of the rectum and posterior vaginal wall through relaxed or weakened musculature of the vagina.

red reflex Red glow over the pupil created by light illuminating the retina.

refraction Deviation of light rays as they pass from one transparent medium into another of different density.

remission Disappearance or diminishment of signs or symptoms.

reticular Describes a netlike pattern or structure of veins on a tissue surface.

retraction Shortening or drawing backward of the skin.

rheumatoid arthritis Chronic, autoimmune inflammatory disease of connective tissue characterized by localized inflammation, thickening, and edema of the joints and systemic symptoms such as fatigue.

rhino Combining form that denotes the nose.

rhonchus Loud, low-pitched, coarse sound similar to a snore heard on auscultation of an airway obstructed by thick secretions, muscular contraction, neoplasm, or external pressure; also called a *sonorous wheeze*.

Romberg's test Test of cerebellar function that evaluates an individual's ability to maintain a given position when standing erect with feet together and eyes closed.

S

scale Small, thin flake of epithelial cells.

schizoid Exhibiting behaviors or having characteristics that resemble schizophrenia.

school age Refers to children between ages 6 and 12 years.

scoliosis Lateral curvature of the spine.

scotoma Defined area of blindness within the visual field; can involve one or both eyes.

sebaceous glands Secretory dermal structures that produce sebum, an oily substance; puberty stimulates production of sebum; the primary areas for secretion are in the face, chest, and upper part of the back.

seborrhea Group of skin conditions characterized by noninflammatory, excessively dry scales or by excessive oiliness.

sensorium Status of level of consciousness and orientation to surroundings.

shifting dullness Change in the dull sounds heard with palpation; at first the dull sound is heard in one location, then in a different location.

shotty node Small lymph node that feels hard and nodular; generally moveable and nontender; may show evidence of having been infected many times in the past.

sign Objective finding perceived by the nurse.

Skene's glands (periurethral) Mucus-secreting glands that lie just inside the urethral orifice of women; not visible during examination.

sleep apnea Breathing abnormalities that occur during sleep ranging from a reduction in airflow to complete cessation of airflow.

smegma Secretion of sebaceous glands, especially the cheesy, foul-smelling secretion sometimes found under the foreskin of the penis and at the base of the labia minora near the glans clitoris.

spasticity Increased tone or contractions of muscles causing stiff and awkward movements; seen with upper motor neuron lesions.

spermatocele (epididymal cyst) Painless, fluid-filled epididymal mass that contains spermatozoa.

spinothalamic tract Sensory nerve tract that carries impulses of pain, pressure, and temperature from the spinal cord to the thalamus.

spiritual state Individual's version of his or her effectiveness in developing and sustaining a belief and value system that assists in self-acceptance and in his or her relationship to others and to a higher being.

spondylitis Inflammation of one or more of the spinal vertebrae; usually characterized by stiffness and pain.

sprain Traumatic injury to the tendon; characteristics are pain, swelling, and discoloration of the skin over the joint.

stapes One of the ossicles in the middle ear; resembles a tiny stirrup and transmits sound vibrations from the incus to the internal ear.

stereognosis Ability to recognize objects by the sense of touch.

sternocleidomastoid muscle Major muscle that rotates and flexes the head; originates by two heads from the sternum and clavicle and inserts on the mastoid process and the occipital bone.

stoma General term that means opening or mouth.

strabismus Condition in which the eyes are not directed at the same object or point.

strain Temporary damage to the muscles usually caused by excessive physical effort.

striae Streaks of linear scars that often result from rapidly developing tension in the skin; also called *stretch marks*.

stridor   Shrill, harsh sound heard during inspiration and caused by laryngeal obstruction.

subjective data   Data obtained from a health history or provided to the nurse by the client.

subluxation   Partial or incomplete dislocation of a joint.

superior   Upper surface of an organ; also refers to a position that is higher in relation to another.

supernumerary nipple   Extra nipple.

supinate   To turn the forearm so that the palm faces upward, or to rotate the foot and leg outward.

symptom   Subjective indicator or sensation perceived by the client.

syncope   Sudden, temporary loss of consciousness; fainting.

systole   Period of time within the cardiac cycle in which the ventricles contract and eject blood into the aorta and pulmonary arteries.

T

tachycardia   Rapid heart rate (more than 100 beats per minute).

tachypnea   Rapid breathing; a respiratory rate that is faster than 20 breaths per minute.

tactile fremitus   Vibratory sensations of the spoken voice felt through the chest wall on palpation.

tail of Spence   Upper outer tail of the breast that extends into the axillary region.

telangiectasia   Dilation of a superficial capillary or network of small capillaries that produces fine, irregular, red lines on the skin surface.

tendinitis   Inflammation of a tendon.

thrill   Palpable murmur; feels like the throat of a purring cat.

thrombophlebitis   Inflammation of a vein; often associated with clot formation.

thrombus   Blood clot attached to the inner wall of a vessel; usually causes some degree of occlusion.

tic   Spasmodic muscular contraction most commonly involving the face, head, neck, or shoulder muscles.

tinnitus   Tinkling or ringing sound heard in one or both ears.

toddlerhood   Refers to ages 12 to 36 months.

tophus   Calculus that contains sodium urate deposits; develops in periauricular fibrous tissue; associated with gout.

torsion (of spermatic cord)   Twisting of the spermatic cord that results in an infarction of the testis.

tragus   Cartilaginous projection in front of the exterior meatus of the ear.

transduction   The first step in the pain process involving the conversion of mechanical, thermal, chemical, or electrical stimuli that damage tissues.

transmission   The second step in the pain process that begins with stimulation of one of the four types of afferent nerves by the nociceptors and ends by closing or opening the "gate" (substantia gelatinosa).

trapezius muscle   Major muscle that rotates and extends the head; originates along the superior curved line of the occiput and the spinous processes of the seventh cervical and all thoracic vertebrae and inserts at the clavicle, acromion, and base of the scapula.

tremor   Continuous involuntary trembling movement of a part or parts of the body.

trimester   Refers to a period of time during pregnancy. There are three trimesters during pregnancy; each trimester lasts a period of 3 months.

tumor   Solid skin elevation that extends into the dermal layer and that is more than 1 cm in diameter.

turbinates   Extensions of the ethmoid bone located along the lateral wall of the nose; these fingerlike projections are covered with erectile mucosal membranes that become swollen or inflamed in response to allergy or viral invasion.

turgor   Normal resiliency of the skin.

two-point discrimination   Ability to identify being touched by two sharp objects simultaneously.

tympany   Low-pitched note heard on percussion of a hollow organ such as the stomach.

U

ulcer   Circumscribed crater on the surface of the skin or mucous membrane that leaves an uncovered wound.

umbo   Central depressed portion of the concavity of the lateral surface of the tympanic membrane; marks the spot where the malleus is attached to the inner surface.

unilateral   Relating to or referring to one side.

upper motor neurons   Nerve cells that originate in the frontal lobe of the cerebral cortex and project downward; make up the corticobulbar and pyramidal tracts and end in the anterior horn of the spinal cord; responsible for the fine and discrete conscious movements.

urticaria (hives)   Pruritic wheals; often transient and allergic in origin.

uvula   A small, cone-shaped tissue suspended midline from the soft palate.

V

vaginitis   Inflammation of the vaginal vault; has various causes.

valgus   Bending outward.

varicocele   Abnormal tortuosity and dilation of spermatic veins; spermatic cord is described as feeling like a bag of worms; condition is not painful but involves a pulling or dragging sensation.

varus   Turning inward.

vellus hair   Soft nonpigmented hair that covers the body.

verge (anal)   External ring at the opening of the anus.

vermilion border   Demarcation point between the mucosal membrane of the lips and the skin of the face; common site for recurrent infections such as herpes infections and carcinoma; blurring of this border may be an early sign of lesion development.

vertigo   Sensation of moving around in space (whirling motion; subjective vertigo) or of objects moving about oneself (objective vertigo); results in disturbance of the individual's equilibrium.

vesicle Fluid-filled, elevated, superficial lesion 1 cm or less in diameter.

vesicular breath sounds Normal breath sounds heard over most of the lungs.

vestibule Middle part of the inner ear located behind the cochlea and in front of the semicircular canals.

vocal fremitus Vibratory sensations of the spoken voice felt through the chest wall on palpation; also known as tactile fremitus.

volar Referring to or denoting the palmar aspect of the hand or the plantar aspect of the foot.

vulva External female genitalia; also referred to as the *pudendum.*

W

wheal Elevated, solid, transient lesion; often irregularly shaped but well demarcated; an edematous response.

wheeze High-pitched, musical noise that sounds like a squeak; heard during auscultation of a narrowed airway.

whispered pectoriloquy Transmission of whispered words through the chest wall, heard during auscultation; indicates solidification of the lungs.

X

xerostomia Dryness of the mouth.

Illustration Credits

American Academy of Dermatology and Institute of Dermatologic Communication and Education, Schaumburg, Ill.

American College of Rheumatology: *Clinical slide collection of the rheumatic diseases,* Atlanta, 1991, 1995, 1997, American College of Rheumatology.

American Medical Association, 1997.

American Nurses Association: *Standards of clinical nursing practice,* Kansas City, 1991, The Association.

Baden HP: *Diseases of the hair and nails,* Chicago, 1987, Year Book.

Baran R, Dawber RR, Levene GM: *Color atlas of the hair, scalp, and nails,* St Louis, 1991, Mosby.

Barkauskas VH et al: *Health and physical assessment,* ed 2, St Louis, 1998, Mosby.

Beaven DW, Brooks SE: *Color atlas of the nail in clinical diagnosis,* ed 2, London, 1994, Times Mirror International Publishers.

Beck AT, Beck RW: Screening depressed patients in family practice: a rapid technique, *Postgrad Med* 52:81, 1972.

Bedford MA: *Color atlas of ophthalmological diagnosis,* ed 2, London, 1986, Wolfe.

Belcher AE: *Cancer nursing,* St Louis, 1992, Mosby.

Bingham BJG, Hawke M, Kwok P: *Atlas of clinical otolaryngology,* St Louis, 1992, Mosby.

Black JM, Mattassarin-Jacobs E: *Medical-surgical nursing: clinical management for continuity of care,* ed 5, Philadelphia, 1997, WB Saunders.

Bluestone C et al: *Pediatric otolaryngology*, ed 4, Philadelphia, 2003, WB Saunders.

Callen JP et al: *Color atlas of dermatology*, Philadelphia, 1993, WB Saunders.

Canobbio MM: *Cardiovascular disorders,* St Louis, 1990, Mosby.

Chipps EM, Clanin NJ, Campbell VG: *Neurologic disorders,* St Louis, 1992, Mosby.

Cohen BA: *Atlas of pediatric dermatology,* London, 1993, Wolfe.

Cutler WP: *Degenerative and hereditary disorders*, ed 7, Washington, DC, 1995, Scientific American Medicine.

Diagnostic picture tests in clinical medicine, St Louis, 1984, Mosby.

Doughty DB, Jackson DB: *Gastrointestinal disorders,* St Louis, 1993, Mosby.

Dunlap C, Barker BF: *Oral lesions,* ed 3, New York, 1991, Colgate-Hoyt.

Farrar WE et al: *Infectious diseases: text and color atlas,* ed 2, London, 1992, Gower.

Forbes CD, Jackson WF: *Color atlas and text of clinical medicine,* ed 3, St. Louis, 2003, Elsevier Limited.

Fortunato N, McCullough SM: *Plastic and reconstructive surgery,* St Louis, 1998, Mosby.

400 self-assessment picture tests in clinical medicine, London, 1984, Wolfe.

Francis CC, Martin AH: *Introduction to human anatomy,* ed 7, St Louis, 1975, Mosby.

Frankenburg WK et al: *Denver II: training manual,* Denver, 1992, Denver Developmental Materials, Inc.

Gallager HS et al: *The breast,* St Louis, 1978, Mosby.

GI series, 1981, Whitehall-Robbins Healthcare.

Goldman MP, Fitzpatrick RE: *Cutaneous laser surgery: the art and science of selective photothermolysis,* 1994, Mosby.

Goldstein BG, Goldstein AO: *Practical dermatology,* ed 2, St Louis, 1997, Mosby.

Greenberger NJ, Hinthorn DR: *History taking and physical examination,* St Louis, 1993, Mosby.

Grimes DE: *Infectious diseases,* St Louis, 1991, Mosby.

Grossman SA et al: A comparison of the Hopkins pain rating scales in patients with standard visual analogue and verbal descriptor scales in patients with cancer pain, *Pain Symptom Manage* 7:196, 1992.

Habif TP: *Clinical dermatology: a color guide to diagnosis and therapy,* ed 2, Philadelphia, 1990, Mosby.

Habif TP: *Clinical dermatology: a color guide to diagnosis and therapy,* ed 3, Philadelphia, 1996, Mosby.

Habif TP: *Clinical dermatology: a color guide to diagnosis and therapy,* ed 4, St Louis, 2004, Mosby.

Habif TP et al: *Skin disease: diagnosis and treatment*, ed 2, Philadelphia, 2005, Mosby.

Harkreader H, Hogan M: *Fundamentals of nursing: caring and clinical judgment,* St Louis, 2000, Mosby.

Herbst AL et al: *Comprehensive gynecology,* ed 2, St Louis, 1992, Mosby.

Herlihy B, Maebius N: *The human body in health and illness,* St Louis, 2000, Mosby.

Hill MJ: *Skin disorders,* St Louis, 1994, Mosby.

Hockenberry MJ et al: *Wong's nursing care of infants and children,* ed 7, St Louis, 2003, Mosby.

Hockenberry MJ et al: *Wong's nursing care of infants and children,* ed 8, St Louis, 2007, Mosby.

Hockenberry MJ: *Wong's essentials of pediatric nursing,* ed 7, St. Louis, 2005, Mosby.

Jellinek MS et al: Screening 4- and 5-year-old children for psychosocial dysfunction: a preliminary study with the pediatric symptom checklist, *Journal of Development and Behavioral Pediatrics* 15:191-197, 1994.

Kamal A, Brockelhurst JC: *Color atlas of geriatric medicine,* London, 1991, Wolfe.

Korting GW: *Practical dermatology of the genital region,* Philadelphia, 1980, WB Saunders.

Lemmi F, Lemmi C: *Physical assessment findings CD-ROM,* Philadelphia, 2001, WB Saunders.

Lewis SM, Heitkemper MM, Dirksen SR: *Medical-surgical nursing: assessment and management of clinical problems,* ed 5, St Louis, 2000, Mosby.

Lewis SM, Heitkemper MM, Dirksen SR: *Medical-surgical nursing: assessment and management of clinical problems,* ed 6, St Louis, 2004, Mosby.

Lewis SM, Heitkemper MM, Dirksen SR: *Medical-surgical nursing: assessment and management of clinical problems,* ed 7, St Louis, 2007, Mosby.

Lloyd-Davies RW et al: *Color atlas of urology,* ed 2, London, 1994, Wolfe.

Lowdermilk DL, Perry SE: *Maternity and women's health care,* ed 8, St Louis, 2004, Mosby.

Lowdermilk DL, Perry SE: *Maternity and women's health care,* ed 9, St Louis, 2007, Mosby.

Lowdermilk DL, Perry SE, Bobak IM: *Maternity nursing,* ed 5, St Louis, 1999, Mosby.

Mansel R, Bundred N: *Color atlas of breast disease,* St Louis, 1995, Mosby-Wolfe.

Marks JG, DeLeo VA: *Contact and occupational dermatology,* St Louis, 1992, Mosby.

Marshall WA, Tanner JM: Variations in pattern of pubertal changes in girls, *Arch Dis Child* 44:291, 1969.

Mashburn J, Scharbo-DeHaan M: A clinician's guide to Pap smear interpretation, *Nurse Pract* 22(4):115, 1997.

McCaffery M, Pasero C: *Pain: clinical manual,* ed 2, St Louis, 1999, Mosby.

McCance KL, Huether SE: *Pathophysiology: the biologic basis for disease in adults and children,* ed 4, St Louis, 2002, Mosby.

McCullough DC: *Pediatric neurosurgery,* Philadelphia, 1989, WB Saunders.

McKenry LM, Salerno E: *Mosby's pharmacology in nursing,* ed 21, St Louis, 2003, Mosby.

McLaren DS: *A colour atlas and text of diet-related disorders,* ed 2, St Louis, 1992, Wolfe.

Melzack R, Katz J: Pain measurement in persons with pain. In Wall PD, Melzack R, editors: *Textbook of pain,* ed 3, New York, 1994, Churchill-Livingstone.

Monteleone JA: *Recognition of child abuse for the mandated reporter,* ed 2, London, 1996, GW Medical Publishing.

Mourad LA: *Orthopedic disorders,* St Louis, 1991, Mosby.

Nesi FA et al: *Smith's ophthalmic plastic and reconstructive surgery,* ed 2, St Louis, 1998, Mosby.

Newell FW: *Ophthalmology: principles and concepts,* ed 7, St Louis, 1992, Mosby.

Nutrition Screening Initiative: A Project of the American Academy of Family Physicians, American Diatetic Association, and National Council on Aging, Inc.

Palay D, Krachmer J: *Ophthalmology for the primary care physician,* St Louis, 1998, Mosby.

Phipps W et al: *Medical-surgical nursing: health and illness perspectives,* ed 7, St Louis, 2003, Mosby.

Phipps WJ, Sands JK, Marek JF: *Medical-surgical nursing: concepts and clinical practice,* ed 6, St Louis, 1999, Mosby.

Polaski A, Tatro S: *Transparencies to accompany Luckmann's core principles and practice of medical-surgical nursing and Luckmann's medical-surgical nursing,* St Louis, 1996, Mosby.

Potter PA, Perry AG: *Basic nursing: essentials for practice,* ed 5, St Louis, 2003, Mosby.

Potter PA, Perry AG: *Basic nursing: essentials for practice,* ed 6, St Louis, 2006, Mosby.

Prior JA, Silberstein JS, Stang JM: *Physical diagnosis: the history and examination of the patient,* ed 6, St Louis, 1981, Mosby.

Raj PP: *Practical management of pain,* ed 2, St Louis, 1992, Mosby.

Regezi J, Sciubba J, Jordan RC: *Oral pathology: clinical pathologic correlations,* ed 4, Philadelphia, 2003, WB Saunders.

Rudy EB: *Advanced neurological and neurosurgical nursing,* St Louis, 1984, Mosby.

Scully C, Welbury R: *Color atlas of oral diseases in children and adolescents,* London, 1994, Wolfe.

Seeley RR, Stephens TD, Tate P: *Anatomy and physiology,* ed 3, St Louis, 1995, Mosby.

Seidel HM et al: *Mosby's guide to physical examination,* ed 4, St Louis, 1999, Mosby.

Seidel HM et al: *Mosby's guide to physical examination,* ed 5, St Louis, 2003, Mosby.

Seidel HM et al: *Mosby's guide to physical examination,* ed 6, St Louis, 2006, Mosby.

Stein HA, Slatt BJ, Stein RM: *The ophthalmic assistant: fundamentals and clinical practice,* ed 5, St Louis, 1988, Mosby.

Stenchever M et al: *Comprehensive gynecology,* ed 4, St Louis, 2001, Mosby.

Swartz MH: *Textbook of physical diagnosis: history and examination,* ed 4, Philadelphia, 2002, WB Saunders.

Swartz MH: *Textbook of physical diagnosis: history and examination,* ed 5, Philadelphia, 2006, WB Saunders.

Symonds EM, MacPhearson MBA: *Color atlas of obstetrics and gynaecology,* London, 1994, Mosby-Wolfe.

Tanner C: Thinking like a nurse: a research-based model of clinical judgment in nursing, *Nurs Educ* 45:204-211, 2006.

Tanner JM: *Growth at adolescence,* ed 2, Oxford, England, 1962, Blackwell Scientific Publications.

Taylor PK: *Diagnostic picture tests in sexually transmitted diseases,* London, 1995, Mosby.

Thibodeau GA, Patton KT: *Anatomy and physiology,* St Louis, 1987, Mosby.

Thibodeau GA, Patton KT: *Anatomy and physiology,* ed 4, St Louis, 1999, Mosby.

Thibodeau GA, Patton KT: *Anatomy and physiology,* ed 5, St Louis, 2003, Mosby.

Thibodeau GA, Patton KT: *Anatomy and physiology,* ed 6, St Louis, 2007, Mosby.

Thiboadeau GA, Patton KT: *The human body in health and disease,* ed 3, St Louis, 2002, Mosby.

Thompson JM et al: *Mosby's clinical nursing,* ed 3, St Louis, 1993, Mosby.

Thompson JM et al: *Mosby's clinical nursing,* ed 4, St Louis, 1997, Mosby.

Thompson JM et al: *Mosby's clinical nursing,* ed 5, St Louis, 2002, Mosby.

US Department of Agriculture, Center for Nutrition Policy and Promotion, *www.mypyramid.gov.*

Van Wieringen JC et al: *Growth diagrams 1965 Netherlands. Second national survey on 0-24-year-olds,* Groningen, Netherlands, 1971, Wolters-Noordhoff.

von Noorden GK: *Binocular vision and ocular motility: theory and management of strabismus,* ed 4, St Louis, 1990, Mosby.

Weston WL, Lane AT: *Color textbook of pediatric dermatology,* ed 2, St Louis, 1996, Mosby.

Weston WL, Lane AT, Morelli JG: *Color textbook of pediatric dermatology,* ed 3, St Louis, 2002, Mosby.

White GM: *Color atlas of regional dermatology,* St Louis, 1994, Mosby-Wolfe.

White GM, Cox N: *Diseases of the skin: a color atlas and text,* St Louis, 2000, Mosby.

Wong DL et al: *Whaley and Wong's essentials of pediatric nursing,* ed 6, St Louis, 2001, Mosby.

Wong DL et al: *Whaley and Wong's nursing care of infants and children,* ed 6, St Louis, 1999, Mosby.

Yesavage JA, Brink TL: Development and validation of a geriatric depression screening scale: a preliminary report, *J Psychiatr Res* 17:37, 1983.

Zitelli BJ, Davis HW: *Atlas of pediatric physical diagnosis,* ed 3, 1997, Mosby.

Zitelli BJ, Davis HW: *Atlas of pediatric physical diagnosis,* ed 4, 2002, Mosby.

Zitelli BJ, Davis HW: *Atlas of pediatric physical diagnosis,* ed 5, 2007, Mosby.

References

Chapter 1

American Nurses Association: *Nursing: scope and standards of practice*, Washington, DC, 2004, *www.nursebooks.org.*

Giddens JF: A survey of physical assessment techniques performed by RNs: lessons for nursing education, *J Nurs Educ* 46:83-87, 2007.

Gordon MJ: *Nursing diagnosis: process and application,* ed 3, St. Louis, 1994, Mosby.

North American Nursing Diagnosis Association: *Nursing diagnosis: definitions and classification 2007-2008*, Philadelphia, 2007, North American Nursing Diagnosis Association.

Pender NJ, Murdaugh CL, Parsons MA: *Health promotion in nursing practice*, ed 5, Upper Saddle River, NJ, 2006, Prentice Hall.

Tanner C: Thinking like a nurse: a research-based model of clinical judgment in nursing. *J Nurs Educ* 45:204-211, 2006.

U.S. Department of Health and Human Services: *Healthy People 2010: understanding and improving health*, ed 2, Washington, DC, 2000, U.S. Government Printing Office.

Chapter 2

Dreher M, MacNaughton N: Cultural competence in nursing: foundation or fallacy? *Nurs Outlook* 50:181-186, 2002.

Lowe J, Struthers R: A conceptual framework of nursing in Native American culture, *J Nurs Scholarsh* 33:279-283, 2001.

McNaughton A: Cultural competency and the primary care provider, *J Pediatr Health Care* 16:105-111, 2002.

Purnell L, Paulanka B: *Guide to culturally competent care*, Philadelphia, 2005, FA Davis.

Spector RE: *Cultural diversity in health and illness*, ed 6, Upper Saddle River, NJ, 2004, Prentice Hall Health.

U.S. Department of Health and Human Services, Office of Public Health, Office of Minority Health: *National standards for culturally and linguistically appropriate services in health care: final report*, Washington, DC, 2001, U.S. Government Printing Office: *www.omhrc.gov.* Accessed July 28, 2008.

Chapter 3

American Nurses Association: *Nursing: scope and standards of practice,* Washington, DC, 2004, *www.nursebooks.org.*

Dreher M, MacNaughton N: Cultural competence in nursing: foundation or fallacy? *Nurs Outlook* 50:181-186, 2002.

Dunn AM: Culture competence and the primary care provider, *J Pediatr Health Care* 16:105-111, 2002.

Gordon MJ: *Nursing diagnosis: process and application,* ed 3, St Louis, 1994, Mosby.

Riley JB: *Communication in nursing,* ed 5, St Louis, 2003, Mosby.

Smith RC: *Patient-centered interviewing,* Philadelphia, 2002, Lippincott Williams & Wilkins.

U.S. Department of Health and Human Services. *Healthy people 2010: understanding and improving health,* ed 2, Washington, DC, 2000, U.S. Government Printing Office.

Chapter 4

Armstrong RS: Nurses' knowledge of error in blood pressure measurement technique, *Int J Nurs Pract* 8:118-126, 2002.

Braun CA: Accuracy of pacifier thermometers in young children, *Pediatr Nurs* 32:413-418, 2006.

Centers for Disease Control and Prevention: Guideline for hand hygiene in health-care settings: recommendations of the Healthcare Infection Control Practices Advisory Committee and the HICPAC/SHEA/APIC/IDSA Hand Hygiene Task Force, *MMWR* 51(RR016):1-45, 2002.

El-Rahdi AS: An evaluation of tympanic thermometry in a paediatric emergency department, *Emerg Med J* 23: 40-41, 2006.

Fallis WM, Hamelin K, Wang X, Symonds J: A multimethod approach to evaluate chemical dot thermometers for oral temperature measurement, *J Nurs Meas* 14: 151-162, 2006.

Farnell S: Temperature measurement: comparison of noninvasive methods used in adult critical care. *J Clin Nurs* 14:632-639, 2005.

Frohlich E et al: Recommendations for human blood pressure determination by sphygmomanometers: American Heart Association Committee Report, *Hypertension* 11:210-222A, 1988.

Garner JS: Guideline for isolation precaution in hospital practice, *Infect Control Hosp Epidemiol* 17:53, 1996.

Korniewicz DM et al: Performance of latex and nonlatex medical examination gloves during simulated use, *Am J Infect Control* 30:133-138, 2002.

Leon C: Infrared ear thermometry in the critically ill patient: an alternative to axillary thermometry, *J Crit Care* 20:106-110, 2005.

Milam MW et al: Bacterial contamination of fabric stethoscope covers: the velveteen rabbit of health care? *Infect Control Hosp Epidemiol* 22:653-655, 2001.

National Institute for Occupational Safety and Health: *NIOSH alert preventing allergic reactions to natural rubber latex in the workplace,* NIOSH pub no 97-135, Cincinnati, OH, 1997, National Institute for Occupational Safety and Health.

National Institute for Occupational Safety and Health: *Latex allergy: a prevention guide,* NIOSH pub no 98-113, Cincinnati, OH, 1998, National Institute for Occupational Safety and Health.

National Institutes of Health, National High Blood Pressure Education Program, National Heart, Lung, and Blood Institute: *The 7th report of the Joint National Committee on Prevention, Detection, Evaluation and Treatment of High Blood Pressure,* NIH pub no 03-5233, Bethesda, MD, 2003, National Institutes of Health.

Rego A, Roley L: In-use barrier integrity of gloves: latex and nitril superior to vinyl, *Am J Infect Control* 27: 405-410, 1999.

Chapter 5

Angeli F et al: Validation of the A&D wrist-cuff UB-511 (UB-512) device for self-measurement of blood pressure, *Blood Press Monit* 11:349-354, 2006.

Armstrong RS: Nurses knowledge of error in blood pressure measurement technique, *Int J Nurs Pract* 8:118-126, 2002.

Carney SL et al: Hospital blood pressure measurement: staff and device assessment, *J Qual Clin Pract* 19:95-98, 1999.

Howell M: Pulse oximetery: an audit of nursing and medical staff understanding, *Br J Nurs* 11:191-197, 2002.

Jensen B et al: Accuracy of digital tympanic, oral, axillary and rectal thermometers compared with standard rectal mercury thermometers, *Eur J Surg* 166:848-851, 2002.

Lockwood C, Conroy-Hiller T, Page T: Vital signs, *JBI Reports* 2:207-30, 2004.

Thomas K et al: Axillary and thoracic skin temperatures poorly comparable to core body temperature circadian rhythm: results from 2 adult populations, *Biol Res Nurs* 5:187-194, 2004.

Chapter 6

Acute Pain Management Guideline Panel: *Acute pain management,* AHCPR Pub No. 02-0032, Rockville, MD, 1992, Agency for Health Care Policy and Research, Public Health Service, U.S. Department of Health and Human Services.

Hockenberry MJ, Wilson D, Winkelstein ML, Kline NE: *Wong's nursing care of infants and children,* ed 7, St Louis, 2003, Mosby.

Huether S, McCance K: *Understanding pathophysiology,* ed 2, St Louis, 2004, Mosby.

McCaffery M, Pasero C: *Pain: clinical manual,* ed 2, St Louis, 1999, Mosby.

The Joint Commission, formerly the Joint Commission on Accreditation of Healthcare Organizations: *Pain standards for 2001,* 2000. *www.jcaho.org.* Accessed December 12, 2001.

Chapter 7

American Psychiatric Association: *Diagnostic and statistical manual of mental disorders,* ed 4, Arlington, VA, 2000, American Psychiatric Association.

Bernstein KS: Clinical assessment and management of depression, *Medsurg Nurs* 15:333-342, 2006.

Compton P: Caring for an alcohol dependent patient, *Nursing* 32:58-63, 2002.

McHenry LM, Salerno E: *Pharmacology in nursing,* ed 21, St Louis, 2003, Mosby.

Naimi T et al: Binge drinking among US adults, *JAMA* 289:70-74, 2003.

National Institute of Mental Health: *Health and outreach* (website): *www.nimh.nih.gov/health.* Accessed July 28, 2008.

Townsend MC: *Psychiatric mental health nursing: concepts of care,* ed 4, Philadelphia, FA Davis.

Varcarolis EM: *Foundations of psychiatric mental health nursing: a clinical approach,* ed 4, Philadelphia, 2002, WB Saunders.

Chapter 8

Chasens ER, Umlauf MG: Nocturia: a problem that disrupts sleep and predicts obstructive sleep apnea, *Geriatr Nurs* 24:76-81, 2003.

Eisendrath SJ, Lichmacher JE: Psychiatric disorders. In Tierney LM, McPhee SJ, Papadakis MA, editors: *Current medical diagnosis and treatment,* ed 42, New York, 2003, Lange.

Colten HR, Altevogt BM, editors: *Sleep disorders and sleep deprivation: An unmet public health problem,* Washington, DC, 2006, Institute of Medicine.

Mayo Clinic (website): *www.mayoclinic.com.* Accessed July 28, 2008.

Neubauer D, Smith P, Earley C: Sleep disorders. In Barker LR et al, editors: *Principles of ambulatory medicine,* ed 6, Baltimore, 2002, Lippincott Williams & Wilkins.

Sleep Foundation (website): *www.sleepfoundation.org.* Accessed July 28, 2008.

Swedish Medical Center: *Risk factors for insomnia*, Seattle, WA, 2007, *www.swedish.org/body*. Accessed May 5, 2007.

Chapter 9

American Psychiatric Association Work Group on Eating Disorders: Practice guideline for the treatment of patients with eating disorders (revision), *Am J Psychiatry* 157(suppl 1):1-39, 2000.

Grodner M, Long S, DeYong S: *Foundations and clinical applications of nutrition: a nursing approach,* St Louis, 2004, Mosby.

Institute of Medicine: *Dietary reference intakes for energy, carbohydrate, fiber, fat, fatty acids, cholesterol, protein and amino acids,* Washington, DC, 2002, National Academy Press.

National Center for Health Statistics: *National health and nutrition examination survey 2003-2004* (report online): *www.cdc.gov/nchs/about/major/nhanes/nhanes2003-2004/nhanes03_04.htm*. Accessed July 28, 2008.

Pagana KD, Pagana TJ: *Mosby's diagnostic and laboratory test reference,* ed 8, St Louis, 2007, Mosby.

U.S. Department of Health and Human Services and U.S. Department of Agriculture: *Dietary guidelines for Americans, 2005,* ed 6, Washington, DC, 2005, U.S. Government Printing Office.

Willimas SR, Schlenker E: *Essentials of nutrition and diet therapy,* ed 8, St Louis, 2003, Mosby.

Chapter 10

American Cancer Society: *Cancer facts and figures,* Atlanta, 2007, American Cancer Society. Centers for Disease Control and Prevention: *Lyme disease statistics* (website). *www.cdc.gov/ncidod/dvbid/lyme/ld_statistics.htm*. Accessed July 28, 2008.

Etter L, Meyers SA: Pruritis in systemic disease: mechanisms and management, *Dermatol Clin* 20:459-472, 2002.

Ferringer T, Miller OF: Cutaneous manifestations of diabetes mellitus, *Dermatol Clin* 20:483-492, 2002.

Giardino AP, Giardino ER: *Recognition of child abuse for the mandated reporter,* ed 3, St. Louis, 2002, Mosby.

Leonhardt JM, Heymann WR: Thyroid disease and the skin, *Dermatol Clin* 20:473-481, 2002.

Monteleone JA. *Child abuse: quick reference for health care professionals, social services, and law enforcement,* St Louis, 2003, Mosby.

Sperling LC: Hair and systemic disease, *Dermatol Clin* 19:711-726, 2002.

Whitelaw SE: Ehlers-Danlos Syndrome classical type: case management. *Dermatol Nurs* 16:433-436, 2004.

Chapter 11

American Cancer Society: *Cancer facts and figures, 2007.* Atlanta, 2007, American Cancer Society.

Braverman L, Utiger R: *The thyroid,* ed 9, Philidelphia, 2005, Lippincott Williams & Wilkins.

Dodick DW, Campbell JK: Cluster headache: diagnosis, management, and treatment. In Silberstein SD, Liptoin RB, Dalessio DJ: *Wolff's headache,* ed 7, New York, 2001, Oxford Press.

Gallichan M: Managing long-term health risks in diabetes, *Practice Nurse* 31:29-30, 2006.

Ivker RS: Chronic sinusitis. In Rakel D: *Integrative Medicine,* Philadelphia, 2003, Elsevier.

Johnson BC, Aijax A: Cost effective workup for tonsillitis, *Postgrad Med* 113:115-121, 2003.

Kanner E, Tsai JC: Glaucoma medications: use and safety in the elderly population, *Drugs Aging* 23:321-332, 2006.

Kucik CJ, Klenny T: Management of epistaxis, *Am Fam Physician* 71:305-311, 2005.

Marx RE, Stern D: *Oral and maxillofacial pathology: a rationale for diagnosis and treatment,* Chicago, 2002, Quintessence.

Okeson JP: *Management of temporomandibular disorders and occlusion,* St Louis, 2003, Mosby.

National Center for Health Statistics: *Health, United States, 2006,* Pub. No. 2006-1232, Hyattsville, MD, 2006, U.S. Government Printing Office.

National Eye Institute: *Cataract Resource Guide* (website), *www.nei.nih.gov/health/cataract/cataract_facts.asp*. Accessed July 28, 2008.

Rovers MM, Glasziou P, Applemen CL et al: Antibiotics for acute otitis media: a meta-analysis with individual patient data, *Lancet* 368:1429-1435, 2006.

Sandhaus S: Stop the spinning: diagnosing and managing vertigo, *Nurse Pract* 27:11-23, 2002.

Silvers WS: Allergic rhinitis. In Rakel D: *Integrative Medicine,* Philadelphia, 2003, Elsevier.

Weeks BH: Graves Disease: the importance of early diagnosis, *Nurse Pract* 30:34-36, 2005.

Williams SR, Schlenker E: *Essentials of nutrition and diet therapy,* ed 8, St Louis, 2003, Mosby.

Yueh B et al: Screening and management of adult hearing loss in primary care, *JAMA* 289:1976-1984, 2003.

Zadeh MH, Selesnick SH: Evaluation of hearing impairment, *Compr Ther* 27:302-310, 2001.

Zunt SL: Recurrent apthous stomatitis, *Dermatol Clin* 21:22-29, 2003.

Chapter 12

American Cancer Society (website): *www.cancer.org*. Accessed July 28, 2008.

American Lung Association (website): *www.lungusa.org*. Accessed July 28, 2008.

Occupational Safety and Health Administration: *Respiratory protection* (website): *www.osha.gov/SLTC/respiratoryprotection/index.html*. Accessed July 28, 2008.

Environmental Protection Agency: *Smoke-free homes and cars program* (website): *www.epa.gov/smokefree/*. Accessed July 28, 2008.

Spiro CE: Evaluating chronic cough, *Clin Rev* 13:52-57, 2003.

Chapter 13

American Heart Association (website): *www.americanheart.org*. Accessed July 28, 2008.

Centers for Disease Control and Prevention (website): *www.cdc.gov*. Accessed July 28, 2008.

Church V: Staying on guard for DVT and PE, *Nursing* 30:34-38, 2000.

Family Practice Notebook (website): *www.fpnotebook.com*. Accessed July 28, 2008.

Massie B, Amidon T: Heart. In Tierney L, McPhee S, Papadakis M, editors: *Current medical diagnosis & treatment*, New York, 2004, Lange McGraw Hill.

National Heart, Lung, and Blood Institute: The seventh report of the Joint Commission on Prevention, Detection, Evaluation and Treatment of High Blood Pressure (JNC VII) (report online): *www.nhlbi.nih.gov/guidelines*. Accessed July 28, 2008.

National Institutes of Health (website): *www.nih.gov/*. Accessed July 28, 2008.

Swartz MH: *Textbook of physical diagnosis: history and examination*, ed 5, Philadelphia, 2006, WB Saunders.

Wipke-Tevis D, Rich K: Nursing management: vascular disorders. In Lewis et al, editors: *Medical-surgical nursing assessment and management of clinical problems*, ed 6, St. Louis, 2004, Mosby.

Chapter 14

Dougherty MC et al: *Evidence-based clinical practice guidelines: incontinence for women*. Washington, DC, 2000, Association of Women's Health, Obstetric, and Neonatal Nurses.

Swartz MH: *Textbook of physical diagnosis: history and examination*, ed 5, Philadelphia, 2006, WB Saunders.

Chapter 15

Biomedical Laboratories: *Osteoarthritis* (website): *www.biomedicalabs.com/osteoarthritis.htm*. Accessed July 28, 2008.

Hellmann D, Stone J: Arthritis and musculoskeletal disorders. In Tierney L, McPhee S, Papadakis M, editors: *Current medical diagnosis and treatment*, New York, 2004, Lange Medical Book/McGraw Hill.

Mayo Clinic: *Gout* (website): *www.mayoclinic.com/health/gout/DS00090http://*. Accessed July 28, 2008.

National Osteoporosis Foundation: *Risk factors for osteoporosis* (website): *www.nof.org/prevention/risk.htm*. Accessed July 28, 2008.

TMJ Association, LTD (website): *www.tmj.org*. Accessed July 28, 2008.

Chapter 16

American Heart Association (website): *www.americanheart.org*. Accessed July 28, 2008.

Hickey JV: *The clinical practice of neurological and neurosurgical nursing*, ed 5, Philadelphia, 2003, Lippincott Williams & Wilkins.

Lower J: Using Pain to assess neurologic response, *Nursing* 33:56-57, 2003.

National Institute on Deafness and Other Communication Disorders: *Balance* (website): *www.nidcd.nih.gov/health/balance*. Accessed July 28, 2008.

O'Hanlon-Nichols T: Neurologic assessment, *Am J Nurs* 99:44-50, 1999.

Seidel H, Ball J, Dains J, Benedict GW: *Mosby's guide to physical examination*, ed 6, St. Louis, 2006, Mosby.

Swartz M: *Textbook of physical diagnosis: history and examination*, ed 5, Philadelphia, 2006, WB Saunders.

Chapter 17

American Cancer Society: *Cancer facts and figures, 2007*, Atlanta, 2007, American Cancer Society.

Barbosa-Cesnik C, Schwartz K, Foxman B: Lactation mastitis, *JAMA* 289:1609-1612, 2003.

Bennett BB, Steinbach BG, Hardt NS, Haigh LS: *Breast disease for clinicians*, New York, 2001, McGraw-Hill.

Hussain AN, Policarpio C, Vincent MT: Evaluating nipple discharge, *Obstet Gynecol Surv* 61:278-283, 2006.

Marchant DJ: Benign breast disease, *Obstet Gynecol Clin North Am* 29:1-20, 2002.

O'Malley CD et al: Socioeconomic status and breast carcinoma survival in four racial ethnic groups, *Cancer* 97:1303-1311, 2003.

Rahal RM, de Freitas-Júnior R, Paulinelli, R: Risk factors for duct ectasia, *Breast J* 11;262-265, 2005.

Chapter 18

Albaugh J: Health care clinicians in sexual health medicine: focus of erectile dysfunction, *Urol Nurs* 22:217-231, 2002.

American Cancer Society: *Cancer facts and figures, 2007*, Atlanta, 2007, American Cancer Society.

Bostwick DG, Quian J, Schlesinger C: Contemporary pathology of prostate cancer, *Urol Clin North Am* 30:181-207, 2003.

Centers for Disease Control and Prevention: Sexually transmitted diseases treatment guidelines 2006, *MMWR* 55 (RR-11), 2006.

Clayton AH et al: Exploratory study of premenstrual symptoms and serotonin variability, *Arch Womens Ment Health* 9:51-57, 2006.

Grisso JA et al: Racial difference in menopause information and the experiences of hot flashes, *J Gen Intern Med* 14:98-103, 1999.

Jass JR: Pathogenesis of colorectal cancer, *Surg Clin North Am* 82:891-904, 2002.

Katz VL et al: *Comprehensive gynecology*, ed 5, St Louis, 2007, Mosby.

Koci A, Strickland O: Relationship of adolescent physical and sexual abuse to perimenstrual symptoms (PMS) in adulthood, *Issues Ment Health Nurs* 28:75-87, 2007.

Lewis JA, Black JJ: Sexuality in women of childbearing age, *J Perinat Educ* 15:29-35, 2006.

Lloyd TD et al: Women presenting with lower abdominal pain: a missed opportunity for Chlamydia screening? *Surgeon* 4:15-19, 2006.

March CM: Uterine leiomyomas. In Mishell DR, Goodwin TM, Brenner PF, editors: *Management of common problems in obstetrics and gynecology,* ed 4, Oxford, 2002, Blackwell Science.

Modugno R et al: Oral contraceptive use, reproductive history, and risk of epithelial ovarian cancer in women with and without endometriosis, *Am J Obstet Gynecol* 191:733-740, 2004.

Monroe LM, Kinney LM, Weist MD et al: The experience of sexual assault: findings from a statewide victim needs assessment, *J Interpers Violence* 20:767-776, 2005.

Nelson R: Anorectal abscess fistula: what do we know? *Surg Clin North Am* 82:1139-1151, 2002.

Nickel JC: Inflammatory conditions of the male genitourinary tract: prostatis and related conditions, orchitis, and epididymitis. In Wein A, editor: *Campbell-Walsh Urology,* ed 9, Philadelphia, 2007, WB Saunders.

Schneck F, Bellinger M: Abnormalities of the testes and scrotum and their surgical management. In Wein A, editor: *Campbell-Walsh Urology,* ed 9, Philadelphia, 2007, WB Saunders.

Sommer B et al: Attitudes towards menopause and aging across ethnic/racial groups, *Psychosom Med* 61:868-875, 1999.

Ward KD et al: Testicular cancer awareness and self-examination among adolescent males in a community-based youth organization, *Prev Med* 41:386-398, 2005.

Zheng H et al: Predictors for erectile dysfunction among diabetics, *Diabetes Res Clin Pract* 71: 313-319, 2006.

Chapter 19

American Academy of Pediatrics (website): *www.aap.org.* Accessed July 28, 2008.

Centers for Disease Control and Prevention (CDC): Catch-up immunization schedule for persons aged 4 months-18 years who start late or who are more than 1 month behind (table online): *www.cispimmunize.org/IZSchedule_Catchup.pdf.* Accessed July 28, 2008.

Boeree CG: *Erik Erikson,* 1997 (website): *http://webspace.ship.edu/cgboer/erikson.html.* Accessed July 28, 2008.

Brown M: *Readings in gerontology,* St Louis, 1984, Mosby.

Centers for Disease Control and Prevention (CDC): Catch-up immunization schedule for persons aged 4 months-18 years who start late or who are more than 1 month behind (table online): *www.cispimmunize.org/IZSchedule_Catchup.pdf.* Accessed July 28, 2008.

Denver Developmental Materials: *Catalog of screening and training materials,* Denver, 1994, DDM.

Dewey KG et al: Height and weight of Southeast Asian preschool children in Northern California, *Am J Public Health* 76:806-808, 1986.

Duvall EM, Miller BC: *Marriage and family development,* ed 6, New York, 1985, Harper & Row.

Erickson EH: *Childhood and society,* ed 2, New York, 1963, Norton.

Frankenburg WK et al: The Denver II: a major revision and restandardization of the Denver Developmental Screening Test, *Pediatrics* 89:91-97, 1992.

Hamill PV, Johnston FE, Lemeshow S: Body weight statute, and sitting height: white and Negro youths 12-17 years, *Vital Health Stat* 11:1, 1973.

Lin WS et al: Physical growth of Chinese school children 7-18 years, in 1985, *Ann Hum Biol* 19:41-55, 1992.

Lueckenotte AG: *Gerontologic nursing,* ed 2, St Louis, 2000, Mosby.

Malina RM, Zavaleta AN, Little BB: Body size, fatness, and leanness of Mexican American children in Brownsville, Texas: changes between 1872 and 1983, *Am J Public Health* 77:573-577, 1987.

Merriam SB, Cafferella RS: *Learning in adulthood: a comprehensive guide,* ed 2, San Francisco, 1999, Jossey-Bass.

Neinstein LS: *Adolescent health care: a practical guide,* ed 2, Baltimore, 1991, Lippencott Williams & Wilkins.

Piaget J, Inhelder B: *The psychology of the child,* New York, 1969, Basic Books (Translated by H Weaver).

Purnell LD, Paulanka BJ: *Transcultural health care: a culturally competent approach,* ed 2, Philadelphia, 2003, FA Davis.

Ryan AS, Martinez GA, Baumgartner RN et al: Median skinfold thickness distributions and fat-wave patterns in Mexican-American children from the Hispanic Health and Nutrition Survey (HHANES 1982-1984), *Am J Clin Nutr* 51:925S-935S, 1990.

Seidel H et al: *Mosby's guide to physical examination,* ed 6, St Louis, 2006, Mosby.

Shaie KW: Intellectual development in adulthood. In Birren JE, Shaie KW, editors: *Handbook of the psychology of aging,* ed 2, Orlando, FL, 1996, Academic Press.

Sternberg RJ: *The triarchic mind: a new theory of human intelligence,* New York, 1988, Viking Penguin.

Strauss KF: American Indian school children height and weight survey, *Provider* 18:8, 1993.

Chapter 20

Chobanian AV et al: The seventh report of the Joint National Committee on Prevention, Detection, Evaluation, and Treatment of High Blood Pressure: the JNC 7 report, *JAMA* 289:2560-2571, 2003.

Cunningham M, Cox E: Hearing assessment in infants and children: recommendations beyond neonatal screening, *Pediatrics* 111:436-439, 2003.

Giardino AP, Giardino ER: *Recognition of child abuse for the mandated reporter,* ed 3, St Louis, 2002, Mosby.

Harlan WR, Harlan EA, Grillo GP: Secondary sex characteristic of girls 12-17 years of age: the U.S. health examination survey, *J Pediatr* 96:1074-1078, 1980.

Hockenberry MJ, Wilson D: *Wong's nursing care of infants and children,* ed 8, St Louis, 2007, Mosby.

Johnson BC, Aijaz A: Cost effective workup for tonsillitis, *Postgrad Med* 113:115-121, 2003.

McGee S, Burkett KW: Identifying common pediatric neurosurgical conditions in the primary care setting, *Nurs Clin North Am* 35:61-85, 2000.

Pena KS, Rosenfeld JA: Evaluation and treatment of galactorrhea, *Am Fam Physician* 63:1763-1770, 2001.

Plewig G, Kligman AM: *Acne and rosacea,* New York, 2002, Springer.

Riddell A, Eppich W: Should tympanic temperature measurement be trusted? *Arch Dis Child* 85:433-434, 2001.

Rovers MM, Glasziou P, Applemen CL et al: Antibiotics for acute otitis media: a meta-analysis with individual patient data, *Lancet* 368:1429-1435, 2006.

Tanner JM: *Growth at adolescence,* ed 2, Oxford, England, 1962, Blackwell Scientific Publications.

Williams CL et al: Cardiovascular health in childhood: a statement for health professionals from the Committee on Atherosclerosis, Hypertension and Obesity in the Young (AHOY) of the Council on Cardiovascular Disease in the Young, American Heart Association, *Circulation* 106:143-160, 2002.

Chapter 21

Sibai BM: Caring for women with hypertension in pregnancy, *JAMA* 298:1566-1568, 2007.

Benedetti T: Obstetric hemorrhage. In Gabbe S, Niebyl J, Simpson J, editors: *Obstetrics: normal and problem pregnancies,* ed 4, New York, 2002, Churchill Livingstone.

Crane J et al: Maternal complications with placenta previa, *Am J Perinatol* 17:101-105, 2000.

Cunningham F et al: *Williams obstetrics,* ed 22, New York, 2005, McGraw-Hill.

Eustace LW, Kang DH, Coombs D: Fetal alcohol syndrome: a growing concern for health care professionals, *J Obstet Gynecol Neonatal Nurs* 32:215-221, 2003.

Ma Y et al: Predictors of smoking cessation in pregnancy and maintenance postpartum in low-income women, *Matern Child Health J* 9:393-402, 2005.

Maloni JA: Preventing low birth weight: how smoking cessation counseling can help, *AWHONN Lifelines* 5:32-35, 2001.

Newburn-Cook CV et al: Where and to what extent is prevention of low birth weight possible? *West J Nurs Res* 24:887-904, 2002.

Tillett J, Kostich LM, VandeVusse L: Use of over-the-counter medications during pregnancy, *J Perinat Neonatal Nurs* 17:3-18, 2003.

Wells CS et al: Factors influencing inadequate and excessive weight gain in pregnancy: Colorado, 2000-2002, *Matern Child Health J* 10:55-62, 2006.

Chapter 22

Aud MA: Sleep and activity. In Leuckenotte AG, editor: *Gerontologic nursing,* ed 2, St Louis, 2000, Mosby.

Cole C, Richards K: Sleep disruption in older adults: harmful and by no means inevitable, it should be assessed and treated, *Am J Nurs* 107:40-49, 2007.

Eddy L, Hricko J: Introduction to differential diagnosis in management of abdominal pain across the life span, *Am J Nurse Pract* 5:10-13, 2001.

Gates GA et al: Screening for handicapping hearing loss in the elderly, *J Fam Pract* 52:56-62, 2003.

Holmes B, Dickinson K: Join the growing number who will live till age 100, *The Senior New Source* 9:7, 2007.

Kamel HK et al: Utilizing pain assessment scales increases frequency of diagnosing pain among elderly nursing home residents, *J Pain Symptom Manage* 21:450-455, 2001.

Lichtenstein MJ, Bess FH, Logan SA: Validation of screening tools for identifying hearing impaired elderly in primary, *JAMA* 259:2875-2878, 1988.

Lueckenotte A: *Gerontological nursing,* ed 2, St. Louis, 2000, Mosby.

National Institute of Mental Health: *Older adults: depression and suicide facts* (website): *www.nimh.nih.gov/publicat/elderlydepsuicide.* Accessed July 28, 2008.

Tabloski PA: *Clinical handbook for gerontological nursing,* Upper Saddle River, NJ, 2007, Pearson Prentice Hall.

Yueh B et al: Screening and management of adult hearing loss in primary care, *JAMA* 289:1976-1984, 2003.

Index